EMERGING RESEARCH AND TREATMENTS IN RENAL CELL CARCINOMA

Edited by **Robert J. Amato**

Emerging Research and Treatments in Renal Cell Carcinoma
Edited by Robert J. Amato

Published by InTech

Janeza Trdine 9, 51000 Rijeka, Croatia

Publishing Process Manager Vedran Greblo

Technical Editor Teodora Smiljanic

Cover Designer InTech Design Team

Additional hard copies can be obtained from orders@intechopen.com

Emerging Research and Treatments in Renal Cell Carcinoma, Edited by Robert J. Amato
p. cm.
ISBN 978-953-51-0022-5

For EU product safety concerns:
IN TECH d.o.o., Prolaz Marije Krucifikse Kozulić 3, 51000 Rijeka, Croatia,
info@intechopen.com or visit our website at intechopen.com.

Meet the editor

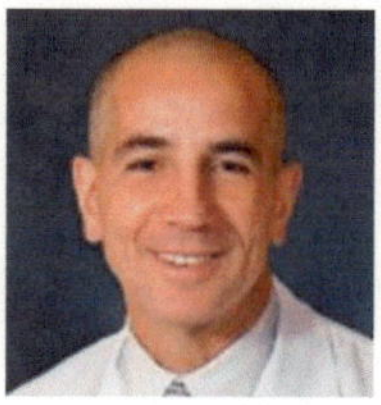

Professor Robert Amato is the Chief of the Oncology Division and a Professor at the University of Texas Medical School at Houston and Director of Oncology at the Memorial Hermann Cancer Center. He obtained his Doctor of Osteopathic Medicine from the University of North Texas before becoming a fellow in Medical Oncology at MD Anderson Cancer Center. Dr. Amato is one of the world's leading experts in the treatment of genitourinary cancer. Early in his career, his research helped make testicular cancer a highly treatable disease. His current research focuses on molecular-targeted therapeutics, halting the progression of metastatic kidney and prostate cancers, the further development of immunotherapies, and determining how his studies may be used to treat genitourinary cancer.

Contents

Preface

Genitourinary cancers are a diverse and challenging set of neoplasms for physicians and scientists to diagnose and manage. The field of renal cell cancer has undergone a significant resurgence. This book is an attempt to summarize, collate, and display this rapidly changing field, which encompasses medicine, surgery, radiation oncology, basic science, pathology, radiology, and supportive care. This text represents an up-to-date look at the issues and answers regarding present knowledge and innovative ideas for the future.

I have assembled a stellar faculty to highlight the latest information of an ever changing disease. This includes tumor biology, molecular biology, surgery techniques, radiation therapy, personal testimonies, and present and future treatments of the disease that are on the horizon.

This book is aimed at the clinician and scientist who has an interest in renal cell cancer. My goal is to produce a textbook that can be read and used by practicing physicians, whether they are academic or nonacademic. The second goal was to produce a textbook that basic scientists working in this diverse and divergent field would be able to reference and read as an authoritative source. And finally, the third goal was to interpret the field for trainees in surgery, medicine, radiation oncology, and pathology. My hope is that this book reflects the increasing knowledge within the field of renal cell cancer treatments and research.

Robert J. Amato, D.O.
Professor and Director, Division of Oncology, University of Texas Medical School/Memorial Hermann Cancer Center, Chief of the Division of Oncology, Memorial Hermann Hospital TMC,
USA

Part 1

Translational

1

Molecular Pathogenesis of Renal Cell Carcinoma: A Review

Israel Gomy and Wilson Araújo Silva Jr.
University of São Paulo, Medical School of Ribeirão Preto, Genetics Department, Ribeirão Preto, Brazil

1. Introduction

Renal cell carcinomas (RCC) represent almost 90% of all kidney cancers and in about 2% of cases there is a family history of RCC (McLaughlin et al, 1984). Despite their rare incidences, Mendelian hereditary syndromes with RCC have provided important insights into the molecular pathogenesis of this tumor. The cloning of susceptibility genes that are involved in familial predisposition has offered entry points into the signaling pathways that are deregulated in sporadic RCC. Sporadic RCC are extremely heterogeneous and are classified into many histolological subtypes. The most frequent form is clear cell or conventional RCC, accounting for approximately 75% of all cases, whereas the most common non-clear cell tumor is papillary RCC (12% of cases), which is subdivided into types 1 and 2. Other subtypes include chromophobe and oncocytomas, each of them occurring in 4% of patients, collecting-duct (<1%) and rare forms or yet to be classified (< 2%). The correlation between histopathological features and genetic alterations in RCC has been introduced in 1997 with the Heidelberg classification (Kovacs et al, 1997). More recently, expression profiles through microarrays have been done for many of the kidney tumor subtypes and provide the evidence that their expression patterns reflect their histological classifications and demonstrate that various renal tumor subtypes are genetically distinct entities (Higgins et al, 2003).

Generally, there is a good correlation between the genetic causes of familial RCC and their histopathological features as exemplified by the commonest form of hereditary RCC, von Hippel-Lindau (VHL) disease, which invariably presents a clear cell type. Moreover, germline mutations in the *MET* proto-oncogene cause type 1 papillary RCC, whereas type 2 is correlated with germline mutations in the fumarate hidratase gene, which cause hereditary leiomyomatosis. Birt-Hogg-Dubè syndrome is also characterized by susceptibility to RCC but with a mixed chromophobe-oncocytoma histopathology, and is associated with germline mutations in the *BHD* tumor suppressor gene.

All the genes identified so far, which are involved in the molecular pathogenesis of hereditary and sporadic RCC comprise a diverse set of complex biochemical and cell metabolism pathways, such as iron, energy, nutrient and oxygen-sensing (Linehan et al., 2010a). A plenty of biochemical and molecular studies of the numerous signalling pathways disrupted in RCC have already provided reasonable translational approaches and clinical applications of target therapy RCC with promising results (Iliopoulos, 2006). The histopathological and molecular features of RCC are summarized in table 1.

Tumor type	Locus	Gene	Pathway	Syndrome
Clear cell	3p25 3p14 3p21 17p11	*VHL* *FHIT* *RASSF1A* *BHD*	VEGF TGF-β AMPK-mTOR	von Hippel-Lindau Familial clear cell RCC Birt-Hogg-Dube
Papillary **type 1** **type 2**	7q31 1q42 7q31.1 9q34 16p13 1q25	*MET* *FH* *FRA7G* *TSC1* *TSC2* *HRPT2*	MET-HGF VEGF TGF-β mTOR mTOR	Hereditary papillary RCC Hereditary leiomatosis Tuberous sclerosis complex Tuberous sclerosis complex Hyperparathyroidism -jaw tumor
Chromophobe	17p11	*BHD*	AMPK-mTOR	Birt-Hogg-Dube
Oncocytoma	17p11 9q34 16p13	*BHD* *TSC1* *TSC2*	AMPK-mTOR mTOR mTOR	Birt-Hogg-Dube Tuberous complex Tuberous complex
Collecting duct carcinoma	-1q32,-6p,-8p, -9p,-13q,- 19q32,-21q	unknown	unknown	none
Renal carcinoma associated with Xp11.2 translocation	1p34 1q21 17q23 17q25 3q23 Xq12	*PSF-TFE3* *PRCC-TFE3* *CTLC-TFE3* *ASPL-TFE3* *?* *NonO-TFE3*	none	none
Mucinous tubular and spindle cell carcinoma	-8p,-9p,- 11q,+12q,+16 q+17,+20q	unknown	unknown	none

Table 1. Histopathological and genetic characteristics of RCC

2. The oxygen-sensing pathway: HIF-VHL interaction and clear-cell RCC pathogenesis

Hypoxia-inducible factors (HIF) are oxygen-sensitive basic helix–loop–helix transcription factors, which regulate biological processes that facilitate both oxygen delivery and cellular adaptation to oxygen deprivation. HIF is a heterodimer consisting of unstable a-subunits and stable constitutively expressed b-subunits. HIF-α, together with HIF-β bind to hypoxia-response elements in gene promoters to regulate the expression of genes that are involved in energy metabolism, angiogenesis, erythropoiesis, iron metabolism, cell proliferation, apoptosis and other biological processes. HIF1-α and HIF2-α mediate transcription of a number of downstream genes thought to be important in cancer, including transforming growth factor alpha (*TGF-α*), platelet-derived growth factor (*PDGF*), and vascular endothelial growth factor (*VEGF*) (Linehan et al., 2010a).

In clear-cell renal-cell carcinoma, HIF-α accumulates, resulting in the overexpression of proteins that are normally inducible with hypoxia, acting on neighboring vascular cells and promoting tumor angiogenesis. The augmented tumor vasculature provides additional nutrients and oxygen to promote the growth of tumor cells (Cohen & McGovern, 2005).

Germline mutations in the VHL gene are found in almost all families with VHL disease, an autosomal dominant condition characterized by a plenty of benign and malignant tumors (Figure 1). The most common cancer is clear cell RCC, which affects 25-30% of patients and is a major concern in disease morbity and mortality (Maher et al., 1990). Remarkably, up to

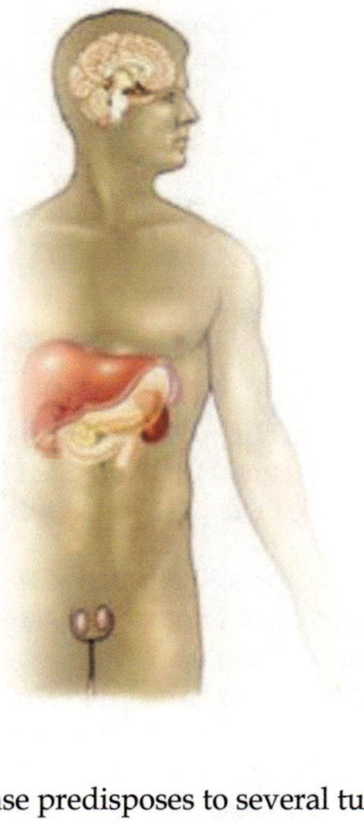

Fig. 1. von Hippel-Lindau disease predisposes to several tumors in brain, spinal cord, eyes, liver, pancreas, kidneys, testes.

91% of patients with sporadic clear cell RCC harbor biallelic VHL inactivation (Gnarra et al, 1994). Somatic mutations are found in approximately 50% of these tumors, whereas inactivation due to promoter hypermethylation has been identified in 10-20% of sporadic clear-cell RCC (Kim & Kaelin, 2004). Therefore, defects in the VHL gene are the major responsible for all cases of RCC.

The product of the VHL gene, VHL protein (pVHL), is part of an intracellular multiprotein complex that contains elongin C and B, Cul2 and Rbx1 and functions as the substrate recognition component of an E3-ubiquitin ligase. This complex selects specific substrates for ubiquitination and targets them for destruction through the proteasome, mainly HIF-α. In normoxia, the a-subunits are the target for prolyl hydroxylation that generates a binding site for pVHL. The interaction between the two proteins causes the polyubiquitynation and subsequent proteosomal degradation of HIF-α. When the cell is hypoxic or iron levels are low, the VHL complex cannot target and degrade HIF and HIF overaccumulates, driving the transcription of a number of genes important in cancer, such as *VEGF*, *PDGF*, and *GLUT1*(Figure 2a). In cells with normal VHL function, the α subunits of HIF are rapidly degraded by the proteasome, whereas in VHL-defective cells HIF-α subunits are constitutively stabilized (Maxwell et al, 1999). When the *VHL* gene is mutated, as in clear cell RCC, the complex cannot target and degrade the α subunits of HIF leading to upregulation of their targets genes (Figure 2b). Therefore, the absence of pVHL mimics hypoxia and results in a constitutive up-regulation of HIF that produces a transcriptional activation of several target genes, such as VEGF, PDGF-B, erythropoietin, TGF-α, and glucose-transporter-1 (GLUT-1).

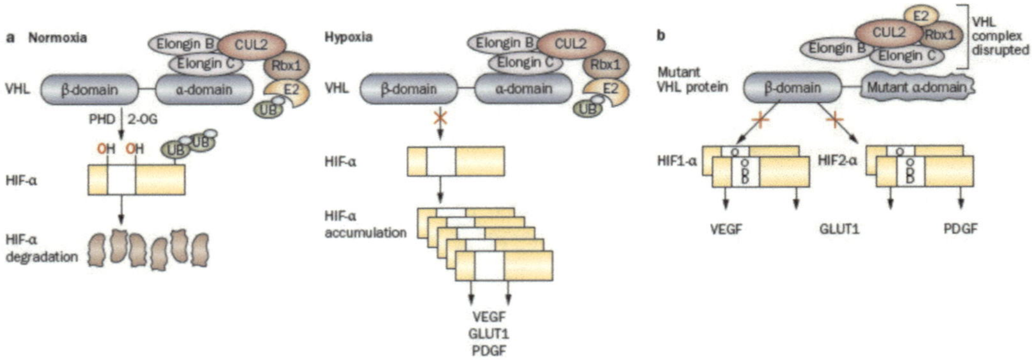

Fig. 2. The HIF-VHL-VEGF pathway. a. HIF- α degradation in normoxic cells and stabilization in hypoxic cells. b. HIF1- α and HIF2- α are not degraded and upregulate the expression of their target genes (VEGF, PDGF, GLUT1)(with permission).

It has been shown that VEGF protein expression in VHL-defective renal cancer cells is mainly induced by HIF-2α activity. The expression of other HIF targets, such as GLUT-1, urokinase-type plasminogen activator receptor (uPAR), and plasminogen activator inhibitor-1 (PAI-1), was also regulated by HIF-2a in these cells. Thus, HIF-2α seems to play a critical role in tumorigenesis of clear-cell RCC mediated by loss of VHL (Kondo et al, 2002). Clear cell kidney cancers (with or without *VHL* mutation) that express both HIF1-α and HIF2-α exhibit enhanced signaling via the mitogen-activated protein kinase (MAPK) and mTOR pathways. Constitutive activation of the Raf/MEK/Erk pathway has been demonstrated in approximately 50% of RCC samples (ref.14. EJC). Conversely, clear cell tumors that express only HIF2-α have elevated activity of the oncogene c-myc (Gordan et al, 2008).

VHL substrates other than HIF have been reported, and although their exact role in kidney carcinogenesis has not been proved to be the same as HIF's, it is possible that they may contribute directly or indirectly to VHL-deficient RCC and/or other solid tumors. VHL has been shown to interact with the RNA polymerase II subunits Rpb1, Rbp6, and Rpb7 at domains that present sequence and structural similarity to the HIF binding domain. Binding of these subunits to pVHL was shown to promote their ubiquitination and decrease transcriptional activity of Pol II (Kuznetsova et al, 2003).

Moreover, pVHL has been shown to influence the content of the extracellular matrix. Fibronectin coimmunoprecipitates with wild type but not mutant pVHL, and pVHL-deficient RCC cell lines fail to assemble extracellular fibronectin, most likely because of a defect in fibronectin maturation (Ohh et al, 1998).

Finally, it was recently shown that VHL is linked to the DNA damage response pathway. pVHL binds directly to p53, inhibits its mdm2-mediated ubiquitination, suppresses p53 nuclear export, and promotes its acetylation by p300 and overall p53 transcriptional activity. Reintroduction of pVHL in VHL-deficient RCC lines enhances p53-mediated G1 arrest and promotes their apoptotic response to genotoxic stress (Roe et al, 2006).

2.1 Therapeutic perspectives

The better understanding of VHL signaling pathway has provided the foundation for the development of therapeutic approaches that target this pathway in patients with advanced clear cell kidney cancer.

Most therapeutic agents currently approved to treat clear cell kidney cancer target either the downstream targets of HiF activity (such as the VEGF receptor) or inhibit mtorC1, which provides translational control of HiF1-α (Thomas et al., 2006). The responses to these agents observed in patients with advanced clear cell kidney cancer is proof of principle that targeting the VHL–HIF pathway can induce tumor regression in humans. However, these agents target only a small proportion of the downstream genes regulated by HIFs. An approach to target HIF transcriptional activity or translation of HIFs themselves—that is, to affect all the genes regulated by HIFs—could potentially provide more-effective therapy. Targeting the HIF2-α pathway is likely to be more successful than solely targeting the HIF1-α pathway. Efforts are currently underway to identify agents that down regulate HIF2-α-induced gene expression (Linehan et al., 2010a). Tyrosine kinase receptors trigger activation of signal transduction pathways involved in cell proliferation and survival of RCCs (Patel et al, 2006). Growth factors, such as VEGF and TGF-a, might bind to the respective tyrosine kinase receptors (EGFR and VEGFR-1) that are expressed in renal cancer cells. Thus, these receptors could potentially be targets of small molecules inhibitors. Nevertheless, many chemotherapeutic and targeted tyrosine kinase approaches are limited by their toxic effects on non-tumor cells. An alternative therapy, might be done by targeting autophagy, a central component of the cell response to nutrient and energy deprivation (Turcotte et al, 2008). By this approach, only those cells with no VHL product would be affected, whereas cells with a wild-type copy of the *VHL* gene would not. Therefore, this would provide a less-toxic and more-effective form of therapy for patients with advanced renal cancer.

3. The MET-HGF pathway and type-1 papillary renal cancer

Papillary renal-cell carcinoma occurs in several familial syndromes. Hereditary papillary renal carcinoma (HPRC) is an autosomal dominant disorder associated with multifocal papillary renal-cell carcinoma with type 1 histological features and is caused by germline activating mutations in the MET proto-oncogene (Schmidt et al, 1997) (Figure 3).

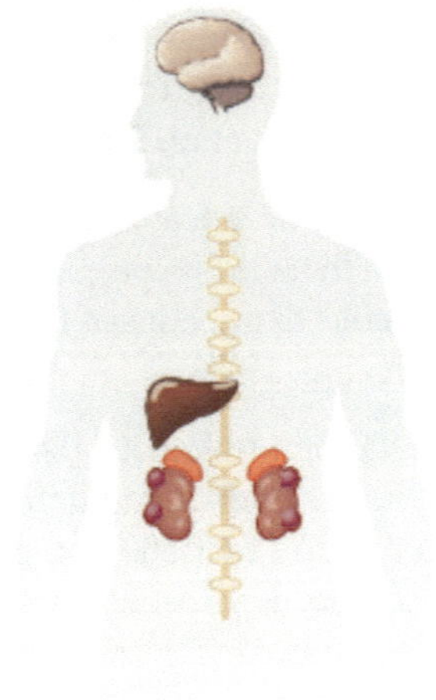

Fig. 3. Hereditary Papillary Renal Carcinoma leads to multiple (even thousands) of papillary tumors. (with permission)

The MET proto-oncogene encodes a receptor tyrosine kinase that is physiologically activated by hepatocyte growth factor (HGF). Binding of HGF to the extracellular portion of the MET receptor triggers autophosphorylation of critical tyrosines in the intracellular tyrosine kinase domain, thus activating a downstream signaling cascade. Activation of the MET/HGF signaling pathway has been shown to be involved in a number of biological activities including cell proliferation, cell motility, branching morphogenesis and epithelial-mesenchymal transition (Boccaccio & Comoglio, 2006).

Mutations of the MET proto-oncogene were detected in germline of all HPRC patients but only in a small subset of cases with sporadic type 1- papillary RCC (Schmidt et al, 1999). Thus, the pathogenesis of hereditary papillary renal carcinoma is usually different from that of sporadic papillary RCC. Tumorigenesis of most sporadic papillary RCCs are not be induced only by MET mutations, but mostly by MET and chromosome 7-related genes dosage. Since the frequency of MET mutations in sporadic papillary RCCs is low, it is possible that other genes might be involved in this form of renal cancer. In this respect, mutations of the KIT proto-oncogene have been described in 68% of papillary RCC patients (Lin et al, 2004). However, the role of KIT in the pathogenesis of this disease needs to be confirmed by functional studies. Furthermore, nutrient-stimulated HGF–MET signaling induces phosphorylation of serine–threonine protein kinase 11 (STK11or LKB1) through the RAS–ERK pathway, implicating *MET* in the LKB1–AMPK–mTOR nutrient and energy sensing pathway (Figure 4).

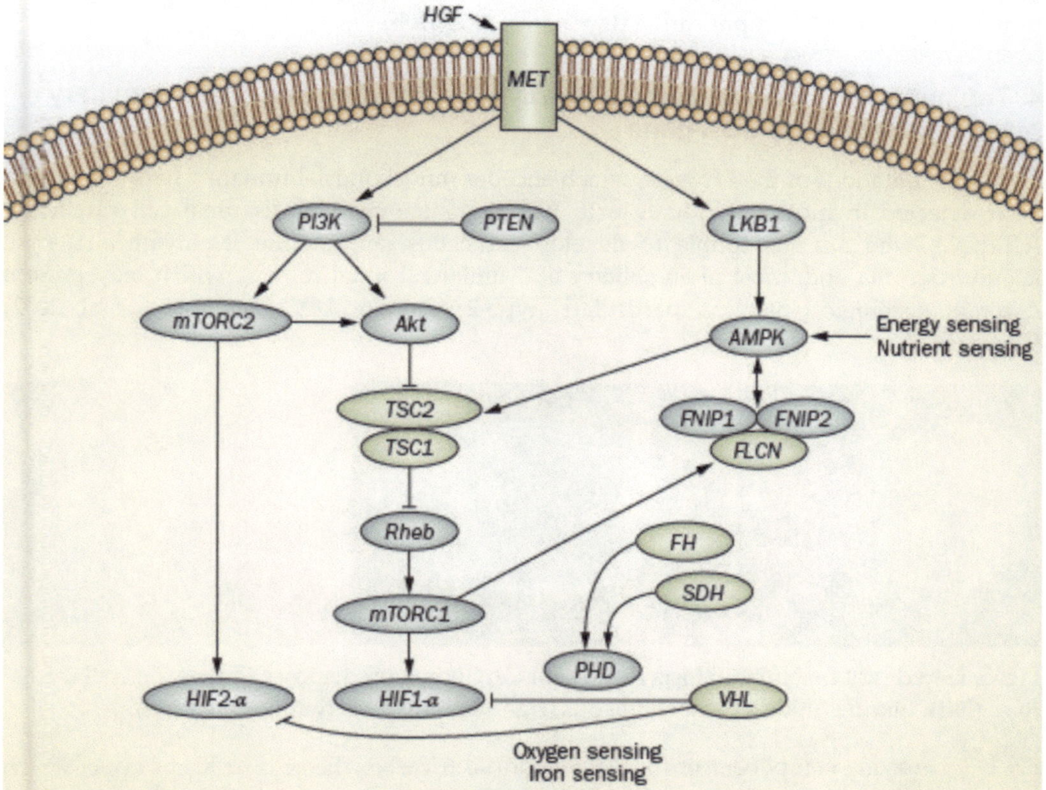

Fig. 4. HGF-MET pathway. Crosslinks between other energy, iron and oxygen-sensing pathways. (with permission)

Of particular interest for renal carcinogenesis is the observation that MET and VHL signaling pathways intersect via pVHL-mediated regulation of HIF function. HIF stabilization through hypoxia or loss of VHL function results in transcriptional upregulation, and therefore promotion of the transforming potential of the *c-MET* receptor (Pennacchietti et al, 2003). This crosstalk between VHL and c-MET pathways may explain why clear-cell and papillary histologies often coexist in the same tumor (Iliopoulos et al, 2006).

3.1 Therapeutic perspectives

The therapeutic implications of inhibiting *c-MET* signaling are promising, as activating mutations or copy number–overexpression of *c-MET* underlies a significant subset of type 1 papillary RCC.

A clinical trial is currently underway to determine the effect of foretinib, a kinase inhibitor of both *MET* and *VEGF* receptors, in patients with either hereditary or sporadic papillary kidney cancer. Early evidence shows the efficacy of this agent in patients with germline mutations in the tyrosine kinase domain of *MET* (Srinivasan et al, 2009). Response to such an agent with activity against *MET* might be seen in tumors that are characterized by a mutation in the tyrosine kinase domain of *MET*; this drug might also have some activity in tumors that have *MET* amplification (Linehan et al., 2010b).

4. The mitochondrial metabolic pathway: The FH gene and type-2 papillary renal cancer and the SDH gene

Germline mutations of the *FH* gene, which encodes mitochondrial fumarate hydratase, have been detected in most individuals with hereditary leiomyomatosis renal cell carcinoma (HLRCC), who are susceptible to develop cutaneous and uterine leiomyomas, uterine leiomyosarcoma and, most often solitary and unilateral renal tumors, which may present different histological patterns, particularly type-2 papillary RCC (Tomlinson et al, 2002) (Figure 5).

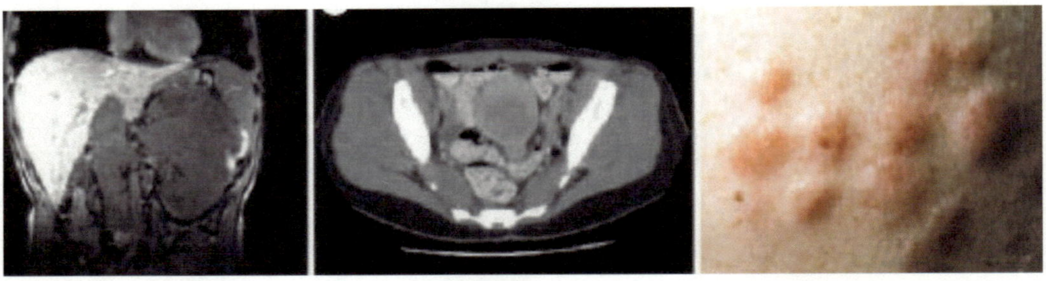

Fig. 5. Hereditary Leiomyomatosis Renal Cell Carcinoma predisposes to type-2 papillary RCC (left), uterine (middle) and cutaneous (right) leiomyomas (with permission).

FH is an enzyme component of the mitochondrial tricarboxylic acid or Krebs cycle, which has an important role in energy metabolism. In patients with FH deficient cells, it has been proposed that the inactivation of this enzyme might lead to a hypoxic environment that can favour renal carcinogenesis. FH inactivating mutations increase fumarate levels, and consequently the concentration of the fumarate precursor succinate. The high levels of succinate in the cytoplasm lead to stabilization of HIF-1α subunits and transcriptional upregulation of hypoxia-inducible genes, such as *VEGF* and *GLUT1* (which encodes the glucose transporter type 1) (Figure 6). Thus, these factors are critically important to increase vasculature and glucose transport in RCC cells, thereby contributing to the highly aggressive nature of HLRCC-associated renal tumors (Iliopoulos et al, 2006).

The inhibition of HIF-1α by the increased levels of fumarate provides a VHL-independent mechanism for dysregulation of HIF degradation in FH-deficient HLRCC-associated kidney cancers. FH-deficient kidney cancer cell lines are glucose-dependent and have significantly impaired oxidative phosphorylation. The glucose-mediated generation of cellular reactive oxygen species in an FH-deficient kidney cancer cell line results in stabilization of HIF1-α (Sudarshan et al, 2009). The impaired oxidative phosphorylation in FH-deficient kidney cancer results in a nearly total dependence on glycolysis for energy production.

Succinate dehydrogenase *(SDH)* is another Krebs cycle enzyme gene that has been associated with the development of familial tumors. Familial paraganglioma/ pheochromocytoma kindreds have been found to have germline mutations in the mitochondrial complex II genes *SDHB*, *SDHC*, and *SDHD*. Renal carcinoma, along with pheochromocytoma/paraganglioma, has been found to be a component of the familial pheochromocytoma/paraganglioma complex associated with germline *SDHB* mutations (Neumann et al, 2004), and a recent report described germline *SDHB* mutations in a family with renal cancer with no history of pheochromocytoma (Ricketts et al, 2008). The inactivation of SDH increases levels of succinate, which has been shown to affect HIF stability (Isaacs et al, 2005). It would be expected to severely impair oxidative phosphorylation and lead to glucose dependence of SDH-deficient kidney tumors, which are likely to be as sensitive to glucose as FH-deficient tumors (Linehan et al., 2010a) (Figure 6).

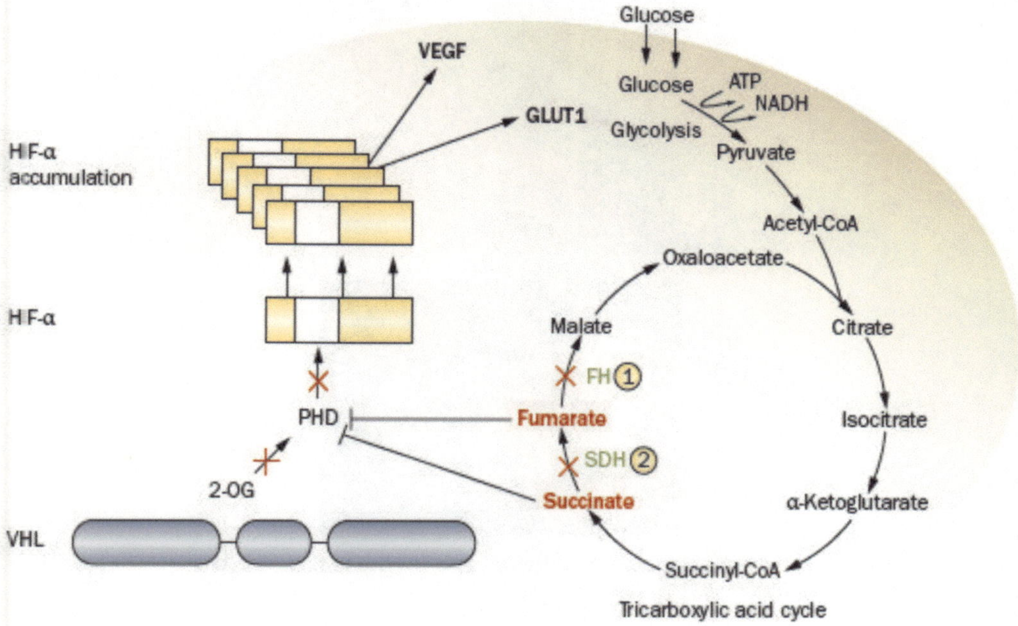

Fig. 6. FH and SDH genes and the metabolic mitochondrial pathway crosslinking with the HIF-VHL pathway (with permission).

4.1 Therapeutic perspectives

Both enhanced tumor angiogenesis and glucose transport could be the best targets for the treatment of either FH-deficient or SDH-deficient renal tumors, because they are extremely dependent on glucose transport for energy production. Whereas targeting the vasculature in patients with advanced VHL-deficient clear cell kidney cancer has only resulted in modest success, targeting the vasculature in both FH and SDH-deficient tumors could provide a powerful and effective approach to disrupt the fundamental metabolic machinery of these aggressive cancers (Linehan et al., 2010a).

5. The *FLCN* gene and chromophobe renal cell carcinomas-oncocytomas

The *FLCN* gene is impaired in Birt-Hogg-Dubè syndrome, a rare autosomal dominant disorder characterized by hair-follicle hamartomas (fibrofolliculomas) of the face and neck, spontaneous pneumotorax, lung cysts and RCCs, particularly chromophobe RCC (33%), hybrid oncocytic renal cell carcinoma (50%), clear-cell RCC (9%) and oncocytomas (5%) (De Luca et al, 2008) (Figure 7).

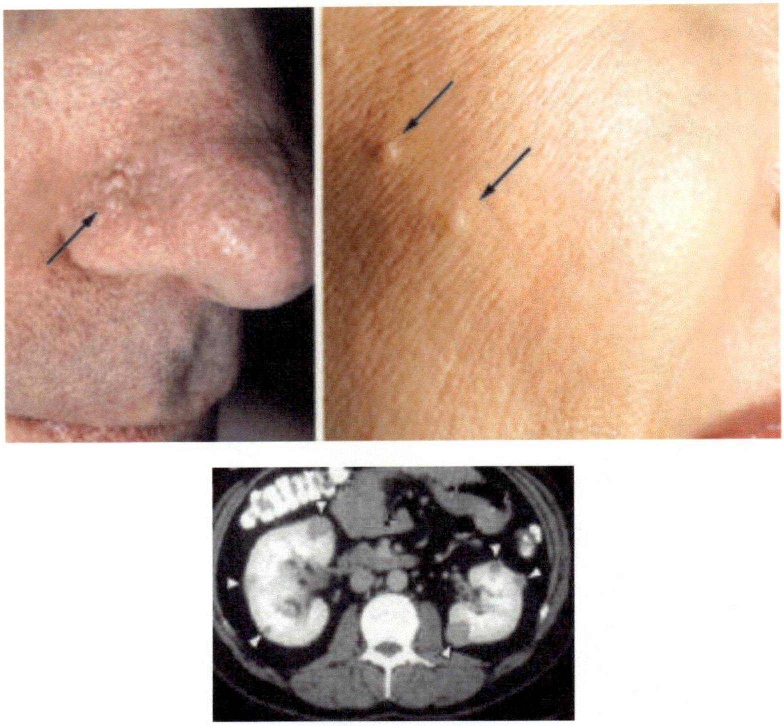

Fig. 7. Birt-Hogg-Dubè syndrome. Fibrofolliculomas on the face and bilateral RCC (with permission).

The *FLCN* gene encodes a protein called folliculin, which has no significant homology to any known human protein, although it is highly conserved across species (Nickerson et al, 2002). All described germline *FLCN* mutations are insertions, deletions, nonsense and splice-site mutations that predict truncation of the protein (Schmidt et al, 2005). In addition, somatic mutations in the second copy of BHD or loss of heterozygosity at the FLCN locus were observed in 70% of patients with germline mutations, thus suggesting *FLCN* to play a role as a tumor suppressor gene (Vocke et al, 2005).

In sporadic cases, somatic mutations are rare, but promoter methylation has been observed, indicating the involvement of *FLCN* in sporadic RCC tumorigenesis (Khoo et al, 2003).The function of folliculin has not been completely elucidated yet, but recent findings have showed that folliculin interacts with FNIP1, which binds to the 5′ AMP-activated protein kinase (AMPK), an energy sensor that negatively regulates mammalian target of rapamycin (mTOR) (Baba et al, 2006). When folliculin functions normally, the FLCN–FNIP1–FNIP2 complex binds to AMPK so *FLCN* is phosphorylated by a rapamycin-sensitive kinase (mTORC1). Conversely, when folliculin is deficient, AKT, mTORC1 and mTORC2 are activated, thus stimulating tumorigenesis (Figure 8). These findings suggest a potential role of folliculin in regulating the activation of this cell survival pathway.

The research in murine models of Birt-Hogg-Dube syndrome would suggest that rapamycin analogs such as sirolimus might be potential therapeutic agents against renal tumors (Linehan et al, 2010a).

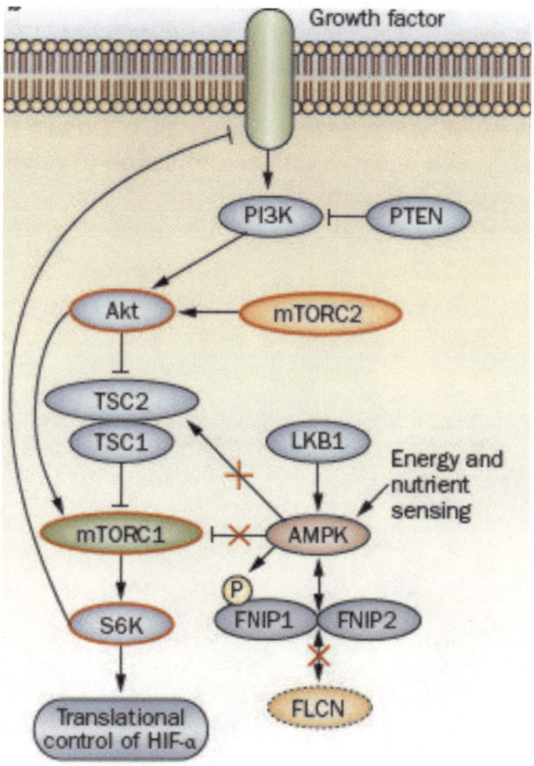

Fig. 8. FLCN interacts with AMPK-mTOR pathway. FLCN deficiency allows activation of proto-oncogenes (red circles) (with permission).

6. The AMPK-mTOR nutrient and energy sensing pathway and Tuberous Sclerosis Complex

Germline mutations in either TSC1 or TSC2 genes lead to the Tuberous Sclerosis Complex, an autosomal dominant genodermatosis characterized by multiple hamartomatous lesions that affect the skin, retina, brain, lungs and kidneys (Figure 9).

Eighty percent of children with TSC have renal lesions including benign angiomyolipomas (70%), cysts (20%), and oncocytoma (<1%) (Ewalt et al, 1998). Renal angiomyolipomas are most often multiple and bilateral, but rarely transform to a malignant tumor (<1%). The cumulative renal cancer incidence is 2.2%–4.4% (4,5) and the average age at diagnosis is 28 years, with occasional early childhood cases (Washecka et al, 1991). The renal abnormalities in TSC are unusual in patients that develop epithelial lesions, such as cysts, oncocytomas and clear cell, papillary, or chromophobe carcinomas as well as mesenchymal lesions (angiomyolipomas), suggesting that TSC genes regulate early differentiation and proliferation of renal precursor cells (Henske, 2004).

The TSC1 gene encodes hamartin and TSC2 encodes tuberin. Both proteins form a heterodimer, which interacts with many cellular pathways, including the AMPK-mTOR nutrient and energy sensing pathway. TSC1-TSC2 acts as a GTPase-activating protein toward rheb, a ras-family GTPase that activates mMTORC1. GTPase activity of the TSC1–TSC2 complex on rheb results in inhibition of mTOR activity. *TSC1*-deficient and *TSC2*-deficient tumors exhibit increased phosphorylation of p70s6 kinase, s6 ribosomal protein and 4e-BP1, downstream effectors of mtorC1 activation, and readouts for initiation of mRNA translation and protein synthesis (Crino et al, 2006). Lack of TSC1–TSC2 inhibition of mTOR would presumably also result in HIF accumulation through increased *HIF* mRNA translation by activated mTORC1 (Figure 10).

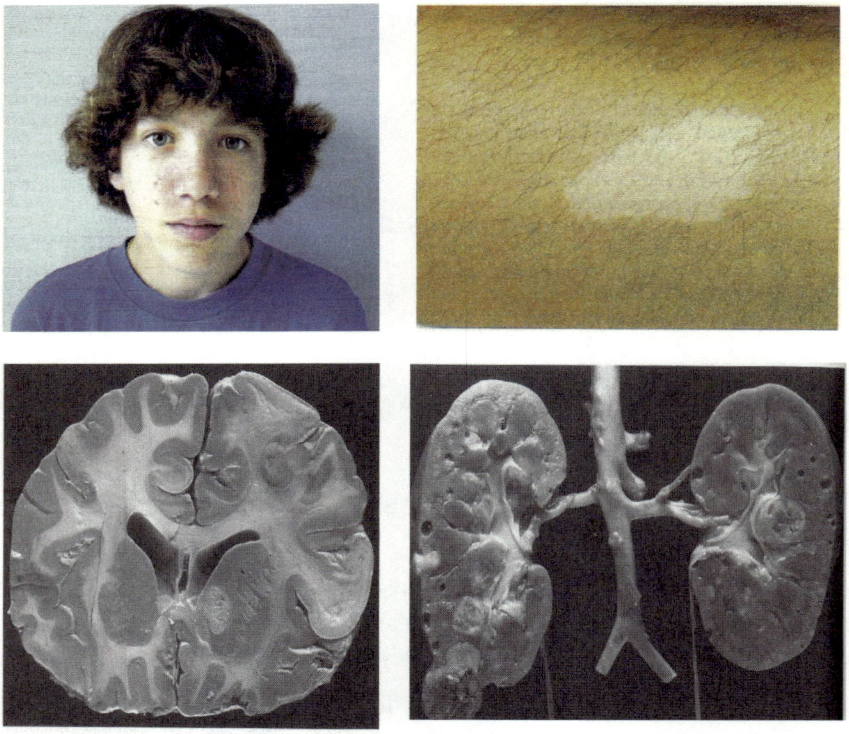

Fig. 9. Tuberous Sclerosis Complex. Hamartomatous lesions on skin (top left), hypomelanotic macules (top right), cortical tubers (bottom left) and angiomyolipomas (bottom right).

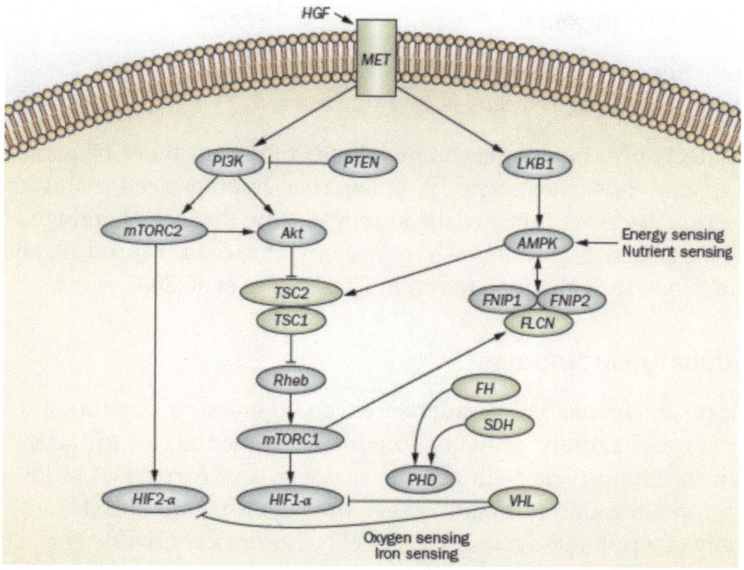

Fig. 10. TSC1-TSC2 tumor suppressor complex interacts with AMPK-mTOR nutrient and energy sensing pathway (with permission).

6.1 Therapeutic perspectives

Currently, there are a number of trials that evaluate the role of sirolimus in patients with Tuberous Sclerosis Complex. This agent has been demonstrated to cause the regression of angiomyolipomas, through the inhibition of the mTOR signaling pathway. Nevertheless, after the treatment was stopped, most renal tumors tended to growth again. In spite of that, this study provided the grounds for a molecular approach to the treatment of renal tumors associated with the *TSC1–TSC2* pathway (Linehan et al., 2010b).

7. Collecting-duct carcinomas

Collecting duct carcinomas (CDC) are uncommon and aggressive tumors thought to arise from cells of the distal nephron.

Their genetic defects have not been completely elucidated; however, they have shown cytogenetic and molecular alterations different from other renal tumors (Kennedy et al, 1990).

Nonetheless, some molecular findings suggest that these cancers are heterogeneous and can exhibit features similar to more common types of RCC as well as to urothelial carcinoma.

Genetic studies have shown monosomy of chromosomes 1, 6, 14, 15 and 22 and frequent allelic loss of 1q, 6p, 8p, 13q and 21q. Monosomy of 8p has been associated with high stage and aggressive behavior and might be responsible for the poor prognosis of CDC (Fuzesi et al, 1992). Loss of heterozygosity (LOH) of 3p is rarely detectable in these tumors, although *VHL* allelic loss has been occasionally reported. Moreover, some studies have found 9p LOH in half of CDC cases, whereas other studies have not. Mutations of the *RB* gene and LOH of 13q have also been observed in some CDC but its role in the pathogenesis of CDC needs to be clarified (Fogt et al, 1998).

8. Tubulocystic carcinomas

The molecular pathogenesis of tubulocystic carcinoma, a rare renal tumor composed of tubular and cystic structures, remains poorly understood.

The genomic defects of tubulocystic carcinoma are similar to those of papillary RCC, as it often exhibits trisomy of chromosome 17. It has been hypothesized that it may represent a lowgrade collecting duct carcinoma of the kidney despite the lack of enough citogenetic and molecular evidence, such as trisomy of 7, monosomy of 1, 6, 14, 15, and 22, allelic loss on 1q, 6p, 8p, 13q, and 21q, which are often found in CDC (Yang et al, 2008).

9. Renal medullary carcinomas

Renal medullary carcinoma is considered as an aggressive variant of collecting duct carcinoma, a rare and rapidly growing tumor of the medulla of kidneys. This tumor is frequently seen in young male with African ancestry and carriers of sickle cell trait. In a study of nine tumors through comparative genomic hybridization (CGH), eight depicted no changes and only one presented monosomy of chromosome 22 (Swartz et al, 2002).

10. TFE translocation carcinomas family

Accordingly with the WHO classification of renal tumors (Eble et al, 2004), an entity recently defined by chromosomal translocations involving the Xp11.2 region is responsible for about one third of renal carcinomas in children and young adults. These cancers resemble clear cell RCC and seems to have a benign evolution, even with metastasis, while others may behave aggressively. They are also known as the TFE translocation carcinoma family (MTTCF) (Tomlinson et al, 1991).

All translocations result in the production of quimeric proteins containing the *TFE3* product , such as those from *PRCC, ASPL, PSF,* and *NonO (p54nrb)* genes. For instance, translocation of Xp to chromosome 1 forms an in-frame fusion of the *TFE3* gene on Xp11.2 to a novel gene *PRCC* on chromosome 1(Camparo et al, 2008).

Because the normal TFE3 protein has a DNA-binding domain, fusion proteins composed of this gene product and the ubiquitously expressed PRCC and ASPL proteins result in the overexpression of an abnormal transcription factor that causes aberrant expression of cellular genes. Another subset of renal tumors are associated with a translocation t(6;11)(p21;q12) involving the transcription factor TFEB(Camparo et al, 2008).

Some gene expression profiling studies indicated a distinct subgroup of tumors. For example, TRIM 63 glutathione S-transferase A1 and alanyl aminopeptidase are the main differentially expressed genes for MTTCF (Camparo et al, 2008).

Therefore, the correct classification of these tumors may pose important prognostic and therapeutical implications. For instance, tumors with the ASPL-TFE3 translocation particularly present at an advanced stage associated with lymph node metastases. In addition, some tumors with *PRCC-TFE3* fusion have been shown to lack a normal mitotic checkpoint control, which may turn them more sensitive to chemotherapeutic agents that target microtubules, such as vincristine and paclitaxel (Lopez-Beltran et al, 2010).

11. Mucinous tubular and spindle renal cell carcinomas

These are rare and morphologically distinctive tumors, although they share some features of type I papillary RCC.

The main molecular differences between them have been studied through CGH expression microarrays. Two studies found multiple genetic abnormalities in all cases, such as losses of chromosomes 1, 4, 6, 8, 9,13, 14, 15, 18 and 22. The major differential diagnosis is papillary RCC with solid growth, whose gains of chromosomes 7 and 17 and losses of chromosome Y are typical, but lack in mucinous tubular and spindle RCC (Rakozy et al, 2002).

12. Renal cell carcinomas with sarcomatoid transformation

Sarcomatoid transformation has been seen in all of the common types of RCC: clear cell, papillary, chromophobe and collecting duct, but its specific molecular mechanisms remain poorly understood.

It is hypothesized that the sarcomatoid components of RCCs represent areas of dedifferentiation, and it seems that the genomic changes associated with a specific type of RCC should be conserved within the dedifferentiated sarcomatoid RCC component. In a recent study, the allelic loss profile between clear cell and sarcomatoid components of RCCs was compared and showed the same pattern of nonrandom X-chromosome inactivation in most cases. The results suggested that both clear cell and sarcomatoid components of RCCs are derived from the same progenitor cell. Some other studies suggest a link between mutation of the *TP53* tumor suppressor gene and sarcomatoid morphology. Major differential diagnosis is poorly differentiated urothelial carcinoma of the renal pelvis, which presents peculiar genetic profiles, specifically, gains of chromosome 3, 7, 17 and losses of 9p21 (Lopez-Beltran et al, 2010).

13. Acquired cystic disease-associated renal tumors

Interestingly, in kidneys that have developed acquired cystic disease and, consequently, resulting in end-stage renal disease, two distinctive types of renal neoplasm have been found to occur: 'acquired cystic disease-associated RCC' and 'clear cell papillary RCC' (Cossu-Rocca et al, 2010).

Acquired cystic disease-associated RCCs are morphologically heterogeneous with abundant eosinophilic cytoplasm and variably solid , cribriform, tubulocystic with papillary architecture. Chromosomal aberrations have been found in these tumors in few studies, such as gains of chromosomes 1, 2, 6, 7, 10 and 17 (Cossu-Rocca et al, 2010).

Clear cell papillary RCC presents with papillary structures proliferating within cystic spaces, both lined by cells with clear cytoplasm. Through interphase FISH analysis, a study found all tumors to lack the gains of chromosome 7 and loss of Y, which are peculiar for papillary RCC and, in addition, there was no 3p deletion, which is typical of clear cell RCC.

The other major differential diagnoses are: tubulocystic carcinoma (trisomic for 17 but not for 7), chromophobe RCC (multiple chromosomal losses) and oncocytoma (loss of chromosome 1) (Lopez-Beltran et al, 2010).

14. Thyroid-like follicular renal cell carcinoma

Recently, there have been reports of an uncommon renal tumor, which had not been classified under a known subtype of RCC (Lopez-Beltran et al, 2010). It shows similar histology to thyroid follicular carcinoma and seems to affect more often women without previous lesions in the thyroid.

Chromosomal gains of 7q36, 8q24, 12, 16, 17p11-q11, 17q24, 19q, 20q13, 21q22.3, and Xp and losses of 1p36, 3, and 9q21-33 were identified through CGH. However, a recent report did not found any chromosomal alterations on CGH analysis. It is speculated that thyroid-like follicular RCC may represent a unique histological subtype of RCC of low malignant potential (Lopez-Beltran et al, 2010).

15. Conclusion

Currently, there is sufficient evidence that kidney cancer is essentially a disease of dysregulated cellular metabolism (Linehan et al, 2010a).

Germline mutations in each of the seven genes involved in inherited kidney cancer syndromes lead to the dysregulation of at least one metabolic pathway that is mediated by oxygen, iron, energy or nutrient sensing (Figure 11).

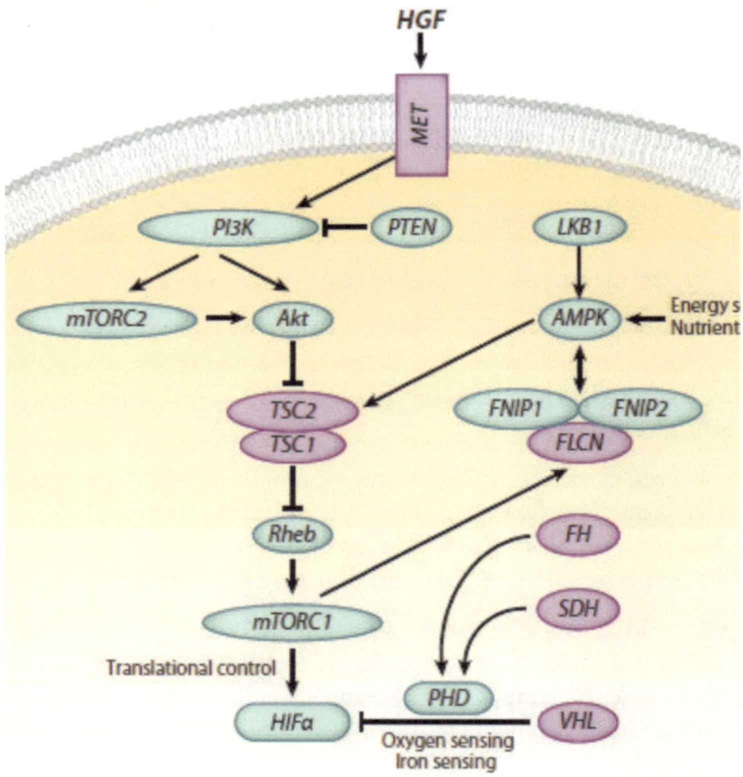

Fig. 11. The metabolic pathways mediated by the seven tumor suppressor genes mutated in hereditary cancer syndromes (with permission)

The shared consequence of *VHL, FH* and *SDH* mutations is the stabilization of HIFs through inactivation of the prolyl-hydroxilase domain, which leads to the transcriptional activation of genes that stimulate tumor growth, neovascularization, invasion and metastasis. HIF overexpression is also triggered by the upregulation of the mTOR pathway, either through inactivating mutations in the tumor suppressor genes *TSC1,TSC2* and *FLCN,* or activating oncogenic "signalling pathways".

By targeting HIF and its downstream genes, a first-line therapeutic approach to VHL-deficient renal tumors may be feasible and can also be applied to FH-deficient and SDH-deficient tumors. To date, novel agents focusing on the VHL pathway have been approved for the treatment of patients with advanced kidney cancer (Table 2) (Linehan et al, 2010b). Unfortunately, however, most of them occasionally present progression and rarely promote long-term complete responses.

In conclusion, the pursuit of a thorough understanding of the molecular pathogenesis and the intricate metabolic pathways of advanced renal cell carcinoma may provide the foundation for the development of novel approaches that might possibly increase the response and survival rates of patients with this extremely heterogeneous disease.

Histology	**Gene**	**Drug**
Clear cell	VHL	Sunitinib, sorafenib, bevacizumab, temsirolimus, everolimus, axitinib
Type 1 papillary	MET	Foretinib
Type 2 papillary	FH	Targeting VEGF
Chromophobe Oncocytoma Hibrid oncocytic	FLCN or BHD	Rapamycin
Angiomyolipoma	TSC1, TSC2	Sirolimus

Table 2. Targeted therapies for the most common renal cell carcinomas

16. References

Baba, M.; Hong, S.; Sharma, N. (2006). Folliculin Encoded by the BHD Gene Interacts with a Binding Protein, FNIP1, and AMPK, and is Involved in AMPK and mTOR Signaling. *Proc Natl Acad Sci U S A*, Vol.103, pp. 15552–15557.

Boccaccio, C. & Comoglio, P. (2006). Invasive Growth: a MET-driven Genetic Programme for Cancer and Stem Cells. *Nat Rev Cancer*, Vol.6, pp. 637–645.

Camparo, P.; Vasiliu, V.; Molinie, V. (2008). Renal Translocation Carcinomas: Clinicopathologic, Immunohistochemical, and Gene Expression Profiling Analysis of 31 Cases with a Review of the Literature. *Am. J.Surg. Pathol.*, Vol.32, pp. 656–670.

Cohen, H. & McGovern, F. (2005). Renal-Cell Carcinoma. *N Engl J Med,* Vol.353, pp. 2477-2490.

Cossu-Rocca, P.; Eble, J.; Zhang, S.; Martignoni, G.; Brunelli, M. & Cheng, L. (2010). Acquired Cystic Disease-associated Renal Tumors: an Immunohistochemical and Fluorescence in situ Hybridization Study. *Mod. Pathol.*, Vol.19, pp.780–787.

Crino, P. B.; Nathanson, K. L. & Henske, E. P.(2006). The Tuberous Sclerosis Complex. *N. Engl. J.Med.* Vol.355, pp. 1345–1356.

De Luca, A.; Carotenuto, P.; D´Alessio, A.; Normanno, N. (2008). Molecular Biology of Renal-Cell Carcinoma. *European Journal of Cancer,* Vol.6, pp. 30-34.

Eble, J.; Sauter, G.; Epstein, J. & Sesterhenn, I. (2004). *Pathology and Genetics. Tumors of the Urinary System and Male Genital Organs.* IARC Press, Lyon, France.

Ewalt, D.; Sheffield, E.; Sparagana, S.; Delgado, M. & Roach, E. (1998). Renal Lesion Growth in Children with Tuberous Sclerosis Complex. *J Urol.*, Vol.160, No.1, pp. 141–145.

Fogt, F.; Zhuang, Z.; Linehan, W. & Merino, M. (1998). Collecting Duct Carcinomas of the Kidney: a Comparative Loss of Heterozygosity Study with Clear Cell Renal Cell Carcinoma. *Oncol. Rep.*, Vol.5, pp. 923–926.

Fuzesi, L.; Cober, M. & Mittermayer, C. (1992). Collecting Duct Carcinoma: Cytogenetic Characterization. *Histopathology* vol.21, pp. 155–160.

Gnarra, J.; Tory, K.; Weng, Y. (1994). Mutations of theVHL Tumor Suppressor Gene in Renal Carcinoma. *Nat. Genet,* Vol.7, pp. 85–90.

Gordan, J. D. *et al.* (2008). HIF-alpha Effects on c-Myc Distinguish Two Subtypes of Sporadic VHL-deficient Clear Cell Renal Carcinoma. *Cancer Cell,* Vol.14, pp. 435–446.

Henske, E. (2004). The genetic basis of kidney cancer: why is tuberous sclerosis complex often overlooked? *Curr Mol Med.* Vol. 4, No.8, pp. 825–831.

Higgins, J.; Shinghal, R.; Gill, H. (2003). Gene Expression Patterns in Renal Cell Carcinoma Assessed by Complementary DNA Microarray. *Am J Pathol,* Vol.162, pp. 925–932.

Iliopoulos O. (2006). Molecular Biology of Renal Cell Cancer and the Identification of Therapeutic Targets. *J Clin Oncol.*, Vol.24, pp. 5593–5600.

Isaacs, J.; Jung, Y.; Mole, D. (2005). HIF Overexpression Correlates with Biallelic Loss of Fumarate Hydratase in Renal Cancer: Novel Role of Fumarate in Regulation of HIF Stability. *Cancer Cell,* Vol. 8, pp. 143–153.

Kennedy, S.; Merino, M.; Linehan, W.; Roberts, J.; Robertson, C. & Neumann, R.(1990). Collecting Duct Carcinoma of the Kidney. *Hum. Pathol.*, Vol.21, pp. 449–456.

Khoo, S.; Kahnoski, K.; Sugimura, J. (2003). Inactivation of BHD in Sporadic Renal Tumors. *Cancer Res,* Vol.63, pp. 4583–4587.

Kim, W. & Kaelin, W. (2004). Role of VHL Gene Mutation in Human Cancer. *J Clin Oncol,* Vol.22, pp. 4991–5004.

Kondo, K., Klco, J., Nakamura, E., Lechpammer, M. & Kaelin, W. G. Jr. (2002). Inhibition of HIF is Necessary for Tumor Suppression by the von Hippel–Lindau Protein. *Cancer Cell,* Vol.1, pp. 237–246.

Kovacs G.; Akhtar, M.; Beckwith, B. (1997). The Heidelberg Classification of Renal Cell Tumours. *J Pathol* Vol.183, pp.131-133.

Kuznetsova, A.; Meller, J.; Schnell, P. (2003). Von Hippel-Lindau Protein Binds Hyperphosphorylated Large Subunit of RNA Polymerase II Through a Proline Hydroxylation Motif and Targets it for Ubiquitination. *Proc Natl Acad Sci USA* Vol.100, pp. 2706-2711.

Lin, Z.; Han, E.; Lee, E. (2004). A Distinct Expression Pattern and Point Mutation of c-kit in Papillary Renal Cell Carcinomas. *Mod Pathol,* Vol.17, pp. 611–616.

Linehan, W.; Srinivasan, R. & Schmidt, L. (2010a). The Genetic Basis of Kidney Cancer: a Metabolic Disease. *Nature Reviews Urology,* Vol.7, (May 2010), pp. 277-285.

Linehan, W.; Bratslavsky, G. ; Pinto, P. ; Schmidt, L. ; Neckers, L. ; Bottaro, D. & Srinivasan, R. (2010b). Molecular Diagnosis and Therapy of Kidney Cancer. *Annual Review of Medicine,* Vol.61, pp. 329-343.

Lopez-Beltran, A.; Montironi, R. ; Egevad, L. ; Caballero-Vargas, M. ; Scarpelli, M. ; Kirkali, Z. & Cheng, L. (2010). Genetic Profiles in Renal Tumors. *Internation Journal of Urology,* Vol.17, pp. 6-19.

Maher, E.; Yates, J.; Harries, R. (1990). Clinical Features and Natural History of von Hippel-Lindau Disease. *Q.J.Med,* Vol.77, pp. 1151-1163.

Maxwell, P.; Wiesener, M.; Chang, G. (1999). The Tumour Suppressor Protein VHL Targets Hypoxia-inducible Factors for Oxygen-dependent Proteolysis. *Nature,* Vol.399, pp. 271–275.

McLaughlin, J.; Mandel, J.; Blot, W.; Schuman, L.; Mehl, E. & Fraumeni, J. (1984). A Population-based Case-control Study of Renal Cell Carcinoma. *J Natl Cancer Inst,* Vol.72, pp. 275-284.

Neumann, H.; Pawlu, C.; Peczkowska, M. (2004). Distinct Clinical Features of Paraganglioma Syndromes Associated with SDHB and SDHD Gene Mutations. *JAMA* Vol.292, pp. 943–951.

Nickerson, M.; Warren, M.; Toro, J. (2002). Mutations in a Novel Gene Lead to Kidney Tumors, Lung Wall Defects, and Benign Tumors of the Hair Follicle in Patients with the Birt–Hogg–Dube Syndrome. *Cancer Cell,* Vol.2, pp. 157–164.

Ohh, M.; Yauch, R.; Lonergan, K. (1998). The von Hippel-Lindau Tumor Suppressor Protein is Required for Proper Assembly of an Extracellular Fibronectin Matrix. *Mol Cell,* Vol.1, pp. 959-968.

Patel, P.; Chadalavada, R.; Chaganti, R. (2006). Targeting von Hippel-Lindau Pathway in Renal Cell Carcinoma. *Clin Cancer Res,* Vol.12, pp. 7215–7220.

Pennacchietti, S.; Michieli, P.; Galluzzo M. (2003). Hypoxia Promotes Invasive Growth by Transcriptional Activation of the MET Protooncogene. *Cancer Cell,* Vol.3, pp. 347-361.

Rakozy, C.; Schmahl, G.; Bogner, S. & Storkel, S. (2002). Low-grade Tubular-mucinous Renal Neoplasms: Morphologic, Immunohistochemical, and genetic features. *Mod. Pathol.,* Vol.15, pp. 1162–1171.

Ricketts, C.; Woodward, E.; Killick, P. (2008). Germline SDHB Mutations and Familial Renal Cell Carcinoma. *J. Natl. Cancer Inst.,* Vol.100, pp. 1260–12662.

Roe, J.; Kim, H.; Lee, S. (2006). p53 Stabilization and Transactivation by a von Hippel-Lindau Protein. *Mol Cell,* Vol.22, pp. 395-405.

Schmidt, L.; Duh, F.; Chen, F. (1997). Germline and Somatic Mutations in the Tyrosine Kinase Domain of the MET Protooncogene in Papillary Renal Carcinomas. *Nat Genet,* Vol.16, pp. 68–73.

Schmidt, L.; Junker, K.; Nakaigawa, N. (1999). Novel Mutations of the MET Proto-oncogene in Papillary Renal Carcinomas. *Oncogene,* Vol.18, pp. 2343–2350.

Schmidt, L.; Nickerson, M.; Warren, M. (2005). Germline BHD Mutation Spectrum and Phenotype Analysis of a Large Cohort of Families with Birt–Hogg–Dube Syndrome. *Am J Hum Genet,* Vol.76, pp. 1023–1033.

Srinivasan, R.; Choueiri, T.; Vaishampayan, U. (2008). A Phase II Study of the Dual MET/VEGFR2 Inhibitor XL880 in Patients with Papillary Renal Carcinoma. *J. Clin. Oncol.* Vol.27 (Suppl), pp.15s.

Sudarshan, S.; Sourbier, C.; Kong, H. (2009). Fumarate Hydratase Deficiency in Renal Cancer Induces Glycolytic Addiction and HIF-1α Stabilization by Glucose-dependent Generation of Reactive Oxygen Species. *Mol. Cell Biol.* Vol.15, pp. 4080–4090.

Swartz, M.; Karth, J.; Schneider, D.; Rodriguez, R.; Beckwith, J. & Perlman, E. (2002). Renal Medullary Carcinoma: Clinical, Pathologic, Immunohistochemical, and Genetic Analysis with Pathogenetic Implications. *Urology,* Vol.60, pp. 1083–1089.

Thomas, G.; Tran, C.; Mellinghoff, I. (2006). Hypoxia-inducible Factor Determines Sensitivity to Inhibitors of mTOR in Kidney Cancer. *Nat. Med.,* Vol.12, pp. 122–127.

Tomlinson, G.; Nisen, P.; Timmons, C. & Schneider, N. (1991). Cytogenetics of a Renal Cell Carcinoma in a 17-month-old Child. Evidence for Xp11.2 as a Recurring Breakpoint. *Cancer Genet. Cytogenet.,* Vol.57, pp. 11–17.

Tomlinson, I.; Alam, N.; Rowan, A. (2002). Germline Mutations in FH Predispose to Dominantly Inherited Uterine Fibroids, Skin Leiomyomata and Papillary Renal Cell Cancer. *Nat. Genet.* Vol.30, pp. 406–410.

Turcotte, S. *et al.* (2008). A Molecule Targeting VHL-deficient Renal Cell Carcinoma that Induces Autophagy. *Cancer Cell* Vol.14, pp. 90–102.

Vocke, C.; Yang, Y.; Pavlovich, C. (2005). High Frequency of Somatic Frameshift BHD Gene Mutations in Birt–Hogg–Dube Associated Renal Tumors. *J Natl Cancer Inst,* Vol.97, pp. 931–935.

Washecka, R. & Hanna, M. (1991). Malignant Renal Tumors in Tuberous Sclerosis. *Urology,* Vol.37, No.4, pp. 340–343.

Yang, X.; Zhou, M.; Hes, O. (2008). Tubulocystic Carcinoma of the Kidney: Clinicopathologic and Molecular Characterization. *Am. J. Surg. Pathol.,* Vol.32, pp. 177–187.

2

Molecular Portrait of Clear Cell Renal Cell Carcinoma: An Integrative Analysis of Gene Expression and Genomic Copy Number Profiling

Cristina Battaglia et al.*
Dept. of Biomedical Sciences and Technologies, University of Milano, Milano, Doctoral School of Molecular Medicine, University of Milano, Milano, Italy

1. Introduction

Renal cell carcinoma (RCC) incidence accounts for about 3 to 10 cases per 100,000 individuals with a predilection for adult males over 60 year old (1.6:1 male/female ratio) (Chow, 2010; Nese, 2009). In Europe, about 60,000 individuals are affected by RCC every year, with a mortality rate of about 18,000 subjects and an incidence rate for all stages steadily rising over the last three decades. Although inherited forms occur in a number of familial cancer syndromes, as the well-known von Hippel-Lindau (VHL) syndrome, RCC is commonly sporadic (Cohen & McGovern, 2005; Kaelin, 2007) and, as recently highlighted by the National Cancer Institute (NCI), influenced by the interplay between exposure to environmental risk factors and genetic susceptibility of exposed individuals (Chow et al., 2010). Being poorly symptomatic in early phases, many cases become clinically detectable only when already advanced and, as such, therapy-resistant (Motzer, 2011). Based on histology, RCC can be classified into several subtypes, i.e., clear cell (80% of cases), papillary (10%), chromophobe (5%) and oncocytoma (5%), each one characterized by specific histo-pathological features, malignant potential and clinical outcome (Cohen & McGovern, 2005). Patient stratification is normally achieved using prognostic algorithms and nomograms based on multiple clinico-pathological factors such as TNM stage, Fuhrman nuclear grade, tumor size, performance status, necrosis and other hematological indices (Flanigan et al., 2011), although the most efficient predictors of survival and recurrence are based on nuclear grade alone (Nese et al., 2009). As recently reviewed by Brannon et al. (Brannon & Rathmell, 2010), a finer RCC subtype classification could be obtained exploiting the vast amount of

* Eleonora Mangano[3], Silvio Bicciato[4], Fabio Frascati[3], Simona Nuzzo[4], Valentina Tinaglia[1,2], Cristina Bianchi[5], Roberto A. Perego[5] and Ingrid Cifola[3]
[1]*Dept. of Biomedical Sciences and Technologies, University of Milano, Milano, Italy;*
[2]*Doctoral School of Molecular Medicine, University of Milano, Milano, Italy*
[3]*Institute for Biomedical Technologies, National Research Council, Segrate, Italy*
[4]*Center for Genome Research, University of Modena and Reggio Emilia, Modena, Italy;*
[5]*Dept. of Experimental Medicine, University of Milano-Bicocca, Milano, Italy*

genomic and transcriptional data that have been presented in numerous studies. For instance, several authors proposed a molecular classification of RCC based on differential gene expression profiles, with any subtype characterized by the activation of distinct gene sets (Brannon, 2010; Furge, 2004; Skubitz, 2006; Sültmann, 2005; Zhang, 2008), while others identified RCC-specific biomarkers (e.g. CA9, ki67, VEGF proteins, phosphorylated AKT, PTEN, HIF-1α). Lately, it has been reported that microRNAs, a small class of non coding RNA molecules, could contribute to RCC development at different levels and may represent a new group of potential tumor biomarkers (Redova et al., 2011). Despite the numerous efforts in dissecting the molecular features of RCC through functional genomics, not a single transcriptional signature or biomarker has gained approval for clinical application yet (Arsanious, 2009; Eichelberg, 2009; Lam, 2007; Yin-Goen, 2006), so that the identification of novel molecular markers to improve early diagnosis and prognostic prediction and of candidate targets to develop new therapeutic approaches remains of primary importance for this pathology.

Among the RCC histotypes, clear cell renal carcinoma (ccRCC) is the most frequent and aggressive subtype and is characterized by a specific pattern of chromosomal alterations (Yoshimoto et al., 2007) that represents a molecular fingerprint potentially useful for diagnostic and prognostic applications (Klatte et al., 2007). Nowadays, the standard clinical treatment comprises surgical resection followed by IFN- and/or IL2-based immunotherapy, although therapy toxicity still represents a major problem (Molina & Motzer, 2011). The development of approaches targeting specific biological pathways, typically deregulated in this tumor, is opening the way to new opportunities for therapeutic intervention (Pal et al., 2010). One of the most investigated processes is the hypoxia pathway (Cohen & McGovern2005; Kaelin, 2007; Wouters & Koritzinsky, 2008) that is genetically linked to ccRCC through one of its key players, i.e., the VHL (von Hippel-Lindau) gene, completely inactivated in all inherited forms and in 80% of sporadic cases. Cloned in 1993, the VHL gene (located at the 3p25.3 locus) is currently known as the main tumor suppressor gene involved in the very early steps of RCC pathogenesis (Banks et al., 2006). Normally, the VHL function is to ubiquinate the two hypoxia-inducible factors HIF-1α and HIF-2α, addressing them to proteasome degradation (Kaelin, 2008). In ccRCC, the bi-allelic VHL inactivation, by combination of deletion and mutation/methylation (Banks et al., 2006), prevents the degradation of HIF-1α and HIF-2α that, in turn, can activate the transcription of a series of hypoxia-inducible genes, such as VEGF, VEGFR, EGFR, PDGF, IGF, GLUT-1, CXCR4, TGF-α, CA9 and EPO, involved in processes like angiogenesis, survival, cell motility, pH-regulation and glucose metabolism (Baldewijns et al., 2010). The complete loss of VHL function results in the up-regulation of a panel of genes that contributes to the ccRCC phenotype and represents a list of potential prognostic markers (Klatte et al., 2007) and/or therapeutic targets (Gong et al., 2010). Additionally, the transcription factor HIF-1α is commonly activated in cancer (Semenza, 2008) and is linked to oncogenic/tumor suppressor molecules implicated in cross-communication, such as the tubular sclerosis complex (TSC) and the mammalian target of rapamycin (mTOR) (Maxwell, 2005). As such, ccRCC represents an ideal model for developing novel targeted therapies directed against the hypoxia pathway and many molecules are already used in clinical trials targeting either HIF-1α, or the upstream pathways regulating HIF (as the Akt-mTOR signal transduction pathway), or the downstream genes induced by HIF (e.g., VEGF and VEGFR) (Baldewijns et al., 2010). Intriguingly, recent evidences indicate that also 20% of RCC sporadic cases with wild-type VHL (and active VHL function) present a peculiar pattern of altered genes, suggesting the involvement of other, still partially unknown, alternative regulatory mechanisms (Gordan et al., 2008).

At DNA level, studies based on traditional cytogenetic and comparative genomic hybridization (CGH) techniques identified a panel of chromosomal aberrations typical of ccRCC (Höglund, 2004; Klatte, 2009). Moreover, high-density single nucleotide polymorphism (SNP) array technology, interrogating thousands of SNP markers distributed throughout the whole human genome, has significantly improved the detection of chromosomal aberrations and offered the opportunity to detect regions with loss of heterozygosity (LOH), an important information for the identification of novel tumor suppressor genes. SNP-arrays have been widely applied to characterize tumor genomic instability (Brenner & Rosenberg, 2010; Lisovich, 2011) and recently to perform the genome-wide DNA profiling of ccRCC tissue samples (Beroukhim, 2009; Chen, 2009; Cifola, 2008). Overall, ccRCC is characterized by recurrent genetic anomalies at characteristic chromosomes, such as deletions with LOH on chromosomes 3p (involving also the VHL locus), 6q, 8p, 9p, and 14q, and duplications of chromosomes 5q and 7. Many evidences suggest that this peculiar pattern of genomic instability represents a tumor-specific molecular fingerprint that has a role in cancer pathogenesis and may be useful in diagnostic and prognostic applications (Gunawan, 2001; Klatte, 2009; Perego, 2008). Furthermore, a comprehensive study showed that cytogenetic alterations could be associated to ccRCC tumorigenesis and malignant progression (Zhang et al., 2010b).

Advances in high-throughput genome-wide profiling technologies allowed an unprecedented comprehensive view of the cancer genome landscape. In particular, high-density microarrays and sequencing-based strategies have been widely used to identify genetic (gene dosage, allelic status, and mutations in gene sequence) and epigenetic (DNA methylation, histone modification, and microRNA) aberrations in cancer (Majewski & Bernards, 2011). The integrative approach of analyzing parallel dimensions has enabled the identification of genes that are often disrupted by multiple mechanisms but at low frequencies by any one mechanism and of pathways that are often disrupted at multiple components but at low frequencies at individual components (Chari et al., 2010). In these last years, there is an increasing tendency to combine genome-wide DNA copy number (CN) analysis with transcriptional profiles to investigate how alterations in DNA content (aneuploidy) can influence global expression patterns. In cancer research, this combined approach helps filtering the large amount of array-based data and, by narrowing down the hundreds of differentially expressed genes to those whose altered expression is attributable to underlying chromosomal alterations, allows highlighting candidate genes that are actively involved in the causation or maintenance of the malignant phenotype. This approach was applied in a wide range of tumor types, including breast (Hyman, 2002; Pollack, 2002), bladder (Harding et al., 2002), prostate (Saramäki et al., 2006), pancreas (Heidenblad et al., 2005), rectal (Grade et al., 2006) and melanoma (Akavia et al., 2010), demonstrating a strong genome-wide correlation between aneuploidy-associated genomic imbalances and global gene expression levels. Most studies focused on amplified and over-expressed genes and calculated that a fraction ranging from 44% to 62% of amplified genes showed concomitant up-regulated expression levels (Hyman et al., 2002). This suggests the presence of an aneuploidy-induced deregulation of the cancer transcriptome that occurs in addition to the transcriptional and mutational deregulation of oncogenes and tumor suppressor genes. This combined approach is exemplified in the study by Garraway et al., in which the analysis of CN data obtained by SNP arrays drives the investigation of pre-existing gene expression profiles (Garraway et al., 2005). Specifically, CN data were used to organize cancer samples into subgroups characterized by specific chromosomal aberrations associated to contiguous SNP chromosomal clusters. This genomic-based sub-grouping constituted the new phenotypic labeling of the samples in the gene expression analysis, i.e. samples from the NCI-60 cancer cell lines panel were re-grouped into two new classes based on the presence or absence of amplification at 3p14-p13 before performing the supervised analysis. The differential expression profiles, inside the SNP cluster characterizing the amplification at 3p14-p13, identified MITF gene as a novel melanoma-specific oncogene. This study clearly demonstrated the usefulness of an integrative approach to investigate candidate regions and genes specifically involved in tumor etiology and potentially useful as novel specific cancer biomarkers.

Clearly, to allow the rapid development of these innovative analytical procedures, it is necessary to implement novel and even more sophisticated mathematical and statistical algorithms. For instance, an important issue is to understand how combining and comparing microarray expression data of single genes with DNA copy number data of whole chromosomal regions. Thus, there is an increasing interest for developing computational tools able to link single differentially expressed genes to their chromosomal location, in order to calculate differentially expressed chromosomal regions and thus assemble regional transcriptional activity maps (Akavia, 2010; Schäfer, 2009). To address the integrative analysis of gene expression and copy number data in tumor samples, we recently developed a computational tool named Position RElated Data Analysis (*preda*, Ferrari et al., 2011). *preda* is particularly suited for the identification of chromosomal regions with concomitant and coordinated copy number and transcriptional imbalances (SODEGIRs, Bicciato et al., 2009), thus providing an opportunity for upgrading the information content of genomic data and for discovering novel cancer biomarkers.

In this chapter, we describe a general framework for depicting the molecular portrait of ccRCC through the integrative analysis of gene expression and copy number profiles obtained from publicly available datasets. The chapter is structured in Methods, Results and Discussion and addresses three major issues: i) the analysis and the functional characterization of a large compendium of gene expression data; ii) the identification of chromosomal alterations in ccRCC samples from SNP copy number data; iii) the integrative analysis of gene expression and copy number data.

2. Methods

2.1 Gene expression analysis of ccRCC

To characterize the transcriptional portrait of ccRCC, we retrieved 12 datasets containing microarray gene expression data of clear cell renal carcinoma and normal samples annotated with clinical information. All data were measured on several releases of the Affymetrix Human Genome HG-U133 arrays (i.e., HG-U133A; HG-U133 Plus 2.0, HG-U133A 2.0 and HT-HG-U133A) and have been downloaded from the public microarray data repositories Gene Expression Omnibus (GEO, http://www.ncbi.nlm.nih.gov/geo/; 11 datasets) and

ArrayExpress (http://www.ebi.ac.uk/arrayexpress/; 1 dataset). Prior to analysis, we re-organized all datasets by manually annotating and tagging all samples, and re-named any original dataset after the first author's name of the corresponding publication. This re-organization resulted in a compendium of 426 samples comprising 320 ccRCCs and 106 normal renal tissues (Table 1). ccRCC samples have been further annotated according to nuclear grade and divided into a low-grade (n=197) and a high-grade (n=123) class, with the low-grade class comprising 29 G1 and 168 G2 samples and the high-grade class including 97 G3 and 26 G4 samples.

Microarray repository code	Dataset name	Samples		References
		ccRCC	*normal*	
GSE781[a]	Lenburg	9	8	Lenburg et al., 2003
GSE15641[a]	Jones	---	23	Jones et al., 2005
GSE6344[a]	Gumz	---	10	Gumz et al., 2007
GSE7023[b]	Furge	---	13	Furge et al., 2007
GSE14762[b]	Wang	---	12	Wang et al., 2009
GSE2109[b]	Bittner	188	---	International Genomics Consortium
GSE11151[b]	Yusenko	---	3	Yusenko et al., 2009
E-TAM-282[b]	Cifola	16	11	Cifola et al., 2008
GSE17895[b]	Dalgliesh	83	13	Dalgliesh et al., 2010
GSE12606[b]	Stickel	3	3	Stickel et al., 2009
GSE11904[c]	Gordan	21	---	Gordan et al., 2008
GSE14994[d]	Beroukhim	26[e]	11	Beroukhim et al., 2009

Table 1. Independent datasets included in the ccRCC compendium. The Affymetrix platforms used to obtain the original data are: [a]HG-U133A, [b]HG-U133 Plus 2.0, [c]HG-U133A 2.0, and [d]HT-HG-U133A. Samples from Beroukhim dataset ([e]) were used only in the integrative analysis of gene expression and copy number, since no grading annotation was available.

The integration and normalization of gene expression signals, obtained using different types of microarray in different experiments, is the most critical step for the meta-analysis of public available data since their direct integration may result in misleading results, due to dissimilar experimental conditions, laboratory-dependent bias, etc. Although Robust Multiarray Analysis (RMA; Irizarry et al., 2003) is the most effective signal quantification method, it cannot be applied to data obtained from different platforms (e.g., the HG-U133A and the HG-U133 Plus 2.0 arrays), due to differences in number, type and physical position of probes. As such, we implemented a procedure, called the Virtual Chip, to create a custom and virtual microarray grid that integrates the geometry and probe content of two or more types of Affymetrix arrays (Fallarino et al., 2010). Once defined the virtual grid, all raw data (represented by the so called CEL files) are re-organized to match a single platform, i.e. the virtual chip. At this point, raw data, originally from different types of microarrays, become homogeneous in terms of platform and can be preprocessed and normalized adopting standard approaches, as RMA. The Virtual Chip method allows combining data directly at the level of probe fluorescence intensity and presents the advantage that gene expression signals are generated with a single step of background correction, normalization and summarization. The construction of the virtual grid is inspired by the generation of custom Chip Definition Files (CDFs), i.e., of ad-hoc probe designs and array topologies. In custom CDFs, probes matching the same transcript, but belonging to different probe sets, are aggregated into putative custom-probe sets, each one including only those probes with a unique and exclusive correspondence with a single transcript. Similarly, probes matching the same transcript but located at different coordinates on different types of arrays may be merged in custom-probe sets and arranged in a virtual platform grid, whose geometry can be arbitrarily set. As for any other microarray geometry, this virtual grid may be used as a reference to create a virtual CDF file containing the probes of the Virtual Chip and their coordinates on the virtual platform. The probes included in the virtual CDF are those shared among the platforms of interest, with the additional condition of generating custom probe set of at least 4 probes. The virtual CDF can be derived from any custom CDF, e.g., those developed by Dai and publicly accessible at the Molecular and Behavioral Neuroscience Institute Microarray Lab (Dai et al., 2005). Finally, the virtual CDF can be used as the geometry file in RMA as far as the original CEL files are properly re-mapped to match the topology described in the virtual CDF. Re-mapped CEL files, called virtual CEL files, are homogeneous in terms of platform and gene expression data can be generated with a single step of background correction, normalization and summarization directly from the fluorescence signals of all microarrays composing the meta-dataset. In this particular case, expression values of the meta-dataset were generated from intensity signals using the combined HG-U133A/HG-U133 Plus 2.0/HG-U133A 2.0/HT-HG-U133A virtual-CDF file, the custom definition files for Affymetrix human arrays based on Entrez (version 12.1.0; http://brainarray.mbni.med.umich.edu/Brainarray/Database/CustomCDF/12.1.0/entrezg.asp), and the transformed virtual-CEL files. Intensity values of meta-probe sets have been background adjusted, normalized using quantile normalization, and gene expression levels calculated using median polish summarization (RMA algorithm; Irizarry et al., 2003). The final meta-dataset comprised gene expression values for a total of 11809 Entrez gene IDs and 426 samples.

The meta-dataset was analyzed using the Analysis of Variance (ANOVA) package of Partek Genomics Suite software (Version 6.5, http://www.partek.com/; Partek Inc., St Louis, MO, USA) to identify a list of differentially expressed genes (DEGs) between ccRCC samples and normal renal tissues. Specifically, genes have been defined as differentially expressed if the average expression values in the two groups differed of at least 2-folds and the False Discovery Rate (FDR; Benjamini-Hochberg method) of the statistical comparison was less than 0.05. Differentially expressed genes have been functionally characterized in term of Gene Ontology (GO) biological process (BP) using DAVID tool (http://david.abcc.ncifcrf.gov/; (Huang, 2009a, 2009b) with an FDR≤0.001. Ingenuity Pathways Analysis (IPA, version 9.0) has been applied to assess functional connections that are statistically overrepresented among the differentially expressed genes. Briefly, in IPA, a p-value, calculated by a right tailed Fisher's Exact Test, quantifies the probability of observing the fraction of the focus genes in the canonical pathway as compared to the fraction expected by chance in the reference set, with the assumption that each gene is equally likely to be picked by chance. Finally, we investigated whether expression levels in ccRCCs and normal tissues were associated with elevated expression of biologically relevant gene sets using Gene Set Enrichment Analysis (GSEA, http://www.broadinstitute.org/gsea/index.jsp; Subramanian et al., 2005) on the meta-dataset. In particular, 217 BioCarta and 186 KEGG gene sets were taken from the Molecular Signatures Database (http://www.broadinstitute.org/gsea/msigdb/index.jsp; version 3.0) and a list of 145 genes associated to HIF and VHL genes was downloaded from the NCBI Pathway Interaction Database (http://pid.nci.nih.gov). Gene sets have been considered significantly enriched at FDR≤0.25 when using Signal2Noise as metric and 1,000 permutations of phenotype labels.

2.2 Genomic copy number analysis of ccRCC

To assess copy number alterations in ccRCC, we used two datasets composed of 27 sporadic ccRCC samples profiled by Affymetrix Human Mapping 100K SNP arrays and downloaded from AE (E-TAM-283, E-TAM-284; Cifola et al., 2008) and 26 sporadic ccRCC samples profiled by Affymetrix Human Mapping 250K Sty SNP array and downloaded from GEO (GSE14994; Beroukhim et al., 2009). The genomic copy number values were quantified using Partek Genomics Suite and the presence of copy number alterations, i.e., chromosomal segments affected by amplification or deletion, was calculated using Partek Genomic Segmentation (GS) algorithm. Partek baseline generated from 90 Mapping 100K Hind/Xba HapMap trio samples (available at Affymetrix website; http://www.affymetrix.com/support/technical/sample_data/hapmap_trio_data.affx) and 270 Mapping 250K Sty HapMap samples (available at GEO, GSE5173) were used as diploid reference. In the Genomic Segmentation analysis, the cut-off values to identify gains and losses were set to 2.3 and 1.7, respectively, each segment was computed using a minimum of 10 consecutive filtered probe sets, and the threshold p-value and the signal to noise ratio were set to 0.001 and 0.5, respectively.

2.3 Integrative analysis of gene expression and genomic copy number in ccRCC

To address the integrative analysis of gene expression and copy number data we applied *preda* (Position RElated Data Analysis) tool, an R package for detecting regional variations of genomic features from high-throughput data (Ferrari et al., 2011). *preda* is particularly suited for the identification of chromosomal regions with coordinated copy number and transcriptional imbalances (SODEGIRs, Bicciato et al., 2009). In *preda*, custom-designed data structures allow to efficiently manage different types of genomics signals and annotations, different choices of smoothing functions and statistics empower a variety of flexible and robust workflows, and tabular and graphical representations facilitate downstream biological interpretation of results. The computational framework directly integrates copy number and gene expression profiles at genome-wide level, by statistically assessing the gene dosage and transcription statuses on common genomic positions. We applied *preda* to both Cifola and Beroukhim datasets (Table 1). Briefly, Cifola dataset comprises a subset of 11 ccRCC cases profiled by both Affymetrix Human Mapping 100K and HG-U133 Plus 2.0 arrays (Cifola et al., 2008), while Beroukhim dataset includes 26 ccRCC and 11 normal samples analyzed using both Affymetrix Human Mapping 250K and HT-HG-U133A arrays (Beroukhim et al., 2009). Copy number log-ratios were calculated using CNAG software (version 3.3.0.1, http://www.genome.umin.jp/; Nannya, 2005; Yamamoto, 2007), while gene expression levels were estimated using RMA algorithm. Both types of data were used as input to *preda* to identify regions harboring both down-regulated genes and CN loss or both up-regulated genes and CN gain (SODEGIR deleted and SODEGIR amplified signatures, respectively). To further validate the presence of areas of deletion and amplification in a larger panel of samples, we intersected the list of genes associated to the SODEGIR signatures with the list of differentially expressed genes obtained from the ANOVA comparison of the 320 ccRCCs with the 106 normal samples of the meta-dataset (Table 1). Differentially expressed genes and genes comprised in the SODEGIR signatures were annotated using GeneDistiller 2 tool (http://www.genedistiller.org; Seelow et al., 2008). Literature mining was performed using PubMatrix tool (http://pubmatrix.grc.nia.nih.gov/; Becker et al., 2003) and applying specific keywords such as *cancer, renal cell carcinoma, amplification, methylation, oncogene, tumor suppressor and biomarker.*

3. Result

3.1 Differential gene expression profiling of ccRCC

The aim of this analysis was to functionally characterize the transcriptional profiles that differentiate cancer specimens from normal tissues. We based our initial analysis on the weight of gene expression data, taking advantage of bioinformatics techniques that allow direct interrogation of differentially expressed genes for activation of specific signaling pathways. The cohort of 426 samples composing the meta-dataset was analyzed by ANOVA to identify a list of differentially expressed genes between ccRCC and normal renal tissues. This comparison resulted in 1036 genes specifically modulated more than 2 folds in ccRCC cancers and that showed 95% of statistical confidence for differential expression. The fold change distribution ranged from -210 to 41, although the majority of DEGs showed an expression modulation varying from 2 to 4 folds. As depicted in the clustering map of Figure 1, the 534 up-regulated and 502 down-regulated genes grouped the meta-dataset samples into two clearly defined differential patterns of transcriptional activation in tumor samples as compared to normal tissues.

The functional and biological characterization of the 1036 differentially expressed genes using Gene Ontology (GO) annotation highlighted that the most significant processes and pathways altered in ccRCC are consistent with the important role of aerobic metabolism typically associated to epithelial cancers (Figure 2). In particular, we observed a down regulation of genes associated to metabolism and transport counteracted by the up regulation of genes associated to signal transduction and cell communication. The GO functional characterization indicated that ccRCC decrements the expression of genes related to oxido-reductase activity, amine catabolism, amine and exose biosynthesis, fatty acid metabolism, excretion and secretion, response to hormone, ion transport (Figure 2, panel A) while induces the transcription of genes related to the immune response, response to wounding, defense response, angiogenesis, response to oxygen level, cell proliferation, chemotaxis, cell adhesion and motility, and T-cell activation (Figure 2, panel B).

A further functional characterization of the differentially expressed genes using the knowledge database of Ingenuity Pathway Analysis (IPA) pointed out *cancer* and *genetic disorder* as the most significant enriched categories ($p\text{-value} \leq 0.0001$ and more than 200 genes). Specifically, IPA analysis associated the modulated genes to the categories of *renal cancer* (ACAT1, BTG2, C7orf68, CA9, CD70, CDH6, CLCNKB, CP, CSF1R, DEFB1, EDNRA, EGF, EPCAM, FGFR3, GPC3, IGF2BP3, IGFBP2, INHBB, KDR, KNG1, MME, MMP9, MUC1, MYC, NR3C1, PDGFRA, RRM2, SFRP1, SLC6A3, TIMP1, TOP2A, TUBA1A, TUBB2A, VEGFA), *cancer progression* (AHR, BCL6, CCND1, CDKN1B, CXCL12, IFI16, KIF2A, MYC, NR4A1, PLAGL1, TGFB1), *angiogenesis* (ANGPTL3, ANGPTL4, ANXA3, APOH, AQP1, ARHGAP24, BTG1, COL4A2, COL4A3, CXCR4, EGF, ITGA5, KDR, MTDH, SERPINE1, SPARC, VASH1, VEGF), *cell cycle* (AHR, CCND1, DEGS1, NEFL, CDKN1B, MMP9), *cell binding* (ABCA1, CAV1, CD2, COL4A3, CXCL12, CXCR4, FGF1, GPC3, IGFBP3, ITGA5, ITGAM, ITGB2, KNG1, SCARB1, SDC1, SERPINE1, SLC6A3, SPARC, ST6GAL1, TGFB1, TLR2, UMOD, VCAM1, VEGFA, VWF), *cell adhesion* (ADAM10, ADAM9, ANGPT2, C3, CCL5, CD93, CDH13, CR2, CXCL12, CYFIP2, FXYD5, INHBB, ITGA4, ITGA5, ITGAM, ITGB2, KDR, KLK6, MARCKS, PECAM1, PLAU, PLXND1, POSTN, ROCK1, SERPINE1, SLIT2, TGFB1, TIMP1, VCAM1, VEGFA, ZEB2), *chemotaxis* (ADAM10, CCL20, CCL5, CD36, CDH13, CXCL11, CXCL12, CXCR4, EGF, HMGB2, KDR, PDGFRA, PLAU, RARRES2, SERPINE1, SLIT2, TGFB1, TLR2, VEGFA), and *fragmentation of DNA* (ABCB1, AIFM1, BNIP3, CLU, DNASE1L3, EGF, FAS, NOX4, SFRP1, SOD2). Moreover, the IPA network analysis resulted in 20 networks including, each one, more than 13 focus molecules and confirmed the previous GO findings of functional activities in mechanisms related to *cell death, cell to cell signaling and interaction, cellular movement,* and *cancer.* Table 2 enlists the top four networks that are mainly enriched in up regulated genes.

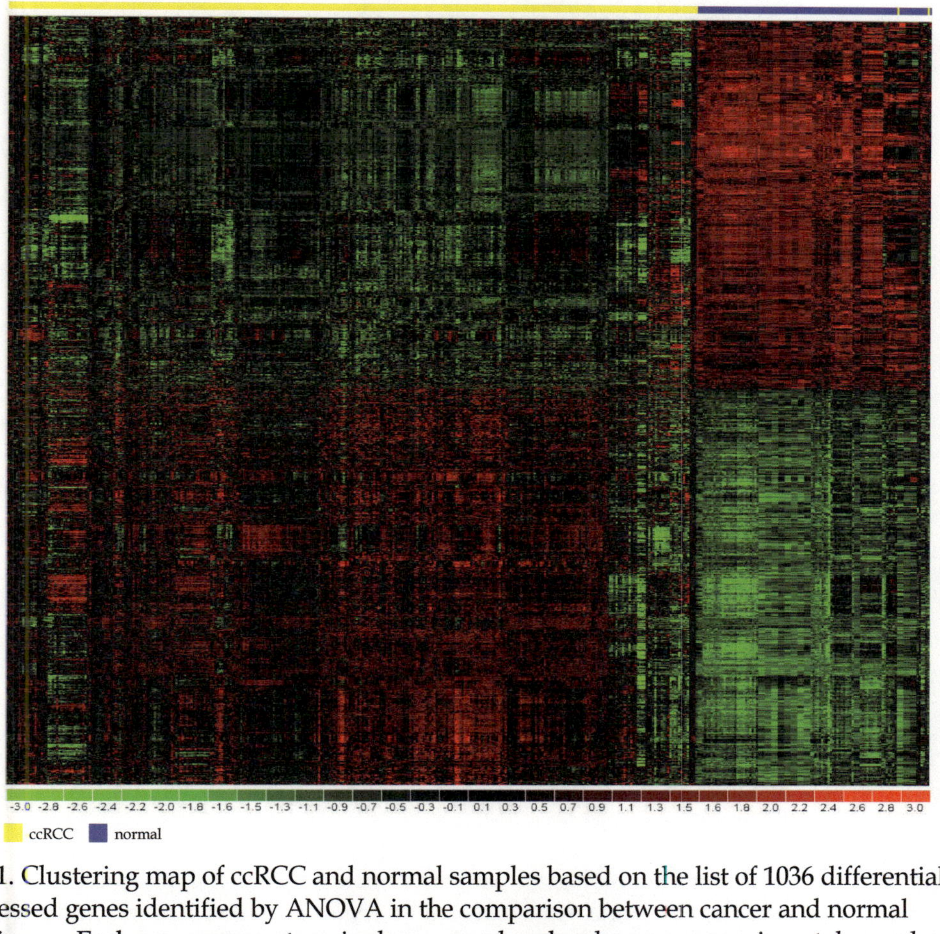

Fig. 1. Clustering map of ccRCC and normal samples based on the list of 1036 differentially expressed genes identified by ANOVA in the comparison between cancer and normal specimens. Each row represents a single gene and each column an experimental sample. Samples are separated into two main groups enriched for ccRCC (upper yellow bar) and normal tissues (upper blue bar). The map has been obtained using the hierarchical clustering of dChip (Li & Wong, 2001) with Pearson correlation and centroid as distance metric and linkage, respectively.

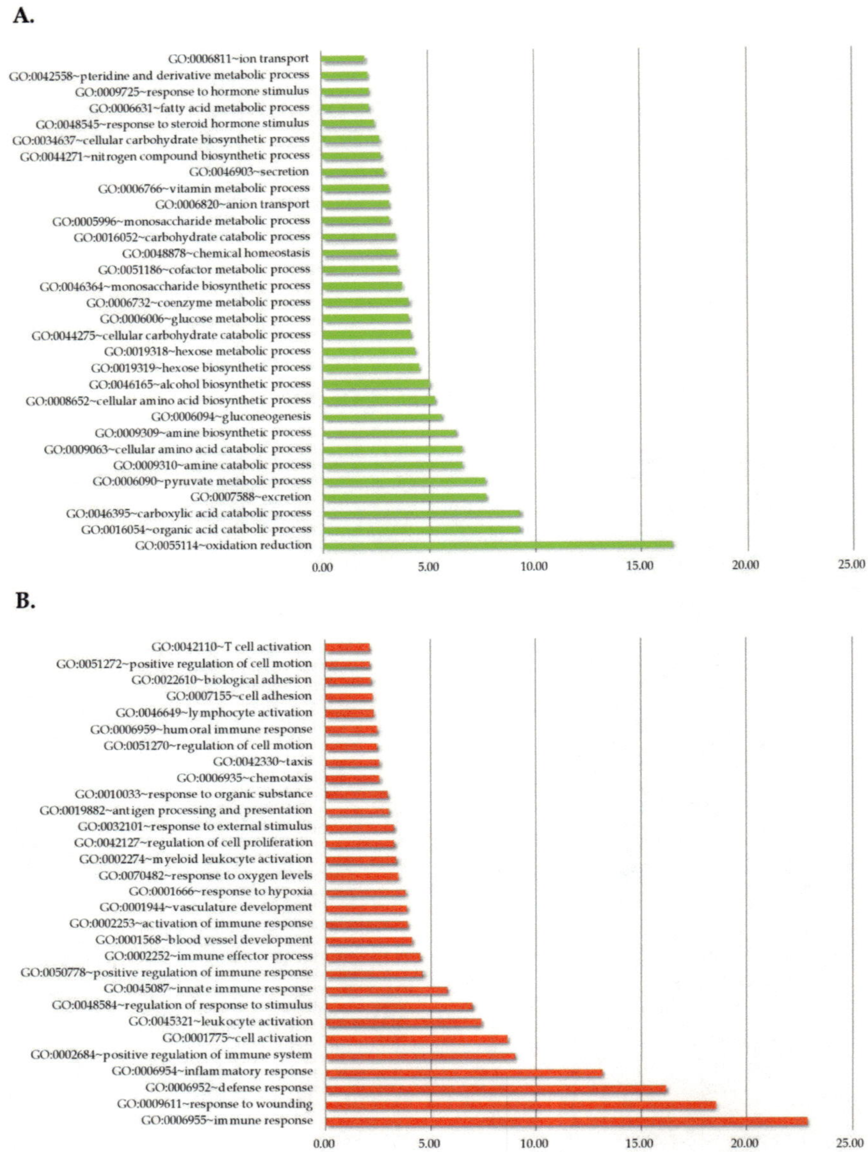

Fig. 2. Functional characterization in terms of GO Biological Process of the 502 down-regulated genes (panel A) and of the 534 up-regulated genes (panel B). On the X-axis the log(FDR) of DAVID enrichment test is reported.

To gain further insight into the biological pathways engaged in ccRCC phenotype, we used bioinformatics classifiers, or gene signatures, that register a modulated activity (either activation or inactivation) of specific signaling pathways in tumor samples. In particular, Gene Set Enrichment Analysis (GSEA) allowed identifying 25 inactivated and 50 activated pathways in cancer samples. The inactivated signaling modules relate to aminoacid metabolism, glucose and lipid metabolism, molecule transport, drug metabolism, glycolysis and gluconeogenesis, oxidative metabolism and immune signaling (Table 3).

Molecules in Network	Score[a]	Focus Molecules[b]	Top Functions
ACTN1, ANGPTL4, ARPC1B, BARD1, BTG1, CASP1, CASP4, CD2, CD70, CLU, CORO1C, CSTA, DNASE1L3, EDN1, GLIPR1, GLUL, GPR65, IFIH1, IL7, IL7R, KDM3A, LGALS1, MAL, NOL3, NR3C1, PLAGL1, PLP2, SCARB1, SERPINB1, SERPINE1, STAT5a/b, TMSB10/TMSB4X, TNFAIP6, TNFAIP8, TNFRSF1B	34	34	Cell Death, Inflammatory Response, Cellular Growth and Proliferation
APOH, BCR, CCL5, CD14, COL4A1, COL4A2, DDX58, Fibrinogen, HLA-F, IFN Beta, IL12 (complex), ISG15, ITGAM, ITGB2, KNG1, LY96, MMP9, NFkB (complex), P38 MAPK, PLAT, PLAU, POSTN, PYCARD, ROCK1, TAP1, TGFB1, TIMP1, TLR1, TLR2, TLR3, TLR7, TNIP1, TRAF3IP2, TRIB3, VCAM1	26	30	Cell-To-Cell Signaling and Interaction, Inflammatory Response, Hematological System Development and Function
ADAM10, AHR, Akt, ANXA1, BAZ1A, C3, C3AR1, CASR, CDH13, CR2, CXCL12, CXCR4, EGF, EIF4EBP1, ERBB4, ERK1/2, GJB1, IGFBP2, IGFBP3, IL1RL1, ITGA5, KDR, KL, LDL, MYOF, PI3K (complex), PLG, PRKCZ, PTPRC, Ras homolog, RCAN1, SLC6A3, TCF4, VDR, VEGFA	26	30	Cellular Movement, Inflammatory Disease, Cellular Growth and Proliferation
ACTG2, AGTR1, ANK2, AUH, BDKRB2, CCNDBP1, CLMN, COL5A1, COL5A2, COL5A3, CSDA, CTH, FBL, GNL2, ID2, IL7, MYH10, NAP1L1, NCL, NTRK2, PLK2, PMP22, PTPN3, RB1, RRAD, S100A2, SPTBN1, TNFRSF1B, TOP2A, TP53, TP73, TP53I3, TSPAN1, TUBA1A, UBE2D1	16	23	Cancer, Neurological Disease, Cellular Development

Table 2. Top four significant networks identified by the IPA network analysis on the list of differentially expressed genes (red, up-regulated DEG; green, down-regulated DEG; black, not regulated). [a] The score column indicates the -log(p-value), while [b] the focus molecules column quantifies the number of modulated genes in the network.

Among the most activated pathways (Table 4), we found association to cancer (renal cell carcinoma and chronic myeloid leukemia) and oncogenic signatures characterized by the presence of several well-known cancer genes (CCND1, MYC, RB1, TP53, RUNX1, AKT2, KRAS, CRKL, CSK, MDM2, NRAS, MET, RAP1A, APC, SHC1, PTEN, ATR, ATM, VAV1, LYN, ROCK1). Some of these signatures are inter-connected through key genes, as the tumor suppressor gene TP53 and the oncogene MYC. As expected, given the fundamental role of hypoxia in renal cell carcinoma, the *HIF and VHL* gene set resulted activated in ccRCC, as illustrated by the high ES score and by the clear-cut pattern of expression of HIF- and VHL- regulated genes in ccRCCs and normal tissues (Table 4 and Figure 3). Among the most active players of this signature, there are genes associated to *angiogenesis* (EDN1, VEGFA), *cell survival* (ATM, MYC), *glucose influx* (SLC2A1), *pH control* (CA9), *oxidative and iron metabolism* (PGK1, HK2, CP, HMOX1) and *HIF processing* (EGLN3, EGLN1). Additional gene sets were related to *cell fate and survival, cell to cell signaling* and *kinase signaling.* Furthermore, several pathways activated in ccRCC are associated to *immune signaling,*

Biological context	GSEA gene set	ES	FDR
Amino acid metabolism	Valine leucine and isoleucine degradation	-0.807	0.141
	Propanoate metabolism	-0.804	0.168
	Beta alanine metabolism	-0.769	0.138
	Glycine serine and threonine metabolism	-0.723	0.133
	Arginine and proline metabolism	-0.695	0.153
	Tryptophan metabolism	-0.655	0.152
	Histidine metabolism	-0.654	0.157
	Alanine aspartate glutamate metabolism	-0.604	0.144
	Lysine degradation	-0.580	0.140
	Selenoamino acid metabolism	-0.572	0.145
	Cysteine and methionine metabolism	-0.492	0.174
Differentiation	Taste transduction	-0.601	0.227
	Cardiac muscle contraction	-0.462	0.198
Drug metabolism	Drug metabolism cytochrome P450	-0.662	0.137
	Metabolism of xenobiotics by cytochrome P450	-0.638	0.139
Glyco-metabolism	Pyruvate metabolism	-0.624	0.141
	Glycolysis and gluconeogenesis	-0.504	0.227
Immuno signaling	Vibrio cholerae infection	-0.465	0.185
Lipid metabolism	Glycerolipid metabolism	-0.517	0.152
	Fatty acid metabolism	-0.691	0.150
Mitochondrial metabolism	Citrate cycle TCA cycle	-0.718	0.196
Molecule transport	Aldosterone regulated sodium reabsorption	-0.612	0.213
	Peroxisome	-0.588	0.143
Oxidative metabolism	Butanoate metabolism	-0.763	0.171
	Retinol metabolism	-0.641	0.168

Table 3. List of pathways identified as inactivated in the cancer phenotype by GSEA. All pathways belong to gene sets derived from the KEGG pathway database. The ES and FDR columns indicate the enrichment score (i.e., the degree to which a gene set is overrepresented at the top or bottom of a ranked list of genes) and the statistical significance (i.e., the estimated probability that a gene set with a given ES represents a false positive finding).

including for instance NFKB, TOLL like receptor, T cell receptor, and NK cell, in which also many cytokines (i.e. IL18, CCL5, IL8, CCL4, IL7) and their receptors (i.e. IL7R, IL2RG) are involved. Finally, the enrichment analysis evidenced a role for genes involved in *DNA repair and replication* (e.g. MSH2, POLD2, RFC2, RFC4, RFC5, PCNA, SSBP1, LIG1).

Biological context	GSEA gene set	ES	FDR
Angiogenesis	VEGF pathway	0.478	0.222
Cancer	Chronic myeloid leukemia	0.410	0.216
	Renal cell carcinoma	0.441	0.206
Cell differentiation	Notch signaling pathway	0.388	0.245
	Calcineurin pathway	0.539	0.235
	Dorso ventral axis formation	0.586	0.232
Cell fate and survival	Apoptosis	0.372	0.232
	Raccycd pathway	0.479	0.243
	PTEN pathway	0.550	0.220
	Chemical pathway	0.555	0.246
	PML pathway	0.601	0.192
Cell to cell signaling	Systemic lupus erythematosus	0.510	0.233
	Viral myocarditis	0.544	0.155
	Leishmania infection	0.621	0.196
	Graft versus host disease	0.682	0.148
	Asthma	0.687	0.166
	Allograft rejection	0.711	0.180
DNA repair	Nucleotide excision repair	0.513	0.152
	DNA replication	0.682	0.205
	Mismatch repair	0.687	0.242
Glyco-metabolism	Type I diabetes mellitus	0.636	0.173
	Glycosaminoglycan biosynthesis chondroitin sulfate	0.666	0.157
Hypoxia	HIF and VHL	0.518	0.197
Immuno signaling	T cell receptor signaling pathway	0.413	0.227
	NFKB pathway	0.449	0.232
	Natural killer cell mediated cytoxicity	0.457	0.211
	HIVNEF pathway	0.460	0.240
	TOLL like receptor signaling pathway	0.486	0.224
	HCMV pathway	0.503	0.241
	NOD like receptor signaling pathway	0.510	0.235
	Cytosolic DNA sensing pathway	0.540	0.230
	IL7 pathway	0.565	0.239
	CSK pathway	0.577	0.248
	Autoimmune Thyroid disease	0.596	0.237
	Intestinal immune network for IGA production	0.609	0.207
	NKT pathway	0.618	0.227
	NKCELLS pathway	0.645	0.219
	NO2IL12 pathway	0.684	0.237
	TH1TH2 pathway	0.733	0.221

Kinase signaling	PAR1 pathway	0.419	0.241
	P38MAPK pathway	0.459	0.219
Molecule transport	Snare interactions in vesicular transport	0.455	0.232
Oncogenic signaling	MTOR signaling pathway	0.431	0.226
	FCER1 pathway	0.443	0.239
	WNT pathway	0.458	0.230
	GCR pathway	0.471	0.245
	P53 signaling pathway	0.559	0.166
	GSK3 pathway	0.566	0.236
	ARF pathway	0.572	0.231
	ATRBRCA pathway	0.627	0.185
Transcription	RNA degradation	0.482	0.231

Table 4. List of pathways identified as activated in the cancer phenotype by GSEA. All pathways belong to gene sets derived from BioCarta and KEGG pathway databases, with the exception of the HIF and VHL list that has been derived from NCBI Pathway Interaction Database. The ES and FDR columns indicate the enrichment score (i.e., the degree to which a gene set is overrepresented at the top or bottom of a ranked list of genes) and the statistical significance (i.e., the estimated probability that a gene set with a given ES represents a false positive finding).

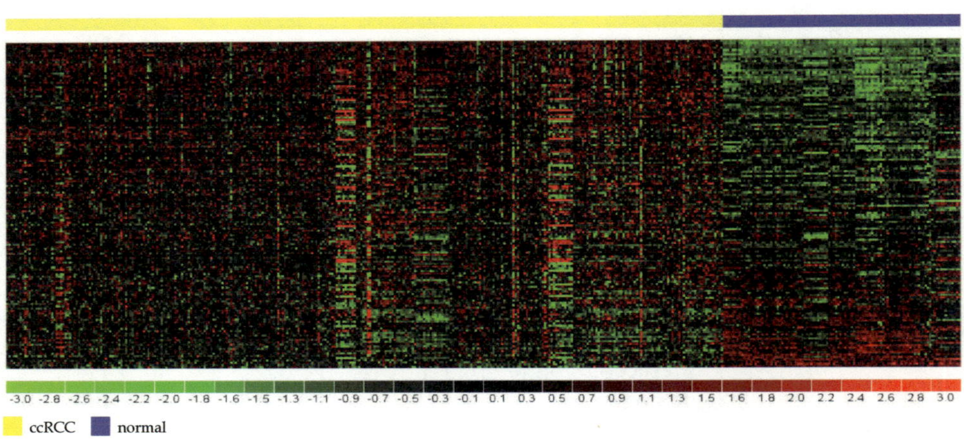

Fig. 3. Standardized gene expression levels of the 145 genes composing the HIF and VHL signaling pathway in ccRCC (upper yellow bar) and normal samples (upper blue bar). Each row represents a single gene and each column an experimental sample. Genes are ordered according to GSEA enrichment score. The map has been obtained using the hierarchical clustering of dChip (Li & Wong, 2001).

We finally investigated whether exists a grade-dependent specific transcriptional signature and compared the two groups of ccRCC cases previously classified as high (G3 and G4) and low grade (G1 and G2) classes. ANOVA differential analysis identified 44 differentially expressed genes (10 up-regulated and 34 down-regulated genes in high grade) that have been grouped according to their cellular localization to highlight putative grade-dependent clinical biomarkers (Table 5). Among the modulated genes, we found *transporters* (COPG, SLC27A2, FABP4, SLCO2A1, SLC17A4, SLC47A1, SLC17A3, SLC6A3), *enzymes* (SOD2,

BHMT, HAO2, ADH1B, MGAM, FMO2, ALDOB, GBA3, BBOX1, ABP1, DNASE1L3), *G-protein coupled receptors* (EDNRB, AGTR1, RGS5), *growth factors* (IGFBP1, PDGFD), *transmembrane receptors* (TMEM204, OSMR) and five *transcription regulators* (TFPI2, PPP1R1A, EMX2, NAT8, RCAN2).

Cellular location	Up-regulated	Down-regulated
Cytoplasm	PPP1R1A, COPG, KRT19, SOD2	PCK1, FABP4, BBOX1, GBA3, C13orf15, C5orf23, ALDOB, SCGN, ADH1B, HAO2, BHMT, APOLD1
Endoplasmic Reticulum Membrane		FMO2, SLC27A2, SLC17A3
Extracellular Space	SPOCK1, IGFBP1, TFPI2, MT1X	EMCN, ABP1, PDGFD, UMOD
Nucleus		DNASE1L3, EMX2, XIST, AUTS2, RCAN2
Plasma Membrane	RARRES, OSMR	SLC6A3, AGTR1, RGS5, SLC47A1, SLC17A4, EDNRB, SLCO2A1, TMEM204, MGAM, NAT8

Table 5. Cellular location of the 44 differentially expressed genes identified between high and low grade samples.

Despite the intrinsic heterogeneity of the meta-dataset (due to the combination of different experimental sets), when applied to cluster the 320 ccRCC samples, the grade-dependent specific transcriptional signature was able to segregate the high-grade phenotypes in an homogenous group characterized by a general down regulation of gene expression (Figure 4).

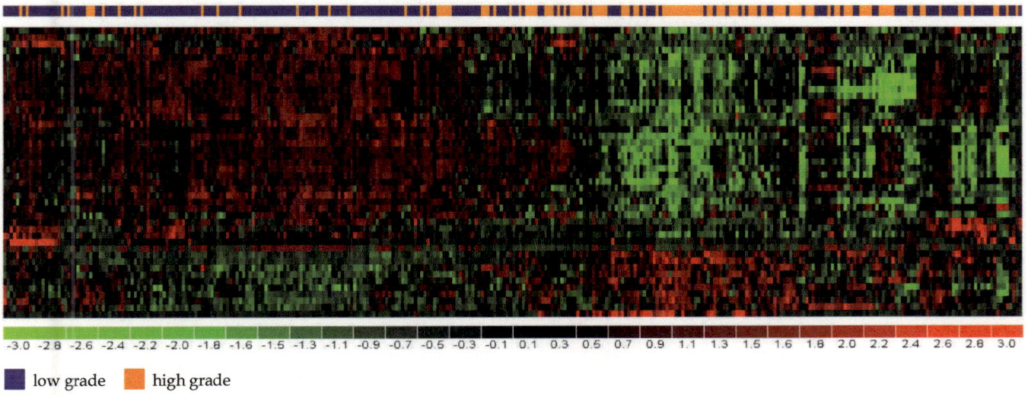

Fig. 4. Clustering map of high and low grade ccRCC samples based on the list of 44 differentially expressed genes identified by ANOVA in the comparison between high and low grade samples. Each row represents a single gene and each column an experimental sample. Samples are separated into two main groups enriched for low (upper blue bars) and high grade (upper orange bars). The map has been obtained using the hierarchical clustering of dChip (Li and Wong2001) with Pearson correlation and centroid as distance metric and linkage, respectively.

3.2 Copy number profiling of ccRCC

Genetic studies on ccRCC clinical samples characterized some recurrent alterations in precise chromosomal regions (i.e. deletions of chromosomes 3p, 6q, 8p, 9p, 14q, and amplifications of chromosomes 5q and 7). To confirm the copy number signature of ccRCC, we analyzed the CN profile of two independent datasets by SNP array technology with different resolution level. As showed in Figure 5, the genome-wide assessment of copy number alterations characterizing 27 and 26 sporadic ccRCC samples profiled by Affymetrix Human Mapping 100K and 250K Sty Array, respectively, revealed that all autosomes were affected by either CN gain or loss or both of them. In Cifola dataset (panel A), the most frequently amplified regions were on chromosomes 4q, 5 (p and q arms), 7 (p and q arms), 11p and 12q, whereas the most recurrent deleted region was identified on chromosome 3p. The longest recurrent amplifications resulted on chromosomes 1 (p and q arms), 2 (p and q arms), 3q, 11q, 16q, 18q and 19p, often spanning two or more consecutive megabases. These DNA alterations presented frequencies ranging from 6 to 12 samples. Similarly, the CN profile of Beroukhim dataset (panel B), obtained with a denser SNP array, showed that the most frequently amplified regions were on chromosomes 5 (p and q arms), 7 (p and q arms), 11p, 12q, 19 and 20, whereas the most recurrent deleted regions were identified on chromosomes 3p, 6, 8q, 9 and 14. Overall, we observed that the CNA profile obtained from the two datasets were globally overlapping, so confirming the typical ccRCC genomic signature. Due to the higher density of SNP array used in their study, Beroukhim et al. were able to better discriminate some CNAs as compared to Cifola dataset (i.e. the loss on chromosomes 8p, 11q, 14q, 15, and the gain on chromosomes 11p, 12, 19, 20).

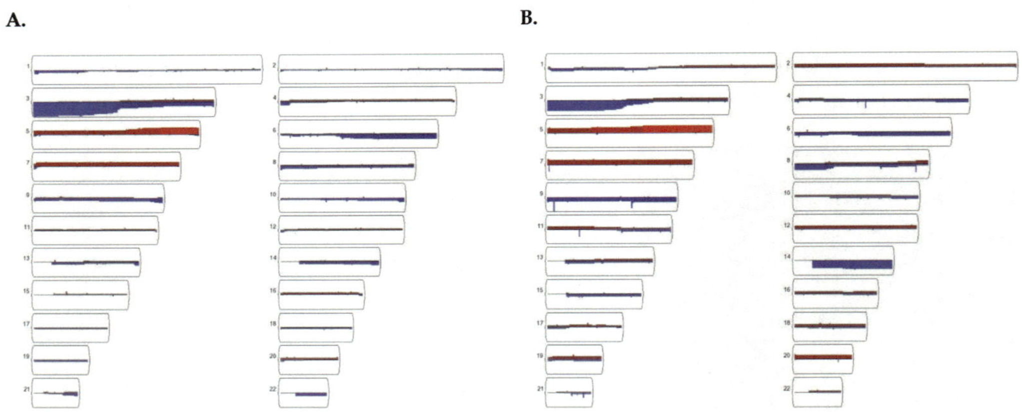

Fig. 5. Visualization of the CNA frequencies occurring in Cifola (panel A) and Beroukhim datasets (panel B). Regions of DNA copy number gain (red bar) and copy number loss (blue bar) are represented along each chromosome (from 1 to 22, ordered horizontally). X chromosome was omitted from this analysis.

3.3 Integrative analysis of gene expression and copy number data

In order to identify chromosomal regions with coordinated copy number and transcriptional imbalances (SODEGIRs), we performed the integrative analysis on the two independent datasets with paired gene expression and copy number data (namely, Cifola and Beroukhim). In Cifola dataset, *preda* analysis revealed segments of amplified

SODEGIR located at 5q21.3-q35.3 (from 130 to 180Mb) and a single deleted SODEGIR at 3p14.1-p22.3 (from 35 to 60 Mb) (Figure 6, panel A). Similar imbalanced regions were found for chromosomes 3 and 5 in Beroukhim dataset (Figure 6, panel B), although the lower probe density of the gene expression platform utilized in this study (i.e., the HG-U133A arrays) did not allow a finer resolution of the chromosomal segments as compared to Cifola dataset.

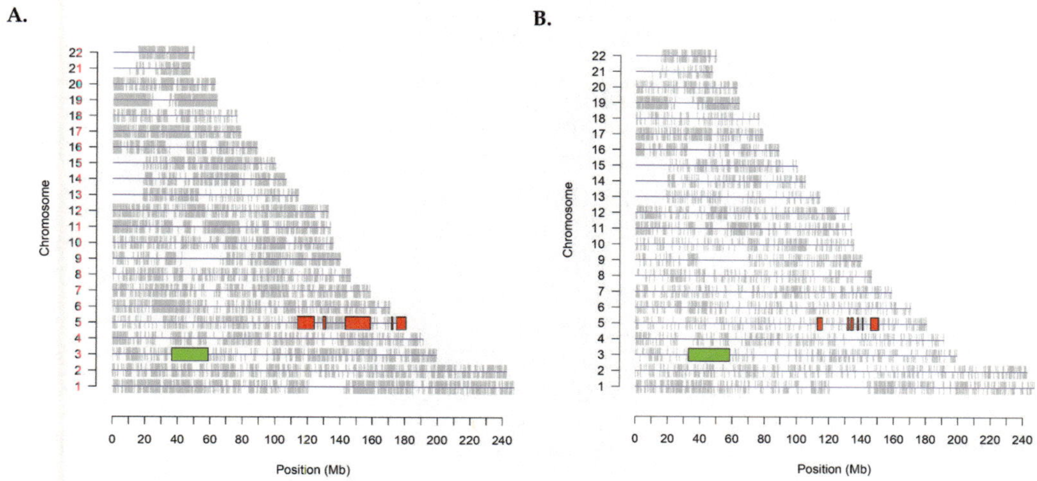

Fig. 6. SODEGIR amplified (red) and deleted (green) chromosomal regions identified by *preda* in the integrative analysis of gene expression and copy number data for Cifola (panel A) and Beroukhim dataset (panel B).

To further study the influence of gene dosage associated to structural position as one of the mechanism of transcriptional regulation, the genes located at SODEGIR signature (199 and 147 genes in deleted and amplified SODEGIRs, respectively) were intersected with the list of differentially expressed genes, identified by ANOVA in the comparison between ccRCC and normal tissues of meta-dataset. Overall, we found that 68% of the genes associated to the deleted signature (136 out of 199 genes) resulted down-regulated in the meta-dataset, while 61% of the genes associated to amplified signature (90 out of 147 genes) were up regulated at a statistically significant level. The most differentially down-regulated genes ranged from -2 to -10 fold changes (PTH1R, ACY1, ACOX2, IL17RB, HYAL1, UQCRC1, ACAA1, DNASE1L3, SEMA3G, ABHD14A, AMT, APEH, ALS2CL, CISH, MYL3, SEMA3B, HIGD1A, PLXNB1, PDHB), while the most up regulated ranged from 2 to 3.5 fold changes (TNFAIP8, LOX, SPARC, CSF1R, TCERG1, LOXL2, SPARCL1, YIPF5, RPS14, ABLIM3, TNIP1, STK10, CLK4). IPA annotation grouped these genes in the biological categories of *transcription and translation regulator, transmembrane receptor, enzyme* and *kinase* (Table 6), while Gene Distiller and PubMatrix highlighted that genes of the deleted SODEGIR are associated to *tumor suppressor function* (DLEC1, TMEM158, PTHR1, SEDT2, LIMD19, FAM107A, BAP1), *epigenetic modification* (STAC, CTDSPL, DLEC1, PRSS50, SEDT2, IP6K1, SEMA3B, TUSC2, PARP3, PRKCD) and *chromosomal deletion* (DLEC1, LIMD1, LTF, RBM6, IRFd2, TUSC2, COL7A1), and genes of the amplified SODEGIR are enriched in *oncogenes* (CSF1R, PDGFRB, LOX, DUSP1, SPARC, ITK, FLT4, GNB2L1, LARS, CD74, F12, MAML1, SQSTM1) and associated to *gene amplification* (CSF1R, PDGFRB, LOX, NSD1).

Biological category	Deleted SODEGIR 3p14.1-p22	Amplified SODEGIR 5q21.3-q35.3
Transcription and translation regulator	RAD54L2, LIMD1, ZNF197, ZNF35, SMARCC1, EIF1B	TCERG1, FEM1C, CNOT8, ZNF354A, NSD1, SQSTM1, MED7, MAML1, SOX30, MXD3, RPS14
Transmembrane receptor	DAG1, NISCH, PLXNB1, IL17RB	CD74, FLT4
Enzyme	HEMK1, ARIH2, TKTL1, GMPPB, PARP3, MLH1, DHX30, SETD2, LARS2, ABHD5, P4HTM, ABHD6, CYB561D2, RPP14, ENTPD3, PLCD1, EXOSC7, ALAS1, PDHB, AMT, ABHD14A, DNASE1L3, ACAA1, UQCRC1, HYAL1, ACOX2	LOX, LOXL2, DDX41, LTC4S, GM2A, THG1L, GNB2L1, DPYSL3, MGAT1, LARS, MGAT4B, HINT1, HNRNPAB, PGGT1B, G3BP1, GFPT2, PPIC, B4GALT7
Kinase	MAP4K2, PRKAR2A, MST1R, OXSR1, ULK4, PRKCD, CAMKV, ACVR2B, NPRL2, MAPKAPK3, NME6, IP6K1	CSF1R, STK10, CLK4, ITK, PDGFRB, CSNK1A1, HK3, CSNK1G3, MAPK9

Table 6. Biological function of the subset of differentially expressed genes located into SODEGIRs.

4. Discussion

In this chapter we illustrated the identification of distinct molecular profiles in ccRCC samples using experimental data available in public repositories and published in peer-reviewed articles (Brannon & Rathmell, 2010). To exemplify how genomic data can be exploited to functionally characterize the molecular characteristics of renal carcinoma, we downloaded more than 500 ccRCC samples from public repositories of genomic data and, after manual selection, we created a compendium (meta-dataset) of gene expression and copy number profiles in 320 ccRCCs, annotated with the nuclear grade information, and 106 normal samples mainly representing adjacent renal tissues from the same surgical specimen. The bioinformatics analysis of gene expression profiles allowed the identification of lists of differentially expressed genes and of gene signatures activated in the cancer phenotype. Additionally, the comprehensive analysis of copy number profiles highlighted characteristic chromosomal aberrations affecting ccRCC cases and the integration of gene expression and copy number data revealed the presence of chromosomal regions with concomitant transcriptional and gene dosage imbalances.

As recently reviewed by Pal et al. (Pal et al., 2010), several gene expression and proteomic studies carried out on fresh and archival ccRCC tissues (Perroud, 2009; Seliger, 2009) evidenced a series of molecular processes and pathways involved in ccRCC tumorigenesis (Banumathy & Cairns, 2010) and indicated that ccRCC progression is strictly associated to the adaptation of cancer cells to low oxygen levels (Baldewijns, 2010; Bristow & Hill, 2008) and to their continuous proliferation even in the presence of compromised DNA repair mechanisms (Semenza, 2008). These results find an additional confirmation from the analysis of genomic data presented in this chapter. Indeed, the application of different bioinformatics tools resulted in a list of genes (e.g., VEGFA, MYC, CA9, SLC2A1, BNIP3, CXCR4, EGLN3 alias PDH3, SERPINA1, KDR, ATM, CP) highly activated in ccRCC and related to hypoxia signaling, known to be targets of the transcription factor HIF-1α or involved in cancer and pathways (as apoptosis and angiogenesis) which have been already targeted for therapeutic intervention in RCC (Pantuck et al., 2003). As expected, among the up-regulated genes, there is the well-known cancer gene MYC (Gordan, 2007, 2008) that several studies indicated as modulated by HIF-1α (Dang, 2008; Gordan, 2007; Podar & Anderson, 2010) and playing a fundamental role in ccRCC proliferation (Tang et al., 2009).

Focusing the investigation to genes and pathways more specifically associated to ccRCC, the analysis of molecular profiles confirmed the presence of the *adipogenic signature* characterized by the up-regulation of genes such as FABP7, NR3C1, ANGPTL4, CAV2, CAV1, and the down-regulation of FABP1 and of the transcription factors TFCP2L1 and GATA3, as previously reported by Tun et al. (Tun et al., 2010). Loss of cell-cell adhesion and cell polarity is commonly observed in epithelial tumors and correlates with their invasion into adjacent tissues and generation of metastases. Many evidences indicate that loss of cell polarity and cell-cell adhesion may also be important in early stages of neoplastic transformation (Coradini et al., 2011). Disruption of intercellular junctions and alterations in cell polarity are specific hallmarks of epithelial cancer cells. In fact, most human tumors arising in epithelial tissues gradually lose their polarized morphology and acquire a mesenchymal phenotype (*epithelial-mesenchymal transition*, EMT) (Thiery, 2003, 2009). Accordingly, and in concordance with Tun et al. (Tun et al., 2010), we observed the up-regulation of several EMT-associated genes (TGFB1, SPARC, VIM, MTHFD2, HSPG2, PROCR, COL3A1, ZEB2), indicating the involvement of this biological process in cancer cell progression and spreading in host tissues, as confirmed very recently by a study on the protein expression of important EMT mediators in ccRCC (Mikami et al., 2011). Among the other up-regulated genes and pathways (Table 4), the up regulation of gene transcription factor 4 (TCF4) confirmed previous evidences of the interplay between Wnt/β-catenin and PI3K/Akt signaling cascades and its involvement in tumor development and progression (Chen et al., 2011). Furthermore, the activation of a series of *immuno pathways*, especially antigen presenting and processing pathways, is quite striking in ccRCC and has been recently demonstrated by the proteomic identification of tumor antigen-derived peptides in RCC (Seliger et al., 2011). In particular, the CD74 up-regulation is suggested to be linked to the PI3K/Akt- and MEK/ERK-dependent intracellular signaling cascades, both associated with NF-kB nuclear translocation and DNA-binding activity (Liu et al., 2008).

Overall, the elucidation of the functional role of the ccRCC activated signaling pathways could be useful for the identification of novel cancer markers or for the development of molecular-targeted therapeutic agents. Taking into account the biological localization and functional roles of genes up regulated in ccRCC, we propose a series of genes that could represent candidate biomarkers for further investigations (Table 7).

Symbol	Description	References
ANXA4	annexin A4	Shi et al., 2004; Jones et al., 2005; Seliger et al., 2009
CA9	carbonic anhydrase IX	Atkins et al., 2004; Pantuck et al., 2005; Zhao et al., 2006; Osunkoya et al., 2009; Zhou et al., 2010
CAV1	caveolin-1	Campbell et al., 2003; Waalkes et al., 2011
CD70	CD70 molecule	Junker et al., 2005; Law et al., 2009
CD74	class II major histocompatibility complex-associated invariant chain	Young et al., 2001; Liu et al., 2008
CDH6	cadherin 6, type 2, K-cadherin (fetal kidney)	Shimazui et al., 2004; Paul et al., 2004
CP	ceruloplasmin (ferroxidase)	Osunkoya et al., 2009;
CXCR4	CXC chemokine receptor-4	Staller et al., 2003; Struckmann et al., 2008
ENGL3	prolyl hydroxylase-3 (PHD3)	Zhao et al., 2006; Sato et al., 2008; Tanaka et al., 2011; Dalgliesh et al., 2010
IGFBP3	insulin-like growth factor binding protein 3	Yao et al., 2005; Takahashi et al., 2005; Chuang et al., 2008
MMP9	matrix metallopeptidase 9 (gelatinase B, 92kDa gelatinase, 92kDa type IV collagenase)	Struckmann et al., 2008; Mikami et al., 2011
NNMT	nicotinamide N-methyltransferase	Yao et al., 2005; Seliger et al., 2009; Kim et al., 2010; Teng et al., 2011
STC2	stanniocalcin 2	Meyer et al., 2009
VEGFA	vascular endothelial growth factor A	Skubitz & Skubitz, 2002; Lam et al., 2005; Liu et al., 2010; Zhou et al., 2010

Table 7. List of candidate biomarker genes up regulated in ccRCC.

In particular, *Annexin A4* (ANXA4) is a member of the annexin family of calcium-dependent phospholipid binding proteins and can exist as a soluble protein as well as a membrane-associated protein. ANXA4 could play an important role in regulating the cellular functions at the level of cell–cell interaction, cell adhesion and motility and, although increased protein expression level of ANXA4 has been confirmed in ccRCC by global proteomic analysis (Seliger et al., 2009), its possible implication in the carcinogenesis of RCC deserves further studies. *Carbonic anhydrase 9* (CA9) is a transmembrane member of the carbonic anhydrase family that catalyses the reversible hydration of carbon dioxide into bicarbonate and a proton, thus enabling tumor cells to maintain a neutral pH despite an acidic microenvironment. CA9 is not expressed in healthy renal tissue but is expressed in most ccRCCs through HIF-1α accumulation driven by hypoxia and inactivation of the VHL gene.

CA9 expression can be detected in the tumor by immunohistochemistry (IHC) and in blood and tissue by ELISA assay and RT-PCR (Truong & Shen, 2011). In metastatic disease, high CA9 expression reported by IHC was indicated as a powerful prognostic marker for better survival and sensitivity to IL-2 treatment, although the robustness of this association is still debated (Atkins, 2004; Pantuck, 2005). Almost no data are currently available about the association of CA9 expression and response to targeted drugs. The prognostic value of CA9 in ccRCC could be explained by the frequent VHL gene inactivation driving an early activation of the HIF pathway. The poorer prognosis associated with low CA9 expressing tumors could be attributed to the simultaneous over-expression of EGFR contributing to the activation of Akt-mTOR pathways. Targeting CA9 by inhibitors, radioimmunotherapy, monoclonal antibodies or vaccination is promising and offers new avenues for clinical research (Tostain et al., 2010). Recently, it was reported that serum CA9 levels are significantly higher in ccRCC than in non-ccRCC samples and may help in the differential diagnosis of RCC. Serum CA9 levels also correlate with tumor size in ccRCC patients (Zhou et al., 2010). The role of *caveolin-1* (CAV1) in RCC pathogenesis is still controversial, as it is considered involved in both suppression and promotion of tumor growth and development. However, its increased expression has been used as marker of less favorable outcome in patients with both clinically confined ccRCC (Campbell et al., 2003) and distant metastasis (Waalkes et al., 2011), thus suggesting to be a candidate prognostic marker for RCC aggressiveness. *CD70 protein* (CD70) is a type II transmembrane protein belonging to the tumor necrosis factor family. It represents the ligand for CD27, a glycosylated transmembrane protein of the tumor necrosis factor receptor family. CD70 protein has been found expressed at a high level in ccRCCs by IHC (Junker et al., 2005). The role of this protein in tumorigenesis and its utility as diagnostic marker in serum and urine or as therapeutic tool certainly deserves further studies. *Cadherin-6* (CDH6) is an adhesion molecule that was proved to be marker of poor prognosis and metastases development in ccRCC (Paul, 2004; Shimazui, 2004). *Ceruroplasmin* (CP) is a protein involved in iron metabolism, is regulated by HIF-1α (Martin et al., 2005) and has been associated to metastatic potential and tumor progression. Serum CP protein level has been found elevated in RCC and other malignancies as compared to healthy controls, indicating its potentiality as a cancer biomarker (Osunkoya et al., 2009). *CXC chemokine receptor-4* (CXCR4) is a target of the VHL-HIF pathway and Staller et al. (Staller, 2003; Struckmann, 2008) demonstrated that its high expression is associated to poor survival. *Prolyl hydroxylase-3* (PHD3/ENGL3) is a member of the PHD family, which is involved in the degradation of HIF proteins in cooperation with VHL protein under normoxic conditions. PHD3 was found frequently over-expressed in RCC tissues, with high specificity to cancer samples (Zhao et al., 2006) and its usefulness as a novel tumor antigen for RCC immunotherapy has been recently demonstrated in clinical serum samples from RCC patients (Sato, 2008; Tanaka, 2011). *Insulin-like growth factor binding protein 3* (IGFBP3) is one of the most over-expressed genes in ccRCC (Takahashi, 2005; Yao, 2005) and its increased protein expression has been demonstrated in 74% of ccRCCs by IHC and associated with higher Fuhrman nuclear grade (Chuang et al., 2008). *Matrix metallopeptidase 9* (MMP9) has been reported increased in ccRCC and associated to survival. Statistical analysis indicated that elevated Snail, MMP2 and MMP9 protein expression are significantly correlated to worse disease-free and disease-specific survival of RCC patients (Mikami et al., 2011). MMP9, TIMP1 and CXCR4 have been studied both in vitro and in vivo and the data strongly indicated that VHL coordinately regulates the expression of metastasis-associated genes CXCR4/CXCL12 and

MMP2/MMP9, but the exact regulatory molecular mechanism remains to be determined (Struckmann et al., 2008). Some of the genes here mentioned have been validated at protein level, as *nicotinamide n-methyltransferase* (NNMT) and *enolase 2* (ENO2) proteins whose expression was found increased in RCC by Western blot (Teng et al., 2011). Increased cytoplasmic expression of *stanniocalcin 2* (STC2) was found correlated to other conventional indicators of RCC aggressiveness and to shorter overall survival. STC2 could become an additional tissue biomarker that may be useful in the post-operative risk stratification of RCC patients (Meyer et al., 2009). The increased expression of vascular *endothelial growth factor A* (VEGFA) was predictive of distant metastases development and lymph node involvement and was significantly associated with poor survival (Lam et al., 2005). These studies have paved the way for the development of new therapeutic agents to block VEGF signaling and the cascade of events leading to tumor formation. In a randomized phase II clinical trial on 116 metastatic ccRCC patients, the use at high doses of a neutralizing antibody against VEGFA (bevacizumab) resulted in a significant prolongation of the time to progression of disease (Yang et al., 2003).

According to the canonical classification of ccRCC (Flanigan et al., 2011), the Furhman nuclear grade is one of the most important parameters for RCC prognosis prediction (Nese et al., 2009), together with stage, age, tumor position and size, necrosis and other few molecular biomarkers (e.g., CA9). Noticeably, recent grade-dependent proteomic characterization reported that MYC, HIF-1α and p53 are the major hubs of the network obtained analyzing formalin-fixed paraffin embedded ccRCC tissues (Perroud et al., 2009). Chen et al (Chen et al., 2009) analyzed the correlation between chromosome aberrations and clinical pathological variables, including tumor stage and nuclear grade, and observed a significant association between LOH at chromosomes 9, 14q and 18q and higher nuclear grade. In the present study, we identified SOD2, KRT19 and OSM as potential grade-dependent ccRCC biomarkers. Briefly, *manganese superoxide dismutase* (SOD2) belongs to the antioxidant gene family and has emerged as a key enzyme with a dual role in tumorigenic progression (Hempel et al., 2011). Recently, SOD2 has been indicated as marker for circulating tumor cells in prostate cancer (Giesing et al., 2010) and potentially predictive for lymph node metastasis in tongue squamous cell carcinoma (Liu et al., 2010). *Keratin 19* (KRT19) encodes for one of the cytoskeleton cytokeratins and has been identified as a novel candidate tumor suppressor gene epigenetically inactivated in RCC cell lines and primary tumors (Morris et al., 2008). This gene was found to be functionally related to miR-492 and crucially involved in neoplastic progression of malignant embryonic liver tumors (von Frowein et al., 2011). *Oncostatin M* (OSM) is a member of the IL-6 cytokine family implicated in signal transduction; its receptor (OSMR) was found increased at both gene copy number and expression levels in gastric cancer (Junnila et al., 2010) and cervical squamous cell carcinomas, in association with poor survival (Scotto et al., 2008). However, to our knowledge, no previous studies exist that link OSMR to renal carcinogenesis. The clinical application of these genes as potential ccRCC grade-dependent biomarkers deserves further investigation in well curate and extensive collections of ccRCC cases.

The analysis of copy number levels in a total of 53 ccRCC samples profiled with SNP arrays (Beroukhim, 2009; Cifola, 2008) identified and confirmed the typical genomic signature of ccRCC, as recently showed by higher density SNP arrays (Dalgliesh et al., 2010). The most frequent CN alterations in ccRCC samples are the deletion of 3p and the amplification of 5q.

Similarly, Chen et al. detected gains of chromosome 5q33.1-qter and losses of chromosome 3p21.31-p22.3 in 58% and 80% of the 80 RCC samples analyzed using Illumina 317K SNP arrays (Chen et al., 2009), respectively. Noticeably, these regions have great influence on the expression levels of the resident genes as previously demonstrated by integrative genomic studies (Beroukhim, 2009; Bicciato, 2009; Cifola, 2008; Furge, 2004). In accordance, the comprehensive integrative analysis pinpointed that the two most significant chromosomal regions with coordinated copy number and transcriptional imbalances (SODEGIRs) are localized at the same chromosomal arms (Figure 6). Although the integrative analysis presented here was conducted using a completely different approach from that applied by Beroukhim et al. (Beroukhim et al., 2009), both studies identified 12 over-expressed genes located at the 5q peak region (GNB2L1, MGAT1, RUFY, RNF130, MAPK9, CANX, SQSTM1, LTC4S, TBC1D9B, HNRPH1, FLT4). Among them, the ubiquitin-binding protein *sequestosome 1* (SQSTM1) was found also in the focal amplification region at 5q35.3 by Chen et al. (Chen et al., 2009) and was reported over-expressed in breast and prostate tumors (Kitamura, 2006; Thompson, 2003). Moreover, we confirmed that, as previously evidenced by Cifola and co-workers (Cifola et al., 2008) and recently confirmed at proteomic level (Liu et al., 2010), *lyxyl oxidase* (LOX) is over-expressed in ccRCC. LOX is one of the critical HIF-1α targets mediating tumor progression and catalyzes the cross-linking of collagens and elastin in the extracellular matrix, thereby regulating tissue tensile strength (Erler & Giaccia, 2006). Paradoxically, LOX has been reported to be both up-regulated and down-regulated in cancer cells, especially in colorectal cancer (Baker, 2011; Pez, 2011). Mechanistic investigations revealed that LOX activates the PI3K-Akt signaling pathway, thereby up-regulating HIF-1α protein synthesis in a manner requiring LOX-mediated hydrogen peroxide production. Concordantly with these results, cancer cell proliferation was stimulated by secreted and active LOX in a HIF-1α-dependent fashion (Pez et al., 2011). Our data suggest that the transcriptional modulation of LOX might be also driven by genomic imbalance. Among the significant down-modulated genes located at the deleted SODEGIR on chromosome 3p14.1-p22, it is worthwhile mentioning two potential tumor suppressor genes, i.e. *deleted in lung cancer* (DLEC1), previously reported as candidate tumor suppressor silenced by methylation in RCC cell lines and primary tumors and with growth inhibitory function tested in in vitro experiments (Zhang et al., 2010a), and *SET domain containing 2* (SETD2), encoding for an histone H3 methyltransferase and found affected by inactivating mutations in 12-17% of ccRCCs, together with other components of the chromatin modification machinery (Dalgliesh et al., 2010).

Although some of these genes could represent novel candidate biomarkers, their role in ccRCC etiology requires further investigations and, given the heterogeneity of tumor tissues, the functional analysis of molecular mechanisms associated to ccRCC progression should be likely conducted on primary cultures as in vitro model of ccRCC. Indeed, primary cultures from RCC and normal tissues at early passages retain the phenotypic features (Bianchi,2010; Perego, 2005) and genomic profile (Cifola et al., 2011) of corresponding original tissues, while providing a more homogeneous cytological material. The integrative analysis of molecular profiles of RCC primary cultures may be particularly useful to elucidate the role of some of the many genes and pathways found typically deregulated in this pathology and to highlight key players in RCC biology.

5. Conclusion

As showed in this chapter, the availability of high-density molecular data as gene expression and copy number profiles, and of bioinformatics approaches for their analysis, allows depicting a finer molecular portrait of ccRCC and confirming previous findings about important genes and gene regulatory pathways associated to this renal cancer subtype. The genome-wide integration of DNA copy number data and transcriptional profiles elucidates the interplay between DNA content and global expression patterns and highlights candidate genes that are actively involved in the causation or maintenance of the malignant phenotype. Altogether, these data indicate the presence of candidate *driver* genes important for ccRCC development that undoubtedly deserve further investigation since they may constitute novel specific cancer biomarkers.

6. Acknowledgment

This work was supported by grants from the Italian Ministry of University and Research: FIRB 2003 (n. RBLA03ER38_004); PRIN 2008 (GDB); FIRB 2007 (Rete nazionale per lo studio del proteoma umano, n. RBRN07BMCT); AIRC Special Program Molecular Clinical Oncology "5 per mille".VT is recipient of a fellow of Scuola di dottorato di medicina molecolare,Università degli Studi di Milano. SN is a PhD student of the School of Biosciences and Biotechnology, curriculum Genetics and Molecular Biology of Development, University of Padova.

7. References

Akavia, U. D., Litvin, O., Kim, J., Sanchez-Garcia, F., Kotliar, D., Causton, H. C., Pochanard, P., Mozes, E., Garraway, L. A., & Pe'er, D. (2010). *An integrated approach to uncover drivers of cancer.* Cell, 143(6):1005–1017.

Arsanious, A., Bjarnason, G. A., & Yousef, G. M. (2009). *From bench to bedside: current and future applications of molecular profiling in renal cell carcinoma.* Mol Cancer, 8:20.

Atkins, M., Regan, M., Stanbridge, E., Upton, M., Youmans, A., Febbo, P., Lechpammer, M., & Signoretti S. (2004). *Carbonic anhydrase IX (CAIX) expression predicts for renal cell cancer (RCC) patient response and survival to IL-2 therapy.* In Journal of Clinical Oncology. 22(Supplement 14):4512.

Baker, A. M., Cox, T. R., Bird, D., Lang, G., Murray, G. I., Sun, X. F., Southall, S. M., Wilson, J. R., & Erler, J. T. (2011). *The role of lysyl oxidase in src-dependent proliferation and metastasis of colorectal cancer.* J Natl Cancer Inst, 103(5):407–424.

Baldewijns, M. M., van Vlodrop, I. J. H., Vermeulen, P. B., Soetekouw, P. M., van Engeland, M., & de Bruïne, A. P. (2010). *VHL and HIF signalling in renal cell carcinogenesis.* J Pathol, 221(2):125–138.

Banks, R. E., Tirukonda, P., Taylor, C., Hornigold, N., Astuti, D., Cohen, D., Maher, E. R., Stanley, A. J., Harnden, P., Joyce, A., Knowles, M., & Selby, P. J. (2006). *Genetic and epigenetic analysis of von Hippel-Lindau (VHL) gene alterations and relationship with clinical variables in sporadic renal cancer.* Cancer Res, 66(4):2000–2011.

Banumathy, G. & Cairns, P. (2010). *Signaling pathways in renal cell carcinoma.* Cancer Biol Ther, 10(7):658–664.

Becker, K. G., Hosack, D. A., Dennis, G., Lempicki, R. A., Bright, T. J., Cheadle, C., & Engel, J. (2003). *PubMatrix: a tool for multiplex literature mining*. BMC Bioinformatics, 4:61.

Beroukhim, R., Brunet, J. P., Napoli, A. D., Mertz, K. D., Seeley, A., Pires, M. M., Linhart, D., Worrell, R. A., Moch, H., Rubin, M. A., Sellers, W. R., Meyerson, M., Linehan, W. M., Kaelin, W. G., & Signoretti, S. (2009). *Patterns of gene expression and copy-number alterations in von-Hippel Lindau disease-associated and sporadic clear cell carcinoma of the kidney*. Cancer Res, 69(11):4674–4681.

Bianchi, C., Bombelli, S., Raimondo, F., Torsello, B., Angeloni, V., Ferrero, S., Stefano, V. D., Chinello, C., Cifola, I., Invernizzi, L., Brambilla, P., Magni, F., Pitto, M., Zanetti, G., Mocarelli, P., & Perego, R. A. (2010). *Primary cell cultures from human renal cortex and renal-cell carcinoma evidence a differential expression of two spliced isoforms of annexin A3*. Am J Pathol, 176(4):1660–1670.

Bicciato, S., Spinelli, R., Zampieri, M., Mangano, E., Ferrari, F., Beltrame, L., Cifola, I., Peano, C., Solari, A., & Battaglia, C. (2009). *A computational procedure to identify significant overlap of differentially expressed and genomic imbalanced regions in cancer datasets*. Nucleic Acids Res, 37(15):5057–5070.

Brannon, A. R. & Rathmell, W. K. (2010). *Renal cell carcinoma: where will the state-of-the-art lead us?* Curr Oncol Rep, 12(3):193–201.

Brannon, A. R., Reddy, A., Seiler, M., Arreola, A., Moore, D. T., Pruthi, R. S., Wallen, E. M., Nielsen, M. E., Liu, H., Nathanson, K. L., Ljungberg, B., Zhao, H., Brooks, J. D., Ganesan, S., Bhanot, G., & Rathmell, W. K. (2010). *Molecular stratification of clear cell renal cell carcinoma by consensus clustering reveals distinct subtypes and survival patterns*. Genes Cancer, 1(2):152–163.

Brenner, B. M. & Rosenberg, D. (2010). *High-throughput SNP/CGH approaches for the analysis of genomic instability in colorectal cancer*. Mutat Res, 693(1-2):46–52.

Bristow, R. G. & Hill, R. P. (2008). *Hypoxia and metabolism. hypoxia, DNA repair and genetic instability*. Nat Rev Cancer, 8(3):180–192.

Campbell, L., Gumbleton, M., & Griffiths, D. F. R. (2003). *Caveolin-1 overexpression predicts poor disease-free survival of patients with clinically confined renal cell carcinoma*. Br J Cancer, 89(10):1909–1913.

Chari, R., Thu, K. L., Wilson, I. M., Lockwood, W. W., Lonergan, K. M., Coe, B. P., Malloff, C. A., Gazdar, A. F., Lam, S., Garnis, C., MacAulay, C. E., Alvarez, C. E., & Lam, W. L. (2010). *Integrating the multiple dimensions of genomic and epigenomic landscapes of cancer*. Cancer Metastasis Rev, 29(1):73–93.

Chen, L., Huang, K., Han, L., Shi, Z., Zhang, K., Pu, P., Jiang, C., & Kang, C. (2011). *β-catenin/tcf-4 complex transcriptionally regulates AKT1 in glioma*. Int J Oncol, 39(4):883–890.

Chen, M., Ye, Y., Yang, H., Tamboli, P., Matin, S., Tannir, N. M., Wood, C. G., Gu, J., & Wu, X. (2009). *Genome-wide profiling of chromosomal alterations in renal cell carcinoma using high-density single nucleotide polymorphism arrays*. Int J Cancer, 125(10):2342–2348.

Chow, W. H., Dong, L. M., & Devesa, S. S. (2010). *Epidemiology and risk factors for kidney cancer*. Nat Rev Urol, 7(5):245–257.

Chuang, S. T., Patton, K. T., Schafernak, K. T., Papavero, V., Lin, F., Baxter, R. C., Teh, B. T., & Yang, X. J. (2008). *Over expression of insulin-like growth factor binding protein 3 in clear cell renal cell carcinoma*. J Urol, 179(2):445–449.

Cifola, I., Bianchi, C., Mangano, E., Bombelli, S., Frascati, F., Fasoli, E., Ferrero, S., Stefano, V. D., Zipeto, M. A., Magni, F., Signorini, S., Battaglia, C., & Perego, R. A. (2011). *Renal cell carcinoma primary cultures maintain genomic and phenotypic profile of parental tumor tissues*. BMC Cancer, 11:244.

Cifola, I., Spinelli, R., Beltrame, L., Peano, C., Fasoli, E., Ferrero, S., Bosari, S., Signorini, S., Rocco, F., Perego, R., Proserpio, V., Raimondo, F., Mocarelli, P., & Battaglia, C. (2008). *Genome-wide screening of copy number alterations and LOH events in renal cell carcinomas and integration with gene expression profile*. Mol Cancer, 7:6.

Cohen, H. T. & McGovern, F. J. (2005). *Renal-cell carcinoma*. N Engl J Med, 353(23):2477–2490.

Coradini, D., Casarsa, C., & Oriana, S. (2011). *Epithelial cell polarity and tumorigenesis: new perspectives for cancer detection and treatment*. Acta Pharmacol Sin, 32(5):552–564.

Dai, M., Wang, P., Boyd, A. D., Kostov, G., Athey, B., Jones, E. G., Bunney, W. E., Myers, R. M., Speed, T. P., Akil, H., Watson, S. J., & Meng, F. (2005). *Evolving gene/transcript definitions significantly alter the interpretation of GeneChip data*. Nucleic Acids Res, 33(20):e175.

Dalgliesh, G. L., Furge, K., Greenman, C., Chen, L., Bignell, G., Butler, A., Davies, H., Edkins, S., Hardy, C., Latimer, C., Teague, J., Andrews, J., Barthorpe, S., Beare, D., Buck, G., Campbell, P. J., Forbes, S., Jia, M., Jones, D., Knott, H., Kok, C. Y., Lau, K. W., Leroy, C., Lin, M. L., McBride, D. J., Maddison, M., Maguire, S., McLay, K., Menzies, A., Mironenko, T., Mulderrig, L., Mudie, L., O'Meara, S., Pleasance, E., Rajasingham, A., Shepherd, R., Smith, R., Stebbings, L., Stephens, P., Tang, G., Tarpey, P. S., Turrell, K., Dykema, K. J., Khoo, S. K., Petillo, D., Wondergem, B., Anema, J., Kahnoski, R. J., Teh, B. T., Stratton, M. R., & Futreal, P. A. (2010). *Systematic sequencing of renal carcinoma reveals inactivation of histone modifying genes*. Nature, 463(7279):360–363.

Dang, C. V., Kim, J. W., Gao, P., & Yustein, J. (2008). *The interplay between MYC and HIF in cancer*. Nat Rev Cancer, 8(1):51–56.

Eichelberg, C., Junker, K., Ljungberg, B., & Moch, H. (2009). *Diagnostic and prognostic molecular markers for renal cell carcinoma: a critical appraisal of the current state of research and clinical applicability*. Eur Urol, 55(4):851–863.

Erler, J. T. & Giaccia, A. J. (2006). *Lysyl oxidase mediates hypoxic control of metastasis*. Cancer Res, 66(21):10238–10241.

Fallarino, F., Volpi, C., Fazio, F., Notartomaso, S., Vacca, C., Busceti, C., Bicciato, S., Battaglia, G., Bruno, V., Puccetti, P., Fioretti, M. C., Nicoletti, F., Grohmann, U., & Marco, R. D. (2010). *Metabotropic glutamate receptor-4 modulates adaptive immunity and restrains neuroinflammation*. Nat Med, 16(8):897–902.

Ferrari, F., Solari, A., Battaglia, C., & Bicciato, S. (2011). *Preda: an R-package to identify regional variations in genomic data*. Bioinformatics, 27(17):2446–2447.

Flanigan, R. C., Polcari, A. J., & Hugen, C. M. (2011). *Prognostic variables and nomograms for renal cell carcinoma*. Int J Urol, 18(1):20–31.

Furge, K. A., Chen, J., Koeman, J., Swiatek, P., Dykema, K., Lucin, K., Kahnoski, R., Yang, X. J., & Teh, B. T. (2007). *Detection of DNA copy number changes and oncogenic signaling abnormalities from gene expression data reveals MYC activation in high-grade papillary renal cell carcinoma*. Cancer Res, 67(7):3171–3176.

Furge, K. A., Lucas, K. A., Takahashi, M., Sugimura, J., Kort, E. J., Kanayama, H., Kagawa, S., Hoekstra, P., Curry, J., Yang, X. J., & Teh, B. T. (2004). *Robust classification of renal cell carcinoma based on gene expression data and predicted cytogenetic profiles.* Cancer Res, 64(12):4117–4121.

Garraway, L. A., Widlund, H. R., Rubin, M. A., Getz, G., Berger, A. J., Ramaswamy, S., Beroukhim, R., Milner, D. A., Granter, S. R., Du, J., Lee, C., Wagner, S. N., Li, C., Golub, T. R., Rimm, D. L., Meyerson, M. L., Fisher, D. E., & Sellers, W. R. (2005). *Integrative genomic analyses identify MITF as a lineage survival oncogene amplified in malignant melanoma.* Nature, 436(7047):117–122.

Giesing, M., Suchy, B., Driesel, G., & Molitor, D. (2010). *Clinical utility of antioxidant gene expression levels in circulating cancer cell clusters for the detection of prostate cancer in patients with prostate-specific antigen levels of 4-10 ng/ml and disease prognostication after radical prostatectomy.* BJU Int, 105(7):1000–1010.

Gong, K., Zhang, N., Zhang, K., & Na, Y. (2010). *The relationship of erythropoietin overexpression with von hippel-lindau tumour suppressor gene mutations between hypoxia-inducible factor-1(and -2(in sporadic clear cell renal carcinoma.* Int J Mol Med, 26(6):907–912.

Gordan, J. D., Lal, P., Dondeti, V. R., Letrero, R., Parekh, K. N., Oquendo, C. E., Greenberg, R. A., Flaherty, K. T., Rathmell, W. K., Keith, B., Simon, M. C., & Nathanson, K. L. (2008). *HIF-alpha effects on c-MYC distinguish two subtypes of sporadic VHL-deficient clear cell renal carcinoma.* Cancer Cell, 14(6):435–446.

Gordan, J. D., Thompson, C. B., & Simon, M. C. (2007). *HIF and c-MYC: sibling rivals for control of cancer cell metabolism and proliferation.* Cancer Cell, 12(2):108–113.

Grade, M., Ghadimi, B. M., Varma, S., Simon, R., Wangsa, D., Barenboim-Stapleton, L., Liersch, T., Becker, H., Ried, T., & Difilippantonio, M. J. (2006). *Aneuploidy-dependent massive deregulation of the cellular transcriptome and apparent divergence of the Wnt/beta-catenin signaling pathway in human rectal carcinomas.* Cancer Res, 66(1):267–282.

Gumz, M. L., Zou, H., Kreinest, P. A., Childs, A. C., Belmonte, L. S., LeGrand, S. N., Wu, K. J., Luxon, B. A., Sinha, M., Parker, A. S., Sun, L. Z., Ahlquist, D. A., Wood, C. G., & Copland, J. A. (2007). *Secreted frizzled-related protein 1 loss contributes to tumor phenotype of clear cell renal cell carcinoma.* Clin Cancer Res, 13(16):4740–4749.

Gunawan, B., Huber, W., Holtrup, M., von Heydebreck, A., Efferth, T., Poustka, A., Ringert, R. H., Jakse, G., & Füzesi, L. (2001). *Prognostic impacts of cytogenetic findings in clear cell renal cell carcinoma: gain of 5q31-qter predicts a distinct clinical phenotype with favorable prognosis.* Cancer Res, 61(21):7731–7738.

Harding, M. A., Arden, K. C., Gildea, J. W., Gildea, J. J., Perlman, E. J., Viars, C., & Theodorescu, D. (2002). *Functional genomic comparison of lineage-related human bladder cancer cell lines with differing tumorigenic and metastatic potentials by spectral karyotyping, comparative genomic hybridization, and a novel method of positional expression profiling.* Cancer Res, 62(23):6981–6989.

Heidenblad, M., Lindgren, D., Veltman, J. A., Jonson, T., Mahlamäki, E. H., Gorunova, L., van Kessel, A. G., Schoenmakers, E. F., & Höglund, M. (2005). *Microarray analyses reveal strong influence of DNA copy number alterations on the transcriptional patterns in pancreatic cancer: implications for the interpretation of genomic amplifications*. Oncogene, 24(10):1794–1801.

Hempel, N., Carrico, P. M., & Melendez, J. A. (2011). *Manganese superoxide dismutase (SOD2) and redox-control of signaling events that drive metastasis*. Anticancer Agents Med Chem, 11(2):191–201.

Höglund, M., Gisselsson, D., Soller, M., Hansen, G. B., Elfving, P., & Mitelman, F. (2004). *Dissecting karyotypic patterns in renal cell carcinoma: an analysis of the accumulated cytogenetic data*. Cancer Genet Cytogenet, 153(1):1–9.

Huang, D. W., Sherman, B. T., & Lempicki, R. A. (2009). *Bioinformatics enrichment tools: paths toward the comprehensive functional analysis of large gene lists*. Nucleic Acids Res, 37(1):1–13.

Huang, D. W., Sherman, B. T., & Lempicki, R. A. (2009a). *Systematic and integrative analysis of large gene lists using DAVID bioinformatics resources*. Nat Protoc, 4(1):44–57.

Hyman, E., Kauraniemi, P., Hautaniemi, S., Wolf, M., Mousses, S., Rozenblum, E., Ringnér, M., Sauter, G., Monni, O., Elkahloun, A., Kallioniemi, O. P., & Kallioniemi, A. (2002). *Impact of DNA amplification on gene expression patterns in breast cancer*. Cancer Res, 62(21):6240–6245.

Irizarry, R. A., Hobbs, B., Collin, F., Beazer-Barclay, Y. D., Antonellis, K. J., Scherf, U., & Speed, T. P. (2003). *Exploration, normalization, and summaries of high density oligonucleotide array probe level data*. Biostatistics, 4(2):249–264.

Jones, J., Otu, H., Spentzos, D., Kolia, S., Inan, M., Beecken, W. D., Fellbaum, C., Gu, X., Joseph, M., Pantuck, A. J., Jonas, D., & Libermann, T. A. (2005). *Gene signatures of progression and metastasis in renal cell cancer*. Clin Cancer Res, 11(16):5730–5739.

Junker, K., Hindermann, W., von Eggeling, F., Diegmann, J., Haessler, K., & Schubert, J. (2005). *CD70: a new tumor specific biomarker for renal cell carcinoma*. J Urol, 173(6):2150–2153.

Junnila, S., Kokkola, A., Karjalainen-Lindsberg, M. L., Puolakkainen, P., & Monni, O. (2010). *Genome-wide gene copy number and expression analysis of primary gastric tumors and gastric cancer cell lines*. BMC Cancer, 10:73.

Kaelin, W. G. (2007). *The von Hippel-Lindau tumor suppressor protein and clear cell renal carcinoma*. Clin Cancer Res, 13(2 Pt 2):680s–684s.

Kaelin, W. G. (2008). *The von Hippel-Lindau tumour suppressor protein: O2 sensing and cancer*. Nat Rev Cancer, 8(11):865–873.

Kim, D. S., Choi, Y. P., Kang, S., Gao, M. Q., Kim, B., Park, H. R., Choi, Y. D., Lim, J. B., Na, H. J., Kim, H. K., Nam, Y. P., Moon, M. H., Yun, H. R., Lee, D. H., Park, W. M., & Cho, N. H. (2010). *Panel of candidate biomarkers for renal cell carcinoma*. J Proteome Res, 9(7):3710–3719.

Kitamura, H., Torigoe, T., Asanuma, H., Hisasue, S. I., Suzuki, K., Tsukamoto, T., Satoh, M., & Sato, N. (2006). *Cytosolic overexpression of p62 sequestosome 1 in neoplastic prostate tissue*. Histopathology, 48(2):157–161.

Klatte, T., Rao, P. N., de Martino, M., LaRochelle, J., Shuch, B., Zomorodian, N., Said, J., Kabbinavar, F. F., Belldegrun, A. S., & Pantuck, A. J. (2009). *Cytogenetic profile predicts prognosis of patients with clear cell renal cell carcinoma*. J Clin Oncol, 27(5):746–753.

Klatte, T., Seligson, D. B., Riggs, S. B., Leppert, J. T., Berkman, M. K., Kleid, M. D., Yu, H., Kabbinavar, F. F., Pantuck, A. J., & Belldegrun, A. S. (2007). *Hypoxia-inducible factor 1 alpha in clear cell renal cell carcinoma.* Clin Cancer Res, 13(24):7388–7393.

Lam, J. S., Pantuck, A. J., Belldegrun, A. S., & Figlin, R. A. (2007). *Protein expression profiles in renal cell carcinoma: staging, prognosis, and patient selection for clinical trials.* Clin Cancer Res, 13(2 Pt 2):703s–708s.

Lam, J. S., Yu, H., Seligson, D. B., Dong, J., Horvath, S., Pantuck, A. J., Figlin, R. A. & Belldegrun A. S. (2005). *Expression of the vascular endothelial growth factor family in tumor dissemination and disease free survival in clear cell renal cell carcinoma.* In Journal of Clinical Oncology, 23(Supplement 16):4538.

Law, C. L., McEarchern, J. A., & Grewal, I. S. (2009). *Novel antibody-based therapeutic agents targeting CD70: a potential approach for treating Waldenström's macroglobulinemia.* Clin Lymphoma Myeloma, 9(1):90–93.

Lenburg, M. E., Liou, L. S., Gerry, N. P., Frampton, G. M., Cohen, H. T., & Christman, M. F. (2003). *Previously unidentified changes in renal cell carcinoma gene expression identified by parametric analysis of microarray data.* BMC Cancer, 3:31.

Li, C. & Wong, W. H. (2001). *Model-based analysis of oligonucleotide arrays: model validation, design issues and standard error application.* Genome Biol, 2(8):RESEARCH0032.

Lisovich, A., Chandran, U. R., Lyons-Weiler, M. A., LaFramboise, W. A., Brown, A. R., Jakacki, R. I., Pollack, I. F., & Sobol, R. W. (2011). *A novel SNP analysis method to detect copy number alterations with an unbiased reference signal directly from tumor samples.* BMC Med Genomics, 4:14.

Liu, X., Wang, A., Muzio, L. L., Kolokythas, A., Sheng, S., Rubini, C., Ye, H., Shi, F., Yu, T., Crowe, D. L., & Zhou, X. (2010). *Deregulation of manganese superoxide dismutase (SOD2) expression and lymph node metastasis in tongue squamous cell carcinoma.* BMC Cancer, 10:365.

Liu, Y. H., Lin, C. Y., Lin, W. C., Tang, S. W., Lai, M. K., & Lin, J. Y. (2008). *Up-regulation of vascular endothelial growth factor-D expression in clear cell renal cell carcinoma by CD74: a critical role in cancer cell tumorigenesis.* J Immunol, 181(9):6584–6594.

Majewski, I. J. & Bernards, R. (2011). *Taming the dragon: genomic biomarkers to individualize the treatment of cancer.* Nat Med, 17(3):304–312.

Martin, F., Linden, T., Katschinski, D. M., Oehme, F., Flamme, I., Mukhopadhyay, C. K., Eckhardt, K., Tröger, J., Barth, S., Camenisch, G., & Wenger, R. H. (2005). *Copper-dependent activation of hypoxia-inducible factor (HIF)-1: implications for ceruloplasmin regulation.* Blood, 105(12):4613–4619.

Maxwell, P. H. (2005). *The HIF pathway in cancer.* Semin Cell Dev Biol, 16(4-5):523–530.

Meyer, H. A., Tölle, A., Jung, M., Fritzsche, F. R., Haendler, B., Kristiansen, I., Gaspert, A., Johannsen, M., Jung, K., & Kristiansen, G. (2009). *Identification of stanniocalcin 2 as prognostic marker in renal cell carcinoma.* Eur Urol, 55(3):669–678.

Mikami, S., Katsube, K. I., Oya, M., Ishida, M., Kosaka, T., Mizuno, R., Mukai, M., & Okada, Y. (2011). *Expression of snail and slug in renal cell carcinoma: E-cadherin repressor snail is associated with cancer invasion and prognosis.* Lab Invest .

Molina, A. M., & Motzer, R. J. (2011). *Clinical practice guidelines for the treatment of metastatic renal cell carcinoma: today and tomorrow.* Oncologist, 16 Suppl 2:45–50.

Morris, M. R., Gentle, D., Abdulrahman, M., Clarke, N., Brown, M., Kishida, T., Yao, M., Teh, B. T., Latif, F., & Maher, E. R. (2008). *Functional epigenomics approach to identify methylated candidate tumour suppressor genes in renal cell carcinoma.* Br J Cancer, 98(2):496–501.

Motzer, R. J. (2011). *New perspectives on the treatment of metastatic renal cell carcinoma: an introduction and historical overview.* Oncologist, 16 Suppl 2:1–3.

Nannya, Y., Sanada, M., Nakazaki, K., Hosoya, N., Wang, L., Hangaishi, A., Kurokawa, M., Chiba, S., Bailey, D. K., Kennedy, G. C., & Ogawa, S. (2005). *A robust algorithm for copy number detection using high-density oligonucleotide single nucleotide polymorphism genotyping arrays.* Cancer Res, 65(14):6071–6079.

Nese, N., Paner, G. P., Mallin, K., Ritchey, J., Stewart, A., & Amin, M. B. (2009). *Renal cell carcinoma: assessment of key pathologic prognostic parameters and patient characteristics in 47,909 cases using the national cancer data base.* Ann Diagn Pathol, 13(1):1–8.

Teng, P. N., Hood, B. L., Sun, M., Dhir, R., & Conrads, T. P. (2011). *Differential proteomic analysis of renal cell carcinoma tissue interstitial fluid.* J Proteome Res, 10(3):1333–1342.

Osunkoya, A. O., Yin-Goen, Q., Phan, J. H., Moffitt, R. A., Stokes, T. H., Wang, M. D., & Young, A. N. (2009). *Diagnostic biomarkers for renal cell carcinoma: selection using novel bioinformatics systems for microarray data analysis.* Hum Pathol, 40(12):1671–1678.

Pal, S. K., Kortylewski, M., Yu, H., & Figlin, R. A. (2010). *Breaking through a plateau in renal cell carcinoma therapeutics: development and incorporation of biomarkers.* Mol Cancer Ther, 9(12):3115–3125.

Pantuck, A. J., Zeng, G., Belldegrun, A. S., & Figlin, R. A. (2003). *Pathobiology, prognosis, and targeted therapy for renal cell carcinoma: exploiting the hypoxia-induced pathway.* Clin Cancer Res, 9(13):4641–4652.

Pantuck, A. J., Fang, Z., Liu, X., Seligson, D. B., Horvath, S., Leppert, J. T., Belldegrun, A. S., & Figlin, R. A. (2005). *Gene expression and tissue microarray analysis of interleukin-2 complete responders in patients with metastatic renal cell carcinoma.* In Journal of Clinical Oncology. *23(Supplement 16):4535.*

Paul, R., Necknig, U., Busch, R., Ewing, C. M., Hartung, R., & Isaacs, W. B. (2004). *Cadherin-6: a new prognostic marker for renal cell carcinoma.* J Urol, 171(1):97–101.

Perego, R. A., Bianchi, C., Corizzato, M., Eroini, B., Torsello, B., Valsecchi, C., Fonzo, A. D., Cordani, N., Favini, P., Ferrero, S., Pitto, M., Sarto, C., Magni, F., Rocco, F., & Mocarelli, P. (2005). *Primary cell cultures arising from normal kidney and renal cell carcinoma retain the proteomic profile of corresponding tissues.* J Proteome Res, 4(5):1503–1510.

Perego, R. A., Corizzato, M., Brambilla, P., Ferrero, S., Bianchi, C., Fasoli, E., Signorini, S., Torsello, B., Invernizzi, L., Bombelli, S., Angeloni, V., Pitto, M., Battaglia, C., Proserpio, V., Magni, F., Galasso, G., & Mocarelli, P. (2008). *Concentration and microsatellite status of plasma DNA for monitoring patients with renal carcinoma.* Eur J Cancer, 44(7):1039–1047.

Perroud, B., Ishimaru, T., Borowsky, A. D., & Weiss, R. H. (2009). *Grade-dependent proteomics characterization of kidney cancer.* Mol Cell Proteomics, 8(5):971–985.

Pez, F., Dayan, F., Durivault, J., Kaniewski, B., Aimond, G., Provost, G. S. L., Deux, B., Clézardin, P., Sommer, P., Pouysségur, J., & Reynaud, C. (2011). *The HIF-1-inducible lysyl oxidase activates HIF-1 via the AKT pathway in a positive regulation loop and synergizes with HIF-1 in promoting tumor cell growth*. Cancer Res, 71(5):1647–1657.

Podar, K. & Anderson, K. C. (2010). *A therapeutic role for targeting c-MYC/HIF-1-dependent signaling pathways*. Cell Cycle, 9(9):1722–1728.

Pollack, J. R., Sørlie, T., Perou, C. M., Rees, C. A., Jeffrey, S. S., Lonning, P. E., Tibshirani, R., Botstein, D., Børresen-Dale, A. L., & Brown, P. O. (2002). *Microarray analysis reveals a major direct role of dna copy number alteration in the transcriptional program of human breast tumors*. Proc Natl Acad Sci U S A, 99(20):12963–12968.

Redova, M., Svoboda, M., & Slaby, O. (2011). *MicroRNAs and their target gene networks in renal cell carcinoma*. Biochem Biophys Res Commun, 405(2):153–156.

Saramäki, O. R., Porkka, K. P., Vessella, R. L., & Visakorpi, T. (2006). *Genetic aberrations in prostate cancer by microarray analysis*. Int J Cancer, 119(6):1322–1329.

Sato, E., Torigoe, T., Hirohashi, Y., Kitamura, H., Tanaka, T., Honma, I., Asanuma, H., Harada, K., Takasu, H., Masumori, N., Ito, N., Hasegawa, T., Tsukamoto, T., & Sato, N. (2008). *Identification of an immunogenic ctl epitope of HIFPH3 for immunotherapy of renal cell carcinoma*. Clin Cancer Res, 14(21):6916–6923.

Schäfer, M., Schwender, H., Merk, S., Haferlach, C., Ickstadt, K., & Dugas, M. (2009). *Integrated analysis of copy number alterations and gene expression: a bivariate assessment of equally directed abnormalities*. Bioinformatics, 25(24):3228–3235.

Scotto, L., Narayan, G., Nandula, S. V., Subramaniyam, S., Kaufmann, A. M., Wright, J. D., Pothuri, B., Mansukhani, M., Schneider, A., Arias-Pulido, H., & Murty, V. V. (2008). *Integrative genomics analysis of chromosome 5p gain in cervical cancer reveals target over-expressed genes, including Drosha*. Mol Cancer, 7:58.

Seelow, D., Schwarz, J. M., & Schuelke, M. (2008). *GeneDistiller–distilling candidate genes from linkage intervals*. PLoS One, 3(12):e3874.

Seliger, B., Dressler, S. P., Massa, C., Recktenwald, C. V., Altenberend, F., Bukur, J., Marincola, F. M., Wang, E., Stevanovic, S., & Lichtenfels, R. (2011). *Identification and characterization of human leukocyte antigen class I ligands in renal cell carcinoma cells*. Proteomics, 11(12):2528–2541.

Seliger, B., Dressler, S. P., Wang, E., Kellner, R., Recktenwald, C. V., Lottspeich, F., Marincola, F. M., Baumgärtner, M., Atkins, D., & Lichtenfels, R. (2009). *Combined analysis of transcriptome and proteome data as a tool for the identification of candidate biomarkers in renal cell carcinoma*. Proteomics, 9(6):1567–1581.

Semenza, G. L. (2008). *Hypoxia-inducible factor 1 and cancer pathogenesis*. IUBMB Life, 60(9):591–597.

Shi, T., Dong, F., Liou, L. S., Duan, Z. H., Novick, A. C., & DiDonato, J. A. (2004). *Differential protein profiling in renal-cell carcinoma*. Mol Carcinog, 40(1):47–61.

Shimazui, T., Yoshikawa, K., Uemura, H., Hirao, Y., Saga, S., & Akaza, H. (2004). *The level of cadherin-6 mRNA in peripheral blood is associated with the site of metastasis and with the subsequent occurrence of metastases in renal cell carcinoma*. Cancer, 101(5):963–968.

Skubitz, K. M. & Skubitz, A. P. N. (2002). *Differential gene expression in renal-cell cancer*. J Lab Clin Med, 140(1):52–64.

Skubitz, K. M., Zimmermann, W., Zimmerman, W., Kammerer, R., Pambuccian, S., & Skubitz, A. P. N. (2006). *Differential gene expression identifies subgroups of renal cell carcinoma*. J Lab Clin Med, 147(5):250–267.

Sültmann, H., von Heydebreck, A., Huber, W., Kuner, R., Buness, A., Vogt, M., Gunawan, B., Vingron, M., Füzesí, L., & Poustka, A. (2005). *Gene expression in kidney cancer is associated with cytogenetic abnormalities, metastasis formation, and patient survival*. Clin Cancer Res, 11(2 Pt 1):646–655.

Staller, P., Sulitkova, J., Lisztwan, J., Moch, H., Oakeley, E. J., & Krek, W. (2003). *Chemokine receptor CXCR4 downregulated by von Hippel-Lindau tumour suppressor pVHL*. Nature, 425(6955):307–311.

Stickel, J. S., Weinzierl, A. O., Hillen, N., Drews, O., Schuler, M. M., Hennenlotter, J., Wernet, D., Müller, C. A., Stenzl, A., Rammensee, H.-G., & Stevanović, S. (2009). *HLA ligand profiles of primary renal cell carcinoma maintained in metastases*. Cancer Immunol Immunother, 58(9):1407–1417.

Struckmann, K., Mertz, K., Steu, S., Storz, M., Staller, P., Krek, W., Schraml, P., & Moch, H. (2008). *pVHL co-ordinately regulates CXCR4/CXCL12 and MMP2/MMP9 expression in human clear-cell renal cell carcinoma*. J Pathol, 214(4):464–471.

Subramanian, A., Tamayo, P., Mootha, V. K., Mukherjee, S., Ebert, B. L., Gillette, M. A., Paulovich, A., Pomeroy, S. L., Golub, T. R., Lander, E. S., & Mesirov, J. P. (2005). *Gene set enrichment analysis: a knowledge-based approach for interpreting genome-wide expression profiles*. Proc Natl Acad Sci U S A, 102(43):15545–15550.

Takahashi, M., Papavero, V., Yuhas, J., Kort, E., Kanayama, H. O., Kagawa, S., Baxter, R. C., Yang, X. J., Gray, S. G., & Teh, B. T. (2005). *Altered expression of members of the IGF-axis in clear cell renal cell carcinoma*. Int J Oncol, 26(4):923–931.

Tanaka, T., Kitamura, H., Torigoe, T., Hirohashi, Y., Sato, E., Masumori, N., Sato, N., & Tsukamoto, T. (2011). *Autoantibody against hypoxia-inducible factor prolyl hydroxylase-3 is a potential serological marker for renal cell carcinoma*. J Cancer Res Clin Oncol, 137(5):789–794.

Tang, S. W., Chang, W. H., Su, Y. C., Chen, Y. C., Lai, Y. H., Wu, P. T., Hsu, C. I., Lin, W. C., Lai, M. K., & Lin, J. Y. (2009). *MYC pathway is activated in clear cell renal cell carcinoma and essential for proliferation of clear cell renal cell carcinoma cells*. Cancer Lett, 273(1):35–43.

Thiery, J. P. (2003). *Epithelial-mesenchymal transitions in development and pathologies*. Curr Opin Cell Biol, 15(6):740–746.

Thiery, J. P., Acloque, H., Huang, R. Y. J., & Nieto, M. A. (2009). *Epithelial-mesenchymal transitions in development and disease*. Cell, 139(5):871–890.

Thompson, H. G. R., Harris, J. W., Wold, B. J., Lin, F., & Brody, J. P. (2003). *p62 overexpression in breast tumors and regulation by prostate-derived ETS factor in breast cancer cells*. Oncogene, 22(15):2322–2333.

Tostain, J., Li, G., Gentil-Perret, A., & Gigante, M. (2010). *Carbonic anhydrase 9 in clear cell renal cell carcinoma: a marker for diagnosis, prognosis and treatment*. Eur J Cancer, 46(18):3141–3148.

Truong, L. D. & Shen, S. S. (2011). *Immunohistochemical diagnosis of renal neoplasms*. Arch Pathol Lab Med, 135(1):92–109.

Tun, H. W., Marlow, L. A., von Roemeling, C. A., Cooper, S. J., Kreinest, P., Wu, K., Luxon, B. A., Sinha, M., Anastasiadis, P. Z., & Copland, J. A. (2010). *Pathway signature and cellular differentiation in clear cell renal cell carcinoma*. PLoS One, 5(5):e10696. von Frowein, J., Pagel, P., Kappler, R., von Schweinitz, D., Roscher, A., & Schmid, I.

(2011). *MicroRNA-492 is processed from the keratin 19 gene and up-regulated in metastatic hepatoblastoma*. Hepatology, 53(3):833–842.

Waalkes, S., Eggers, H., Blasig, H., Atschekzei, F., Kramer, M. W., Hennenlotter, J., Tränkenschuh, W., Stenzl, A., Serth, J., Schrader, A. J., Kuczyk, M. A., & Merseburger, A. S. (2011). *Caveolin 1 mRNA is overexpressed in malignant renal tissue and might serve as a novel diagnostic marker for renal cancer*. Biomark Med, 5(2):219–225.

Wang, Y., Roche, O., Yan, M. S., Finak, G., Evans, A. J., Metcalf, J. L., Hast, B. E., Hanna, S. C., Wondergem, B., Furge, K. A., Irwin, M. S., Kim, W. Y., Teh, B. T., Grinstein, S., Park, M., Marsden, P. A., & Ohh, M. (2009). *Regulation of endocytosis via the oxygen-sensing pathway*. Nat Med, 15(3):319–324.

Wouters, B. G. & Koritzinsky, M. (2008). *Hypoxia signalling through mTOR and the unfolded protein response in cancer*. Nat Rev Cancer, 8(11):851–864.

Yamamoto, G., Nannya, Y., Kato, M., Sanada, M., Levine, R. L., Kawamata, N., Hangaishi, A., Kurokawa, M., Chiba, S., Gilliland, D. G., Koeffler, H. P., & Ogawa, S. (2007). *Highly sensitive method for genomewide detection of allelic composition in nonpaired, primary tumor specimens by use of Affymetrix single-nucleotide-polymorphism genotyping microarrays*. Am J Hum Genet, 81(1):114–126.

Yang, J. C., Haworth, L., Sherry, R. M., Hwu, P., Schwartzentruber, D. J., Topalian, S. L., Steinberg, S. M., Chen, H. X., & Rosenberg, S. A. (2003). *A randomized trial of bevacizumab, an anti-vascular endothelial growth factor antibody, for metastatic renal cancer*. N Engl J Med, 349(5):427–434.

Yao, M., Tabuchi, H., Nagashima, Y., Baba, M., Nakaigawa, N., Ishiguro, H., Hamada, K., Inayama, Y., Kishida, T., Hattori, K., Yamada-Okabe, H., & Kubota, Y. (2005). *Gene expression analysis of renal carcinoma: adipose differentiation-related protein as a potential diagnostic and prognostic biomarker for clear-cell renal carcinoma*. J Pathol, 205(3):377–387.

Yin-Goen, Q., Dale, J., Yang, W. L., Phan, J., Moffitt, R., Petros, J. A., Datta, M. W., Amin, M. B., Wang, M ., & Young, A. N. (2006). *Advances in molecular classification of renal neoplasms*. Histol Histopathol, 21(3):325–339.

Yoshimoto, T., Matsuura, K., Karnan, S., Tagawa, H., Nakada, C., Tanigawa, M., Tsukamoto, Y., Uchida, T., Kashima, K., Akizuki, S., Takeuchi, I., Sato, F., Mimata, H., Seto, M., & Moriyama, M. (2007). *High-resolution analysis of DNA copy number alterations and gene expression in renal clear cell carcinoma*. J Pathol, 213(4):392–401.

Young, A. N., Amin, M. B., Moreno, C. S., Lim, S. D., Cohen, C., Petros, J. A., Marshall, F. F., & Neish, A. S. (2001). *Expression profiling of renal epithelial neoplasms: a method for tumor classification and discovery of diagnostic molecular markers*. Am J Pathol, 158(5):1639–1651.

Yusenko, M. V., Zubakov, D., & Kovacs, G. (2009). *Gene expression profiling of chromophobe renal cell carcinomas and renal oncocytomas by Affymetrix genechip using pooled and individual tumours*. Int J Biol Sci, 5(6):517–527.

Zhang, Q., Ying, J., Li, J., Fan, Y., Poon, F. F., Ng, K. M., Tao, Q., & Jin, J. (2010). *Aberrant promoter methylation of DLEC1, a critical 3p22 tumor suppressor for renal cell carcinoma, is associated with more advanced tumor stage*. J Urol, 184(2):731–737.

Zhang, Z., Wondergem, B., & Dykema, K. (2010). *A comprehensive study of progressive cytogenetic alterations in clear cell renal cell carcinoma and a new model for ccRCC tumorigenesis and progression*. Adv Bioinformatics, page 428325.

Zhang, Z. F., Matsuda, D., Khoo, S. K., Buzzitta, K., Block, E., Petillo, D., Richard, S., Anema, J., Furge, K. A., & Teh, B. T. (2008). *A comparison study reveals important features of agreement and disagreement between summarized DNA and RNA data obtained from renal cell carcinoma*. Mutat Res, 657(1):77–83.

Zhao, H., Ljungberg, B., Grankvist, K., Rasmuson, T., Tibshirani, R., & Brooks, J. D. (2006). *Gene expression profiling predicts survival in conventional renal cell carcinoma*. PLoS Med, 3(1):e13.

Zhou, G. X., Ireland, J., Rayman, P., Finke, J., & Zhou, M. (2010). *Quantification of carbonic anhydrase IX expression in serum and tissue of renal cell carcinoma patients using enzyme-linked immunosorbent assay: prognostic and diagnostic potentials*. Urology, 75(2):257–261.

3

The VHL-HIF Signaling in Renal Cell Carcinoma: Promises and Pitfalls

Christudas Morais[1*], David W. Johnson[1,2] and Glenda C. Gobe[1]
[1]*Centre for Kidney Disease Research, School of Medicine, The University of Queensland,*
[2]*Department of Renal Medicine, The University of Queensland at Princess Alexandra Hospital, Brisbane, Australia*

1. Introduction

Renal cell carcinoma (RCC) is the third most common genitourinary cancer behind prostate and bladder cancer, accounting for 3% of all adult malignancies (Curti, 2004). It is a highly metastatic and heterogeneous disease with at least 16 histologic subtypes (Eble et al., 2001; Lopez-Beltran et al., 2006), among which clear cell (70-80%), papillary (10-15%) and chromophobe (5%) are the most common (Curti, 2004). Up to 25% of patients with RCC have distant metastases at presentation. Another 50% develop metastases or local recurrence during follow-up, despite treatment of the primary tumor (Thyavihally et al., 2005). The average survival, following metastatic RCC, is about 4 months, and only 10% of patients survive for one year. The global incidence of RCC per year is close to 300000, with a male to female ratio of 3:2 and an estimated mortality of approximately 100000 (Arai&Kanai, 2010; Ferlay et al., 2010). The incidence of RCC has been rising steadily, probably because of incidental findings from imaging techniques performed for other reasons. It can occur at any age, but is most frequently diagnosed in the 40-70 year old group (Eble et al., 2001; Pascual & Borque, 2008; Arai&Kanai, 2010).

Well before the advent of the modern era of genetics and molecular biology, surgeons and pathologists were aware of the hyper-vascular nature of RCC (Corn, 2007). The subsequent isolation of the von Hippel-Lindau (VHL) gene in 1993 led to the important discoveries that aberrant VHL is the most important risk for RCC and that VHL negatively regulates the hypoxia inducible factor (HIF) and thus the downstream angiogenesis pathway thereby engendering increased vascularity. In this chapter, we will focus on the role of the VHL-HIF pathway in RCC, advancements in novel therapeutics targeting this pathway and future directions.

2. Von Hippel-Lindau syndrome

VHL disease, commonly known as the VHL syndrome, is named after the German ophthalmologist Eugene von Hippel, and the Swedish neuropathologist Arvid Lindau, who

* Corresponding Author

in the early 1900s, described highly vascularised tumors of the retina and the central nervous system (Kim&Kaelin, 2004; Ohh, 2006). VHL syndrome is the result of germ line mutations in VHL, a tumor-suppressor gene located on chromosome 3p25 (Seizinger et al., 1988; Kim&Kaelin, 2004; Clark, 2009; Gossage&Eisen, 2010). It affects 1 in 35,000 individuals and is associated with the development of tumors in multiple organs, including the brain, spinal cord, pancreas, adrenal gland, epididymis (in males), broad ligament (in women) and kidneys (Lonser et al., 2003; Kim&Kaelin, 2004; Grubb et al., 2005; Clark, 2009). Individuals with VHL syndrome carry one wild type VHL allele and one faulty allele. Tumors develop only after the spontaneous somatic loss (loss of heterzygosity [LoH]) or inactivation, or both, of the remaining wild type. Thus, at cellular level, VHL syndrome can be considered as an autosomal recessive disease, whilst clinically, it manifests more like an autosomal dominant disease because the inactivation of the wild type allele is almost guaranteed (Ohh&Kaelin, 2003; Ohh, 2006). Apart from LoH and mutations, hypermethylation of the VHL promoter regions can prevent the wild-type VHL gene from expressing its functional tumor suppressor protein pVHL (Kim&Kaelin, 2004). The VHL gene is mutated in 50-80% (Weiss&Lin, 2006; Arai&Kanai, 2010) and hypermethylated in 19% (Herman et al., 1994; Arai&Kanai, 2010) of sporadic clear cell RCC. Clear cell RCC is the leading cause of death in patients with VHL mutation (Maher et al., 1990; Clark, 2009; Gossage&Eisen, 2010).

The VHL gene, which was isolated in 1993 (Latif et al., 1993), has three exons and encodes for two mRNA transcripts that are translated into three types of pVHL (Ohh&Kaelin, 2003; Ohh, 2006). The first VHL mRNA transcript that contains all three exons, is translated into a larger 213 amino acid protein of approximately 24-30 kDa ($pVHL_{30}$), and a smaller 160 amino acid protein of approximately 18-19 kDa ($pVHL_{19}$) due to alternative translation initiation (Iliopoulos et al., 1998; Schoenfeld et al., 1998; Blankenship et al., 1999; Safran&Kaelin, 2003). In the early days, both $pVHL_{30}$ and $pVHL_{19}$ were considered to be tumor suppressors (Iliopoulos et al., 1995; Ohh, 2006). However, further studies have cast doubt on the tumor suppressive role of $pVHL_{19}$ (Ohh, 2006). Generally, the term 'pVHL' is used to refer to both isoforms (Kim&Kaelin, 2004; Kaelin, 2007). The second VHL mRNA transcript lacks exon 2 due to alternative splicing. Literature on this isoform is scant, although RCCs that exclusively produce this shorter VHL mRNA transcript have been identified (Gnarra et al., 1996; Safran&Kaelin, 2003; Ohh, 2006).

pVHL consists of α and β domains (Fig.1), which are essential for its tumor suppressor activities (Stebbins et al., 1999; Kaelin, 2002). pVHL forms complexes with elonginB, elonginC, Rbx1, and Cullin 2 to form an E3 ubiquitin ligase complex (Stebbins et al., 1999; Ohh et al., 2000; Tanimoto et al., 2000; Kaelin, 2002; Kaelin, 2005a; Kaelin, 2005b; Gossage&Eisen, 2010). The α domain binds to elongin C and the β domain interacts with hydroxylated prolines of HIF (Fig.1). This complex has multiple functions, which can be broadly classified into HIF-independent and HIF-dependent. The HIF-independent functions include maintenance of primary cilia (Hergovich et al., 2003; Baldewijns et al., 2010), assembly of extracellular fibronectin matrix (Guo et al., 2009), regulation of apoptosis (Guo et al., 2009), epithelial mesenchymal transition (EMT) (Koochekpour et al., 1999; Hara et al., 2006), and transcriptional regulation (Yuen et al., 2007; Mikhaylova et al., 2008; Baldewijns et al., 2010). The best studied role is its HIF-dependent function in RCC, which is the degradation of HIF (Ohh, 2006; Baldewijns et al., 2010; Gossage&Eisen, 2010).

3. Hypoxia-inducible factor

A hypoxic tumor microenvironment is one of the characteristics of solid tumors. Cells undergo a variety of adaptive changes that will facilitate their survival under hypoxic conditions. One such change at the molecular level is the activation of the hypoxia-sensitive transcription factor, HIF. HIF is a heterodimer consisting of two subunits: α and β (Wang et al., 1995; Kaluz et al., 2008). The β subunit, also known as aryl hydrocarbon receptor nuclear translocator (ARNT), is constitutively expressed and is independent of intracellular oxygen tension. The oxygen-sensitive α subunit, which has three further subunits, HIF-1α, HIF-2α, and HIF-3α, is also constitutively expressed, but is rapidly degraded under normoxic conditions (Semenza, 1999; Huang&Bunn, 2003; Maynard et al., 2003; Maynard&Ohh, 2004; Kaluz et al., 2008; Baldewijns et al., 2010). At least two mechanisms that negatively regulate the stability of HIF-α under normoxia have been recognized: oxygen-dependent prolyl hydroxylation and asparaginyl hydroxylation (Lando et al., 2002a; Lando et al., 2002b; Ohh, 2006).

HIF-1α and HIF-2α contain an N-terminal transactivation domain (NTAD), a C-terminal transactivation domain (CTAD) and an oxygen-dependent degradation domain (ODDD) [Fig.1] (Pugh et al., 1997; Sang et al., 2002; Baldewijns et al., 2010). The ODDD has a stretch of proline residues. HIF-3α lacks the transactivation domain and has many splice variants. Under normoxic conditions, the proline residues within the ODDD of HIF-α are hydroxylated by prolyl hydroxylases (PH) at positions 402 and 564 (Ivan et al., 2001; Jaakkola et al., 2001; Schofield&Ratcliffe, 2005; Koivunen et al., 2007; Kaluz et al., 2008; Baldewijns et al., 2010). The pVHL-E3 ubiquitin ligase complex binds to the hydroxylated HIF-α through the β domain of pVHL and enables polyubiquitination. The polyubiquitinated HIF-α is degraded by the 26S proteasome (Maxwell et al., 1999; Ohh et al., 2000; Tanimoto et al., 2000; Jaakkola et al., 2001; Baldewijns et al., 2010). While the prolyl hydroxylation enables the binding of pVHL to HIF-α and its eventual degradation, the asparaginyl hydroxylation prevents the transcriptional activation of HIF target genes (Dames et al., 2002; Freedman et al., 2002). For transcriptional activity, HIF-α requires the recruitment of p300/CBP transcriptional coactivators (Arany et al., 1996). The CTAD has a conserved C-terminal asparagine. In normoxia, the factor inhibiting HIF-1 (FIH-1), an oxygenase, hydroxylates asparagine at position 803, which diminishes the recruitment of p300/CBP to HIF-α (Freedman et al., 2002) leading to the transcriptional downregulation of HIF responsive elements (Mahon et al., 2001; Dames et al., 2002; Lando et al., 2002a; Lando et al., 2002b).

In hypoxia, the activity of prolyl hydroxylases and FIH-1 are reduced, leading to the inhibition of proline and asparginyl hydroxylation, respectively. In the absence of a functional pVHL, the binding of the pVHL-E3 ubiquitin ligase complex to HIF-α and the subsequent polyubiquitination and degradation of HIF-α are inhibited even under normoxic conditions. Both events lead to the stabilization and accumulation of HIF-α in cells. As a result, HIF-α is translocated to the nucleus, where it dimerizes with HIF-β. The HIF-α/HIF-β heterodimer binds to hypoxia-responsive elements (HRE) of the DNA, recruits p300/CBP to the CTAD and transactivates over 60 hypoxia-inducible genes of which, vascular endothelial growth factor (VEGF) (angiogenesis), transforming growth factor alpha (TGF-α) and epidermal growth factor receptor (EGFR) (proliferation), carbonic anhydrase IX (CAIX) (pH regulation), erythropoietin (EPO) (erythropoiesis), e-cadherin (EMT) and glucose transporter-1 (GLUT-1) (glucose metabolism) have attracted much attention (Ohh, 2006; Clark, 2009; Baldewijns et al., 2010). Because of the defective VHL-HIF-VEGF pathway, RCC is considered to be one of the most hypervascularized tumors. Hence, it is not surprising that considerable research in the past decade has focused on the angiogenic pathway, which led to the development of some promising novel therapeutics.

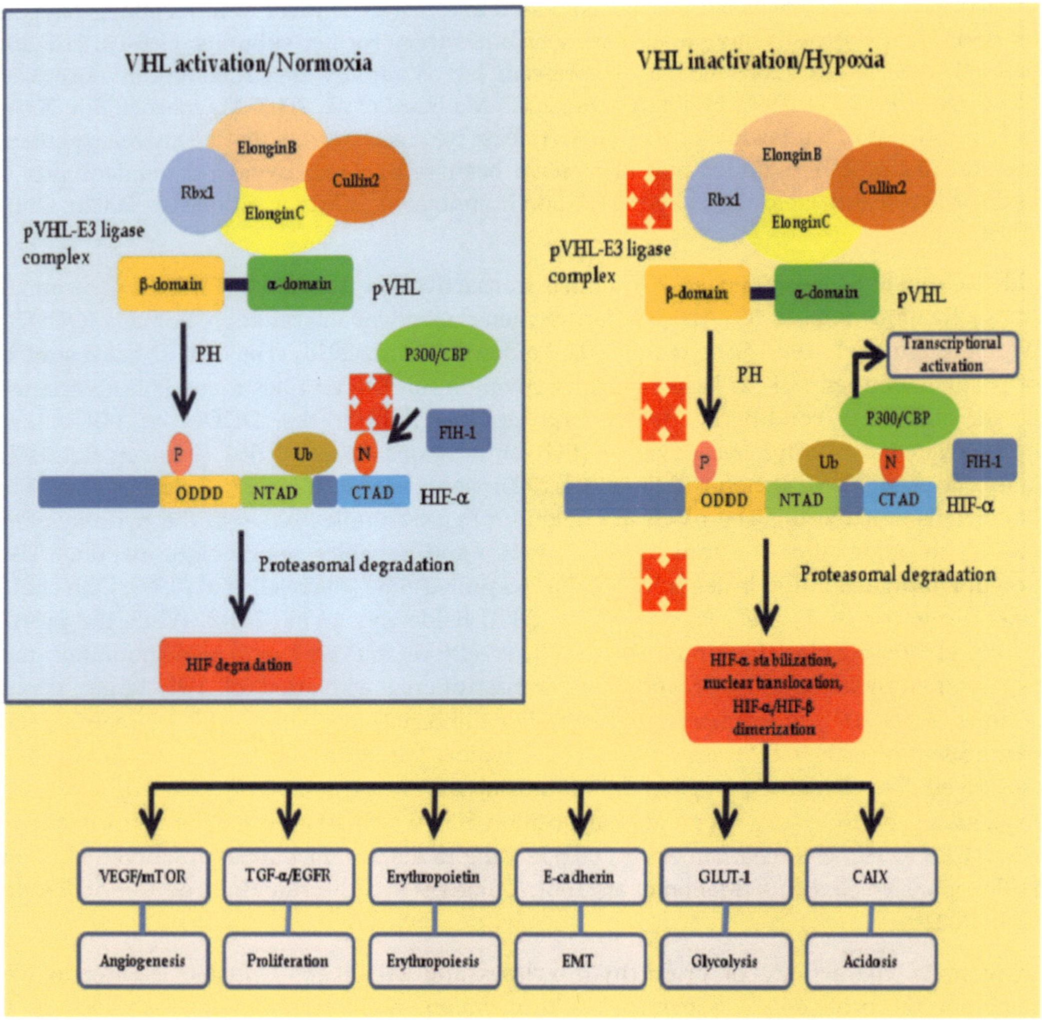

Fig. 1. The von Hippel-Lindau-Hypoxia Inducible Factor (VHL-HIF) pathway. The details are given in text. In brief, under active VHL and normoxic conditions, HIF is degraded. When the VHL gene is inactive due to mutations or hypermethylation, HIF is stabilized, translocated to the nucleus and activates the transcription of over 60 hypoxia-responsive molecules that are involved in oncogenesis and tumor progression. Only selected molecules and their alleged roles in tumor progression that are discussed in this chapter are shown. X, represents inhibition or inactivation. N, asparagine; P, proline; PH, prolyl hydroxylases; Ub, ubiquitination.

4. VHL inactivation and HIF-induced hypoxia responsive genes

4.1 Vascular endothelial growth factor – mammalian target of rapamycin

Of the many HIF-regulated angiogenic molecules, VEGF is perhaps the most studied - not only in RCC but also cancers in general. In humans, the VEGF system consists of five secreted ligands, namely VEGF-A, VEGF-B, VEGF-C, VEGF-D and placenta growth factor-1 (PlGF) and three receptor tyrosine kinases, VEGF-R1 (flt-1), VEGF-R2 (flk1 in the mouse, KDR in the human), and VEGF-R3 (flt4) (Carmeliet, 2005; Hicklin&Ellis, 2005; Tammela et al., 2005; Cebe-Suarez et al., 2006; Donovan&Kummar, 2006; Roy et al., 2006; Thurston&Kitajewski, 2008; Clark, 2009; Stuttfeld&Ballmer-Hofer, 2009; Bates, 2010). VEGF-R1 and VEGF-R2 are predominantly expressed in vascular endothelial cells and VEGF-R3 in lymphatic endothelial cells (Tammela et al., 2005; Thurston&Kitajewski, 2008). Hence, VEGF-R1 and VEGF-R2 are thought to be more important for angiogenesis and VEGF-R3 for lymphangiogenesis (Donovan&Kummar, 2006; Clark, 2009). The binding of the ligands to the receptors is an essential step in the initiation of the VEGF signaling. Generally, VEGF-R1 binds to VEGF-A, VEGF-B and PlGF; VEGF-R2 binds to VEGF-A, VEGF-C and VEGF-D and VEGF-R3 to VEGF-C and VEGF-D (Cebe-Suarez et al., 2006; Stuttfeld&Ballmer-Hofer, 2009). The receptor-ligand binding promotes conformational changes, followed by phosphorylation of specific tyrosine residues of the receptor (Cebe-Suarez et al., 2006; Stuttfeld&Ballmer-Hofer, 2009). Subsequently, a variety of downstream signaling pathways is activated, of which the most studied are the RAF-MEK-ERK series of kinases and the phosphatidylinositol-3 kinase-protein kinase B-mammalian target of rapamycin (PI3K-AKT-mTOR) pathway (Clark, 2009; Banumathy&Cairns, 2010). Increased mTOR, which itself is the result of HIF activation secondary to VHL loss, can in turn lead to an increase in HIF thereby maintaining a positive feedback loop that exacerbates the deleterious effects of VHL inactivation (Cho et al., 2007; Clark, 2009; Banumathy&Cairns, 2010). Both pathways predominantly up-regulate a variety of pro-angiogenic factors, thereby imparting a hyper-angiogenic phenotype to RCC.

There is considerable evidence demonstrating that VEGF is significantly elevated in RCC, with some studies reporting its up-regulation in up to 96% of RCC (Takahashi et al., 1994). There is a direct correlation between VEGF expression, tumor microvascular density, disease progression and metastasis of RCC (Takahashi et al., 1994; Zhang et al., 2002; Fukata et al., 2005; Baldewijns et al., 2007; Rioux-Leclercq et al., 2007; Patard et al., 2009). Apart from VEGF, RCC is reported to over-express several potent pro-angiogenic factors, including basic fibroblast growth factor (bFGF) (Cenni et al., 2007), PlGF (Takahashi et al., 1994), platelet-derived growth factor (PDGF) (Xu et al., 2005a), epidermal growth factor (EGF) (Kedar et al., 2002), the interleukins IL-6 (Angelo et al., 2002) and IL-8 (Konig et al., 1999), leptin (Horiguchi et al., 2006b; Horiguchi et al., 2006a) and various chemokines (Slaton et al., 2001; Fukata et al., 2005).

Hence, it is not surprising that the past decade has placed much emphasis on HIF-regulated downstream pathways, especially angiogenesis. This has resulted in the development of many clinically available novel chemotherapeutic agents. They can be broadly categorized as VEGF inhibitors, multiple tyrosine kinase inhibitors and mTOR inhibitors. The most successful VEGF inhibitor is the humanized VEGF-neutralizing antibody, bevacizumab. Bevacizumab is thought to exert its anti-angiogenic activity by acting against the angiogenic endothelial cells surrounding the tumor rather than the tumor *per se* thus blocking the supply of oxygen and nutrients to the tumors (Ellis&Hicklin, 2008; Ainsworth et al., 2009; Banumathy&Cairns, 2010). The clinically available multiple tyrosine kinase inhibitors are sunitinib, sorafenib, pazopanib and axitinib. As summarized in Table 1, they target multiple tyrosine kinase receptors neutralizing the downstream signaling pathways activated by ligand-receptor binding, as discussed above. Two of the most successful mTOR inhibitors are temsirolimus and everolimus. Both are rapamycin analogues and bind to FK506-binding protein 12 (FKBP12), which in turn binds to mTOR leading to the inhibition of the PI3K/Akt/mTOR pathway (Thomas et al., 2006; Abraham&Gibbons, 2007; Ainsworth et al., 2009; Banumathy&Cairns, 2010). In addition, temsirolimus has been shown to have a direct inhibitory effect on HIF-α and VEGF (Del Bufalo et al., 2006; Motzer et al., 2008; Banumathy&Cairns, 2010; Houghton, 2010).

Drug	Target receptors	Reference
Sunitinib	VEGFR1, VEGFR2, VEGFR3, PDGFR-α, PDGFR-β, FLT3, c-KIT, RET	(Mendel et al., 2003; Faivre et al., 2006; Ainsworth et al., 2009; Banumathy&Cairns, 2010)
Sorafenib	VEGFR-2, PDGFR-β, c-KIT, Raf-1	(Wilhelm&Chien, 2002; Wilhelm et al., 2004; Ainsworth et al., 2009)
Pazopanib	VEGFR1, VEGFR2, VEGFR3, PDGFR-α, PDGFR-β, c-KIT	(Kumar et al., 2007; Ainsworth et al., 2009; Banumathy&Cairns, 2010; Sternberg et al., 2010)
Axitinib	VEGFR1, VEGFR2, VEGFR3, PDGFR-β, c-KIT,	(Rugo et al., 2005; Rixe et al., 2007)

Table 1. Clinically available multiple tyrosine kinase inhibitors for metastatic RCC (Bullock et al., 2010)

4.2 Transforming growth factor-α and epidermal growth factor receptor

TGF-α is an autocrine mitogen for fibroblasts and epithelial cells. It has structural and functional homology to EGF (Derynck, 1986; Everitt et al., 1997). TGF-α is thought to mediate its biological effects through the binding of EGFR, which is a family of four closely related cell membrane receptors, EGFR (HER1; ErbB1), HER2 (ErbB2), HER3 (ErbB3), and HER4 (ErbB4) (Higashiyama et al., 2008; Pu et al., 2009). These receptors are transmembrane glycoproteins with an extracellular ligand-binding domain and an intracellular tyrosine kinase domain (Higashiyama et al., 2008; Pu et al., 2009). Ligand-binding to the extracellular domain of EGFR activates tyrosine kinase, resulting in autophosphorylation of EGFR and subsequent signal transduction leading to cell cycle progression, inhibition of apoptosis, induction of angiogenesis, promotion of invasion and metastasis, and other oncogenic activities (Derynck, 1986; Everitt et al., 1997; Gunaratnam et al., 2003; Black&Dinney, 2008; Lee et al., 2008; Uberall et al., 2008; Pu et al., 2009). TGF-α/EGFR activation in RCC is either independent of, or dependent on the VHL status. While the mechanisms behind VHL-independent activation have not been fully elucidated, the VHL-dependent TGF-α/EGFR follows the classical pattern of HIF-1 up-regulation secondary to loss of VHL function (de

Paulsen et al., 2001; Gunaratnam et al., 2003; Lee et al., 2008). It has been suggested that TGF-α overproduction secondary to VHL deficiency is the consequence of HIF activation and that such activation establishes an autocrine TGF-α/EGFR stimulatory system leading to the oncogenic transformation of normal renal epithelial cells and the formation of RCC (Ishikawa et al., 1990; Atlas et al., 1992; Yoshida et al., 1994; Everitt et al., 1997; de Paulsen et al., 2001; Gunaratnam et al., 2003; Pelletier et al., 2009; Pu et al., 2009). For example, transgenic expression of TGF-α in mice leads to the formation of multiple renal cysts reminiscent of pre-neoplastic lesions of the human kidney, whilst the re-introduction of wild type VHL inhibits TGF-α expression and cyst formation (Lowden et al., 1994; Everitt et al., 1997; Knebelmann et al., 1998; de Paulsen et al., 2001; Kaelin, 2002; Gunaratnam et al., 2003).

Many studies have reported the over expression of TGF-α and EGFR in RCC (Freeman et al., 1989; Gomella et al., 1989; Mydlo et al., 1989; Sargent et al., 1989; Petrides et al., 1990; Lager et al., 1994; Yoshida et al., 1994; Uhlman et al., 1995; Everitt et al., 1997; Yoshida et al., 1997; Ramp et al., 2000; Merseburger et al., 2005; Lee et al., 2008; Pelletier et al., 2009; Pu et al., 2009). The expression pattern of TGF-α in RCC is such that it has been identified as an ideal candidate for immunotherapy (Pelletier et al., 2009). The prognostic association between over-expression of EGFR in RCC, and development of the cancer is controversial. Two distinct patterns of EGFR expression have been observed: a) cytoplasmic in normal renal cells, and b) membranous in RCC. These observations suggest that it is not just the over expression of EGFR, but the location of its over-expression that determines prognosis. Accordingly, RCC patients with positive membranous EGFR expression may have a poorer survival outcome when compared with those with negative expression of membranous EGFR (Pu et al., 2009). However, a previous study casts doubt on this hypothesis (Kallio et al., 2003).

Some studies have explored the therapeutic efficiency of EGFR inhibitors, either as single agents or in combination, with a success rate of around 10% (Motzer et al., 2003; Dawson et al., 2004; Rowinsky et al., 2004; Jermann et al., 2006; Ravaud et al., 2008; Gordon et al., 2009; Pu et al., 2009). Interestingly however, results of anti-EGFR therapy in other cancers show a lack of correlation between EGFR expression and response to therapy, suggesting that differential intracellular signaling events rather than the mere expression of EGFR may also play significant roles in predicting response to anti-EGFR therapy (Marks et al., 2008; Gordon et al., 2009). Furthermore, RCC cells with wild type VHL have been shown to be more sensitive to anti-EGFR treatment than those with mutated VHL (Perera et al., 2000; Gordon et al., 2009).

4.3 Erythropoietin

Paraneoplastic erythrocytosis is a salient feature of many cancers, including RCC in which about 5% of patients are polycythemic (Wiesener et al., 2002; Wiesener et al., 2007; Papworth et al., 2009). In adults, the kidney is the major source of EPO. EPO regulates erythropoiesis and is the only hematopoietic cytokine whose production is regulated by hypoxia (Lacombe&Mayeux, 1999; Fandrey, 2004; Michael et al., 2007; Wiesener et al., 2007). Although RCC is thought to arise from proximal tubular epithelial cells (PTEC), normal PTEC do not express detectable levels of EPO even under hypoxic conditions (Wiesener et al., 2002; Wiesener et al., 2007). This pointed towards the role of molecular mechanisms that transform a non-EPO expressing PTEC to an EPO-expressing RCC , leading to the identification of the link between VHL mutation and the subsequent HIF-mediated EPO upregulation in RCC (Da Silva et al., 1990; Noguchi et al., 1999; Wiesener et al., 2002; Pastore et al., 2003; Lee et al., 2005; Wiesener et al., 2007; Rad et al., 2008; Papworth et al., 2009). Enhanced expression of EPO and its receptor EPOR has been reported in cultured RCC cells and in patient samples, the reported prevalence ranges from 33 - 84% (Murphy et al., 1970; Hagiwara et al., 1984; Da Silva et al., 1990; Ljungberg et al., 1992; Noguchi et al., 1999; Wiesener et al., 2002; Sakamoto et al., 2003; Lee et al., 2005; Michael et al., 2007; Wiesener et al., 2007; Papworth et al., 2009).

Although 33-84% of the RCC patients have elevated plasma level of EPO, only 5% of them are polycythemic (Kazal&Erslev, 1975; Ljungberg et al., 1992; Michael et al., 2007; Wiesener et al., 2007; Papworth et al., 2009). The lack of correlation between paraneoplastic EPO production and paraneoplastic erythrocytosis has led to the suggestion that other cancer-related factors can counterbalance the effect of increased EPO. One of the well studied factors is the reduced iron availability and the resultant anemia in cancer patients. Since recombinant human EPO (rhEPO) is frequently used to treat anemia in patients with cancer, the presence of EPOR in RCC has raised concern (Lai&Grandis, 2006; Papworth et al., 2009). As EPOR is over-expressed in RCC, and EPO exerts its effects through its binding of EPOR, exogenous rhEPO could enhance tumor aggressiveness as reported in breast and head and neck cancers (Henke et al., 2003; Leyland-Jones et al., 2005; Wiesener et al., 2007). Furthermore, EPO has been shown to reduce cisplatin-induced apoptosis in cultured RCC cells (Li et al., 2007). In contrast, EPO sensitized RCC cell lines to vinblastin and daunorubicin-induced apoptosis (Carvalho et al., 2005).

4.4 E-cadherin

Cell-cell adherence, mediated by intercellular junctional complexes, plays an important role in tissue formation and maintenance of cell phenotypes. Intercellular junctional complexes are composed of tight junctions, adherence junctions and desmosomes (Cavallaro & Christofori, 2004; Krishnamachary et al., 2006; Migita et al., 2008). E-cadherin, a transmembrane glycoprotein, is the principal component of adherence junctions and desmosomes in epithelial cells (Cavallaro&Christofori, 2004; Krishnamachary et al., 2006). The extracellular domain of E-cadherin mediates cell-cell adherence through homophilic interaction with the E-cadherin of adjacent cells, whereas the intracellular domain binds with the cytoskeleton *via* a protein complex containing α-, ß- and γ -catenins (Behrens et al., 1989; Cavallaro&Christofori, 2004; Krishnamachary et al., 2006; Russell&Ohh, 2007). EMT is the hallmark of many cancers, in which E-cadherin-mediated cell-cell adherence is lost and the cells attain hyper-proliferative, invasive and metastatic properties (Behrens et al., 1989; Thiery, 2002; Krishnamachary et al., 2006). While the reasons for loss of E-cadherin in cancers are undoubtedly multifactoral, many studies have shown a direct role of VHL in regulating E-cadherin expression in RCC (Esteban et al., 2006; Krishnamachary et al., 2006; Evans et al., 2007; Russell&Ohh, 2007).

The loss of VHL in turn leads to a loss or significant downregulation of E-cadherin and its re-introduction restores E-cadherin expression in RCC (Esteban et al., 2006; Krishnamachary et al., 2006; Russell&Ohh, 2007). Further reports of E-cadherin loss in pre-malignant foci of VHL patients has led to the suggestion that E-cadherin loss is an early step in the pathogenesis of RCC, attributed to VHL inactivation (Esteban et al., 2006; Russell&Ohh,

2007). In line with these observations, tissue microarray of human RCC samples has shown the lack of E-cadherin immunoreactivity in VHL-deficient samples (Gervais et al., 2007). This study also found that low Fuhrman grade samples were positive for E-cadherin and VHL immunostaining and had a better prognosis. Conversely, high-grade tumors were negative for E-cadherin and VHL immunoreactivity and had a worse prognosis. However, these observations have been contradicted by another report, which found no association between E-cadherin expression, tumor grade and prognosis in RCC (Ronkainen et al., 2010).

4.5 Glucose transporter-1

Glucose is the major substrate for energy production in mammalian cells. The intracellular transport of glucose and its oxidative metabolism are vital for normal functioning of cells. Intracellular glucose transport is facilitated by a family of 14 glucose transporters (GLUT), of which GLUT-1 is the most studied (Macheda et al., 2005; Ozcan et al., 2007; Suganuma et al., 2007; Lidgren et al., 2008). Due to rapid proliferative rate relative to vascular support of cancer cells, the tumor microenvironment is in a constant state of hypoxia (Ozcan et al., 2007). In order to counteract the deleterious effects of hypoxia, such as apoptosis and necrosis, malignant cells undergo adaptive and genetic changes. One such change is increased uptake of glucose when compared with normal cells through accelerated glycolysis – often referred to as 'glycolytic switch' or 'Warburg effect' (Warburg, 1956; Airley&Mobasheri, 2007; Singer et al., 2011). This is largely mediated by the up-regulation of GLUT especially GLUT-1 (Binder et al., 1997; Smith, 1999; Medina&Owen, 2002; Airley&Mobasheri, 2007; Ozcan et al., 2007; Suganuma et al., 2007). It is now well established that accelerated glycolysis and increased glucose uptake mediated by GLUT-1 are the hallmarks of many malignant tumors and that these adaptive changes in glucose metabolism favor survival, proliferation and metastasis of tumor cells, even under hypoxic conditions (Airley&Mobasheri, 2007; Ozcan et al., 2007; Singer et al., 2011).

The link between VHL-HIF and GLUT-1 has been well established. GLUT-1 is over-expressed in VHL-mutated mice and the GLUT-1 promoter region has an HRE (Ebert et al., 1995; Park et al., 2007; Lidgren et al., 2008). While the basal level of expression of GLUT-1 in normal PTEC is a subject of debate (Nagase et al., 1995; Ozcan et al., 2007), the over-expression of GLUT-1 in RCC has been demonstrated by many studies (Nagase et al., 1995; Miyakita et al., 2002; Ozcan et al., 2007; Suganuma et al., 2007; Lidgren et al., 2008; Singer et al., 2011). All of these studies concluded that GLUT-1 is over-expressed markedly in clear cell RCC compared with other RCC subtypes, confirming the link between VHL aberration and the subsequent HIF up-regulation. Lactate is one of the byproducts of glycolysis. Due to the enhanced glycolysis, RCC patients are reported to have increased glycolytic enzymes and higher levels of lactate in their serum (Gao et al., 2008). Increased dependence of cancer cells on glycolysis suggests that glycolysis inhibition may be a therapeutic option. Although not well-documented in RCC, experimental glycolysis inhibition has produced anti-cancer effects in certain cancer cell lines (Xu et al., 2005b; Pelicano et al., 2006).

4.6 Carbonic anhydrase IX

CAIX is a membrane-bound glycoprotein belonging to the carbonic anhydrase (CA) family of enzymes and is thought to promote cell proliferation, oncogenesis and tumor progression in response to hypoxia (Grabmaier et al., 2000; Ivanov et al., 2001; Bui et al., 2003; Lawrentschuk et al., 2011). There are at least 15 isoforms of CA. These enzymes play an important role in the regulation of pH of cells by catalyzing one of the vital reactions of biological systems - the reversible hydration of CO_2 into bicarbonate and hydrogen ions, $CO_2+H_2O \Leftrightarrow HCO_3^- + H^+$ (Opavsky et al., 1996; Pastorekova et al., 2008; Stillebroer et al., 2010). As discussed above, enhanced glycolysis is a hallmark of cancer cells, which results in accumulation of lactate and a hypoxic acidic microenvironment. CO_2 is a significant source of hypoxia and acidity in tumors (Pastorekova et al., 2008). Enhanced CAIX expression and the resultant rapid reversible conversion of CO_2 to H^+ helps to maintain an acidic, hypoxic microenvironment thereby sustaining tumor progression (Opavsky et al., 1996; Dorai et al., 2006; Pastorekova et al., 2008; Patard et al., 2008; Stillebroer et al., 2010). CAIX is regulated by HIF and the correlation between VHL-HIF-CAIX is well-established (Wykoff et al., 2000; Grabmaier et al., 2004; Patard et al., 2008; Kaluz et al., 2009; Lawrentschuk et al., 2011). Enhanced expression of CAIX has been well documented in RCC (Bui et al., 2003; Zavada et al., 2003; Atkins et al., 2005; Al-Ahmadie et al., 2008; Jensen et al., 2008; Li et al., 2008; Patard et al., 2008; Patard et al., 2009; Stillebroer et al., 2010; Zhou et al., 2010). However, in contrast to other cancers, enhanced CAIX in RCC is associated with a better prognosis. Furthermore, metastatic patients with higher tumoral CAIX expression showed a better response to interleukin-2 treatment (Atkins et al., 2005). Based on the VHL-CAIX status of RCC, Patard and colleagues (Patard et al., 2008) stratified RCC patients into three distinct groups: patients with both VHL mutation and high CAIX expression had the most favourable prognosis; patients with either VHL mutation or high CAIX expression had an intermediate prognosis; and patients with neither VHL mutation nor high CAIX expression had the worst prognosis.

5. Promises, pitfalls and future directions

The past decade has witnessed an unprecedented increase in the understanding of molecular mechanisms of RCC, of which, the VHL-HIF pathway arguably is the most explored. Not surprisingly, this has resulted in promising, clinically available novel therapeutic agents. Patients were reported to have progression-free survival with these novel therapeutic agents, and many new drugs are under clinical trial, offering hope for better treatment strategies in the future. However, progression-free survival, which occurs in approximately 10% of selected patients, is generally measured in months, rather than years. Moreover, there is currently no compound, either singly or in combination, which is capable of producing a complete response in metastatic RCC. Systemic toxicity and resistance of RCC in response to currently available VEGF/mTOR inhibitors are starting to emerge. Also, the rising costs of therapy associated with these novel drugs are another barrier to effective treatment. These highlight the need for more effective therapeutic agents for metastatic RCC. One approach would be simultaneous targeting of multiple molecular pathways. Pertinent to the molecular mechanism of VHL-HIF, there are at least 60 HIF-regulated molecules that are engaged in tumor development and progression. This means that targeting the VEGF/mTOR pathway could be potentially abrogated by the opposing actions of numerous molecules favoring tumor progression. Therefore, given the heterogeneity of RCC, individualized, targeted treatment based on a preceding 'molecular map' of each tumor might represent an innovative therapeutic approach to achieving improved clinical outcomes. With the rapid advancements in technology, especially microarrays and bioinformatics, the availability of clinically feasible platforms to generate molecular maps of individual tumors and customized treatment strategies may become a reality in the near future.

6. References

Abraham, R.T. & Gibbons, J.J. (2007). The mammalian target of rapamycin signaling pathway: twists and turns in the road to cancer therapy. *Clin Cancer Res* Vol.13, No.11, (Jun 1), pp.3109-14

Ainsworth, N.L., Lee, J.S. & Eisen, T. (2009). Impact of anti-angiogenic treatments on metastatic renal cell carcinoma. *Expert Rev Anticancer Ther* Vol.9, No.12, (Dec), pp.1793-805

Airley, R.E. & Mobasheri, A. (2007). Hypoxic regulation of glucose transport, anaerobic metabolism and angiogenesis in cancer: novel pathways and targets for anticancer therapeutics. *Chemotherapy* Vol.53, No.4, pp.233-56

Al-Ahmadie, H.A., Alden, D., Qin, L.X., Olgac, S., Fine, S.W., Gopalan, A., Russo, P., Motzer, R.J., Reuter, V.E. & Tickoo, S.K. (2008). Carbonic anhydrase IX expression in clear cell renal cell carcinoma: an immunohistochemical study comparing 2 antibodies. *Am J Surg Pathol* Vol.32, No.3, (Mar), pp.377-82

Angelo, L.S., Talpaz, M. & Kurzrock, R. (2002). Autocrine interleukin-6 production in renal cell carcinoma: evidence for the involvement of p53. *Cancer Res* Vol.62, No.3, (Feb 1), pp.932-40

Arai, E. & Kanai, Y. (2010). Genetic and epigenetic alterations during renal carcinogenesis. *Int J Clin Exp Pathol* Vol.4, No.1, pp.58-73

Arany, Z., Huang, L.E., Eckner, R., Bhattacharya, S., Jiang, C., Goldberg, M.A., Bunn, H.F. & Livingston, D.M. (1996). An essential role for p300/CBP in the cellular response to hypoxia. *Proc Natl Acad Sci U S A* Vol.93, No.23, (Nov 12), pp.12969-73

Atkins, M., Regan, M., McDermott, D., Mier, J., Stanbridge, E., Youmans, A., Febbo, P., Upton, M., Lechpammer, M. & Signoretti, S. (2005). Carbonic anhydrase IX expression predicts outcome of interleukin 2 therapy for renal cancer. *Clin Cancer Res* Vol.11, No.10, (May 15), pp.3714-21

Atlas, I., Mendelsohn, J., Baselga, J., Fair, W.R., Masui, H. & Kumar, R. (1992). Growth regulation of human renal carcinoma cells: role of transforming growth factor alpha. *Cancer Res* Vol.52, No.12, (Jun 15), pp.3335-9

Baldewijns, M.M., Thijssen, V.L., Van den Eynden, G.G., Van Laere, S.J., Bluekens, A.M., Roskams, T., van Poppel, H., De Bruine, A.P., Griffioen, A.W. & Vermeulen, P.B. (2007). High-grade clear cell renal cell carcinoma has a higher angiogenic activity than low-grade renal cell carcinoma based on histomorphological quantification and qRT-PCR mRNA expression profile. *Br J Cancer* Vol.96, No.12, (Jun 18), pp.1888-95

Baldewijns, M.M., van Vlodrop, I.J., Vermeulen, P.B., Soetekouw, P.M., van Engeland, M. & de Bruine, A.P. (2010). VHL and HIF signalling in renal cell carcinogenesis. *J Pathol* Vol.221, No.2, (Jun), pp.125-38

Banumathy, G. & Cairns, P. (2010). Signaling pathways in renal cell carcinoma. *Cancer Biol Ther* Vol.10, No.7, (Oct), pp.658-64

Bates, D.O. (2010). Vascular endothelial growth factors and vascular permeability. *Cardiovasc Res* Vol.87, No.2, (Jul 15), pp.262-71

Behrens, J., Mareel, M.M., Van Roy, F.M. & Birchmeier, W. (1989). Dissecting tumor cell invasion: epithelial cells acquire invasive properties after the loss of uvomorulin-mediated cell-cell adhesion. *J Cell Biol* Vol.108, No.6, (Jun), pp.2435-47

Binder, C., Binder, L., Marx, D., Schauer, A. & Hiddemann, W. (1997). Deregulated simultaneous expression of multiple glucose transporter isoforms in malignant cells and tissues. *Anticancer Res* Vol.17, No.6D, (Nov-Dec), pp.4299-304

Black, P.C. & Dinney, C.P. (2008). Growth factors and receptors as prognostic markers in urothelial carcinoma. *Curr Urol Rep* Vol.9, No.1, (Jan), pp.55-61

Blankenship, C., Naglich, J.G., Whaley, J.M., Seizinger, B. & Kley, N. (1999). Alternate choice of initiation codon produces a biologically active product of the von Hippel Lindau gene with tumor suppressor activity. *Oncogene* Vol.18, No.8, (Feb 25), pp.1529-35

Bui, M.H., Seligson, D., Han, K.R., Pantuck, A.J., Dorey, F.J., Huang, Y., Horvath, S., Leibovich, B.C., Chopra, S., Liao, S.Y., Stanbridge, E., Lerman, M.I., Palotie, A., Figlin, R.A. & Belldegrun, A.S. (2003). Carbonic anhydrase IX is an independent predictor of survival in advanced renal clear cell carcinoma: implications for prognosis and therapy. *Clin Cancer Res* Vol.9, No.2, (Feb), pp.802-11

Bullock, A., McDermott, D.F. & Atkins, M.B. (2010). Management of metastatic renal cell carcinoma in patients with poor prognosis. *Cancer Manag Res* Vol.2, pp.123-32

Carmeliet, P. (2005). VEGF as a key mediator of angiogenesis in cancer. *Oncology* Vol.69 Suppl 3, pp.4-10

Carvalho, G., Lefaucheur, C., Cherbonnier, C., Metivier, D., Chapel, A., Pallardy, M., Bourgeade, M.F., Charpentier, B., Hirsch, F. & Kroemer, G. (2005). Chemosensitization by erythropoietin through inhibition of the NF-kappaB rescue pathway. *Oncogene* Vol.24, No.5, (Jan 27), pp.737-45

Cavallaro, U. & Christofori, G. (2004). Cell adhesion and signalling by cadherins and Ig-CAMs in cancer. *Nat Rev Cancer* Vol.4, No.2, (Feb), pp.118-32

Cebe-Suarez, S., Zehnder-Fjallman, A. & Ballmer-Hofer, K. (2006). The role of VEGF receptors in angiogenesis; complex partnerships. *Cell Mol Life Sci* Vol.63, No.5, (Mar), pp.601-15

Cenni, E., Perut, F., Granchi, D., Avnet, S., Amato, I., Brandi, M.L., Giunti, A. & Baldini, N. (2007). Inhibition of angiogenesis via FGF-2 blockage in primitive and bone metastatic renal cell carcinoma. *Anticancer Res* Vol.27, No.1A, (Jan-Feb), pp.315-9

Cho, D., Signoretti, S., Regan, M., Mier, J.W. & Atkins, M.B. (2007). The role of mammalian target of rapamycin inhibitors in the treatment of advanced renal cancer. *Clin Cancer Res* Vol.13, No.2 Pt 2, (Jan 15), pp.758s-63s

Clark, P.E. (2009). The role of VHL in clear-cell renal cell carcinoma and its relation to targeted therapy. *Kidney Int* Vol.76, No.9, (Nov), pp.939-45

Corn, P.G. (2007). Role of the ubiquitin proteasome system in renal cell carcinoma. *BMC Biochem* Vol.8 Suppl 1, pp.S4

Curti, B.D. (2004). Renal cell carcinoma. *Jama* Vol.292, No.1, (Jul 7), pp.97-100

Da Silva, J.L., Lacombe, C., Bruneval, P., Casadevall, N., Leporrier, M., Camilleri, J.P., Bariety, J., Tambourin, P. & Varet, B. (1990). Tumor cells are the site of erythropoietin synthesis in human renal cancers associated with polycythemia. *Blood* Vol.75, No.3, (Feb 1), pp.577-82

Dames, S.A., Martinez-Yamout, M., De Guzman, R.N., Dyson, H.J. & Wright, P.E. (2002). Structural basis for Hif-1 alpha /CBP recognition in the cellular hypoxic response. *Proc Natl Acad Sci U S A* Vol.99, No.8, (Apr 16), pp.5271-6

Dawson, N.A., Guo, C., Zak, R., Dorsey, B., Smoot, J., Wong, J. & Hussain, A. (2004). A phase II trial of gefitinib (Iressa, ZD1839) in stage IV and recurrent renal cell carcinoma. *Clin Cancer Res* Vol.10, No.23, (Dec 1), pp.7812-9

de Paulsen, N., Brychzy, A., Fournier, M.C., Klausner, R.D., Gnarra, J.R., Pause, A. & Lee, S. (2001). Role of transforming growth factor-alpha in von Hippel--Lindau (VHL)(-/-) clear cell renal carcinoma cell proliferation: a possible mechanism coupling VHL tumor suppressor inactivation and tumorigenesis. *Proc Natl Acad Sci U S A* Vol.98, No.4, (Feb 13), pp.1387-92

Del Bufalo, D., Ciuffreda, L., Trisciuoglio, D., Desideri, M., Cognetti, F., Zupi, G. & Milella, M. (2006). Antiangiogenic potential of the Mammalian target of rapamycin inhibitor temsirolimus. *Cancer Res* Vol.66, No.11, (Jun 1), pp.5549-54

Derynck, R. (1986). Transforming growth factor-alpha: structure and biological activities. *J Cell Biochem* Vol.32, No.4, pp.293-304

Donovan, E.A. & Kummar, S. (2006). Targeting VEGF in cancer therapy. *Curr Probl Cancer* Vol.30, No.1, (Jan-Feb), pp.7-32

Dorai, T., Sawczuk, I., Pastorek, J., Wiernik, P.H. & Dutcher, J.P. (2006). Role of carbonic anhydrases in the progression of renal cell carcinoma subtypes: proposal of a unified hypothesis. *Cancer Invest* Vol.24, No.8, (Dec), pp.754-79

Ebert, B.L., Firth, J.D. & Ratcliffe, P.J. (1995). Hypoxia and mitochondrial inhibitors regulate expression of glucose transporter-1 via distinct Cis-acting sequences. *J Biol Chem* Vol.270, No.49, (Dec 8), pp.29083-9

Eble, J., Sauter, G., Epstein, J. & Sesterhenn, I. (2001). *Pathology and genetics. Tumours of the urinary system and male genital organs,* (Editor ed.). Lyon: IARC Press.

Ellis, L.M. & Hicklin, D.J. (2008). VEGF-targeted therapy: mechanisms of anti-tumour activity. *Nat Rev Cancer* Vol.8, No.8, (Aug), pp.579-91

Esteban, M.A., Tran, M.G., Harten, S.K., Hill, P., Castellanos, M.C., Chandra, A., Raval, R., O'Brien T, S. & Maxwell, P.H. (2006). Regulation of E-cadherin expression by VHL and hypoxia-inducible factor. *Cancer Res* Vol.66, No.7, (Apr 1), pp.3567-75

Evans, A.J., Russell, R.C., Roche, O., Burry, T.N., Fish, J.E., Chow, V.W., Kim, W.Y., Saravanan, A., Maynard, M.A., Gervais, M.L., Sufan, R.I., Roberts, A.M., Wilson, L.A., Betten, M., Vandewalle, C., Berx, G., Marsden, P.A., Irwin, M.S., Teh, B.T., Jewett, M.A. & Ohh, M. (2007). VHL promotes E2 box-dependent E-cadherin transcription by HIF-mediated regulation of SIP1 and snail. *Mol Cell Biol* Vol.27, No.1, (Jan), pp.157-69

Everitt, J.I., Walker, C.L., Goldsworthy, T.W. & Wolf, D.C. (1997). Altered expression of transforming growth factor-alpha: an early event in renal cell carcinoma development. *Mol Carcinog* Vol.19, No.3, (Jul), pp.213-9

Faivre, S., Delbaldo, C., Vera, K., Robert, C., Lozahic, S., Lassau, N., Bello, C., Deprimo, S., Brega, N., Massimini, G., Armand, J.P., Scigalla, P. & Raymond, E. (2006). Safety, pharmacokinetic, and antitumor activity of SU11248, a novel oral multitarget tyrosine kinase inhibitor, in patients with cancer. *J Clin Oncol* Vol.24, No.1, (Jan 1), pp.25-35

Fandrey, J. (2004). Oxygen-dependent and tissue-specific regulation of erythropoietin gene expression. *Am J Physiol Regul Integr Comp Physiol* Vol.286, No.6, (Jun), pp.R977-88

Ferlay, J., Shin, H.R., Bray, F., Forman, D., Mathers, C. & Parkin, D.M. (2010). Estimates of worldwide burden of cancer in 2008: GLOBOCAN 2008. *Int J Cancer* Vol.127, No.12, (Dec 15), pp.2893-917

Freedman, S.J., Sun, Z.Y., Poy, F., Kung, A.L., Livingston, D.M., Wagner, G. & Eck, M.J. (2002). Structural basis for recruitment of CBP/p300 by hypoxia-inducible factor-1 alpha. *Proc Natl Acad Sci U S A* Vol.99, No.8, (Apr 16), pp.5367-72

Freeman, M.R., Washecka, R. & Chung, L.W. (1989). Aberrant expression of epidermal growth factor receptor and HER-2 (erbB-2) messenger RNAs in human renal cancers. *Cancer Res* Vol.49, No.22, (Nov 15), pp.6221-5

Fukata, S., Inoue, K., Kamada, M., Kawada, C., Furihata, M., Ohtsuki, Y. & Shuin, T. (2005). Levels of angiogenesis and expression of angiogenesis-related genes are prognostic for organ-specific metastasis of renal cell carcinoma. *Cancer* Vol.103, No.5, (Mar 1), pp.931-42

Gao, H., Dong, B., Liu, X., Xuan, H., Huang, Y. & Lin, D. (2008). Metabonomic profiling of renal cell carcinoma: high-resolution proton nuclear magnetic resonance spectroscopy of human serum with multivariate data analysis. *Anal Chim Acta* Vol.624, No.2, (Aug 29), pp.269-77

Gervais, M.L., Henry, P.C., Saravanan, A., Burry, T.N., Gallie, B.L., Jewett, M.A., Hill, R.P., Evans, A.J. & Ohh, M. (2007). Nuclear E-cadherin and VHL immunoreactivity are prognostic indicators of clear-cell renal cell carcinoma. *Lab Invest* Vol.87, No.12, (Dec), pp.1252-64

Gnarra, J.R., Zhou, S., Merrill, M.J., Wagner, J.R., Krumm, A., Papavassiliou, E., Oldfield, E.H., Klausner, R.D. & Linehan, W.M. (1996). Post-transcriptional regulation of vascular endothelial growth factor mRNA by the product of the VHL tumor suppressor gene. *Proc Natl Acad Sci U S A* Vol.93, No.20, (Oct 1), pp.10589-94

Gomella, L.G., Sargent, E.R., Wade, T.P., Anglard, P., Linehan, W.M. & Kasid, A. (1989). Expression of transforming growth factor alpha in normal human adult kidney and enhanced expression of transforming growth factors alpha and beta 1 in renal cell carcinoma. *Cancer Res* Vol.49, No.24 Pt 1, (Dec 15), pp.6972-5

Gordon, M.S., Hussey, M., Nagle, R.B., Lara, P.N., Jr., Mack, P.C., Dutcher, J., Samlowski, W., Clark, J.I., Quinn, D.I., Pan, C.X. & Crawford, D. (2009). Phase II study of erlotinib in patients with locally advanced or metastatic papillary histology renal cell cancer: SWOG S0317. *J Clin Oncol* Vol.27, No.34, (Dec 1), pp.5788-93

Gossage, L. & Eisen, T. (2010). Alterations in VHL as potential biomarkers in renal-cell carcinoma. *Nat Rev Clin Oncol* Vol.7, No.5, (May), pp.277-88

Grabmaier, K., MC, A.d.W., Verhaegh, G.W., Schalken, J.A. & Oosterwijk, E. (2004). Strict regulation of CAIX(G250/MN) by HIF-1alpha in clear cell renal cell carcinoma. *Oncogene* Vol.23, No.33, (Jul 22), pp.5624-31

Grabmaier, K., Vissers, J.L., De Weijert, M.C., Oosterwijk-Wakka, J.C., Van Bokhoven, A., Brakenhoff, R.H., Noessner, E., Mulders, P.A., Merkx, G., Figdor, C.G., Adema, G.J.

& Oosterwijk, E. (2000). Molecular cloning and immunogenicity of renal cell carcinoma-associated antigen G250. *Int J Cancer* Vol.85, No.6, (Mar 15), pp.865-70

Grubb, R.L., 3rd, Choyke, P.L., Pinto, P.A., Linehan, W.M. & Walther, M.M. (2005). Management of von Hippel-Lindau-associated kidney cancer. *Nat Clin Pract Urol* Vol.2, No.5, (May), pp.248-55

Gunaratnam, L., Morley, M., Franovic, A., de Paulsen, N., Mekhail, K., Parolin, D.A., Nakamura, E., Lorimer, I.A. & Lee, S. (2003). Hypoxia inducible factor activates the transforming growth factor-alpha/epidermal growth factor receptor growth stimulatory pathway in VHL(-/-) renal cell carcinoma cells. *J Biol Chem* Vol.278, No.45, (Nov 7), pp.44966-74

Guo, Y., Schoell, M.C. & Freeman, R.S. (2009). The von Hippel-Lindau protein sensitizes renal carcinoma cells to apoptotic stimuli through stabilization of BIM(EL). *Oncogene* Vol.28, No.16, (Apr 23), pp.1864-74

Hagiwara, M., Chen, I.L., McGonigle, R., Beckman, B., Kasten, F.H. & Fisher, J.W. (1984). Erythropoietin production in a primary culture of human renal carcinoma cells maintained in nude mice. *Blood* Vol.63, No.4, (Apr), pp.828-35

Hara, S., Nakashiro, K., Klosek, S.K., Ishikawa, T., Shintani, S. & Hamakawa, H. (2006). Hypoxia enhances c-Met/HGF receptor expression and signaling by activating HIF-1alpha in human salivary gland cancer cells. *Oral Oncol* Vol.42, No.6, (Jul), pp.593-8

Henke, M., Laszig, R., Rube, C., Schafer, U., Haase, K.D., Schilcher, B., Mose, S., Beer, K.T., Burger, U., Dougherty, C. & Frommhold, H. (2003). Erythropoietin to treat head and neck cancer patients with anaemia undergoing radiotherapy: randomised, double-blind, placebo-controlled trial. *Lancet* Vol.362, No.9392, (Oct 18), pp.1255-60

Hergovich, A., Lisztwan, J., Barry, R., Ballschmieter, P. & Krek, W. (2003). Regulation of microtubule stability by the von Hippel-Lindau tumour suppressor protein pVHL. *Nat Cell Biol* Vol.5, No.1, (Jan), pp.64-70

Herman, J.G., Latif, F., Weng, Y., Lerman, M.I., Zbar, B., Liu, S., Samid, D., Duan, D.S., Gnarra, J.R., Linehan, W.M. & et al. (1994). Silencing of the VHL tumor-suppressor gene by DNA methylation in renal carcinoma. *Proc Natl Acad Sci U S A* Vol.91, No.21, (Oct 11), pp.9700-4

Hicklin, D.J. & Ellis, L.M. (2005). Role of the vascular endothelial growth factor pathway in tumor growth and angiogenesis. *J Clin Oncol* Vol.23, No.5, (Feb 10), pp.1011-27

Higashiyama, S., Iwabuki, H., Morimoto, C., Hieda, M., Inoue, H. & Matsushita, N. (2008). Membrane-anchored growth factors, the epidermal growth factor family: beyond receptor ligands. *Cancer Sci* Vol.99, No.2, (Feb), pp.214-20

Horiguchi, A., Sumitomo, M., Asakuma, J., Asano, T., Zheng, R., Nanus, D.M. & Hayakawa, M. (2006a). Increased serum leptin levels and over expression of leptin receptors are associated with the invasion and progression of renal cell carcinoma. *J Urol* Vol.176, No.4 Pt 1, (Oct), pp.1631-5

Horiguchi, A., Sumitomo, M., Asakuma, J., Asano, T., Zheng, R., Nanus, D.M. & Hayakawa, M. (2006b). Leptin promotes invasiveness of murine renal cancer cells via extracellular signal-regulated kinases and rho dependent pathway. *J Urol* Vol.176, No.4 Pt 1, (Oct), pp.1636-41

Houghton, P.J. (2010). Everolimus. *Clin Cancer Res* Vol.16, No.5, (Mar 1), pp.1368-72

Huang, L.E. & Bunn, H.F. (2003). Hypoxia-inducible factor and its biomedical relevance. *J Biol Chem* Vol.278, No.22, (May 30), pp.19575-8

Iliopoulos, O., Kibel, A., Gray, S. & Kaelin, W.G., Jr. (1995). Tumour suppression by the human von Hippel-Lindau gene product. *Nat Med* Vol.1, No.8, (Aug), pp.822-6

Iliopoulos, O., Ohh, M. & Kaelin, W.G., Jr. (1998). pVHL19 is a biologically active product of the von Hippel-Lindau gene arising from internal translation initiation. *Proc Natl Acad Sci U S A* Vol.95, No.20, (Sep 29), pp.11661-6

Ishikawa, J., Maeda, S., Umezu, K., Sugiyama, T. & Kamidono, S. (1990). Amplification and overexpression of the epidermal growth factor receptor gene in human renal-cell carcinoma. *Int J Cancer* Vol.45, No.6, (Jun 15), pp.1018-21

Ivan, M., Kondo, K., Yang, H., Kim, W., Valiando, J., Ohh, M., Salic, A., Asara, J.M., Lane, W.S. & Kaelin, W.G., Jr. (2001). HIFalpha targeted for VHL-mediated destruction by proline hydroxylation: implications for O2 sensing. *Science* Vol.292, No.5516, (Apr 20), pp.464-8

Ivanov, S., Liao, S.Y., Ivanova, A., Danilkovitch-Miagkova, A., Tarasova, N., Weirich, G., Merrill, M.J., Proescholdt, M.A., Oldfield, E.H., Lee, J., Zavada, J., Waheed, A., Sly, W., Lerman, M.I. & Stanbridge, E.J. (2001). Expression of hypoxia-inducible cell-surface transmembrane carbonic anhydrases in human cancer. *Am J Pathol* Vol.158, No.3, (Mar), pp.905-19

Jaakkola, P., Mole, D.R., Tian, Y.M., Wilson, M.I., Gielbert, J., Gaskell, S.J., Kriegsheim, A., Hebestreit, H.F., Mukherji, M., Schofield, C.J., Maxwell, P.H., Pugh, C.W. & Ratcliffe, P.J. (2001). Targeting of HIF-alpha to the von Hippel-Lindau ubiquitylation complex by O2-regulated prolyl hydroxylation. *Science* Vol.292, No.5516, (Apr 20), pp.468-72

Jensen, H.K., Nordsmark, M., Donskov, F., Marcussen, N. & von der Maase, H. (2008). Immunohistochemical expression of carbonic anhydrase IX assessed over time and during treatment in renal cell carcinoma. *BJU Int* Vol.101 Suppl 4, (Jun), pp.41-4

Jermann, M., Stahel, R.A., Salzberg, M., Cerny, T., Joerger, M., Gillessen, S., Morant, R., Egli, F., Rhyner, K., Bauer, J.A. & Pless, M. (2006). A phase II, open-label study of gefitinib (IRESSA) in patients with locally advanced, metastatic, or relapsed renal-cell carcinoma. *Cancer Chemother Pharmacol* Vol.57, No.4, (Apr), pp.533-9

Kaelin, W.G. (2005a). The von Hippel-Lindau tumor suppressor protein: roles in cancer and oxygen sensing. *Cold Spring Harb Symp Quant Biol* Vol.70, pp.159-66

Kaelin, W.G., Jr. (2002). Molecular basis of the VHL hereditary cancer syndrome. *Nat Rev Cancer* Vol.2, No.9, (Sep), pp.673-82

Kaelin, W.G., Jr. (2005b). The von Hippel-Lindau protein, HIF hydroxylation, and oxygen sensing. *Biochem Biophys Res Commun* Vol.338, No.1, (Dec 9), pp.627-38

Kaelin, W.G., Jr. (2007). The von Hippel-Lindau tumor suppressor protein and clear cell renal carcinoma. *Clin Cancer Res* Vol.13, No.2 Pt 2, (Jan 15), pp.680s-4s

Kallio, J.P., Hirvikoski, P., Helin, H., Kellokumpu-Lehtinen, P., Luukkaala, T., Tammela, T.L. & Martikainen, P.M. (2003). Membranous location of EGFR immunostaining is associated with good prognosis in renal cell carcinoma. *Br J Cancer* Vol.89, No.7, (Oct 6), pp.1266-9

Kaluz, S., Kaluzova, M., Liao, S.Y., Lerman, M. & Stanbridge, E.J. (2009). Transcriptional control of the tumor- and hypoxia-marker carbonic anhydrase 9: A one transcription factor (HIF-1) show? *Biochim Biophys Acta* Vol.1795, No.2, (Apr), pp.162-72

Kaluz, S., Kaluzova, M. & Stanbridge, E.J. (2008). Does inhibition of degradation of hypoxia-inducible factor (HIF) alpha always lead to activation of HIF? Lessons learnt from the effect of proteasomal inhibition on HIF activity. *J Cell Biochem* Vol.104, No.2, (May 15), pp.536-44

Kazal, L.A. & Erslev, A.J. (1975). Erythropoietin production in renal tumors. *Ann Clin Lab Sci* Vol.5, No.2, (Mar-Apr), pp.98-109

Kedar, D., Baker, C.H., Killion, J.J., Dinney, C.P. & Fidler, I.J. (2002). Blockade of the epidermal growth factor receptor signaling inhibits angiogenesis leading to regression of human renal cell carcinoma growing orthotopically in nude mice. *Clin Cancer Res* Vol.8, No.11, (Nov), pp.3592-600

Kim, W.Y. & Kaelin, W.G. (2004). Role of VHL gene mutation in human cancer. *J Clin Oncol* Vol.22, No.24, (Dec 15), pp.4991-5004

Knebelmann, B., Ananth, S., Cohen, H.T. & Sukhatme, V.P. (1998). Transforming growth factor alpha is a target for the von Hippel-Lindau tumor suppressor. *Cancer Res* Vol.58, No.2, (Jan 15), pp.226-31

Koivunen, P., Tiainen, P., Hyvarinen, J., Williams, K.E., Sormunen, R., Klaus, S.J., Kivirikko, K.I. & Myllyharju, J. (2007). An endoplasmic reticulum transmembrane prolyl 4-hydroxylase is induced by hypoxia and acts on hypoxia-inducible factor alpha. *J Biol Chem* Vol.282, No.42, (Oct 19), pp.30544-52

Konig, B., Steinbach, F., Janocha, B., Drynda, A., Stumm, M., Philipp, C., Allhoff, E.P. & Konig, W. (1999). The differential expression of proinflammatory cytokines IL-6, IL-8 and TNF-alpha in renal cell carcinoma. *Anticancer Res* Vol.19, No.2C, (Mar-Apr), pp.1519-24

Koochekpour, S., Jeffers, M., Wang, P.H., Gong, C., Taylor, G.A., Roessler, L.M., Stearman, R., Vasselli, J.R., Stetler-Stevenson, W.G., Kaelin, W.G., Jr., Linehan, W.M., Klausner, R.D., Gnarra, J.R. & Vande Woude, G.F. (1999). The von Hippel-Lindau tumor suppressor gene inhibits hepatocyte growth factor/scatter factor-induced invasion and branching morphogenesis in renal carcinoma cells. *Mol Cell Biol* Vol.19, No.9, (Sep), pp.5902-12

Krishnamachary, B., Zagzag, D., Nagasawa, H., Rainey, K., Okuyama, H., Baek, J.H. & Semenza, G.L. (2006). Hypoxia-inducible factor-1-dependent repression of E-cadherin in von Hippel-Lindau tumor suppressor-null renal cell carcinoma mediated by TCF3, ZFHX1A, and ZFHX1B. *Cancer Res* Vol.66, No.5, (Mar 1), pp.2725-31

Kumar, R., Knick, V.B., Rudolph, S.K., Johnson, J.H., Crosby, R.M., Crouthamel, M.C., Hopper, T.M., Miller, C.G., Harrington, L.E., Onori, J.A., Mullin, R.J., Gilmer, T.M., Truesdale, A.T., Epperly, A.H., Boloor, A., Stafford, J.A., Luttrell, D.K. & Cheung, M. (2007). Pharmacokinetic-pharmacodynamic correlation from mouse to human with pazopanib, a multikinase angiogenesis inhibitor with potent antitumor and antiangiogenic activity. *Mol Cancer Ther* Vol.6, No.7, (Jul), pp.2012-21

Lacombe, C. & Mayeux, P. (1999). The molecular biology of erythropoietin. *Nephrol Dial Transplant* Vol.14 Suppl 2, pp.22-8

Lager, D.J., Slagel, D.D. & Palechek, P.L. (1994). The expression of epidermal growth factor receptor and transforming growth factor alpha in renal cell carcinoma. *Mod Pathol* Vol.7, No.5, (Jun), pp.544-8

Lai, S.Y. & Grandis, J.R. (2006). Understanding the presence and function of erythropoietin receptors on cancer cells. *J Clin Oncol* Vol.24, No.29, (Oct 10), pp.4675-6

Lando, D., Peet, D.J., Gorman, J.J., Whelan, D.A., Whitelaw, M.L. & Bruick, R.K. (2002a). FIH-1 is an asparaginyl hydroxylase enzyme that regulates the transcriptional activity of hypoxia-inducible factor. *Genes Dev* Vol.16, No.12, (Jun 15), pp.1466-71

Lando, D., Peet, D.J., Whelan, D.A., Gorman, J.J. & Whitelaw, M.L. (2002b). Asparagine hydroxylation of the HIF transactivation domain a hypoxic switch. *Science* Vol.295, No.5556, (Feb 1), pp.858-61

Latif, F., Tory, K., Gnarra, J., Yao, M., Duh, F.M., Orcutt, M.L., Stackhouse, T., Kuzmin, I., Modi, W., Geil, L. & et al. (1993). Identification of the von Hippel-Lindau disease tumor suppressor gene. *Science* Vol.260, No.5112, (May 28), pp.1317-20

Lawrentschuk, N., Lee, F.T., Jones, G., Rigopoulos, A., Mountain, A., O'Keefe, G., Papenfuss, A.T., Bolton, D.M., Davis, I.D. & Scott, A.M. (2011). Investigation of hypoxia and carbonic anhydrase IX expression in a renal cell carcinoma xenograft model with oxygen tension measurements and (124)I-cG250 PET/CT. *Urol Oncol* Vol.29, No.4, (Jul-Aug), pp.411-20

Lee, S.J., Lattouf, J.B., Xanthopoulos, J., Linehan, W.M., Bottaro, D.P. & Vasselli, J.R. (2008). Von Hippel-Lindau tumor suppressor gene loss in renal cell carcinoma promotes oncogenic epidermal growth factor receptor signaling via Akt-1 and MEK-1. *Eur Urol* Vol.54, No.4, (Oct), pp.845-53

Lee, Y.S., Vortmeyer, A.O., Lubensky, I.A., Vogel, T.W., Ikejiri, B., Ferlicot, S., Benoit, G., Giraud, S., Oldfield, E.H., Linehan, W.M., Teh, B.T., Richard, S. & Zhuang, Z. (2005). Coexpression of erythropoietin and erythropoietin receptor in von Hippel-Lindau disease-associated renal cysts and renal cell carcinoma. *Clin Cancer Res* Vol.11, No.3, (Feb 1), pp.1059-64

Leyland-Jones, B., Semiglazov, V., Pawlicki, M., Pienkowski, T., Tjulandin, S., Manikhas, G., Makhson, A., Roth, A., Dodwell, D., Baselga, J., Biakhov, M., Valuckas, K., Voznyi, E., Liu, X. & Vercammen, E. (2005). Maintaining normal hemoglobin levels with epoetin alfa in mainly nonanemic patients with metastatic breast cancer receiving first-line chemotherapy: a survival study. *J Clin Oncol* Vol.23, No.25, (Sep 1), pp.5960-72

Li, G., Feng, G., Gentil-Perret, A., Genin, C. & Tostain, J. (2008). Serum carbonic anhydrase 9 level is associated with postoperative recurrence of conventional renal cell cancer. *J Urol* Vol.180, No.2, (Aug), pp.510-3; discussion 3-4

Li, J., Vesey, D.A., Johnson, D.W. & Gobe, G. (2007). Erythropoietin reduces cisplatin-induced apoptosis in renal carcinoma cells via a PKC dependent pathway. *Cancer Biol Ther* Vol.6, No.12, (Dec), pp.1944-50

Lidgren, A., Bergh, A., Grankvist, K., Rasmuson, T. & Ljungberg, B. (2008). Glucose transporter-1 expression in renal cell carcinoma and its correlation with hypoxia inducible factor-1 alpha. *BJU Int* Vol.101, No.4, (Feb), pp.480-4

Ljungberg, B., Rasmuson, T. & Grankvist, K. (1992). Erythropoietin in renal cell carcinoma: evaluation of its usefulness as a tumor marker. *Eur Urol* Vol.21, No.2, pp.160-3

Lonser, R.R., Glenn, G.M., Walther, M., Chew, E.Y., Libutti, S.K., Linehan, W.M. & Oldfield, E.H. (2003). von Hippel-Lindau disease. *Lancet* Vol.361, No.9374, (Jun 14), pp.2059-67

Lopez-Beltran, A., Scarpelli, M., Montironi, R. & Kirkali, Z. (2006). 2004 WHO classification of the renal tumors of the adults. *Eur Urol* Vol.49, No.5, (May), pp.798-805

Lowden, D.A., Lindemann, G.W., Merlino, G., Barash, B.D., Calvet, J.P. & Gattone, V.H., 2nd. (1994). Renal cysts in transgenic mice expressing transforming growth factor-alpha. *J Lab Clin Med* Vol.124, No.3, (Sep), pp.386-94

Macheda, M.L., Rogers, S. & Best, J.D. (2005). Molecular and cellular regulation of glucose transporter (GLUT) proteins in cancer. *J Cell Physiol* Vol.202, No.3, (Mar), pp.654-62

Maher, E.R., Yates, J.R., Harries, R., Benjamin, C., Harris, R., Moore, A.T. & Ferguson-Smith, M.A. (1990). Clinical features and natural history of von Hippel-Lindau disease. *Q J Med* Vol.77, No.283, (Nov), pp.1151-63

Mahon, P.C., Hirota, K. & Semenza, G.L. (2001). FIH-1: a novel protein that interacts with HIF-1alpha and VHL to mediate repression of HIF-1 transcriptional activity. *Genes Dev* Vol.15, No.20, (Oct 15), pp.2675-86

Marks, J.L., Broderick, S., Zhou, Q., Chitale, D., Li, A.R., Zakowski, M.F., Kris, M.G., Rusch, V.W., Azzoli, C.G., Seshan, V.E., Ladanyi, M. & Pao, W. (2008). Prognostic and therapeutic implications of EGFR and KRAS mutations in resected lung adenocarcinoma. *J Thorac Oncol* Vol.3, No.2, (Feb), pp.111-6

Maxwell, P.H., Wiesener, M.S., Chang, G.W., Clifford, S.C., Vaux, E.C., Cockman, M.E., Wykoff, C.C., Pugh, C.W., Maher, E.R. & Ratcliffe, P.J. (1999). The tumour suppressor protein VHL targets hypoxia-inducible factors for oxygen-dependent proteolysis. *Nature* Vol.399, No.6733, (May 20), pp.271-5

Maynard, M.A. & Ohh, M. (2004). Von Hippel-Lindau tumor suppressor protein and hypoxia-inducible factor in kidney cancer. *Am J Nephrol* Vol.24, No.1, (Jan-Feb), pp.1-13

Maynard, M.A., Qi, H., Chung, J., Lee, E.H., Kondo, Y., Hara, S., Conaway, R.C., Conaway, J.W. & Ohh, M. (2003). Multiple splice variants of the human HIF-3 alpha locus are targets of the von Hippel-Lindau E3 ubiquitin ligase complex. *J Biol Chem* Vol.278, No.13, (Mar 28), pp.11032-40

Medina, R.A. & Owen, G.I. (2002). Glucose transporters: expression, regulation and cancer. *Biol Res* Vol.35, No.1, pp.9-26

Mendel, D.B., Laird, A.D., Xin, X., Louie, S.G., Christensen, J.G., Li, G., Schreck, R.E., Abrams, T.J., Ngai, T.J., Lee, L.B., Murray, L.J., Carver, J., Chan, E., Moss, K.G., Haznedar, J.O., Sukbuntherng, J., Blake, R.A., Sun, L., Tang, C., Miller, T., Shirazian, S., McMahon, G. & Cherrington, J.M. (2003). In vivo antitumor activity of SU11248, a novel tyrosine kinase inhibitor targeting vascular endothelial growth factor and platelet-derived growth factor receptors: determination of a pharmacokinetic/pharmacodynamic relationship. *Clin Cancer Res* Vol.9, No.1, (Jan), pp.327-37

Merseburger, A.S., Hennenlotter, J., Simon, P., Kruck, S., Koch, E., Horstmann, M., Kuehs, U., Kufer, R., Stenzl, A. & Kuczyk, M.A. (2005). Membranous expression and prognostic implications of epidermal growth factor receptor protein in human renal cell cancer. *Anticancer Res* Vol.25, No.3B, (May-Jun), pp.1901-7

Michael, A., Politi, E., Havranek, E., Corbishley, C., Karapanagiotou, L., Anderson, C., Relph, K., Syrigos, K.N. & Pandha, H. (2007). Prognostic significance of erythropoietin expression in human renal cell carcinoma. *BJU Int* Vol.100, No.2, (Aug), pp.291-4

Migita, T., Oda, Y., Masuda, K., Hirata, A., Kuwano, M., Naito, S. & Tsuneyoshi, M. (2008). Inverse relationship between E-cadherin and p27Kip1 expression in renal cell carcinoma. *Int J Oncol* Vol.33, No.1, (Jul), pp.41-7

Mikhaylova, O., Ignacak, M.L., Barankiewicz, T.J., Harbaugh, S.V., Yi, Y., Maxwell, P.H., Schneider, M., Van Geyte, K., Carmeliet, P., Revelo, M.P., Wyder, M., Greis, K.D., Meller, J. & Czyzyk-Krzeska, M.F. (2008). The von Hippel-Lindau tumor suppressor protein and Egl-9-Type proline hydroxylases regulate the large subunit of RNA polymerase II in response to oxidative stress. *Mol Cell Biol* Vol.28, No.8, (Apr), pp.2701-17

Miyakita, H., Tokunaga, M., Onda, H., Usui, Y., Kinoshita, H., Kawamura, N. & Yasuda, S. (2002). Significance of 18F-fluorodeoxyglucose positron emission tomography (FDG-PET) for detection of renal cell carcinoma and immunohistochemical glucose transporter 1 (GLUT-1) expression in the cancer. *Int J Urol* Vol.9, No.1, (Jan), pp.15-8

Motzer, R.J., Amato, R., Todd, M., Hwu, W.J., Cohen, R., Baselga, J., Muss, H., Cooper, M., Yu, R., Ginsberg, M.S. & Needle, M. (2003). Phase II trial of antiepidermal growth factor receptor antibody C225 in patients with advanced renal cell carcinoma. *Invest New Drugs* Vol.21, No.1, (Feb), pp.99-101

Motzer, R.J., Escudier, B., Oudard, S., Hutson, T.E., Porta, C., Bracarda, S., Grunwald, V., Thompson, J.A., Figlin, R.A., Hollaender, N., Urbanowitz, G., Berg, W.J., Kay, A., Lebwohl, D. & Ravaud, A. (2008). Efficacy of everolimus in advanced renal cell carcinoma: a double-blind, randomised, placebo-controlled phase III trial. *Lancet* Vol.372, No.9637, (Aug 9), pp.449-56

Murphy, G.P., Kenny, G.M. & Mirand, E.A. (1970). Erythropoietin levels in patients with renal tumors or cysts. *Cancer* Vol.26, No.1, (Jul), pp.191-4

Mydlo, J.H., Michaeli, J., Cordon-Cardo, C., Goldenberg, A.S., Heston, W.D. & Fair, W.R. (1989). Expression of transforming growth factor alpha and epidermal growth factor receptor messenger RNA in neoplastic and nonneoplastic human kidney tissue. *Cancer Res* Vol.49, No.12, (Jun 15), pp.3407-11

Nagase, Y., Takata, K., Moriyama, N., Aso, Y., Murakami, T. & Hirano, H. (1995). Immunohistochemical localization of glucose transporters in human renal cell carcinoma. *J Urol* Vol.153, No.3 Pt 1, (Mar), pp.798-801

Noguchi, Y., Goto, T., Yufu, Y., Uike, N., Hasegawa, Y., Fukuda, T., Jimi, A. & Funakoshi, A. (1999). Gene expression of erythropoietin in renal cell carcinoma. *Intern Med* Vol.38, No.12, (Dec), pp.991-4

Ohh, M. (2006). Ubiquitin pathway in VHL cancer syndrome. *Neoplasia* Vol.8, No.8, (Aug), pp.623-9

Ohh, M. & Kaelin, W.G., Jr. (2003). VHL and kidney cancer. *Methods Mol Biol* Vol.222, pp.167-83

Ohh, M., Park, C.W., Ivan, M., Hoffman, M.A., Kim, T.Y., Huang, L.E., Pavletich, N., Chau, V. & Kaelin, W.G. (2000). Ubiquitination of hypoxia-inducible factor requires direct binding to the beta-domain of the von Hippel-Lindau protein. *Nat Cell Biol* Vol.2, No.7, (Jul), pp.423-7

Opavsky, R., Pastorekova, S., Zelnik, V., Gibadulinova, A., Stanbridge, E.J., Zavada, J., Kettmann, R. & Pastorek, J. (1996). Human MN/CA9 gene, a novel member of the carbonic anhydrase family: structure and exon to protein domain relationships. *Genomics* Vol.33, No.3, (May 1), pp.480-7

Ozcan, A., Shen, S.S., Zhai, Q.J. & Truong, L.D. (2007). Expression of GLUT1 in primary renal tumors: morphologic and biologic implications. *Am J Clin Pathol* Vol.128, No.2, (Aug), pp.245-54

Papworth, K., Bergh, A., Grankvist, K., Ljungberg, B. & Rasmuson, T. (2009). Expression of erythropoietin and its receptor in human renal cell carcinoma. *Tumour Biol* Vol.30, No.2, pp.86-92

Park, S.K., Haase, V.H. & Johnson, R.S. (2007). von Hippel Lindau tumor suppressor regulates hepatic glucose metabolism by controlling expression of glucose transporter 2 and glucose 6-phosphatase. *Int J Oncol* Vol.30, No.2, (Feb), pp.341-8

Pascual, D. & Borque, A. (2008). Epidemiology of kidney cancer. *Adv Urol* pp.782381

Pastore, Y., Jedlickova, K., Guan, Y., Liu, E., Fahner, J., Hasle, H., Prchal, J.F. & Prchal, J.T. (2003). Mutations of von Hippel-Lindau tumor-suppressor gene and congenital polycythemia. *Am J Hum Genet* Vol.73, No.2, (Aug), pp.412-9

Pastorekova, S., Ratcliffe, P.J. & Pastorek, J. (2008). Molecular mechanisms of carbonic anhydrase IX-mediated pH regulation under hypoxia. *BJU Int* Vol.101 Suppl 4, (Jun), pp.8-15

Patard, J.J., Fergelot, P., Karakiewicz, P.I., Klatte, T., Trinh, Q.D., Rioux-Leclercq, N., Said, J.W., Belldegrun, A.S. & Pantuck, A.J. (2008). Low CAIX expression and absence of VHL gene mutation are associated with tumor aggressiveness and poor survival of clear cell renal cell carcinoma. *Int J Cancer* Vol.123, No.2, (Jul 15), pp.395-400

Patard, J.J., Rioux-Leclercq, N., Masson, D., Zerrouki, S., Jouan, F., Collet, N., Dubourg, C., Lobel, B., Denis, M. & Fergelot, P. (2009). Absence of VHL gene alteration and high VEGF expression are associated with tumour aggressiveness and poor survival of renal-cell carcinoma. *Br J Cancer* Vol.101, No.8, (Oct 20), pp.1417-24

Pelicano, H., Martin, D.S., Xu, R.H. & Huang, P. (2006). Glycolysis inhibition for anticancer treatment. *Oncogene* Vol.25, No.34, (Aug 7), pp.4633-46

Pelletier, S., Tanguay, S., Lee, S., Gunaratnam, L., Arbour, N. & Lapointe, R. (2009). TGF-alpha as a candidate tumor antigen for renal cell carcinomas. *Cancer Immunol Immunother* Vol.58, No.8, (Aug), pp.1207-18

Perera, A.D., Kleymenova, E.V. & Walker, C.L. (2000). Requirement for the von Hippel-Lindau tumor suppressor gene for functional epidermal growth factor receptor blockade by monoclonal antibody C225 in renal cell carcinoma. *Clin Cancer Res* Vol.6, No.4, (Apr), pp.1518-23

Petrides, P.E., Bock, S., Bovens, J., Hofmann, R. & Jakse, G. (1990). Modulation of pro-epidermal growth factor, pro-transforming growth factor alpha and epidermal growth factor receptor gene expression in human renal carcinomas. *Cancer Res* Vol.50, No.13, (Jul 1), pp.3934-9

Pu, Y.S., Huang, C.Y., Kuo, Y.Z., Kang, W.Y., Liu, G.Y., Huang, A.M., Yu, H.J., Lai, M.K., Huang, S.P., Wu, W.J., Chiou, S.J. & Hour, T.C. (2009). Characterization of membranous and cytoplasmic EGFR expression in human normal renal cortex and renal cell carcinoma. *J Biomed Sci* Vol.16, pp.82

Pugh, C.W., O'Rourke, J.F., Nagao, M., Gleadle, J.M. & Ratcliffe, P.J. (1997). Activation of hypoxia-inducible factor-1; definition of regulatory domains within the alpha subunit. *J Biol Chem* Vol.272, No.17, (Apr 25), pp.11205-14

Rad, F.H., Ulusakarya, A., Gad, S., Sibony, M., Juin, F., Richard, S., Machover, D. & Uzan, G. (2008). Novel somatic mutations of the VHL gene in an erythropoietin-producing renal carcinoma associated with secondary polycythemia and elevated circulating endothelial progenitor cells. *Am J Hematol* Vol.83, No.2, (Feb), pp.155-8

Ramp, U., Reinecke, P., Gabbert, H.E. & Gerharz, C.D. (2000). Differential response to transforming growth factor (TGF)-alpha and fibroblast growth factor (FGF) in human renal cell carcinomas of the clear cell and papillary types. *Eur J Cancer* Vol.36, No.7, (May), pp.932-41

Ravaud, A., Hawkins, R., Gardner, J.P., von der Maase, H., Zantl, N., Harper, P., Rolland, F., Audhuy, B., Machiels, J.P., Petavy, F., Gore, M., Schoffski, P. & El-Hariry, I. (2008). Lapatinib versus hormone therapy in patients with advanced renal cell carcinoma: a randomized phase III clinical trial. *J Clin Oncol* Vol.26, No.14, (May 10), pp.2285-91

Rioux-Leclercq, N., Fergelot, P., Zerrouki, S., Leray, E., Jouan, F., Bellaud, P., Epstein, J.I. & Patard, J.J. (2007). Plasma level and tissue expression of vascular endothelial growth factor in renal cell carcinoma: a prospective study of 50 cases. *Hum Pathol* Vol.38, No.10, (Oct), pp.1489-95

Rixe, O., Bukowski, R.M., Michaelson, M.D., Wilding, G., Hudes, G.R., Bolte, O., Motzer, R.J., Bycott, P., Liau, K.F., Freddo, J., Trask, P.C., Kim, S. & Rini, B.I. (2007). Axitinib treatment in patients with cytokine-refractory metastatic renal-cell cancer: a phase II study. *Lancet Oncol* Vol.8, No.11, (Nov), pp.975-84

Ronkainen, H., Kauppila, S., Hirvikoski, P. & Vaarala, M.H. (2010). Evaluation of myosin VI, E-cadherin and beta-catenin immunostaining in renal cell carcinoma. *J Exp Clin Cancer Res* Vol.29, pp.2

Rowinsky, E.K., Schwartz, G.H., Gollob, J.A., Thompson, J.A., Vogelzang, N.J., Figlin, R., Bukowski, R., Haas, N., Lockbaum, P., Li, Y.P., Arends, R., Foon, K.A., Schwab, G. & Dutcher, J. (2004). Safety, pharmacokinetics, and activity of ABX-EGF, a fully human anti-epidermal growth factor receptor monoclonal antibody in patients with metastatic renal cell cancer. *J Clin Oncol* Vol.22, No.15, (Aug 1), pp.3003-15

Roy, H., Bhardwaj, S. & Yla-Herttuala, S. (2006). Biology of vascular endothelial growth factors. *Febs Letters* Vol.580, No.12, (May 22), pp.2879-87

Rugo, H.S., Herbst, R.S., Liu, G., Park, J.W., Kies, M.S., Steinfeldt, H.M., Pithavala, Y.K., Reich, S.D., Freddo, J.L. & Wilding, G. (2005). Phase I trial of the oral antiangiogenesis agent AG-013736 in patients with advanced solid tumors: pharmacokinetic and clinical results. *J Clin Oncol* Vol.23, No.24, (Aug 20), pp.5474-83

Russell, R.C. & Ohh, M. (2007). The role of VHL in the regulation of E-cadherin: a new connection in an old pathway. *Cell Cycle* Vol.6, No.1, (Jan 1), pp.56-9

Safran, M. & Kaelin, W.G., Jr. (2003). HIF hydroxylation and the mammalian oxygen-sensing pathway. *J Clin Invest* Vol.111, No.6, (Mar), pp.779-83

Sakamoto, S., Igarashi, T., Osumi, N., Imamoto, T., Tobe, T., Kamiya, M. & Ito, H. (2003). Erythropoietin-producing renal cell carcinoma in chronic hemodialysis patients: a report of two cases. *Int J Urol* Vol.10, No.1, (Jan), pp.49-51

Sang, N., Fang, J., Srinivas, V., Leshchinsky, I. & Caro, J. (2002). Carboxyl-terminal transactivation activity of hypoxia-inducible factor 1 alpha is governed by a von Hippel-Lindau protein-independent, hydroxylation-regulated association with p300/CBP. *Mol Cell Biol* Vol.22, No.9, (May), pp.2984-92

Sargent, E.R., Gomella, L.G., Belldegrun, A., Linehan, W.M. & Kasid, A. (1989). Epidermal growth factor receptor gene expression in normal human kidney and renal cell carcinoma. *J Urol* Vol.142, No.5, (Nov), pp.1364-8

Schoenfeld, A., Davidowitz, E.J. & Burk, R.D. (1998). A second major native von Hippel-Lindau gene product, initiated from an internal translation start site, functions as a tumor suppressor. *Proc Natl Acad Sci U S A* Vol.95, No.15, (Jul 21), pp.8817-22

Schofield, C.J. & Ratcliffe, P.J. (2005). Signalling hypoxia by HIF hydroxylases. *Biochem Biophys Res Commun* Vol.338, No.1, (Dec 9), pp.617-26

Seizinger, B.R., Rouleau, G.A., Ozelius, L.J., Lane, A.H., Farmer, G.E., Lamiell, J.M., Haines, J., Yuen, J.W., Collins, D., Majoor-Krakauer, D. & et al. (1988). Von Hippel-Lindau disease maps to the region of chromosome 3 associated with renal cell carcinoma. *Nature* Vol.332, No.6161, (Mar 17), pp.268-9

Semenza, G.L. (1999). Regulation of mammalian O2 homeostasis by hypoxia-inducible factor 1. *Annu Rev Cell Dev Biol* Vol.15, pp.551-78

Singer, K., Kastenberger, M., Gottfried, E., Hammerschmied, C.G., Buttner, M., Aigner, M., Seliger, B., Walter, B., Schlosser, H., Hartmann, A., Andreesen, R., Mackensen, A. & Kreutz, M. (2011). Warburg phenotype in renal cell carcinoma: high expression of glucose-transporter 1 (GLUT-1) correlates with low CD8(+) T-cell infiltration in the tumor. *Int J Cancer* Vol.128, No.9, (May 1), pp.2085-95

Slaton, J.W., Inoue, K., Perrotte, P., El-Naggar, A.K., Swanson, D.A., Fidler, I.J. & Dinney, C.P. (2001). Expression levels of genes that regulate metastasis and angiogenesis correlate with advanced pathological stage of renal cell carcinoma. *Am J Pathol* Vol.158, No.2, (Feb), pp.735-43

Smith, T.A. (1999). Facilitative glucose transporter expression in human cancer tissue. *Br J Biomed Sci* Vol.56, No.4, pp.285-92

Stebbins, C.E., Kaelin, W.G., Jr. & Pavletich, N.P. (1999). Structure of the VHL-ElonginC-ElonginB complex: implications for VHL tumor suppressor function. *Science* Vol.284, No.5413, (Apr 16), pp.455-61

Sternberg, C.N., Davis, I.D., Mardiak, J., Szczylik, C., Lee, E., Wagstaff, J., Barrios, C.H., Salman, P., Gladkov, O.A., Kavina, A., Zarba, J.J., Chen, M., McCann, L., Pandite, L., Roychowdhury, D.F. & Hawkins, R.E. (2010). Pazopanib in locally advanced or metastatic renal cell carcinoma: results of a randomized phase III trial. *J Clin Oncol* Vol.28, No.6, (Feb 20), pp.1061-8

Stillebroer, A.B., Mulders, P.F., Boerman, O.C., Oyen, W.J. & Oosterwijk, E. (2010). Carbonic anhydrase IX in renal cell carcinoma: implications for prognosis, diagnosis, and therapy. *Eur Urol* Vol.58, No.1, (Jul), pp.75-83

Stuttfeld, E. & Ballmer-Hofer, K. (2009). Structure and function of VEGF receptors. *IUBMB Life* Vol.61, No.9, (Sep), pp.915-22

Suganuma, N., Segade, F., Matsuzu, K. & Bowden, D.W. (2007). Differential expression of facilitative glucose transporters in normal and tumour kidney tissues. *BJU Int* Vol.99, No.5, (May), pp.1143-9

Takahashi, A., Sasaki, H., Kim, S.J., Tobisu, K., Kakizoe, T., Tsukamoto, T., Kumamoto, Y., Sugimura, T. & Terada, M. (1994). Markedly increased amounts of messenger RNAs for vascular endothelial growth factor and placenta growth factor in renal cell carcinoma associated with angiogenesis. *Cancer Res* Vol.54, No.15, (Aug 1), pp.4233-7

Tammela, T., Enholm, B., Alitalo, K. & Paavonen, K. (2005). The biology of vascular endothelial growth factors. *Cardiovasc Res* Vol.65, No.3, (Feb 15), pp.550-63

Tanimoto, K., Makino, Y., Pereira, T. & Poellinger, L. (2000). Mechanism of regulation of the hypoxia-inducible factor-1 alpha by the von Hippel-Lindau tumor suppressor protein. *Embo J* Vol.19, No.16, (Aug 15), pp.4298-309

Thiery, J.P. (2002). Epithelial-mesenchymal transitions in tumour progression. *Nat Rev Cancer* Vol.2, No.6, (Jun), pp.442-54

Thomas, G.V., Tran, C., Mellinghoff, I.K., Welsbie, D.S., Chan, E., Fueger, B., Czernin, J. & Sawyers, C.L. (2006). Hypoxia-inducible factor determines sensitivity to inhibitors of mTOR in kidney cancer. *Nat Med* Vol.12, No.1, (Jan), pp.122-7

Thurston, G. & Kitajewski, J. (2008). VEGF and Delta-Notch: interacting signalling pathways in tumour angiogenesis. *Br J Cancer* Vol.99, No.8, (Oct 21), pp.1204-9

Thyavihally, Y.B., Mahantshetty, U., Chamarajanagar, R.S., Raibhattanavar, S.G. & Tongaonkar, H.B. (2005). Management of renal cell carcinoma with solitary metastasis. *World J Surg Oncol* Vol.3, (Jul 20), pp.48

Uberall, I., Kolar, Z., Trojanec, R., Berkovcova, J. & Hajduch, M. (2008). The status and role of ErbB receptors in human cancer. *Exp Mol Pathol* Vol.84, No.2, (Apr), pp.79-89

Uhlman, D.L., Nguyen, P., Manivel, J.C., Zhang, G., Hagen, K., Fraley, E., Aeppli, D. & Niehans, G.A. (1995). Epidermal growth factor receptor and transforming growth factor alpha expression in papillary and nonpapillary renal cell carcinoma: correlation with metastatic behavior and prognosis. *Clin Cancer Res* Vol.1, No.8, (Aug), pp.913-20

Wang, G.L., Jiang, B.H., Rue, E.A. & Semenza, G.L. (1995). Hypoxia-inducible factor 1 is a basic-helix-loop-helix-PAS heterodimer regulated by cellular O2 tension. *Proc Natl Acad Sci U S A* Vol.92, No.12, (Jun 6), pp.5510-4

Warburg, O. (1956). On the origin of cancer cells. *Science* Vol.123, No.3191, (Feb 24), pp.309-14

Weiss, R.H. & Lin, P.Y. (2006). Kidney cancer: identification of novel targets for therapy. *Kidney Int* Vol.69, No.2, (Jan), pp.224-32

Wiesener, M.S., Munchenhagen, P., Glaser, M., Sobottka, B.A., Knaup, K.X., Jozefowski, K., Jurgensen, J.S., Roigas, J., Warnecke, C., Grone, H.J., Maxwell, P.H., Willam, C. & Eckardt, K.U. (2007). Erythropoietin gene expression in renal carcinoma is considerably more frequent than paraneoplastic polycythemia. *Int J Cancer* Vol.121, No.11, (Dec 1), pp.2434-42

Wiesener, M.S., Seyfarth, M., Warnecke, C., Jurgensen, J.S., Rosenberger, C., Morgan, N.V., Maher, E.R., Frei, U. & Eckardt, K.U. (2002). Paraneoplastic erythrocytosis associated with an inactivating point mutation of the von Hippel-Lindau gene in a renal cell carcinoma. *Blood* Vol.99, No.10, (May 15), pp.3562-5

Wilhelm, S. & Chien, D.S. (2002). BAY 43-9006: preclinical data. *Curr Pharm Des* Vol.8, No.25, pp.2255-7

Wilhelm, S.M., Carter, C., Tang, L., Wilkie, D., McNabola, A., Rong, H., Chen, C., Zhang, X., Vincent, P., McHugh, M., Cao, Y., Shujath, J., Gawlak, S., Eveleigh, D., Rowley, B., Liu, L., Adnane, L., Lynch, M., Auclair, D., Taylor, I., Gedrich, R., Voznesensky, A., Riedl, B., Post, L.E., Bollag, G. & Trail, P.A. (2004). BAY 43-9006 exhibits broad spectrum oral antitumor activity and targets the RAF/MEK/ERK pathway and receptor tyrosine kinases involved in tumor progression and angiogenesis. *Cancer Res* Vol.64, No.19, (Oct 1), pp.7099-109

Wykoff, C.C., Beasley, N.J., Watson, P.H., Turner, K.J., Pastorek, J., Sibtain, A., Wilson, G.D., Turley, H., Talks, K.L., Maxwell, P.H., Pugh, C.W., Ratcliffe, P.J. & Harris, A.L. (2000). Hypoxia-inducible expression of tumor-associated carbonic anhydrases. *Cancer Res* Vol.60, No.24, (Dec 15), pp.7075-83

Xu, L., Tong, R., Cochran, D.M. & Jain, R.K. (2005a). Blocking platelet-derived growth factor-D/platelet-derived growth factor receptor beta signaling inhibits human renal cell carcinoma progression in an orthotopic mouse model. *Cancer Res* Vol.65, No.13, (Jul 1), pp.5711-9

Xu, R.H., Pelicano, H., Zhou, Y., Carew, J.S., Feng, L., Bhalla, K.N., Keating, M.J. & Huang, P. (2005b). Inhibition of glycolysis in cancer cells: a novel strategy to overcome drug resistance associated with mitochondrial respiratory defect and hypoxia. *Cancer Res* Vol.65, No.2, (Jan 15), pp.613-21

Yoshida, K., Hosoya, Y., Sumi, S., Honda, M., Moriguchi, H., Yano, M. & Ueda, Y. (1997). Studies of the expression of epidermal growth factor receptor in human renal cell carcinoma: a comparison of immunohistochemical method versus ligand binding assay. *Oncology* Vol.54, No.3, (May-Jun), pp.220-5

Yoshida, K., Tosaka, A., Takeuchi, S. & Kobayashi, N. (1994). Epidermal growth factor receptor content in human renal cell carcinomas. *Cancer* Vol.73, No.7, (Apr 1), pp.1913-8

Yuen, J.S., Cockman, M.E., Sullivan, M., Protheroe, A., Turner, G.D., Roberts, I.S., Pugh, C.W., Werner, H. & Macaulay, V.M. (2007). The VHL tumor suppressor inhibits expression of the IGF1R and its loss induces IGF1R upregulation in human clear cell renal carcinoma. *Oncogene* Vol.26, No.45, (Oct 4), pp.6499-508

Zavada, J., Zavadova, Z., Zat'ovicova, M., Hyrsl, L. & Kawaciuk, I. (2003). Soluble form of carbonic anhydrase IX (CA IX) in the serum and urine of renal carcinoma patients. *Br J Cancer* Vol.89, No.6, (Sep 15), pp.1067-71

Zhang, X., Yamashita, M., Uetsuki, H. & Kakehi, Y. (2002). Angiogenesis in renal cell carcinoma: Evaluation of microvessel density, vascular endothelial growth factor and matrix metalloproteinases. *Int J Urol* Vol.9, No.9, (Sep), pp.509-14

Zhou, G.X., Ireland, J., Rayman, P., Finke, J. & Zhou, M. (2010). Quantification of carbonic anhydrase IX expression in serum and tissue of renal cell carcinoma patients using enzyme-linked immunosorbent assay: prognostic and diagnostic potentials. *Urology* Vol.75, No.2, (Feb), pp.257-61

4

The Next Challenge in the Treatment of Renal Cell Carcinoma: Overcoming the Resistance Mechanisms to Antiangiogenic Agents

Michele Guida and Giuseppe Colucci
Department of Medical Oncology National Cancer Institute Viale Orazio Flacco Bari Italy

1. Introduction

In recent years, important advances have been made in the medical therapy of metastatic renal cell carcinoma (mRCC). These advances are due on the one hand to the availability of many new molecules directed at specific biomolecular targets, and on the other hand to the understanding of both the pathogenetic mechanisms which have led to the identification of the key role of some gene mutations and angiogenesis, fundamental mechanisms in the process of tumour proliferation (1,2). In particular, there have been great developments in molecules capable of inhibiting the activity of the pro-angiogenesis receptors of vascular endothelial growth factor (VEGF) and platelet-derived growth factor (PDGF) such as tyrosine-kinase inhibitors (TKI) sunitinib, sorafenib, pazopanib, and monoclonal antibodies bevacizumab. Also inhibitors of specific pathways correlated with tumour growth such as the mTOR inhibitors temsirolinmus and everolimus have become crucial drugs in the management of mRCC (3).

In the last few years, these drugs have radically changed the course of medical therapy of mRCC and other molecules currently in an advanced stage of clinical development will soon further enrich the therapeutic options of mRCC: axitinib (new, powerful anti-tyrosine kinases inhibitor), dovitinib (multi-target inhibitor particularly active against Beta Fibroblast Growth Factor Receptor (FGFR)), volociximab (new chimeric antibody with powerful anti-angiogenic activity directed towards the α5β1integrin), regorafenib, cediranib etc.

As is known, RCC is a highly vascularized neoplasm which is dependent on VEGF-mediated angiogenesis. In fact, mRCC is among neoplasms showing the highest level of circulating VEGF. The importance of VEGF signaling for tumoral growth is also supported by the high frequency of von Hippel-Lindau *(*VHL*)* gene mutations found in about 70% of clear cell RCC. The VHL gene product regulates VEGF expression through suppression of the HIF transcription factor. Loss of function mutations in VHL lead to unregulated activation of HIF and overexpression of VEGF and other proangiogenic factors. For these reasons, anti-angiogenic drugs are particularly active in clear cell RCC and these drugs are currently considered the standard of care for first-line treatment. They include the monoclonal antibody bevacizumab which binds to the soluble ligand of VEGF, and the inhibitors of multiple receptor TK for vascular endothelial growth factor receptors (VEGFR-

1, VEGFR-2, and VEGFR-3), PDGFR-α and PDGFR-β, FLT3, the stem cell growth factor receptor KIT, and RET (4).

Despite the efficacy of TKI and bevacizumab therapy, the development of resistance is of major clinical concern; in fact, almost all patients with mRCC develop resistance and the disease inexorably progress.

Conventionally, patients are categorised as "early progressors" when they develop resistance within approximately 6 months of the beginning of first-line therapy, and "late progressors" when they develop resistance later. About 30% of patients present a primary resistance to these drugs with a rapid spreading of disease and a very poor survival (primary refractory). Another 40% of patients, after an initial positive response, exhibit disease progression after about 1 year of treatment (5).

Consequently, the number of patients who receive a second line therapy after anti-angiogenic agents is only about half of the total. In the registrative phase III trial which compared sunitinib to interferon alpha, of 375 patients treated in the sunitinib arm, only 182 patients, corresponding to 56% of the total, received a second line therapy with an anti-mTOR or with a second anti-angiogenic drug (6). Similarly, in the AVOREN study with bevacizumab plus interferon *vs* interferon alone, of 325 patients in the bevacizumab plus interferon arm only 180 patients corresponding to 55% received a second line therapy (7). These data have been confirmed in the similar CALGB 90206 study (8). Notably, outside large controlled studies the percentage of patients receiving a second line treatment after anti-angiogenic agents is much lower. In a recent retrospective analysis of 645 patients from 7 centers and recruited in various studies, only 216 (30%) underwent second line therapy with anti-VEGF/anti-mammalian target of rapamycin (mTOR) drugs (9). Of interest, basal performance status resulted the only significant independent predictor of receiving second-line targeted therapy. Moreover, patients who received a second-line anti-VEGF drug appeared to have a similar overall survival to those who receive a second-line anti-mTOR drug (9).

The adoption of alternative angiogenic signaling pathways to compensate for inhibition of VEGF/VEGFR-mediated signaling seems to be the main, but not the only, common mechanism for the development of cancer resistance to VEGF pathway inhibitors. Nevertheless, to date very few data are available in literature about which alternative pathways are involved in resistant disease. Therefore, understanding the escape mechanisms of resistance to anti-angiogenic agents could improve clinical outcomes and the number of responsive patients.

2. Mechanisms of resistance in MRC

Resistance is generally defined as the capability of tumors to evade the antineoplastic effects of various treatments. About 30% of mRCC have an innate resistance to all available treatments independently from the type of anti-angiogenic agent used. Furthermore, treatment with mTORi as second line therapy results in primary resistance in about 20% of patients.

In this chapter we will attempt to give some partial responses to the numerous questions regarding the significance of resistance in mRCC: what is the definition of resistance? Which mechanisms sustain it? How can we overcome the resistance mechanisms?

2.1 Definition of resistance and its clinical implications

Resistance is divided into primary (also "refractoriness" or "intrinsic responsiveness"), which is characterized by a lack of efficacy to anti-angiogenic agents from the start of therapy, and secondary (also "acquired" or "adaptive" or "evasive" or "angiogenesis escape"), which begins after an initial response to TKI lasting for a period of time of variable length. Notably, early treatment failure involves all anti-angiogenic agents and all type of patients with mRCC.

Nevertheless, primary resistance to TKI in mRCC is heavily influenced by the patient risk score (low-intermediate *vs* poor) and by the type of first line therapy used. Primary refractory patients are about 20% in good-intermediate risk patients treated with different TKI, and it arises over 30% in poor risk patients (6, 8, 10, 11). In addition, the mTORi everolimus generally utilized as second line therapy is characterized by a resistance involving about 20% of patients (12). It is not clear if the patients who present primary resistance are the same as those who also present secondary resistance as data on this topic are not available.

The influence of prior therapies on the risk of primary resistance in patients with mRCC treated with sunitinib as first line has recently been reported in a systemic review and meta-analysis of 10 clinical studies including a total of 4,320 (13). The overall incidence of primary resistance to sunitinib was 22.4%. Moreover, the risk of developing primary resistance was significantly lower in patients with clear-cell cancer compared with non-clear-cell cancer. Notably, patients with prior cytokine therapy exhibited a significantly higher risk of primary progressive disease with sunitinib compared with those who had no prior treatment (RR, 1.18, 95% CI, 1.05-1.34, p=0.007). Although not statistically significant, there was a trend supporting that prior treatment with another mTKI sorafenib increased the risk of resistance to sunitinib in comparison with no prior treatment (RR 1.33, 95% CI: 0.98-1.80, p=0.069).

The conclusions of the Authors are that the risk of primary resistance to sunitinib may vary with tumor histology and prior therapies. In particular, previous exposure to cytokines significantly increased the risk of primary resistance suggesting that an immune mechanism may underlie the resistance to this drug.

A similar meta-analysis was done in patients treated with sorafenib as first line therapy (14). A total of 3,269 patients from 20 studies were included for the analysis. The overall incidence of primary resistance was 22.6% without significant difference between clear cell and non-clear cell nor between prior cytokine therapies and no prior treatment. Notably, patients with prior exposure to sunitinib had a significantly higher incidence of resistance when treated with sorafenib (52.2%). The conclusions of the Authors are that prior exposure to sunitinib but not cytokines significantly increased the risk of resistance with sorafenib in mRCC patients, suggesting that initial therapy with angiogenesis inhibitors may promote the development of resistance to sorafenib.

The conclusive considerations regarding the primary resistance to anti-angiogenic agents in mRCC are that about 30% of mRCC have an innate resistance to all available treatments and the resistance to angiogenic drugs seems to be independent from the type of TKI used.

In second line treatment, resistance to mTORi everolimus occurs in about 20% of patients (12), but when a second TKI was used, the risk of resistance increased to about 50%.

Therefore, considering that only 30%-50% of patients receive second line therapy, the re-challenge with a second TKI is an option available for very few and selected patients.

2.2 The resistance mechanisms

Resistance has yet to be thoroughly understood in kidney cancer. The "angiogenic escape" to anti-VEGF treatment may be dependent both on cancer cell phenomena or endothelial cell phenomena. It is believed that multiple factors affect resistance including factors that decrease angiogenesis and factors that increase angiogenesis. Often these mechanisms are present contemporarily in a single patient. Several of these factors need to be accounted for when developing a comprehensive treatment approach and in understanding why a patient may be resistant to any one approach.

Hypoxia is a known inducer of angiogenic response in a wide variety of tumors. Nevertheless, it is strongly believed that hypoxia is also the key mechanism of angiogenic escape. It involves induction of gene expression via HIF transcription factor of various pro-angiogenic factors including VEGF, FGFs and ephrins. When angiogenesis is inhibited, tumors are in a hypoxic state and develop new alternative pathways to guarantee their further growth (15).

2.3 Primary resistance mechanisms

It is thought that patients with primary resistance to TKI have already activated one or more alternative mechanisms of resistance in response to the selective pressure of their microenvironment. Probably these cases are not, or not only, sustained by angiogenesis mechanisms. Moreover, in patients with primary resistance there is frequently an upregulation of alternative pro-angiogenic pathways mediated by FGFR, interleukin-8 (IL-8), insulin-like GFR, ephrins, and angiopoietins. In particular, FGF/FGFR system has been reported as one of the most important escape pathways of anti-VEGFR therapies.

Other possible mechanisms include the pre-existing inflammatory cell-mediated vascular protection (myeloid cell); an hypovascularity status with consequent indifference toward angiogenesis inhibitors (desmoplastic stroma); the co-option of normal vessels without requisite angiogenesis (4, 16-18).

2.4 Secondary resistance mechanisms

Regarding secondary resistance, many Authors believe that it is precisely the state of **hypoxia** determined by anti-angiogenic drugs which is at the root of the onset of the *escape* mechanisms sustained by new HIF, FGF, IL-8, ephrine etc transcript factors, which lead to the activation of alternative pathways which support a "*new angiogenic wave*" (15). It is notable that during therapy with anti-VEGF the expression of new and ever-increasing pro-angiogenic factors is observed. It is known that the early phase of angiogenesis is generally characterized by a response to anti-VEGF treatment. On the contrary, the late phase of angiogenesis is characterized by the escape to anti-VEGF treatment. This late phase is sustained by FGF, IL-8 and other factors. It has been reported that in the presence of sunitinib the tumor is able to produce until 19 pro-angiogenic factors to rescue endothelia cell proliferation (19,20).

Function-blocking antibodies to VEGF receptors R1 and R2 were used to probe their roles in controlling angiogenesis in a mouse model of pancreatic islet carcinogenesis. Inhibition of VEGFR2 but not VEGFR1 markedly disrupted angiogenic switching, persistent angiogenesis, and initial tumor growth. In late-stage tumors, phenotypic resistance to VEGFR2 blockade emerged, as tumors regrew during treatment after an initial period of growth suppression. This resistance to VEGF blockade involves reactivation of tumor angiogenesis, independent of VEGF and associated with hypoxia-mediated induction of other proangiogenic factors, including members of the FGF family. These other proangiogenic signals are functionally implicated in the revascularization and regrowth of tumors in the evasion phase, as FGF blockade impairs progression in the face of VEGF inhibition (15).

Recently, it has been demonstrated that the FGF pathway is important in patients who develop resistance to sunitinib. Welti and collegues (21) reported that FGF2 supports endothelial proliferation and de novo tubule formation in the presence of sunitinib and that FGF2 can suppress sunitinib-induced retraction of tubules. Importantly, these effects of FGF2 were ablated by PD173074, a small molecule inhibitor of FGF receptor signalling. They also showed that FGF2 can stimulate pro-angiogenic signalling pathways in endothelial cells despite the presence of sunitinib. Finally, analysis of clinical renal-cancer samples demonstrated that a large proportion of renal cancers strongly express FGF2. In conclusion, they suggest that therapeutic strategies designed to simultaneously target both VEGF and FGF2 signalling may prove more efficacious than sunitinib in renal cancer patients whose tumours express FGF2.

Interestingly, it has been demonstrated that FGFR is highly expressed in RCC. Tsimafeyeu and collegues analyzed the expression of FGFR1 in 140 patients with mRCC. Expression of FGFR1 was observed in 98% of primary tumors and in 82.5% of lymph node metastases. Moreover, a significant rise in plasma bFGF levels was reported in patients with disease progression but a non-significant fall in patients with response or stable disease. Plasma VEGF-A level increased in patients with response whereas no detectable changes in plasma VEGF-A level was found in patients with progressive disease. The conclusions of the Authors are that plasma levels of bFGF and VEGF-A are altered in MRCC patients receiving sunitinib, and the increases in bFGF levels may represent biomarker of resistance to targeted therapy (22). Recently it has confirmed that the subset of clear cell RCC tumors with increased expression of FGFR1 is associated with a shorter progression free survival (23).

Also the role of IL-8 in resistance mechanisms seems to be determinant. In xenograft models, sunitinib resistance/refractoriness has been reported associated to higher levels of IL-8 (16). Moreover, the resistance to sunitinib was associated with a higher microvessel density, indicating an escape from anti-angiogenesis mechanisms. Finally, the addition of monoclonal antibody anti-IL-8 resensitized the tumor to sunitinib activity. The conclusions of the Authors are that IL-8 mediates resistance to sunitinib and could represent a candidate target to reverse acquired or intrinsic resistance to sunitinib.

Higher levels of IL-8 were associated with shorter progression free survival in mRCC patients treated in phase III trials of pazopanib (24).

Some Authors also demonstrated in pre-clinical models that antiangiogenic drugs could elicit malignant progression of tumors with an increase of local invasion and distant metastasis. In particular, it has been reported that short-term treatment with a potent inhibitor of tumor angiogenesis is able to induce an acceleration of metastasis formation (25). Moreover, other Authors reported that angiogenesis inhibitors targeting the VEGF pathway had antitumor effects in mouse models of pancreatic neuroendocrine carcinoma and glioblastoma, but concomitantly these drugs elicit tumor adaptation and progression to stages of greater malignancy, with heightened invasiveness and in some cases increased lymphatic and distant metastasis (26). Increased invasiveness is also seen by genetic ablation of the VEGF-A gene in both models, substantiating the results of the pharmacological inhibitors. The realization that potent angiogenesis inhibition can alter the natural history of tumors by increasing invasion and metastasis warrants clinical investigation, as the prospect has important implications for the development of enduring antiangiogenic therapies (26).

Other two main mechanisms that could partially explain the ability of the tumor to become resistant to treatment are their capability to epithelial-mesenchimal transformation and the intra-tumoral heterogeneity.

The **epithelial to mesenchymal transition** (EMT) process has been described in different neoplasms and associated with metastatic disease, drug resistance, and develop of angiogenesis (27-30). Treatment-associated tumor hypoxia has been reported to induce an EMT in several tumor models (31). How EMT as a mechanism of acquired resistance occurs in human tumors is unknown and deserves further investigation. In RCC, sarcomatoid phenotype is observed across all histological subtypes, and associated with a poorer prognosis and an increased resistance to VEGF inhibitors. A growing number of interdependent pathways have been linked to the induction of EMT, which, by definition, is a potentially transient/reversible phenotype of epithelial cancers. The reverted histologic phenotype observed in the xenografts also suggests that this escape mechanisms against anti-VEGF therapies may be transient (30, 32, 33).

According to this hypothesis, patients who have initially received clinical benefit from treatment with TKIs and then developed resistant disease may respond again to TKIs following a break from anti-VEGF therapies. The "holiday" period from anti-VEGF therapies may lead to "reset" the tumor microenvironment and reestablish a primarily EGF driven tumor growth. This hypothesis is supported by anecdotic reports of patients who were treated with sunitinib with initial response and subsequent progression who responded again to sunitinib following different targeted therapies such as mTOR inhibitors. The apparent transient/reversible mechanism of resistance to anti-VEGF therapies may also explain why clinical benefit has been reported by sequencing different anti-VEGF therapies despite the fact that these agents target the same VEGF pathway.

Regarding **intratumoral heterogeneity**, it has been demonstrated that mRCC, like other cancer, is characterized by a significant chromosomal instability that creates a selection of multiple clonal tumor subpopulations with an intrinsic multidrug resistance. Multiple intermixed cell subpopulations within one tumour differ by large genomic events as focal amplifications and deletions. For this reason, it is thought that single biopsy is often not representative of mutational landscape of the tumor (34). Recently have been developed methods able to study multiple subpopulations from different anatomic locations of neoplastic tissue (35).

	First line	Second line		Predictive factors
Drug/Author	N. Pts	Type of therapy	N. of Pts (%)	
Sunitinib *Motzer et al, JCO 2009*	375 (sunitinib arm)	Anti-VEGF/ anti-mTOR	182 (56)	-
Beva + IFN *Escudier et al, JCO 2010*	325 (bevacizumab-IFN arm)	TKI	180 (55)	-
TKI* *Vikers et al, Urology 2010*	645	Anti-VEGF/ anti-mTOR	216 (30)	Basal PS

* Multi-institutional studies
Abbreviations: PS: Performance status

Table 1. Percentage of patients who access to a second line treatment after TKi in mRCC

Setting	Author	Drug	% of incidence resistance
1ª line therapy Good-intermediate prognosis	Motzer, 2007 Ranpura, 2010*	Sunitinib	22.4
	Su, 2010*	Sorafenib	22.6
1ª line Poor prognosis	Hudes 2007	Temsirolimus	33
2ª line therapy	Motzer, 2008	Everolimus after TKI	20
	Ranpura, 2010*	Sorafenib after Sunitinib	33
	Su, 2010*	Sunitinib after Sorafenib	52.2

*Meta-analysis

Table 2. Percentage of patients with resistance according to the risk score and treatments in mRCC

Due to this genomic instability, it is strongly believed that resistance is a dynamic mechanism changing in different conditions (treatment pressure, hypoxia pressure, etc) and during the tumor growth. This aspect could explain the response obtained in some patients re-challenged with sunitinib. It thought that during treatment interruption, the selective pressure from drugs is removed and drug-sensitive clones re-growth. Recently, Zama and colleagues reported the results of a retrospective study describing 5 partial response (22%) of 23 mRCC patients re-treated with sunitinib (36, 37).

Also a "holiday" period from anti-VEGF therapies it is thought able to determine a reacquired drug-sensitivity by clones become resistant to TKI drugs.

Various genes associated with resistance have been identified which could become a target for future treatments. Recently, Sanjmyatas and colleagues also reported a specific gene expression signature able to characterize the different metastatic potential in ccRCC (38).

It has been demonstrated that some genes are hyperexpressed when there is resistance, for example the gene which encodes sphingosine kinase, calvasculin, chemokine receptor 4 (CXCR4), NNP1, arginase II, hypoxia-inducible protein-2 (HIG2) and VEGF. Other anti-angiogenic genes, however, show reduced expression in resistant tumors, such as the genes which encode cytokines associated with interferon-gamma, in particular IP10 (CXCL10) and Mig (CXCL9) (39). Sphingosine-1-phosphate (S1P), a pleiotropic bioactive lipid derived from sphingosine through sphingosine kinase (SphK) action, is dysregulated in a variety of disease conditions including cancer. S1P is a tumorigenic and angiogenic growth factor produced normally by blood platelets, mast cells and possibly fibroblasts in the tumour microenvironment. It is capable of determining proliferation and migration of endothelial cells, favouring angiogenesis and tumour proliferation. Notably, several tumors up regulate the expression of SPHK1, which may greatly contribute to the putative increased levels of S1P. In experimental models it has been demonstrated that SphK and S1P expression was increased during sunitinib resistance (39).

In xenografts models Bhatt and colleagues provided evidence that resistance to VEGF receptor therapy is due at least in part to resumption of angiogenesis in association with reduction of IFNγ-related angiostatic chemokines, and that this resistance can be delayed by restoration of angiostatic signalling with the concomitant administration of CXCL9 (40).

An emerging area of drug discovery called lipidomic-based therapeutics is in rapid develop. It directly targets pleiotropic bioactive lipids involved in cancer as well as other disorders. It has been postulated that S1P antibodies could represented a potential therapeutic strategies in the treatment of renal cancer (41).

Other mechanisms, not completely known, sustaining secondary resistance in mRCC include: **secondary mutations in tyrosine kinase receptors** (analogous to EGFR TKI); **recruitment of bone marrow-derived pro-angiogenic cells** which can obviate the necessity of VEGF signalling, thereby affecting re-initiaton and continuance of tumour angiogenesis; **increasing of pericyte** coverage of the tumour vasculature, serving to support its integrity and attenuate the necessity for VEGF-mediated survival signalling has been described; activation and enhancement of invasion and metastasis to provide **access to normal tissue vasculature** without obligate neovascularisation (4).

In table 3 are reported the main mechanisms of primary and secondary resistance in mRCC.

3. How can we overcome resistance to anti-angiogenic agents?

Many attempts have been made in the effort to overcome resistance to anti-VEGF treatments, but so far the results are disappointing. They include the use of non cross-resistant drugs, integrating or combining current treatment, optimization of sequential therapies and TKI re-challenge. Finally, several ongoing studies are trying to clarify the optimal sequence of the different drugs and the significance of the rechallenge with TKI in the treatment strategies.

As regards primary resistance, other than new experimental molecules the main route taken up until now has been to the combination of drugs for different biomolecular targets.

Primary resistance	- Alternative pro-angiogenic pathways mediated by FGFR, interleukin-8 (IL-8), insulin-like GFR, ephrins, and angiopoietins; - Non angiogenic mechanisms -Pre-existing inflammatory cell-mediated vascular protection (myeloid cell); -Hypovascularity status with consequent indifference toward angiogenesis inhibitors (desmoplastic stroma); -Co-option of normal vessels without requisite angiogenesis -Non clear cell histology
Secondary resistance	- New angiogenic wave induced by hypoxia determined by anti-angiogenic drugs - Epithelial to mesenchymal transition - Intra-tumoral heterogeneity - Gene instability and gene iperexpression - Secondary mutations in tyrosine kinase receptors - Bone marrow-derived pro-angiogenic cells which can obviate the necessity of VEGF signalling; - Increasing of pericyte coverage of the tumour vasculature, serving to support its integrity and attenuate the necessity for VEGF-mediated survival; - Access to normal tissue vasculature without obligate neovascularisation

Note: to bibliographic references see the text

Table 3. Main mechanisms of primary and secondary resistance in mRCC

To overcome secondary resistance, various strategies are being explored: increasing the dose of the current drug, the use of non cross-resistant drugs (for example changing to a mTOR inhibitor such as everolimus after a anti-angiogenic drug), changing to another VEGF inhibitor (for example sunitinib after bevacizumab, or sorafenib after sunitinib, or axitinib after sorafenib), the use of a "drug holiday" (12, 42, 43). However, results obtained so far have been modest, above all because in general the choice of strategy has been empirical rather than determined by a strong biological rationale. It is therefore desirable that new studies are founded on convincing preclinical data.

3.1 Drug combinations

As previously mentioned, several studies using combinations of drugs targeted to different biomolecular targets have been started with the aim of increasing clinical activity. Many attempts have been made to verify if the combination of drugs with different mechanisms of action was able to improve the results of single agent therapy. Unfortunately, so far this strategy has given disappointing or negative results with a heavier profile of toxicity.

Figure 1 shows the possible drug combination strategies in mCRC therapy.

Some combinations have proved to be very toxic and relatively inactive and therefore they were quickly abandoned, as was the case of the combination of TKI and bevacizumab (44, 45).

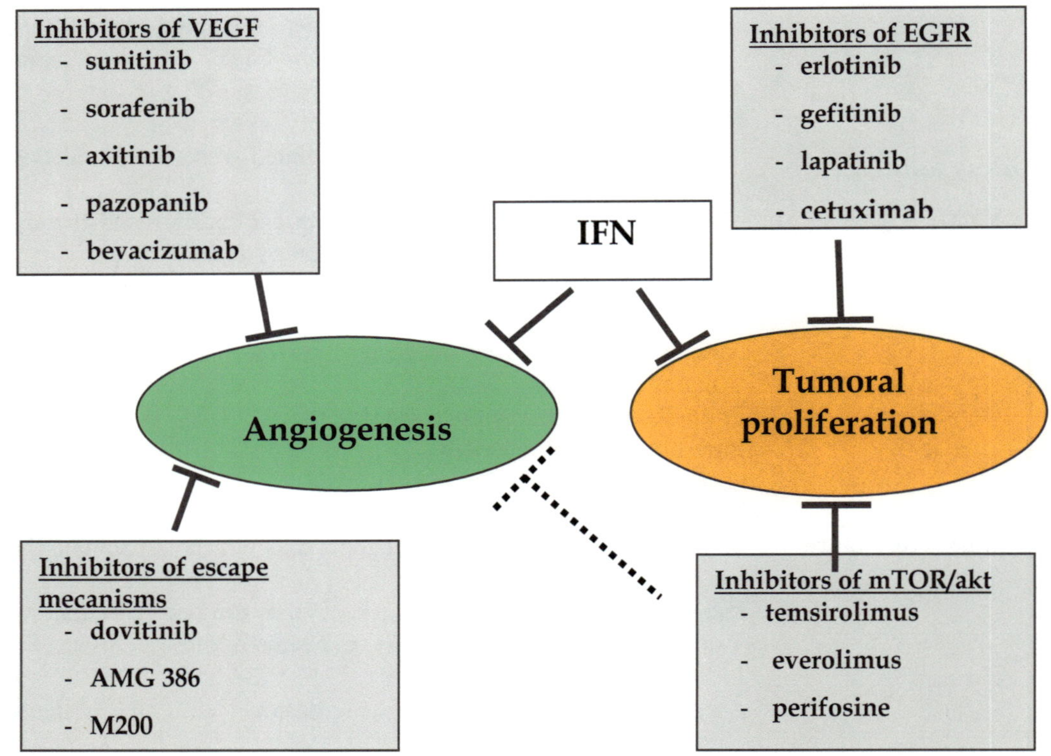

Fig. 1. Possible strategies of drugs association in mRCC

The high expression of EGFR in renal tumours from 50 to 90% (46), has also encouraged the use of anti-EGFR drugs in combination with anti-angiogenic agents. A study has recently been published by Motzer and colleagues at the Memorial Sloan-Kettering Cancer Center in New York in which gefitinib was combined with sunitinib in order to realise a double target. However, the reported results were similar to those obtained with sunitinib alone, but with an increase in toxicity. The Authors therefore discourage further studies on this combination (47).

Another route which seems more promising is the combination of bevacizumab and m-TOR inhibitors. However, after some encouraging early experiences (48-50), more recent studies are re-dimensioning the preliminary results. Of particular note are the results of a randomized phase II trial which compared temsirolimus and bevacizumab *vs* sunitinib *vs* interferon alfa and bevacizumab (TORAVA study). Unfortunately, in view of clearly higher toxicity in the temsirolimus plus bevacizumab arm, superiority of this combination compared to other arms was not reported (51). The conclusions of Authors are that the toxicity of the temsirolimus and bevacizumab combination was much higher than anticipated and limited treatment continuation over time, whereas clinical activity was low compared with the benefit expected from sequential use of each targeted therapy. Thus, this combination cannot be recommended for first-line treatment in patients with mRCC.

The combination of targeted drugs with immunological molecules such as interferon is proving to be more interesting. In particular, encouraging results have been reported on the combination of sorafenib and interferon alpha (52).

Generally speaking, even if it is necessary to wait for definitive results of ongoing phase III trials, the results reported so far do not encourage this therapeutic strategy.

Table 4 shows the most significant experiences of the different drug combinations used.

Drugs combinations/ Authors	Setting	N. of pts	PFS (Mo)	OR/SD	Toxicity	Notes
Sorafenib + Interferone *Gollob et al, JCO 2007*	phase II (1ª e 2ª line)	40	10	33% PR 29% SD	moderate	50% pts in 2ª line Good activity
Beva + Sunitinib* *Garcia et al, ASCO 2008*	phase I	31 (varius histology)	-	3/7 mRCC 1 /3 melanoma 1 surrene	moderate	Good activity
Beva + Sorafenib *Sosman et al, ASCO 2008*	phase I-II	48	14	25% PR 18% SD	high (hypertension, stomatite, hand-foot sindrome)	A negative experience
Sunitinib + Gefitinib *Motzer et al, AJCO 2010*	phase II	42	11	37% OR 34% SD	acceptable (diarrea G3-4 in 14% of pts)	Activity similar to that of sunitinib alone
Beva + Everolimus *Whorf et al, ASCO '08* *Hainsworth, Whorf, JCO 2010*	phase II 1ª e 2ª lines	80	9,1 7,1	30/23% OR 50/64% SD (1ª/2ª linea)	moderate	Good activity
Beva + Temsirolimus *Merchan et al, JCO 2009*	phae I-II	45	18/5.3	14,5%	acceptable	Long PFS
Beva + Temsirolimus *vs* Sunitinib *vs* IFN + Beva *Escudier et al, ASCO 2010* *(TORAVA Trial)*	phase II R Beva + Tem		8,2	27,3% OR 47,7% SD	High (41% of pts stop therapy)	Higher toxicity for experimental arm
	Sunitinib		8,2	23,8% OR 50% SD	As aspected	No confirmed results of phase II studies
	Beva + alpha IFN		16,8	39% OR 34% SD	As aspected	

Abbreviations: PFS: progression free survival.

Table 4. Most significant experiences with drug combinations in mRCC

3.2 New drugs and sequences

Clearly, another approach to overcoming resistance mechanisms is the use of new molecules which have a more powerful anti-angiogenic activity or which are more directly aimed at the targets involved in resistance mechanisms. Axitinib and dovitinib are of particular interest here. In preclinical trials, axitinib has shown much more powerful antiangiogenic activity than other TKIs (53, 54). Furthermore, interesting results have been reported in phase II studies as a second line therapy after sorafenib with an overall response of 23% and a stable disease of 55%; interestingly, the progression free survival was 7.4 months, one of the longest ever reported (42).

Recently, beta FGFR has been identified as a new target for anti-angiogenic therapy. The system FGF/FGF receptor (FGFR) has been frequently reported as one of the most important escape pathways of anti-VEGFR therapies. It is involved in primary and secondary resistance mechanisms. The activation of FGFR3 is associated with cell proliferation and survival in certain cancer cell types. Thus, beta FGFR is proving to be a new interesting target for anti-angiogenic therapy.

Dovitinib, a new small multi-target molecule, is able to strongly binds to FGFR3 and inhibits its phosphorylation, which may result in the inhibition of tumor cell proliferation and the induction of tumor cell death. In addition, this agent may inhibit other members of the TK receptors superfamily, including the VEGFR; FGFR1; PDGFR3; FMS-like tyrosine kinase 3; stem cell factor receptor (c-KIT); and colony-stimulating factor receptor 1; this may result in an additional reduction in cellular proliferation and angiogenesis, and the induction of tumor cell apoptosis. A phase I/II has been recently concluded (55) and a large phase III clinical trial is ongoing to evaluate the efficacy of this drug as third line therapy in mRCC.

Other drugs of great interest are the monoclonal antibody anti-S1P, a molecule directly involved in resistance mechanisms already being developed clinically, and the anti- IL-8 and anti-IL-12 antibodies, which are still being studied in preclinical trials.

Regarding **sequences**, factors that could drive the choice of a more appropriate second line therapy are the response to primary treatment with TKI, the side effects reported in first line therapy, the patient risk score, and the histology of the tumor.

At present, the use of non cross-resistant mTOR inhibitor everolimus is the only registered agent available as second line therapy for mRCC resistant to anti-angiogenic drugs. In fact, the registrative trial showed a significant benefit in terms of PFS of 4.9 months for everolimus *vs* 1.9 months for placebo (12).

A second TKi as second line therapy is another option to consider for patients resistant to antiangiogenetic agents. Nevertheless, it is thought that this treatment must be propose only in carefully selected patients who did not show a rapid progression at the first line TKi. At present, this choice has a weaker recommendation because no definitive data from phase III studies are available yet.

Notably, in the AVOREN study it has been reported a median overall survival of 23.3 months for the sequence alfa interferone/bevacizumab followed by a second antiangiogenetic agent (TKI), with respect to only 21.3 months for the sequence alfa interferone/placebo followed by a TKI (7).

Some Authors believe that better clinical outcomes are correlated with a higher number of lines of treatments used rather than with the sequences utilized. Consequently, they have hypothesize specific sequences with the aim to utilize the maximum of therapeutic options available. Others suppose that the sequence TKI-TKI is to prefer to that with TKI-mTORi on the basis of some preliminary experiences. Also the rechallenge with the same drug has been proposed, especially when a "holiday" period from anti-VEGF therapies is given to the patient. This break could be able to determine a reacquired drug-sensitivity by clones become resistant to TKI. Nevertheless, at present the majority of data are from small and retrospective studies regarding selected patients (36,37,56-61).

Recently, the results of the phase III study with Axitinib as second line therapy have been published (62). Axitinib resulted in significantly longer PFS compared with sorafenib. Nevertheless, in the subgroup of the patients treated previously with the TKI inhibitor the PFS was similar to what has been reported for the mTOR inhibitor everolimus (4.8 vs. 4.9 months).

Of course, further controlled studies are needed to determine the real effect of prior anti-angiogenesis therapy on the development of resistance to further therapies. A series of planned trials are evaluating what are the best sequences and timing.

4. Conclusions

The adoption of alternative angiogenic signaling pathways to compensate for inhibition of VEGF/VEGFR-mediated signaling seems to be the common mechanism for the development of cancer resistance to VEGF pathway inhibitors. Nevertheless, until now very few data are known about which alternative pathways are involved in resistant disease.

Many attempts have been proposed to overcome resistance. These include the use of non cross-resistant drugs, the optimization of sequential therapies, and the use of combined therapies. Unfortunately, all these approaches have given only modest results. Therefore, the overcome resistance mechanisms to antiangiogenic agents remains the next challenge in the treatment of renal cell carcinoma.

5. Acknowledgements

The author would like to thank Caroline Oakley and Silvana Valerio for their assistance with the linguistic revision of this review.

6. References

[1] Rini BI, Small EJ: Biology and clinical development of vascular endothelial growth factor-targeted therapy in renal cell carcinoma. J Clin Oncol 2005; 23:1028-1043.

[2] Motzer RJ, Michaelson MD, Redman BG et al: Activity of SUI 1248, a multitargeted inhibitor of vascular endothelial growth factor receptor and platelet-derived growth factor receptor, in patients with metastatic renal cell carcinoma. J Clin Oncol 2006; 24:1-3.

[3] Schmidinger M, Bellmunt J: Plethora of agents, plethora of targets, plethora of side effects in metastatic renal cell carcinoma. Cancer Treat Rev 2010; 36:416-424.

[4] Bergers G and Hanahan D: Modes of resistance to anti-angiogenic therapy. Nature Reviews 2008; 8(8):592-603.

[5] Rini B, Atkins MB: Resistance to targeted therapy in renal cell carcinoma. Lancet Oncol 2009; 10:992-1000.

[6] Motzer RJ, Hutson TE, Tomczak P, et al: Overall survival and updated results for sunitinib compared with interferon alfa in patients with metastatic renal cell carcinoma. J Clin Oncol. 2009; 27(22):3584-3590.
[7] Escudier B, Bellmunt J, Négrier S et al: Phase III trial of bevacizumab plus interferon alfa-2a in patients with metastatic renai celi carcinoma (AVOREN): final analysis of overall survival. J Clin Oncol 2010; 28:2144-2150.
[8] Rini, BI Halabi S, Rosenberg JE, et al. Phase III trial of bevacizumab plus interferon alfa versus interferon alfa monotherapy in patients with metastatic renal cell carcinoma: final results of CALGB 90206. J Clin Oncol 2010; 28:2137-2143.
[9] Vickers MM, Choueiri TK, Rogers M, et al: Clinical outcome in metastatic renal cell carcinoma patients after failure of initial vascular endothelial growth factor-targeted therapy. Urology 2010; 76(2):430-434.
[10] Hutson, TE, Davis ID, Machiels JP, et al. Efficacy and safety of pazopanib in patients with metastatic renal cell carcinoma.J Clin Oncol 2010 ; 28(3):475-480.
[11] Hudes G, Carducci M, Tomczak P et al: Temsirolimus, interferon alfa, or both for advanced renal-cell carcinoma. N Engl J Med 2007; 356: 2271-2281.
[12] Motzer RJ, Escudier B, Oudard S et al: Efficacy of everolimus in advanced renal cell carcinoma: a double-blind, randomised, placebo-controlled phase III trial. Lancet 2008; 372:449-456.
[13] RanpuraV, Su X, Wu S: Influence of prior therapies on the risk of primary progressive disease in patients with metastatic renal cell carcinoma treated with sunitinib: A meta-analysis. GU ASCO meeting 2010. J Clin Oncol 2011, Abst 347.
[14] Su X, Wu S: Treatment failure secondary to primary progressive disease in patients with metastatic renal cell carcinoma treated with sorafenib: A meta-analysis. GU ASCO 2010, Abst 391.
[15] Casanovas O, Hicklin DJ, Bergers G, Hanahan D: Drug resistance by evasion of antiangiogenic targeting of VEGF signaling in late-stage pancreatic islet tumors. Cancer Cell. 2005; 8(4):299-309.
[16] Sleijfer S, Wiemer E, Seynaeve C, Verweij J: Improved insight into resistance mechanisms to imatinib in gastrointestinal stromal tumors: a basis for novel approaches and individualization of treatment. Oncologist. 2007; 12(6):719-726.
[17] Reichardt P: Novel approaches to imatinib- and sunitinib-resistant GIST. Curr Oncol Rep 2008;10(4):344-349. Review.
[18] Huang D, Ding Y, Zhou M, et al: Interleukin-8 mediates resistance to antiangiogenic agent sunitinib in renal cell carcinoma.. Cancer Res 2010; 70(3):1063-1071.
[19] Folkman J: Principles and practice in Oncology Cancer 2005.
[20] Faivre S, Demetri G, Sargent W, Raymond E: Molecular basis for sunitinib efficacy and future clinical development. Nat Rev Drug Discov. 2007; 6(9):734-745. Review.
[21] Welti JC, Gourlaouen M, Powles T, et al: Fibroblast growth factor 2 regulates endothelial cell sensitivity to sunitinib. Oncogene 2011; 30(10):1183-1193.
[22] Tsimafeyeu I, Demidov L, Ta H, et al: Fibroblast growth factor pathway in renal cell carcinoma. J Clin Oncol 28:15s, 2010 (suppl; abstr 4621).
[23] Ho TH, Wang F, Hoang A, et al: FGFR1) expression and activation in clear cell renal cell carcinoma (ccRCC). ASCO meeting 2011. J Clin Oncol 29: 2011 (suppl; abstr e15015).
[24] Liu Y, Tran HT, Lin Y, et al: Plasma cytokine and angiogenic factors (CAFs) predictive of clinical benefit and prognosis in patients (Pts) with advanced or metastatic renal cell cancer (mRCC) treated in phase III trials of pazopanib (PAZO). ASCO meeting 2011. J Clin Oncol 29: 2011 (suppl 7; abstr 334).

[25] Ebos JM, Lee CR, Cruz-Munoz W, et al: Accelerated metastasis after short-term treatment with a potent inhibitor of tumor angiogenesis. Cancer Cell 2009; 15(3):232-239.
[26] Paez-Ribes M, Allen E, Hudock J, et al: Antiangiogenic therapy elicits malignant progression of tumors to increased local invasion and distant metastasis. Cancer Cell 2009; 3;15(3):220-31. Review.
[27] Frederick BA, Helfrich BA, Coldren CD, et al: Epithelial to mesenchymal transition predicts gefitinib resistance in cell lines of head and neck squamous cell carcinoma and non-small cell lung carcinoma. Mol Cancer Ther 2007; 6:1683–1691.
[28] Shah AN, Summy JM, Zhang J, et al: Development and characterization of gemcitabine-resistant pancreatic tumor cells. Ann Surg Oncol 2007; 14:3629–3637.
[29] Kajiyama H, Shibata K, Terauchi M, et al: Chemoresistance to paclitaxel induces epithelial-mesenchymal transition and enhances metastatic potential for epithelial ovarian carcinoma cells. Int J Oncol 2007; 31:277–283.
[30] Ghersi G: Roles of molecules involved in epithelial/mesenchymal transition during angiogenesis. Front Biosci 2008; 13:2335–2355.
[31] Hugo H, Ackland ML, Blick T, et al: Epithelial-mesenchymal and mesenchymal-epithelial transitions in carcinoma progression. J Cell Physiol 2007; 213:374–383.
[32] Hammers HJ, Verheul HM, Salumbides B, et al: Reversible epithelial to mesenchymal transition and acquired resistance to sunitinib in patients with renal cell carcinoma: evidence from a xenograft study. Mol Cancer Ther 2010; 9:1525-1535.
[33] Klymkowsky MW, Savagner P: Epithelial-mesenchymal transition: A cancer researcher's conceptual friend and foe. Am J Pathol 2009; 174:1588–1593.
[34] Lee AJ, Endesfelder D, Rowan AJ, Walther A, et al: Chromosomal instability confers intrinsic multidrug resistance. Cancer Res. 2011; 71(5):1858-70.
[35] Navin N, Kendall J, Troge J, et al: Tumour evolution inferred by single-cell sequencing. Nature 2011; 472(7341):90-94.
[36] Zama IN, Hutson TE, Elson P, et al: Sunitinib rechallenge in metastatic renal cell carcinoma patients. Cancer 2010; 116(23):5400-5406.
[37] Rini BI, Hutson HE, Elson P et al: Clinical activity of sunitinib rechallenge in metastatic renal cell carcinoma. GU ASCO 2010, J Clin Oncol 2010, Abst 396.
[38] Sanjmyatas J, Steiner T, Wunderlich H, et al: A specific gene expression signature characterizes metastatic potential in clear cell renal cell carcinoma. J Urol 2011; 186(1):289-294.
[39] Sabbadini RA: Targeting sphingosine-1 -phosphate for cancer therapy. Br J Cancer 2006; 95:1131-1135.
[40] Bhatt RS, Wang X, Zhang L, et al: Renal cancer resistance to antiangiogenic therapy is delayed by restoration of angiostatic signaling. Mol Cancer Ther. 2010; 9(10):2793-802.
[41] Sabbadini RA. Sphingosine-1-phosphate antibodies as potential agents in the treatment of cancer and age-related macular degeneration. Br J Pharmacol. 2011; 162(6):1225-1238.
[42] Rini BI, Wilding G, Hudes G et al: Phase II study of axitinib in sorafenib-refractory metastatic renal cell carcinoma. J Clin Oncol 2009; 27:4462-4468.
[43] Rini BI, Hutson HE, Elson P et al: Clinical activity of sunitinib rechallenge in metastatic renal cell carcinoma. GU ASCO meeting 2010, J Clin Oncol 2010, Abst 396.
[44] Rini BI, Garcia JA, Cooney MM, et al: Toxicity of sunitinib plus bevacizumab in renal cell carcinoma. J Clin Oncol. 2010; 10;28(17):284-285.

[45] Sosman JA, Flaherty KT, Atkins MB et al: Updated results of phase I trial of sorafenib (S) and bevacizumab (B) in patients with metastatic renal cell cancer (mRCC). ASCO meeting 2008, abst. 5011.

[46] Yoshida K, Hosoya Y, Sumi S, et al: Studies of the expression of epidermal growth factor receptor in human renal cell carcinoma: a comparison of immunohistochemical method versus ligand binding assay. Oncology. 1997; 54(3):220-225.

[47] Motzer RJ, Hudes GR, Ginsberg MS, et al: Phase I/II trial of sunitinib plus gefitinib in patients with metastatic renal cell carcinoma. Am J Clin Oncol 2010; 33(6):614-618.

[48] Whorf RC, Hainsworth JD, Spigel DR, et al: Phase II study of bevacizumab and everolimus (RAD001) in the treatment of advanced renal cell carcinoma (RCC). ASCO meeting 2008, J Clin Oncol 2008, abst 5010.

[49] Hainsworth JD, Spigel DR, Burris HA, et al: Phase II trial of bevacizumab and everolimus in patients with advanced renal cell carcinoma. J Clin Oncol 2010; 28:2131-2136.

[50] Merchan J R, Pitot HC, Qin R, et al: Phase I/II trial of CCI 779 and bevacizumab in advanced renal cell carcinoma (RCC): Safety and activity in RTKI refractory RCC patients. ASCO meeting 2009, J Clin Oncol 2011, Abst 5039.

[51] Négrier S, Gravis G, Pérol D, et al: Temsirolimus and bevacizumab, or sunitinib, or interferon alfa and bevacizumab for patients with advanced renal cell carcinoma (TORAVA): a randomised phase 2 trial. Lancet Oncol. 2011; 12(7):673-680.

[52] Gollob JA, Rathmell WK, Richmond TM., et al: Phase II trial of sorafenib plus interferon alfa-2b as first- or second-line therapy in patients with metastatic renal cell cancer. J Clin Oncol 2007; 25:3288-3295.

[53] Larkin JM, Chowdhury S, Gore ME: Drug insight: advances in renal cell carcinoma and the role of targeted therapies. Nat Clin Pract Oncol. 2007; 4(8):470-479.

[54] Kelly RJ, Rixe O: Axitinib (AG-013736). Recent Results Cancer Res 2010;184:33-44.

[55] Angevin E, Lopez JA, Pande A, et al: TKI258 (dovitinib lactate) in metastatic renal cell carcinoma (mRCC) patients refractory to approved targeted therapies: A phase I/II dose finding and biomarker study. ASCO meeting 2009, J Clin Oncol 2009, Abst 3563.

[56] Dudek AZ, Zolnierek J, Dham A et al: Sequential therapy with sorafenib and sunitinib in renal cell carcinoma. Cancer 2009; 115: 61-67

[57] Di Lorenzo G, Carteni G, Autorino R et al: Phase II study of sorafenib in patients with sunitinib-refractory metastatic renai celi cancer. J Clin Oncol 2009; 27:4469-4474.

[58] Tamaskar I, Garcia JA, Elson P et al: Antitumor effects of sunitinib or sorafenib in patients with metastatic renal cell carcinoma who received prior antiangiogenic therapy. J Urol 2008; 179:81-86.

[59] Merseburger AS, Simon A, Waalkes S, Kuczyk MA: Sorafenib reveals efficacy in sequential treatment of metastatic renal cell cancer. Expert Rev Anticancer Ther 2009; 9:1429-1434.

[60] Sablin MP, Négrier S, Ravaud A et al: Sequential sorafenib and sunitinib for renai celi carcinoma. J Urol 2009; 182:29-34.

[61] Zimmermann K, Schmittel A, Steiner U et al: Sunitinib treatment for patients with advanced clear-cell renal-cell carcinoma after progression on sorafenib. Oncology 2009; 76:350-354.

[62] Rini BI, Escudier B, Tomczak P, et al: Comparative effectiveness of axitinib versus sorafenib in advanced renal cell carcinoma (AXIS): a randomised phase 3 trial. Lancet. 2011 [Epub ahead of print].

5

Steroid Receptors in Renal Cell Carcinoma

Evgeny Yakirevich, Andres Matoso,
David J. Morris and Murray B. Resnick
Department of Pathology and Laboratory Medicine, Rhode Island Hospital and Alpert Medical School of Brown University, USA

1. Introduction

Renal cell carcinomas (RCCs) are the most common epithelial neoplasms of adult kidney. It has been estimated that there will be about 60,920 new cases of kidney cancer in the United States in 2011 and about 13,120 people will die from this disease (Siegel et al. 2011). Currently, surgery remains the only effective treatment for RCC, since metastatic disease is highly resistant to radiotherapy and chemotherapy. Approximately 20 to 30% of patients with RCCs present with non-resectable metastatic disease and 20 to 40% of patients undergoing nephrectomy for clinically localized RCC will develop metastatic disease. In the past two decades significant advances in the diagnosis and treatment of patients with RCC have resulted in improved survival of a select group of patients. Prior to the availability of targeted therapies, Interferon-α (IFN) was the standard of care but was associated with a low response rate and significant toxicity (Interferon-alpha and survival in metastatic renal carcinoma: early results of a randomized controlled trial. Medical Research Council Renal Cancer Collaborators 1999). High dose interleukin-2 (IL-2) has a similar response rate as IFN, but can cure approximately 3-5% of patients (Yang, Sherry, et al. 2003). Targeted molecular therapies include inhibitors of angiogenesis (Yang, Haworth, et al. 2003), inhibitors of receptor tyrosine kinases with promiscuous targets including VEGFR1 and VEGFR2, PDGFR, C-Kit, Raf kinase, mammalian target of rapamycin (mTOR) (Atkins et al. 2004; Motzer et al. 2006; Porta et al. 2011) and combination treatment modalities (Escudier et al. 2007; Hudes et al. 2007; Motzer et al. 2007). These novel therapies have demonstrated improved outcomes and have become the first line of therapy in patients with advanced metastatic disease or second line of therapy in patients who have failed prior cytokine immunotherapy (Leveridge & Jewett 2011). As new treatment modalities become standard of care, clinical practices in diagnosis and treatment of the primary tumor will undergo revision. For instance, the role of cytoreductive surgery in patients selected for targeted therapy has not yet been established. This could increase the number of cases diagnosed and treated based on core needle biopsies alone, presenting new challenges to surgical pathologists who will likely have to use smaller amounts of tissue to accurately classify the tumor and provide molecular information aimed to personalize clinical care.

RCC is a heterogeneous neoplasm, which includes distinct histological subtypes (Table 1). Among the adult population, clear cell RCC constitutes the most prevalent subtype (70-80%)

Histological Subtype	Incidence	5-Year Survival	Cell of Origin
Clear Cell RCC	70-80%	45-76%	Proximal convoluted tubules
Papillary RCC	10-15%	82-90%	Shared phenotype of proximal and distal tubules
Chromophobe RCC	5%	78-92%	Intercalated cells of collecting tubules and ducts
Oncocytoma	5%	100%	Intercalated cells of collecting tubules and ducts

Table 1. Major Histological Subtypes of Renal Cell Neoplasms with Corresponding Incidence, Survival, and Cell of Origin

and has a relatively unfavorable prognosis (Amin et al. 2002; Eble et al. 2004). Papillary and chromophobe RCCs are less common, comprising 10-15% and 5%, respectively, and have a better prognosis compared to clear cell RCC (Amin et al. 2002). Oncocytoma is a benign renal cell tumor characterized by an extremely favorable prognosis. Renal epithelial tumors are thought to originate in cells of different compartments along the nephron. Clear cell RCC is believed to arise from the proximal tubules. Tumors that originate in the collecting tubules and ducts include chromophobe RCC, oncocytomas, and the more rare collecting duct and medullary carcinomas. The histogenesis of papillary carcinoma is controversial with some studies suggesting a proximal tubule origin while phenotyping by immunohistochemistry supports a distal nephron origin. Renal tumors with papillary growth include papillary RCC types 1 and 2, clear cell RCC with papillary features and the recently described clear cell papillary RCC (CPRCC) (Gobbo et al. 2008). CPRCC is a subtype of renal cell carcinoma characterized by cells with clear cytoplasm arranged in papillary structures which was first described in patients with end stage renal disease, but later also identified in kidneys unaffected by end stage renal disease (Fuzesi et al. 1999; Gobbo et al. 2008).

Immunohistochemistry is useful in distinguishing the different subtypes of renal neoplasms. Clear cell RCCs are frequently CD10 positive but AMACR and CK7 negative; papillary carcinoma, on the other hand, is positive for CK7 and AMACR and usually negative for CD10. Recent studies in CPRCC demonstrate positive immunoreactivity for CK7 but negative AMACR and CD10. These and other immunohistochemical markers are currently used routinely in diagnostic histopathology to help classify tumors. However, this is a constantly evolving field and new immunohistochemical and molecular markers are being investigated to address new clinical needs.

Steroid receptors are a family of ligand dependent transcription factors, which have important roles in control of growth and differentiation in many non-neoplastic and neoplastic cell types. The steroid receptor family is characterized by a unique modular structure, with receptors classically divided into three main domains and several

Steroid Receptor	Expression in Normal Kidney	Tumor Type	Clinical Relevance	References
GR	Proximal tubules, glomeruli	Clear cell RCC	Increased expression is a favorable marker	Yakirevich et al. 2011
MR	Distal tubules, loops of Henle and collecting ducts	Oncocytoma and chromophobe RCC	Diagnostic marker	Yakirevich et al. 2008
ER	Interstitial stromal cells	Cystic nephroma, mixed epithelial and stromal tumor, angiomyolipoma with epithelial cysts	Hormonal mechanism of pathogenesis	Adsay et al. 2000
PR	Interstitial stromal cells	Cystic nephroma, mixed epithelial and stromal tumor, angiomyolipoma with epithelial cysts, chromophobe RCC and oncocytoma	Hormonal mechanism of pathogenesis Diagnostic marker	Adsay et al. 2000 Tickoo et al. 2008 Mai et al. 2008
AR	Proximal and distal tubules	Clear cell, papillary, and chromophobe RCC	Increased expression is a favorable marker	Kimura et al 1993 Langner et al, 2004
VDR	Distal tubules and collecting ducts	Papillary RCC, chromophobe RCC, oncocytoma, collecting duct carcinoma	Diagnostic marker	Obara, Konda et al. 2007 Liu et al. 2006
RAR and RXR	Proximal tubules, interstitial cells	Clear cell RCC, chromophobe RCC (RAR-β)	Increased expression of RXR-γ is a favorable marker	Goelden et al. 2005 Obara, Konda et al. 2007

Table 2. Steroid Receptors in Renal Cell Neoplasms

subdomains or regions. In general, the receptor members share a variable amino-terminal transactivation domain, a central and well-conserved DNA-binding domain (DBD), and a moderately conserved carboxy-terminal domain responsible for ligand binding. The latter domain also contains activating functions. The well known members of the steroid receptor family includes glucocorticoid (GR), mineralocorticoid (MR), progesterone (PR), androgen (AR), estrogen (ER), vitamin D (VDR), thyroid, and retinoic acid (RAR)/retinoid X receptors (RXR) (Fuller 1991).

There is emerging evidence that steroid receptors can induce gene expression through both ligand-dependent and ligand-independent pathways, and distinct families of genes are likely to be regulated depending on the mechanism of nuclear receptor signaling. Until recently, the study of steroid receptors in renal cell neoplasm's (RCNs) has been limited to ER and PR. The employment of novel techniques for studying steroid receptors in RCCs, such as immunohistochemistry, tissue microarray technology, and quantitative real-time PCR has revealed the presence and biologic importance of several steroid receptors in RCNs, including GR, MR, VDR, and others (Table 2). This review will focus on histogenetic, diagnostic, and prognostic implications of steroid receptor expression in RCNs.

2. Glucocorticoid receptor

Glucocorticoids mediate their effects via their intracellular glucocorticoid receptors. Studies of GRs have revealed that there is only one GR gene, but several GR receptor isoforms resulting from alternative splicing or alternative translation initiation (Pujols et al. 2002; Revollo & Cidlowski 2009). Two main human isoforms, GR-α and GR-β, have a different distribution pattern and biologic activity in healthy and diseased human cells and tissues. It has been demonstrated that GR-α is the predominant isoform expressed in a large number of healthy human tissues including brain, liver, kidney, skeletal muscle, lung, and other organs. The GR- α isoform possesses steroid binding activity. In contrast, GR-β expression level is lower than that of the GR- α isoform and is relatively abundant in inflammatory blood cells (Pujols et al. 2002). In non-activated cells, the GR resides in the cytoplasm as a part of a large complex consisting of chaperone and cochaperone proteins including heat shock proteins hsp90, hsp70, immunophilins FKBP51 and FKBP52, and others (De Bosscher et al. 2003). Upon ligand binding, GR undergoes phosphorylation and activation and translocates from the cytoplasm to the nucleus where it converts to a DNA-binding form. Transcriptional responses triggered by activated GR include both positive and negative gene regulation. The direct positive transcriptional regulation of genes (transactivation) requires binding of the GR homodimer to glucocorticoid-response elements (GRE) in gene promoters. The indirect negative regulation (transrepression) is mediated through negative cross-talk with other transcription factors including AP-1, NF-kB and p53 (Beato et al. 1995). As a result, glucocorticoids modulate a variety of physiologic and pathologic processes, including among others cellular differentiation, growth, inflammation, immune response, and carbohydrate metabolism.

2.1 Expression of GR in the normal kidney

In normal human kidneys GRs contribute to the regulation of renal fluid and electrolyte homeostasis. Keeping with their physiologic function, GRs are differentially distributed along the kidney nephron. *In vitro* studies have implicated GRs in the regulation of ammoniagenesis, gluconeogenesis, GFR, Na-H exchange and Na-phosphate co-transport, all of which are proximal renal tubule processes (Baylis et al. 1990; Boross et al. 1986; Campen et al. 1983; Freiberg et al. 1982). Measurement of GRs in normal rat kidney cortical tubules enriched in proximal tubules yielded three to six fold higher GR content as compared to the distal tubules (Mishina et al. 1981). Predominant proximal tubule localization of GR was demonstrated by quantitation of GR mRNA levels in microdissected nephron segments from the rat kidney by a competitive polymerase chain reaction (PCR) technique (Todd-Turla et al. 1993). GR mRNA was twofold more abundant in glomeruli, proximal tubule, and thick ascending limb segments than in the collecting duct segments (Todd-Turla et al. 1993). In an additional study GR mRNA was localized by in-situ hybridization predominantly to renal proximal tubules and cortical collecting tubules with lower levels in distal collecting tubules of the rat kidney (Roland et al. 1995). In a recent study we provided immunohistochemical evidence of GR expression in the proximal tubular epithelium of normal human kidneys and in the epithelial cells of normal renal glomeruli (Yakirevich et al. 2011). However, several *in vitro* and *in vivo* studies have demonstrated that glucocorticoids can exert mineralocorticoid-like effects, such as Na+ reabsorption and K+ secretion, in the distal nephron (Morris & Souness 1992; Naray-Fejes-Toth & Fejes-Toth 1990; Thomas et al. 2006).

2.2 Expression of GR in kidney tumors

Initial studies of GR expression in RCCs based on ligand-binding assays in the early 1980's demonstrated the presence of GRs in kidney tumors (Bojar et al. 1979; Chen et al. 1980; Hemstreet et al. 1980; Liu et al. 1980). In these pioneer studies renal tumors were not subdivided into different histologic subtypes and were all designated as RCCs. Bojar et al. demonstrated GRs in 10 of 15 tumors studied (Bojar et al. 1979). The average dexamethasone binding capacity was calculated and found to be 7.1 fmol/mg of cytosol protein. The ligand specificity experiments clearly indicated that binding to GRs is not restricted to glucocorticoids alone. Progesterone and aldosterone turned out to be moderate competitors for dexamethasone binding. Medroxyprogesterone acetate, the compound widely used in hormone therapy of advanced renal cancer in man, was demonstrated to be one of the strongest inhibitors of [3H] dexamethasone. The binding of medroxyprogesterone acetate to GRs may represent the primary mechanism of action of the compound in causing tumor regression. Hemstreet et al. identified and measured the levels of GRs in 47 autologous pairs of normal and neoplastic renal tissue (Hemstreet et al. 1980). Glucocorticoid receptors were demonstrated in this study in normal and neoplastic tissues of both sexes. The levels of GRs were higher in the tumors (mean 31.3 fmol/mg) than in the normal tissue (18.5 fmol/mg). In an additional study conducted at the same time, Liu et al. reported high concentrations of GRs in four of seven RCC cases (Liu et al. 1980). The levels of GRs in RCCs were comparable to those in the glucocorticoid-responsive rat liver. Furthermore, the GR levels in RCCs were comparable to human acute lymphocytic leukemia cells sensitive (0.03 pmol/mg cytosol protein), in contrast to those that have become resistant (0.015 pmol/mg cytosol protein) to glucocorticoids. Chen et al. detected GRs in cytosol of RCCs (Chen et al. 1980). Competition experiments demonstrated that progestin competed for the GR sites in all renal tumors tested, whereas diethylstilbestrol and testosterone were weak or not competitive.

Development of antibodies against human GR enabled immunohistochemical and Western blot assessment of GR protein expression. In addition, molecular studies utilizing reverse transcriptase polymerase chain reaction (RT-PCR) revealed that most commonly used RCC cell lines express high levels of GR. In a study by Arai et al., two RCC cell lines OUR-10 and NC65 expressed high levels of GR, whereas Caki-1 cell exhibited low levels of GR expression by Western blot (Arai et al. 2008). Iwai et al. demonstrated GR mRNA expression in the A498, RCC270, Caki1, and ACHN renal carcinoma cells. A498 and RCC270 expressed especially high levels of the GR gene (Iwai et al. 2004). Recently, using tissue microarray technology and real-time RT-PCR we described the immunohistochemical and mRNA expression of GRs in different histologic subtypes of RCNs including clear cell RCC, papillary RCC, chromophobe RCC, and oncocytoma (Yakirevich et al. 2011). We found that GRs are strongly expressed in the majority of clear cell RCCs (66%), in 26% of papillary RCCs, and in only 6% of chromophobe RCC and 14% of oncocytomas. Within the clear cell carcinoma group, most positive cases (87%) demonstrated strong expression, whereas only 1 papillary RCC, 1 chromophobe RCC and none of the oncocytomas demonstrated strong immunoreactivity. In this study we used commercially available rabbit-antihuman GR polyclonal antibody PA1-511A from Affinity Bioreagents (Golden, CO) which recognizes both the -α and -β isoforms of GR. In order to recognize specific isoform expressed in RCC, we measured both isoforms by quantitative real-time PCR and demonstrated that RCCs express GR-α isoform. We found that GR expression is associated with tumors of low nuclear grade (Fuhrman grade 1 and 2) and low stage (stage 1 and 2). Although GR expression was demonstrated predominantly in clear cell RCC group, the loss of GR expression in high-grade tumors and overlap with other histologic subtypes of RCCs limit the diagnostic utility of this marker. GR appears to be a marker of less aggressive behavior in RCC as there is significant correlation between GR expression and overall survival in RCC. By the end of follow-up 86% of CRCC patients with tumors expressing GRs were alive as compared to 54% of patients whose tumors were negative.

Since GRs are cytoplasmic receptors, which are translocated to the nuclei upon activation, the predominantly nuclear immunoreactivity of GRs suggests that these receptors are activated in RCCs. Association of GR expression with less aggressive behavior also suggests the tumor-suppressive role of GRs. Signaling through GRs in renal cancer cells involves suppression of other transcription factors, including nuclear factor *k*B, AP-1, CREB, CCAAT enhancer binding protein (C/EBP), signal transduction activator of transcription (STAT), p53, Smad, *etc* (De Bosscher et al. 2003). Treatment of RCC cell lines with glucocorticoids (dexamethasone) inhibits the activation of nuclear factor kB and its downstream products including IL-2, IL-6, IL-8, and vascular endothelial growth factor which have been demonstrated to promote growth of RCC cell lines (Arai et al. 2008; Iwai et al. 2004; Miki et al. 1989; Takenawa et al. 1995). Glucocorticoids have long been used as anti-inflammatory drugs, and have been beneficial in the treatment of hematopoietic neoplasms (multiple myeloma) and solid malignancies such as hormone-refractory prostate cancer (Greenstein et al. 2002; Storlie et al. 1995). Although glucocorticoids have not been implicated in the treatment of patients with renal cancer, there are few case reports describing the beneficial effects of incidental glucocorticoid treatment in metastatic RCC (Christophersen et al. 2006; Omland & Fossa 1989; Tanaka et al. 2003). Palliation treatment with oral dexamethasone was associated with complete regression of pulmonary and brain metastases (Omland & Fossa 1989). In another case, multiple lung and bone metastases of RCC completely regressed after palliative treatment with betamethasone (Tanaka et al. 2003). A 10 year complete remission of metastatic RCC to the liver and retroperitoneal lymph nodes was described in a patient who received palliative cortisone therapy (Christophersen et al. 2006). The mechanism of metastases regression in these cases is unknown and is not likely to be immune related, because glucocorticoids are known to suppress the immune system. These observations suggest that GR and its agonists may have a potential role in novel anti-cancer hormonal therapies in clear cell RCC.

3. Mineralocorticoid receptor

The mineralocorticoid receptor (MR) has long been considered as a secondary glucocorticoid receptor, even though specific roles of its natural ligand, aldosterone, have been well established since the purification of electrocortin more than 50 years ago. Aldosterone was initially restricted to the control of sodium reabsorption in the kidney, thereby being recognized as a major regulator of volume status and blood pressure. The cloning of a specific receptor for aldosterone (Arriza et al. 1987) definitively moved MR out of the shadow of GR and opened a new era of exciting biological, biochemical, and genetic studies that have provided important insights into the complexity of MR action. The MR is closely related to GR and is 94% homologous in the DNA binding domain and 57% homologous in the ligand binding domain, but only 15% homologous in the N-terminal region (Evans 1988). The MR has a similar affinity for the mineralocorticoid aldosterone and the glucocorticoids corticosterone and cortisol (Krozowski & Funder 1983). Although rats and mice synthesize only corticosterone, cortisol is the predominant glucocorticoid in humans and many other mammals, including rodents. Since the circulating levels of glucocorticoids are several orders of magnitude higher than those of aldosterone, the primary mineralocorticoid, glucocorticoid activation of MR may be functionally significant. Specificity is conferred by the enzyme 11β-hydroxysteroid dehydrogenase type II (11β-HSD2) which converts the cortisol to the less active compound cortisone, thus allowing aldosterone binding to MR. In the absence of ligand, MRs are located in both the cytosol and nucleus bound by a variety of chaperone proteins, including hsp90. Upon exposure to either aldosterone or corticosterone, most MRs are found in the nucleus, where they bind to hormone-response elements and mediate gene expression of signaling proteins regulating water and electrolyte transport including K-ras, serine-threonine kinase Sgk1, and corticosteroid hormone-induced factor (Connell & Davies 2005). The most recent role of aldosterone in renal and cardiac fibrosis has indicated a pro-fibrotic role for MR and the product of 11β-HSD2, cortisone or 11-dehydro-corticosterone in the regulation of this process (Brem et al.).

3.1 Expression of MR in the normal kidney

In contrast to GRs which are expressed in a broad variety of cells, expression of MRs is restricted to fewer cell types. The MR is expressed in so-called "classical" aldosterone target tissues, which are sodium-transporting epithelia (kidney, colon, pancreas, salivary, and sweat glands) and in a variety of non-epithelial target tissues such as the central nervous system, mononuclear lymphocytes, large blood vessels, and the heart (Arriza et al. 1987; Sasano et al. 1992). A general agreement exists that the distal nephron is an aldosterone-specific target site. Specific nuclear binding sites for aldosterone exist from the thick ascending limb of Henle's loop (cortical part) to the distal collecting duct in rabbit and rat kidneys (Farman & Bonvalet 1983; Farman et al. 1982). MR is expressed in the distal tubules, the connecting tubules, and along the collecting ducts at the mRNA level in rat and rabbit kidneys (Escoubet et al. 1996; Todd-Turla et al. 1993) and at the protein level in rabbit kidneys (Lombes et al. 1990). Immunohistochemical studies showed that in normal human kidney MR is expressed in the distal convoluted tubules, collecting ducts, and loops of Henle with predominant nuclear localization (Hirasawa et al. 1997; Sasano et al. 1992; Yakirevich et al. 2008).

3.2 Expression of MR in kidney tumors

More than 30 years ago Rafestin-Oblin et al. demonstrated the presence of high-affinity sites for aldosterone in normal human kidneys using a ligand-binding assay. In RCCs the cytosol and nuclear aldosterone binding was significantly lower than in normal tissues (Rafestin-Oblin et al. 1979). However, this study focused exclusively on clear cell RCCs. Recently using immunohistochemistry we analyzed tissue microarray specimens from patients with different histologic subtypes of renal cell neoplasms, and in addition, we quantitated MR mRNA by real time RT-PCR (Yakirevich et al. 2008). Most of the chromophobe RCC (90%) and oncocytomas (93%) strongly expressed MR. No MR immunoreactivity was detected in clear cell RCC, including clear cell carcinoma with predominantly granular cytoplasm, or in papillary RCC. The MR+ immunophenotype of chromophobe carcinoma and oncocytoma reflects their histogenetic origin from phenotypically similar distal convoluted tubules and collecting ducts, whereas absence of immunoreactivity in clear cell RCC is consistent with its origin from proximal convoluted tubules. As we described in the previous section, proximal tubules and histogenetically related clear cell RCCs express high levels of GR. MR appears to be a sensitive and specific marker of the distal nephron and its related neoplasms (chromophobe RCC and oncocytoma) and may be considered in the immunohistochemical panel to more accurately subtype renal cell tumors.

4. Estrogen receptor

The effects of estrogens are mediated by estrogen receptors (ERs). ERs were discovered in the 1960's by Jensen and Jacobson (Jensen et al. 2010). The basic structure of ER protein is similar to other steroid receptors and contains a DNA binding domain, transcription modulating domain, and steroid hormone binding domain. There are two ER types encoded on different chromosomes: ER-α cloned in 1986 and ER-β, which was discovered in 1996 (Greene et al. 1986; Kuiper et al. 1996). ER-α is expressed in a variety of human organs, mainly reproductive, including the mammary gland, ovary, uterus, and vagina (Muramatsu & Inoue 2000). ER-β is expressed in genitourinary human tissues such as prostate, ovary, testis, bladder, uterus, and renal pelvis, in the central nervous system, and is especially increased compared to ER-α in various fetal tissues such as adrenals (Gustafsson 1999). The affinity of ER-β to bind estradiol-17β is similar to the ER-α form. However, ER-β binds both androgens and phytoestrogens with greater affinity. The main physiologic role of ERs is implicated in the control of proliferation, differentiation, and development of many tissues. In contrast to the beneficial physiologic effects, ERs may also promote the development and growth of variety of cancers, including breast, endometrial and ovarian carcinomas in humans (Speirs et al. 1999) and renal tumors in Syrian hamsters (Li et al. 2001).

4.1 Expression of ER in the normal kidney

Expression of ERs was extensively studied in hamster kidneys; however, the distribution of ER in normal hamster kidney is controversial. In a study by Bhat et al. who treated hamsters with estradiol to induce tumors, ER immunolocalization in normal kidneys of estrogen-treated hamsters or in untreated controls was identified only in the renal glomerular pododcytes, mesangial and parietal cells and in several interstitial cell types but not in the tubular epithelia of the cortex (Bhat et al. 1993). In addition, arterial cells, including pericytes and endothelial cells of the arteriolae rectae and endothelial cells of the arterial vasa recta, strongly expressed ER. The receptor distribution in kidneys of untreated female hamsters matched that of males, but the intensity of staining was higher than in male kidneys. Another study confirmed immunohistochemical expression of ER in interstitial cells and localized these cells to the corticomedullary junction (Li et al. 2001). The authors found that estrogen treatment causes a significant increase in ER-α positive interstitial cells compared to untreated controls and hypothesized that renal tumors arise from a subset of multipotential interstitial cells driven to proliferate by estrogens. However, in contrast to the study by Bhat et al., in this study ER expression was consistently demonstrated in nuclei of proximal tubules and disappeared after estrogen treatment.

4.2 Expression of ER in kidney tumors

Initial biochemical studies of ER status in renal tumors were performed in early 1980s by the dextran-coated charcoal method and the sucrose gradient centrifugation assay. These biochemical assays were based on cytosol preparations containing high, but unknown levels of plasma contamination. Furthermore, there was significant inconsistency in the number of tumor cells present within the specimens (Karr et al. 1983). Therefore, the level and frequency of ER expression in human kidney tumors were highly variable. Hemstreet et al. reported detectable ERs in 30% of the tumors compared to 40% of normals, whereas in other studies utilizing similar biochemical techniques ERs were not detected or detected in a rather low percentage of 4-9% of tumors (Hemstreet et al. 1980; Karr et al. 1983; Pearson et al. 1981). In a more recent immunohistochemical analysis of steroid hormone expression in tissue microarrays containing 182 RCCs of different histologic subtypes, Langer et al. demonstrated ER immunoreactivity in less than 10% of tumor cells in only 2 of 182 of patients (1.1%), including one clear cell RCC and one chromophobe RCC (Langner et al. 2004). Thus, the biochemical and immunohistochemical results provide evidence that ER is not expressed or very rare expressed in low levels in RCCs.

Recently, several benign renal tumors, characterized by the presence of stroma that resembles ovarian, endometrial, and mullerian-like, have been described, including cystic nephroma, mixed epithelial and stromal tumor (MEST) and angiomyolipomas with epithelial cysts (AMLEC) (Fine et al. 2006; Turbiner et al. 2007). Adsay et al. detected ERs in nuclei of the spindle cells in seven of 12 MESTs (Adsay et al. 2000). The staining was strong and diffuse and was present predominantly in the areas with long, slender, fibrocyte-like cells. In three of these cases, the epithelial cells also exhibited a cytoplasmic reaction with antibody to ER. Distinctive clinical and pathologic features characterize these lesions. Most of the patients in study of Adsay et al. were middle-aged (perimenopausal) females (mean age, 56 years) who had a long-term history of estrogen use. The only male patient also had a history of diethylstilbestrol exposure for 7 years followed by 4 years of lupron therapy for prostatic adenocarcinoma. These clinical findings, combined with frequent ER expression detected by immunohistochemistry raise the possibility of hormonal mechanism of pathogenesis of these tumors. It is plausible that the spindle cells of these tumors arise from a "periductal fetal mesenchyma" present in epithelial structures of organs such as kidney, pancreas, and liver. The primitive mesenchyme may have the capacity to interact with epithelia. Alterations of hormonal milieu (perimenopausal changes or therapeutic hormones with unopposed estrogens) may induce proliferation of this mesenchyme, which in turn activates the growth of epithelial component.

5. Progesterone receptor

The progesterone receptor (PR) has two predominant isoforms: PR-α, and PR-β, which are produced from a single gene by alternative promoter usage (Jeltsch et al. 1986). These isoforms have similar steroid hormone and DNA binding activities, but PR-β has a much higher transcriptional activating potential. Clinically, PR expression is routinely assessed by immunohistochemistry using an antibody that recognizes both PR-α and PR-β.

5.1 Expression of PR in the normal kidney

No detectable PR staining was seen in renal sections from untreated castrated male hamsters in a study by Bhat et al. (Bhat et al. 1993). However, after estrogen treatment, PR expression was detected in single interstitial cells. The pattern of PR immunoreactivity was largely confined to interstitial cells located at the renal corticomedullary region, similar to ER expressing cells described above. PRs were identified in normal human kidneys by biochemical and more recently immunohistochemical techniques (Hemstreet et al. 1980; McDonald et al. 1983). Interesting, in normal human kidneys PRs were detected by immunohistochemistry in interstitial stromal cells, some tubules, and mesangial cells of glomeruli in two of seven cases (Tickoo et al. 2008).

5.2 Expression of PR in kidney tumors

Expression of PR in kidney tumors was studied in parallel with ER analysis. The level and frequency of PR in human kidney tumors is highly variable when analyzed biochemically varying from 0 to 23% (Hemstreet et al. 1980; Karr et al. 1983; Pearson et al. 1981). Immunohistochemical analysis of steroid hormone expression in tissue microarrays containing 182 RCCs of different histologic subtypes demonstrated PR immunoreactivity in less than 10% of tumor cells in only two of 182 patients, including one clear cell RCC and one papillary RCC (Langner et al. 2004). PRs were found in stromal cells of renal neoplasms with ovarian-like stroma, although less frequently as compared to ER (Adsay et al. 2000). More recently Mai et al. identified PR immunoreactivity of tumor cells and stromal cells within the neoplasm and/or surrounding capsule in renal oncocytoma and chromophobe RCC (Mai et al. 2008). This immunoreactivity was not seen in other tumors with oncocytic/eosinophilic cytoplasm, such as papillary RCC with eosinophilc cytoplasm or clear cell RCC with eosinophilic cytoplasm. PR appears to be a sensitive and highly specific marker for renal oncocytoma and a highly specific marker for chromophobe RCC. It was demonstrated that PR immunoreactivity is more extensive in oncocytoma than in chromophobe RCC, therefore, the extent of PR immunoreactivity could be useful in distinguishing oncocytoma from chromophobe RCC. The presence of PR in oncocytoma and chromophobe RCC provides additional support to the histopathogenetic relationship between renal oncocytoma and chromophobe RCC.

6. Androgen receptor

Androgens are essential for differentiation and growth of male reproductive organs and for various biological effects in the kidney, brain, liver, muscle, bone and skin. Androgens include testosterone and dihydrotestosterone and mediate their biologic effect through the androgen receptor (AR). The *AR* gene is located on chromosome Xq11-12 (Brown et al. 1989; Lubahn et al. 1988). Males have a single copy of the gene allowing phenotypic manifestation of any genetic alteration. Transcription of the *AR* gene is cell-specific and modified by age, androgen and other steroid hormones (Gelmann 2002). Androgen is best known to influence development and growth of prostate cancer. However, its metabolic role in cancer is not limited to the prostate and a number of studies utilizing animal models combined with clinical and epidemiologic data suggest a role for androgen in RCC (Concolino, Marocchi, Conti et al. 1978; Karr et al. 1983).

6.1 Expression of AR in the normal kidney

AR is ubiquitously expressed in the whole body with studies showing detectable levels of protein and mRNA in adrenal glands, uterus, aorta, adipose tissue, kidney, spleen, heart, lung, large intestine, stomach, small intestine and liver (Kimura et al. 1993; Ruizeveld de Winter et al. 1991; Takeda et al. 1990). In normal kidneys AR expression was consistently demonstrated to be present in the nuclei of distal tubule cells (Kimura et al. 1993; Li et al. 2010). Additionally, a study by Takeda et al. showed AR immunoreactivity not only in the distal tubule but also in the proximal tubule and focal parietal expression in the Bowman's capsule (Takeda et al. 1990).

6.2 Expression of AR in kidney tumors

The hormone dependence of RCC has been established in animal models and in humans for many years (Bloom 1973; Concolino, Marocchi, Conti et al. 1978; Concolino, Marocchi, Tenaglia et al. 1978; Li et al. 1977). In humans, extensive research on AR in RCC has shown variable results (Concolino et al. 1981; Jakse & Muller-Holzner 1988; Karr et al. 1983; Klotzl et al. 1987; Nakano et al. 1984; Noronha & Rao 1985) In a case series study by Brown et al., that included 12 primary clear cell RCCs and 5 clear cell RCCs metastatic to the central nervous system, AR immunoreactivity was present in five primary and one metastatic RCC (Brown et al. 1998). A more recent study by Langner et al. demonstrated that AR immunoreactivity was not detectable in non-tumoral kidney tissue (Langner et al. 2004). However, AR was found in 15% of patients with RCC and inversely correlated with histopathologic stage, with 27% of pT1 tumors being positive versus 4% of pT3 tumors. Furthermore, expression of AR was higher in pT1a tumors compared to pT1b (32% vs. 17%). Additionally, AR expression inversely correlated with nuclear grade with 21% positivity in nuclear grades 1 and 2 and 7% in nuclear grades 3 and 4. Univariate analysis showed a longer disease free survival in patients with AR positive tumors compared to patients with

AR negative tumors (Langner et al. 2004). These results reflect similar trends observed with GRs in RCC (Yakirevich et al. 2011), however, the diagnostic, prognostic or therapeutic utility of AR analysis in RCC is uncertain and might require further investigations.

7. Vitamin D receptor

Vitamin D is a lipid-soluble compound whose major function is the maintenance of adequate plasma levels of calcium and phosphorus, important for bone mineralization, neuromuscular transmission and general cellular metabolism. Vitamin D receptor (VDR) is present in various tissues that do not participate in calcium metabolism and regulates the expression of hundreds of genes that control cell proliferation, differentiation and angiogenesis. Low levels of vitamin D have been associated with increased incidence of colon, prostate and breast cancer (Thacher & Clarke 2011). Recent studies suggest that vitamin D may be inversely associated with the risk of RCC. (Bosetti et al. 2007; Ikuyama et al. 2002; Karami et al. 2008; Obara, Suzuki et al. 2007). Vitamin D receptor is expressed in malignant tumors, including RCC, and mediates the biological actions of $1,25(OH)_2D_3$ (Lamprecht & Lipkin 2003). In this section, we will review the current literature on the relevance of vitamin D and its receptor in RCC.

7.1 Expression of VDR in the normal kidney

The kidney is a major organ for vitamin D metabolism and calcium homeostasis. Activation of vitamin D involves conversion of 7-dehydrocholesterol to cholecalciferol by UVB radiation in the skin. Cholecalciferol is metabolized by the 25-hydroxylases (CYP2R1 and CYP27A1) in the liver to 25-hydroxycholecalciferol ($25(OH)D_3$). $25(OH)D_3$ then undergoes glomerular filtration and is subsequently converted to the active form calcitriol ($1,25(OH)_2D_3$) by the 1α-hydroxylase (CYP27B1) located primarily in the proximal tubule. Calcitriol binds to an intracellular receptor (VDR), a ligand dependent transcription factor belonging to the class II nuclear receptor subfamily. The effect of calcitriol is negatively controlled by CYP24A1 (Fleet 2008; Nykjaer et al. 1999). Immunohistochemistry studies of non-tumoral kidney show expression of VDR predominantly in the distal tubules and collecting ducts with only faint or lack of stain in the proximal tubule cells (Blomberg Jensen et al. 2010; Liu et al. 2006; Obara, Konda et al. 2007). This expression pattern is consistent with studies that demonstrate that vitamin-D induced calcium re-absorption occurs in the distal tubules (Li & Christakos 1991).

7.2 Expression of VDR in kidney tumors

In keeping with absence of VDR expression in the proximal tubule, a study by Liu et al. showed that clear cell RCC is generally negative for VDR by immunohistochemistry and showed decreased mRNA level compared to non-tumoral kidney control tissue by RT-PCR (Liu et al. 2006). When whole sections of tumors were stained, expression of VDR was present only focally in the peripheral region of the tumor. Previously, a study by Madej et al. showed that expression of VDR in clear cell RCC was similar to control tissue by Western and Northern blot analysis (Madej et al. 2003). This discrepancy could be due to a difference in the degree of differentiation of the tumors analyzed in each study. While the expression level seems not to be affected by the Fuhrman nuclear grade, increased VDR immunoreactivity was observed in sarcomatous and poorly differentiated areas of RCC and in metastatic tumors or in intravascular tumor islands (Liu et al. 2006).

A different study by Blomberg Jensen et al. showed that VDR mRNA was detected in all normal kidney samples while almost undetectable in clear cell RCC with similar results confirmed by Western blot (Blomberg Jensen et al. 2010). Additionally, in this study, the authors investigated the expression of Vitamin D activating enzymes including CYP2R1, CYP27A1, and CYP27B1. The 1 α-hydroxylase (CYP27B1) was present in all normal samples with varying degrees of expression levels, the lowest expression in atrophic kidneys. By immunohistochemistry and in-situ hybridization, expression of CYP2R1 and CYP27A1 was localized to the distal tubule, collecting ducts and minimal expression in the proximal tubule. Expression of CYP27B1 was more prominent in the proximal tubule. Expression of these enzymes was diminished in clear cell RCC along with decreased expression of VDR (Blomberg Jensen et al. 2010). Papillary RCC is positive for VDR in the great majority of cases. This recapitulates more closely the phenotype of distal tubules. Similarly, chromophobe carcinoma and oncocytomas are also positive for VDR. Staining of chromophobe carcinoma accentuates the cell membrane while in oncocytomas it is stronger in the perinuclear area (Liu et al. 2006). Collecting duct carcinoma is thought to derive from the principal cells of the collecting duct of Bellini. Consistent with other tumors of origin from the distal nephron, three out of three collecting duct carcinomas tested were positive for VDR by immunohistochemistry (Liu et al. 2006).

Currently, immunohistochemistry for vitamin D is not routinely used for diagnostic purposes. However, several findings described above could eventually prove to have diagnostic utility in anatomic pathology. Because almost all clear cell RCC proved to be negative by immunohistochemistry (with the exception of some high grade tumors, or tumor present within vascular lumens), a positive VDR immunohistochemistry result should alert the pathologist about a potential problem in the classification of a tumor thought to be clear cell RCC (Liu et al. 2006).

A frequent problem in the diagnosis of renal tumors is the distinction between oncocytomas and eosinophilic chromophobe carcinoma (Takahashi et al. 2003; Young et al. 2001). This distinction is critical as these tumors have completely different prognostic and therapeutic clinical implications. Results reported in the literature indicate that both tumors are immunoreactive for VDR with a difference in the localization of the stain. While oncocytomas stained preferably in the perinuclear area, chromophobe carcinoma showed accentuated stain of the cell membrane (Liu et al. 2006).

Positive stain for VDR in papillary RCC could help differentiate this tumor from clear cell RCC with papillary features, which will be negative in the great majority of cases. VDR expression in CPRCC has not been tested; however, since these tumors are CK7 positive, it is likely that they are VDR positive as well, consistent with distal nephron phenotype. Only three cases of collecting duct carcinoma have been tested for VDR immunoreactivity and all of them turned positive. Differential diagnosis of these tumors could be challenging due to their infrequent presentations. Main differential diagnoses include adenocarcinoma or urothelial carcinoma with glandular differentiation. Although there is lack of information in the literature regarding expression of VDR receptor in urothelial carcinoma with glandular differentiation, studies on normal urothelium and urothelial neoplasms have shown consistent positivity for VDR for which it seems unlikely that it would have utility in the differential diagnosis on this context (Hermann & Andersen 1997; Konety et al. 2001).

The anti-cancer effect of vitamin D includes inhibition of cell proliferation and induction of apoptosis (Blutt et al. 2000; Rashid et al. 2001; Zhuang & Burnstein 1998). Expression of VDR as detected by immunohistochemistry was not associated with survival in a cohort of 68 RCC patients (Obara, Konda et al. 2007). This could be due to a small number of patients studied or secondary to other possible alterations within the signaling pathway that could interfere with the normal function of the receptor. Different studies have shown consistently that VDR-DNA complexes are decreased in RCC, even in the presence of exogenous vitamin D (Madej et al. 2003; Trydal et al. 1988). This functional impairment could be secondary to suboptimal VDR heterodimerization with its partners in tumor cells. Before binding to DNA, VDR heterodimerizes with retinoid X receptor (RXR), its obligate partner (Barsony & Prufer 2002; Prufer & Barsony 2002). Retinoid X receptors are part of the retinoic acid receptor systems and share with retinoic acid part of the signaling pathways. Notably, positive RXR-γ staining in RCC correlates with prolonged overall 5-years survival (Obara, Konda et al. 2007).

Calcitriol has anti-proliferative properties in a variety of malignant cell types (Getzenberg et al. 1997; Reichel et al. 1989). The anti-neoplastic activity of VDR ligands was first described in 1981 in a study showing differentiating properties of calcitriol in mouse myeloid leukemia cells (Abe et al. 1981). Since then, a number of studies have demonstrated the in-vitro and in-vivo anti-cancer potential of vitamin D in models of bladder, breast, colon, endometrium, lung, pancreas, prostate and squamous cell carcinoma, sarcomas of the soft tissues and bone, neuroblastoma, glioma, melanoma, and other malignancies (Beer & Myrthue 2004; Trump et al. 2004; Trump et al. 2006).

Calcitriol treatment of cells inhibited cell growth and clonogenicity of the RCC cell line derived from a pulmonary metastasis of RCC, (Nagakura et al. 1986). In a different study, BALB/c mice were inoculated with murine renal cancer Renca and graded doses of calcitriol were given intraperitoneally. Vitamin D inhibited tumor growth and prolonged the life span of Renca-bearing mice in a dose-dependent manner. Furthermore, vitamin D treated mice showed reduced pulmonary and hepatic metastates (Fujioka et al. 1998). Despite these and other promising results in cell culture and in murine models, the utility of vitamin D therapy in humans has been challenged by its hypercalcemic toxic effect (Fakih et al. 2007; Muindi et al. 2009). To try to bypass this toxicity, researchers have explored alternative vitamin D like molecules. A recent published study investigated the in-vitro and in-vivo effect of 1,25-dihydroxyvitamin D3-3-bromoacetate [1,25$(OH)_2$D3-3-BE], an alkylating derivative of 1,25$(OH)_2$D3 (Lambert et al. 2010). This study reports that 1,25$(OH)_2$D3-3-BE is significantly more potent than an equivalent concentration of 1,25$(OH)_2$D3 in inhibiting growth of A498 and Caki 1 human kidney cancer cells. The mechanisms behind cell growth inhibition of cell-cycle progression include downregulating cyclin A and induction of apoptosis through caspase activity. When compared to calcitriol, 1,25$(OH)_2$D3-3-BE was more potent at reducing tumor size, which was accompanied by an increase in apoptosis and reduction of cyclin A staining in the tumors. These results show a promising potential of vitamin D derived compounds as targeted therapy for RCC patients (Lambert et al. 2010).

8. Retinoic acid receptors

Retinoids are a family of molecules related to vitamin A that include retinoic acid (RA) and all-trans retinoid. Retinoids participate in diverse functions in many organ systems during development and in adulthood including vision, neural function and immune response. Extensive research also supports a role of retinoids in cell proliferation and differentiation through cell cycle signaling promoting block in G1 phase of cell cycle, by directly or indirectly modulating cyclins, CDKs, and cell-cycle inhibitors (Mongan & Gudas 2007; Tang & Gudas 2011). There are two distinct retinoid nuclear receptor systems, the RARs types -α, -β and -γ, and RXRs types -α, -β and -γ (Pemrick et al. 1994). RARs form heterodimers with RXRs and act by binding to retinoic acid response elements (RARE) located in the promoter regions of RA-target genes and modulate transcription rates (Altucci & Gronemeyer 2001). In addition to its role in senescence and cell differentiation, retinoic acid can follow an alternative pathway by binding to a so-called orphan nuclear receptor, PPAR-β/-δ to promote cell survival under certain conditions (Schug et al. 2007).

8.1 Expression of retinoic acid receptors in the normal kidney

Studies evaluating the expression of RARs and RXRs indicate that expression of a given receptor subtype is cell type specific and that retinoic acid effect in different cell types are linked to specific receptor type (Geradts et al. 1993; Kakizuka et al. 1991; Moasser et al. 1994; Moasser et al. 1995; Sheikh et al. 1994; Swisshelm et al. 1994). Information on expression of RARs in normal kidney derives primarily from normal controls used in studies for various purposes. RAR-β mRNA has consistently been found to be expressed in normal kidney tissue samples (Goelden et al. 2005; Vanderleede et al. 1995). Additionally, expression of RARs and RXRs were studied in podocytes, which expressed most isoforms of retinoic acid receptors (RAR) and RXRs with the exception of RXR-γ (He et al. 2007). Obara et al. detected expression of RXR-α and-γ in nuclei of proximal tubule cells, while RXR-β expression was present in proximal tubule cells and interstitial cells (Obara, Konda et al. 2007).

8.2 Expression of retinoic acid receptors in kidney tumors

Dysregulation of each RA receptor has been found in association with different types of cancer. RAR-α is dysregulated in acute promyelocytic leukemia (APL). Majority of APL cases present a chromosomal translocation that fuses the promyelocytic leukemia gene, *PML* and the *RAR-α* genes [t(15;17)(22;q11.2-12)] which can be effectively treated and cured with a combination of retinoid and chemotherapy. In contrast to RAR-α, RAR-β is involved in solid tumorigenesis including RCC (Argiles et al. 1994; Berg et al. 1999; Goelden et al. 2005; Hoffman et al. 1996). The RAR-β gene maps on the short arm of chromosome 3, a region frequently deleted in cancer (Houle et al. 1993). Several studies demonstrated decreased or undetectable levels of RAR-β mRNA in tissue or cell lines derived from different tumors including lung (Suh et al. 2002; Zhang et al. 1994), prostate (Nakayama et al. 2001), breast (Swisshelm et al. 1994), ovary (Sabichi et al. 1998), colon (Cote et al. 1998), head and neck

(Xu et al. 1994) and cervix (Geisen et al. 1997). RAR-β mRNA was decreased or not detectable in 11 of 12 RCC cell lines (Hoffman et al. 1996). These cell lines were either resistant or minimally inhibited when treated with 13-*cis*-RA (13-CRA). Conversely, chromophobe RCC shows much higher levels of expression of RAR-β with a ratio of tumor/normal of over 36 (Goelden et al. 2005). In clear cell RCC, immunoreactivity for RXR-α was observed in up to 70% of the cases, RXR-β was present in 47% of cases, and RXR-γ stain was seen in 85% of cases, in a study that included 49 CRCCs (Obara, Konda et al. 2007). Only expression of RXR-γ was found to correlate inversely with pathological and clinical stage. While all subtypes of RXRs showed variable nuclear or cytoplasmic stain, subcellular location did not correlate with any prognostic variables. Additionally, this study suggests a prolonged overall 5-year survival of patients with tumors that are RXR-γ positive (Obara, Konda et al. 2007).

In clinical trials, the effect of RA in RCC patients has been tested in patients with metastatic disease. A randomized clinical trial of 284 patients evaluated response to treatment with IFNα2a plus 13-cis-retinoic acid (13-CRA) or treatment with IFNα2a alone (Motzer et al. 2000). This study showed no difference in the overall survival but median duration of response (complete and partial combined) in the group treated with the combination was 33 months versus 22 months for the second group. Nineteen percent of patients treated with IFNα2a plus 13-CRA were progression-free at 24 months, compared with 10% of patients treated with IFNα2a alone (Motzer et al. 2000). However, a separate clinical trial that involved 320 patients concluded that progression-free and overall survival for patients with progressive metastatic RCC treated with IFNα2a plus 13-CRA were significantly longer compared with patients on IFN alone (Aass et al. 2005). Another clinical trial that included three different treatment regimens: *a*) triple combination of IL-2, IFNα2a, and fluorouracil; *b*) triple combination of group *a* and additional 13-CRA; *c*) control group treated with IFN-α and vinblastine. Progression-free and overall survival were significantly longer in groups *a* and *b* but there was no significant survival advantage for patients receiving 13-CRA (Atzpodien et al. 2004). These studies suggest that there is some beneficial effect of retinoids treatment, in at least a subset of patients with RCC.

9. Conclusion

Steroid receptors are differentially expressed in the normal kidney and in renal cell neoplasms. Several steroid receptors, such as MR, PR, and vitamin D receptor may be included in diagnostic immunohistochemical panels in order to more accurately subtype renal cell tumors. Although ER is not detected in significant amounts in RCCs, it is expressed by stromal cells in several benign renal neoplasms and may be involved in their pathogenesis. GR and AR appear to be markers of less aggressive behavior in clear cell RCC. Finally, steroid receptors and their downstream signaling mechanisms may have a potential role in novel anticancer hormonal therapies in RCCs.

10. References

Aass, N., De Mulder, P. H., Mickisch, G. H., Mulders, P., van Oosterom, A. T., van Poppel, H., Fossa, S. D., de Prijck, L., and Sylvester, R. J. 2005. Randomized phase II/III trial of interferon Alfa-2a with and without 13-cis-retinoic acid in patients with progressive metastatic renal cell Carcinoma: the European Organisation for Research and Treatment of Cancer Genito-Urinary Tract Cancer Group (EORTC 30951). *J Clin Oncol* 23 (18):4172-8.

Abe, E., Miyaura, C., Sakagami, H., Takeda, M., Konno, K., Yamazaki, T., Yoshiki, S., and Suda, T. 1981. Differentiation of mouse myeloid leukemia cells induced by 1 alpha,25-dihydroxyvitamin D3. *Proc Natl Acad Sci U S A* 78 (8):4990-4.

Adsay, N. V., Eble, J. N., Srigley, J. R., Jones, E. C., and Grignon, D. J. 2000. Mixed epithelial and stromal tumor of the kidney. *Am J Surg Pathol* 24 (7):958-70.

Altucci, L., and Gronemeyer, H. 2001. The promise of retinoids to fight against cancer. *Nat Rev Cancer* 1 (3):181-93.

Amin, M. B., Tamboli, P., Javidan, J., Stricker, H., de-Peralta Venturina, M., Deshpande, A., and Menon, M. 2002. Prognostic impact of histologic subtyping of adult renal epithelial neoplasms: an experience of 405 cases. *Am J Surg Pathol* 26 (3):281-91.

Arai, Y., Nonomura, N., Nakai, Y., Nishimura, K., Oka, D., Shiba, M., Nakayama, M., Takayama, H., Mizutani, Y., Miki, T., and Okuyama, A. 2008. The growth-inhibitory effects of dexamethasone on renal cell carcinoma in vivo and in vitro. *Cancer Invest* 26 (1):35-40.

Argiles, A., Ootaka, T., Hill, P. A., Nikolic-Paterson, D. J., Hutchinson, P., Kraft, N. E., and Atkins, R. C. 1994. Regulation of human renal adenocarcinoma cell growth by retinoic acid and its interactions with epidermal growth factor. *Kidney Int* 45 (1):23-31.

Arriza, J. L., Weinberger, C., Cerelli, G., Glaser, T. M., Handelin, B. L., Housman, D. E., and Evans, R. M. 1987. Cloning of human mineralocorticoid receptor complementary DNA: structural and functional kinship with the glucocorticoid receptor. *Science* 237 (4812):268-75.

Atkins, M. B., Hidalgo, M., Stadler, W. M., Logan, T. F., Dutcher, J. P., Hudes, G. R., Park, Y., Liou, S. H., Marshall, B., Boni, J. P., Dukart, G., and Sherman, M. L. 2004. Randomized phase II study of multiple dose levels of CCI-779, a novel mammalian target of rapamycin kinase inhibitor, in patients with advanced refractory renal cell carcinoma. *J Clin Oncol* 22 (5):909-18.

Atzpodien, J., Kirchner, H., Jonas, U., Bergmann, L., Schott, H., Heynemann, H., Fornara, P., Loening, S. A., Roigas, J., Muller, S. C., Bodenstein, H., Pomer, S., Metzner, B., Rebmann, U., Oberneder, R., Siebels, M., Wandert, T., Puchberger, T., and Reitz, M. 2004. Interleukin-2- and interferon alfa-2a-based immunochemotherapy in advanced renal cell carcinoma: a Prospectively Randomized Trial of the German Cooperative Renal Carcinoma Chemoimmunotherapy Group (DGCIN). *J Clin Oncol* 22 (7):1188-94.

Barsony, J., and Prufer, K. 2002. Vitamin D receptor and retinoid X receptor interactions in motion. *Vitam Horm* 65:345-76.

Baylis, C., Handa, R. K., and Sorkin, M. 1990. Glucocorticoids and control of glomerular filtration rate. *Semin Nephrol* 10 (4):320-9.

Beato, M., Herrlich, P., and Schutz, G. 1995. Steroid hormone receptors: many actors in search of a plot. *Cell* 83 (6):851-7.

Beer, T. M., and Myrthue, A. 2004. Calcitriol in cancer treatment: from the lab to the clinic. *Mol Cancer Ther* 3 (3):373-81.

Berg, W. J., Nanus, D. M., Leung, A., Brown, K. T., Hutchinson, B., Mazumdar, M., Xu, X. C., Lotan, R., Reuter, V. E., and Motzer, R. J. 1999. Up-regulation of retinoic acid receptor beta expression in renal cancers in vivo correlates with response to 13-cis-retinoic acid and interferon-alpha-2a. *Clin Cancer Res* 5 (7):1671-5.

Bhat, H. K., Hacker, H. J., Bannasch, P., Thompson, E. A., and Liehr, J. G. 1993. Localization of estrogen receptors in interstitial cells of hamster kidney and in estradiol-induced renal tumors as evidence of the mesenchymal origin of this neoplasm. *Cancer Res* 53 (22):5447-51.

Blomberg Jensen, M., Andersen, C. B., Nielsen, J. E., Bagi, P., Jorgensen, A., Juul, A., and Leffers, H. 2010. Expression of the vitamin D receptor, 25-hydroxylases, 1alpha-hydroxylase and 24-hydroxylase in the human kidney and renal clear cell cancer. *J Steroid Biochem Mol Biol* 121 (1-2):376-82.

Bloom, H. J. 1973. Proceedings: Hormone-induced and spontaneous regression of metastatic renal cancer. *Cancer* 32 (5):1066-71.

Blutt, S. E., McDonnell, T. J., Polek, T. C., and Weigel, N. L. 2000. Calcitriol-induced apoptosis in LNCaP cells is blocked by overexpression of Bcl-2. *Endocrinology* 141 (1):10-7.

Bojar, H., Maar, K., and Staib, W. 1979. The endocrine background of human renal cell carcinoma. IV. Glucocorticoid receptors as possible mediators of progestogen action. *Urol Int* 34 (5):330-8.

Boross, M., Kinsella, J., Cheng, L., and Sacktor, B. 1986. Glucocorticoids and metabolic acidosis-induced renal transports of inorganic phosphate, calcium, and NH4. *Am J Physiol* 250 (5 Pt 2):F827-33.

Bosetti, C., Scotti, L., Maso, L. D., Talamini, R., Montella, M., Negri, E., Ramazzotti, V., Franceschi, S., and La Vecchia, C. 2007. Micronutrients and the risk of renal cell cancer: a case-control study from Italy. *Int J Cancer* 120 (4):892-6.

Brem, A. S., Morris, D. J., Ge, Y., Dworkin, L. D., Tolbert, E., and Gong, R. 2010. Direct Fibrogenic Effects of Aldosterone on Normotensive Kidney: An Effect Modified by 11{beta}-HSD Activity. *Am J Physiol Renal Physiol*. 298: F1178–87.

Brown, C. J., Goss, S. J., Lubahn, D. B., Joseph, D. R., Wilson, E. M., French, F. S., and Willard, H. F. 1989. Androgen receptor locus on the human X chromosome: regional localization to Xq11-12 and description of a DNA polymorphism. *Am J Hum Genet* 44 (2):264-9.

Brown, D. F., Dababo, M. A., Hladik, C. L., Eagan, K. P., White, C. L., 3rd, and Rushing, E. J. 1998. Hormone receptor immunoreactivity in hemangioblastomas and clear cell renal cell carcinomas. *Mod Pathol* 11 (1):55-9.

Campen, T. J., Vaughn, D. A., and Fanestil, D. D. 1983. Mineralo- and glucocorticoid effects on renal excretion of electrolytes. *Pflugers Arch* 399 (2):93-101.

Chen, L., Weiss, F. R., Chaichik, S., and Keydar, I. 1980. Steroid receptors in human renal carcinoma. *Isr J Med Sci* 16 (11):756-60.

Christophersen, A. O., Lie, A. K., and Fossa, S. D. 2006. Unexpected 10 years complete remission after cortisone mono-therapy in metastatic renal cell carcinoma. *Acta Oncol* 45 (2):226-8.

Concolino, G., Marocchi, A., Conti, C., Tenaglia, R., Di Silverio, F., and Bracci, U. 1978. Human renal cell carcinoma as a hormone-dependent tumor. *Cancer Res* 38 (11 Pt 2):4340-4.

Concolino, G., Marocchi, A., Tenaglia, R., Di Silverio, F., and Sparano, F. 1978. Specific progesterone receptor in human renal cancer. *J Steroid Biochem* 9 (5):399-402.

Concolino, G., Marocchi, A., Toscano, V., and Di Silverio, F. 1981. Nuclear androgen receptor as marker of responsiveness to medroxyprogesterone acetate in human renal cell carcinoma. *J Steroid Biochem* 15:397-402.

Connell, J. M., and Davies, E. 2005. The new biology of aldosterone. *J Endocrinol* 186 (1):1-20.

Cote, S., Sinnett, D., and Momparler, R. L. 1998. Demethylation by 5-aza-2'-deoxycytidine of specific 5-methylcytosine sites in the promoter region of the retinoic acid receptor beta gene in human colon carcinoma cells. *Anticancer Drugs* 9 (9):743-50.

De Bosscher, K., Vanden Berghe, W., and Haegeman, G. 2003. The interplay between the glucocorticoid receptor and nuclear factor-kappaB or activator protein-1: molecular mechanisms for gene repression. *Endocr Rev* 24 (4):488-522.

Eble, J. N., Sauter, G. , Epstein, J. I., and Sesterhenn, I., eds. 2004. *World Health Organization classification of tumours: pathology and genetics of tumours of the urinary system and male genital organs*. Lyon, France: IARC Press.

Escoubet, B., Coureau, C., Blot-Chabaud, M., Bonvalet, J. P., and Farman, N. 1996. Corticosteroid receptor mRNA expression is unaffected by corticosteroids in rat kidney, heart, and colon. *Am J Physiol* 270 (5 Pt 1):C1343-53.

Escudier, B., Pluzanska, A., Koralewski, P., Ravaud, A., Bracarda, S., Szczylik, C., Chevreau, C., Filipek, M., Melichar, B., Bajetta, E., Gorbunova, V., Bay, J. O., Bodrogi, I., Jagiello-Gruszfeld, A., and Moore, N. 2007. Bevacizumab plus interferon alfa-2a for treatment of metastatic renal cell carcinoma: a randomised, double-blind phase III trial. *Lancet* 370 (9605):2103-11.

Evans, R. M. 1988. The steroid and thyroid hormone receptor superfamily. *Science* 240 (4854):889-95.

Fakih, M. G., Trump, D. L., Muindi, J. R., Black, J. D., Bernardi, R. J., Creaven, P. J., Schwartz, J., Brattain, M. G., Hutson, A., French, R., and Johnson, C. S. 2007. A phase I pharmacokinetic and pharmacodynamic study of intravenous calcitriol in combination with oral gefitinib in patients with advanced solid tumors. *Clin Cancer Res* 13 (4):1216-23.

Farman, N., and Bonvalet, J. P. 1983. Aldosterone binding in isolated tubules. III. Autoradiography along the rat nephron. *Am J Physiol* 245 (5 Pt 1):F606-14.

Farman, N., Vandewalle, A., and Bonvalet, J. P. 1982. Aldosterone binding in isolated tubules I. Biochemical determination in proximal and distal parts of the rabbit nephron. *Am J Physiol* 242 (1):F63-8.

Fine, S. W., Reuter, V. E., Epstein, J. I., and Argani, P. 2006. Angiomyolipoma with epithelial cysts (AMLEC): a distinct cystic variant of angiomyolipoma. *Am J Surg Pathol* 30 (5):593-9.

Fleet, J. C. 2008. Molecular actions of vitamin D contributing to cancer prevention. *Mol Aspects Med* 29 (6):388-96.

Freiberg, J. M., Kinsella, J., and Sacktor, B. 1982. Glucocorticoids increase the Na+-H+ exchange and decrease the Na+ gradient-dependent phosphate-uptake systems in renal brush border membrane vesicles. *Proc Natl Acad Sci U S A* 79 (16):4932-6.

Fujioka, T., Hasegawa, M., Ishikura, K., Matsushita, Y., Sato, M., and Tanji, S. 1998. Inhibition of tumor growth and angiogenesis by vitamin D3 agents in murine renal cell carcinoma. *J Urol* 160 (1):247-51.

Fuller, P. J. 1991. The steroid receptor superfamily: mechanisms of diversity. *FASEB J* 5 (15):3092-9.

Fuzesi, L., Gunawan, B., Bergmann, F., Tack, S., Braun, S., and Jakse, G. 1999. Papillary renal cell carcinoma with clear cell cytomorphology and chromosomal loss of 3p. *Histopathology* 35 (2):157-61.

Geisen, C., Denk, C., Gremm, B., Baust, C., Karger, A., Bollag, W., and Schwarz, E. 1997. High-level expression of the retinoic acid receptor beta gene in normal cells of the uterine cervix is regulated by the retinoic acid receptor alpha and is abnormally down-regulated in cervical carcinoma cells. *Cancer Res* 57 (8):1460-7.

Gelmann, E. P. 2002. Molecular biology of the androgen receptor. *J Clin Oncol* 20 (13):3001-15.

Geradts, J., Chen, J. Y., Russell, E. K., Yankaskas, J. R., Nieves, L., and Minna, J. D. 1993. Human lung cancer cell lines exhibit resistance to retinoic acid treatment. *Cell Growth Differ* 4 (10):799-809.

Getzenberg, R. H., Light, B. W., Lapco, P. E., Konety, B. R., Nangia, A. K., Acierno, J. S., Dhir, R., Shurin, Z., Day, R. S., Trump, D. L., and Johnson, C. S. 1997. Vitamin D inhibition of prostate adenocarcinoma growth and metastasis in the Dunning rat prostate model system. *Urology* 50 (6):999-1006.

Gobbo, S., Eble, J. N., Grignon, D. J., Martignoni, G., MacLennan, G. T., Shah, R. B., Zhang, S., Brunelli, M., and Cheng, L. 2008. Clear cell papillary renal cell carcinoma: a distinct histopathologic and molecular genetic entity. *Am J Surg Pathol* 32 (8):1239-45.

Goelden, U., Ukena, S. N., Pfoertner, S., Hofmann, R., Buer, J., and Schrader, A. J. 2005. RAR-beta(1) overexpression in chromophobe renal cell carcinoma: a novel target for therapeutic intervention? *Exp Oncol* 27 (3):220-4.

Greene, G. L., Gilna, P., Waterfield, M., Baker, A., Hort, Y., and Shine, J. 1986. Sequence and expression of human estrogen receptor complementary DNA. *Science* 231 (4742):1150-4.

Greenstein, S., Ghias, K., Krett, N. L., and Rosen, S. T. 2002. Mechanisms of glucocorticoid-mediated apoptosis in hematological malignancies. *Clin Cancer Res* 8 (6):1681-94.

Gustafsson, J. A. 1999. Estrogen receptor beta--a new dimension in estrogen mechanism of action. *J Endocrinol* 163 (3):379-83.

He, J. C., Lu, T. C., Fleet, M., Sunamoto, M., Husain, M., Fang, W., Neves, S., Chen, Y., Shankland, S., Iyengar, R., and Klotman, P. E. 2007. Retinoic acid inhibits HIV-1-induced podocyte proliferation through the cAMP pathway. *J Am Soc Nephrol* 18 (1):93-102.

Hemstreet, G. P., 3rd, Wittliff, J. L., Sarrif, A. M., Hall, M. L., 3rd, McRae, L. J., and Durant, J. R. 1980. Comparison of steroid receptor levels in renal-cell carcinoma and autologous normal kidney. *Int J Cancer* 26 (6):769-75.

Hermann, G. G., and Andersen, C. B. 1997. Transitional cell carcinoma express vitamin D receptors. *Scand J Urol Nephrol* 31 (2):161-6.

Hirasawa, G., Sasano, H., Takahashi, K., Fukushima, K., Suzuki, T., Hiwatashi, N., Toyota, T., Krozowski, Z. S., and Nagura, H. 1997. Colocalization of 11 beta-hydroxysteroid dehydrogenase type II and mineralocorticoid receptor in human epithelia. *J Clin Endocrinol Metab* 82 (11):3859-63.

Hoffman, A. D., Engelstein, D., Bogenrieder, T., Papandreou, C. N., Steckelman, E., Dave, A., Motzer, R. J., Dmitrovsky, E., Albino, A. P., and Nanus, D. M. 1996. Expression of retinoic acid receptor beta in human renal cell carcinomas correlates with sensitivity to the antiproliferative effects of 13-cis-retinoic acid. *Clin Cancer Res* 2 (6):1077-82.

Houle, B., Rochette-Egly, C., and Bradley, W. E. 1993. Tumor-suppressive effect of the retinoic acid receptor beta in human epidermoid lung cancer cells. *Proc Natl Acad Sci U S A* 90 (3):985-9.

Hudes, G., Carducci, M., Tomczak, P., Dutcher, J., Figlin, R., Kapoor, A., Staroslawska, E., Sosman, J., McDermott, D., Bodrogi, I., Kovacevic, Z., Lesovoy, V., Schmidt-Wolf, I. G., Barbarash, O., Gokmen, E., O'Toole, T., Lustgarten, S., Moore, L., and Motzer, R. J. 2007. Temsirolimus, interferon alfa, or both for advanced renal-cell carcinoma. *N Engl J Med* 356 (22):2271-81.

Ikuyama, T., Hamasaki, T., Inatomi, H., Katoh, T., Muratani, T., and Matsumoto, T. 2002. Association of vitamin D receptor gene polymorphism with renal cell carcinoma in Japanese. *Endocr J* 49 (4):433-8.

Interferon-alpha and survival in metastatic renal carcinoma: early results of a randomised controlled trial. Medical Research Council Renal Cancer Collaborators. 1999. *Lancet* 353 (9146):14-7.

Iwai, A., Fujii, Y., Kawakami, S., Takazawa, R., Kageyama, Y., Yoshida, M. A., and Kihara, K. 2004. Down-regulation of vascular endothelial growth factor in renal cell carcinoma cells by glucocorticoids. *Mol Cell Endocrinol* 226 (1-2):11-7.

Jakse, G., and Muller-Holzner, E. 1988. Hormone receptors in renal cancer: an overview. *Semin Surg Oncol* 4 (3):161-4.

Jeltsch, J. M., Krozowski, Z., Quirin-Stricker, C., Gronemeyer, H., Simpson, R. J., Garnier, J. M., Krust, A., Jacob, F., and Chambon, P. 1986. Cloning of the chicken progesterone receptor. *Proc Natl Acad Sci U S A* 83 (15):5424-8.

Jensen, E. V., Jacobson, H. I., Walf, A. A., and Frye, C. A. 2010. Estrogen action: a historic perspective on the implications of considering alternative approaches. *Physiol Behav* 99 (2):151-62.

Kakizuka, A., Miller, W. H., Jr., Umesono, K., Warrell, R. P., Jr., Frankel, S. R., Murty, V. V., Dmitrovsky, E., and Evans, R. M. 1991. Chromosomal translocation t(15;17) in human acute promyelocytic leukemia fuses RAR alpha with a novel putative transcription factor, PML. *Cell* 66 (4):663-74.

Karami, S., Brennan, P., Hung, R. J., Boffetta, P., Toro, J., Wilson, R. T., Zaridze, D., Navratilova, M., Chatterjee, N., Mates, D., Janout, V., Kollarova, H., Bencko, V., Szeszenia-Dabrowska, N., Holcatova, I., Moukeria, A., Welch, R., Chanock, S., Rothman, N., Chow, W. H., and Moore, L. E. 2008. Vitamin D receptor polymorphisms and renal cancer risk in Central and Eastern Europe. *J Toxicol Environ Health A* 71 (6):367-72.

Karr, J. P., Pontes, J. E., Schneider, S., Sandberg, A. A., and Murphy, G. P. 1983. Clinical aspects of steroid hormone receptors in human renal cell carcinoma. *J Surg Oncol* 23 (2):117-24.

Kimura, N., Mizokami, A., Oonuma, T., Sasano, H., and Nagura, H. 1993. Immunocytochemical localization of androgen receptor with polyclonal antibody in paraffin-embedded human tissues. *J Histochem Cytochem* 41 (5):671-8.

Klotzl, G., Otto, U., Becker, H., and Klosterhalfen, H. 1987. Determination of androgen, progestin and estrogen receptors with two different assays in renal cell carcinoma. *Urol Int* 42 (2):100-4.

Konety, B. R., Lavelle, J. P., Pirtskalaishvili, G., Dhir, R., Meyers, S. A., Nguyen, T. S., Hershberger, P., Shurin, M. R., Johnson, C. S., Trump, D. L., Zeidel, M. L., and Getzenberg, R. H. 2001. Effects of vitamin D (calcitriol) on transitional cell carcinoma of the bladder in vitro and in vivo. *J Urol* 165 (1):253-8.

Krozowski, Z. S., and Funder, J. W. 1983. Renal mineralocorticoid receptors and hippocampal corticosterone-binding species have identical intrinsic steroid specificity. *Proc Natl Acad Sci U S A* 80 (19):6056-60.

Kuiper, G. G., Enmark, E., Pelto-Huikko, M., Nilsson, S., and Gustafsson, J. A. 1996. Cloning of a novel receptor expressed in rat prostate and ovary. *Proc Natl Acad Sci U S A* 93 (12):5925-30.

Lambert, J. R., Eddy, V. J., Young, C. D., Persons, K. S., Sarkar, S., Kelly, J. A., Genova, E., Lucia, M. S., Faller, D. V., and Ray, R. 2010. A vitamin D receptor-alkylating derivative of 1alpha,25-dihydroxyvitamin D3 inhibits growth of human kidney cancer cells and suppresses tumor growth. *Cancer Prev Res (Phila)* 3 (12):1596-607.

Lamprecht, S. A., and Lipkin, M. 2003. Chemoprevention of colon cancer by calcium, vitamin D and folate: molecular mechanisms. *Nat Rev Cancer* 3 (8):601-14.

Langner, C., Ratschek, M., Rehak, P., Schips, L., and Zigeuner, R. 2004. Steroid hormone receptor expression in renal cell carcinoma: an immunohistochemical analysis of 182 tumors. *J Urol* 171 (2 Pt 1):611-4.

Leveridge, M. J., and Jewett, M. A. 2011. Recent developments in kidney cancer. *Can Urol Assoc J* 5 (3):195-203.

Li, H., and Christakos, S. 1991. Differential regulation by 1,25-dihydroxyvitamin D3 of calbindin-D9k and calbindin-D28k gene expression in mouse kidney. *Endocrinology* 128 (6):2844-52.

Li, J. J., Weroha, S. J., Davis, M. F., Tawfik, O., Hou, X., and Li, S. A. 2001. ER and PR in renomedullary interstitial cells during Syrian hamster estrogen-induced tumorigenesis: evidence for receptor-mediated oncogenesis. *Endocrinology* 142 (9):4006-14.

Li, J. Y., Zhou, T., Gao, X., Xu, C., Sun, Y., Peng, Y., Chang, Z., Zhang, Y., Jiang, J., Wang, L., and Hou, J. 2010. Testosterone and androgen receptor in human nephrolithiasis. *J Urol* 184 (6):2360-3.

Li, S. A., Li, J. J., and Villee, C. A. 1977. Significance of the progesterone receptor in the estrogen-induced and -dependent renal tumor of the Syrian golden hamster. *Ann N Y Acad Sci* 286:369-83.

Liu, S. H., Otal-Brun, M., and Webb, T. E. 1980. Glucocorticoid receptors in human tumors. *Cancer Lett* 10 (3):269-75.

Liu, W., Tretiakova, M., Kong, J., Turkyilmaz, M., Li, Y. C., and Krausz, T. 2006. Expression of vitamin D3 receptor in kidney tumors. *Hum Pathol* 37 (10):1268-78.

Lombes, M., Farman, N., Oblin, M. E., Baulieu, E. E., Bonvalet, J. P., Erlanger, B. F., and Gasc, J. M. 1990. Immunohistochemical localization of renal mineralocorticoid receptor by using an anti-idiotypic antibody that is an internal image of aldosterone. *Proc Natl Acad Sci U S A* 87 (3):1086-8.

Lubahn, D. B., Joseph, D. R., Sullivan, P. M., Willard, H. F., French, F. S., and Wilson, E. M. 1988. Cloning of human androgen receptor complementary DNA and localization to the X chromosome. *Science* 240 (4850):327-30.

Madej, A., Puzianowska-Kuznicka, M., Tanski, Z., Nauman, J., and Nauman, A. 2003. Vitamin D receptor binding to DNA is altered without the change in its expression in human renal clear cell cancer. *Nephron Exp Nephrol* 93 (4):e150-7.

Mai, K. T., Teo, I., Belanger, E. C., Robertson, S. J., Marginean, E. C., and Islam, S. 2008. Progesterone receptor reactivity in renal oncocytoma and chromophobe renal cell carcinoma. *Histopathology* 52 (3):277-82.

McDonald, M. W., Diokno, A. C., Seski, J. C., and Menon, K. M. 1983. Measurement of progesterone receptor in human renal cell carcinoma and normal renal tissue. *J Surg Oncol* 22 (3):164-6.

Miki, S., Iwano, M., Miki, Y., Yamamoto, M., Tang, B., Yokokawa, K., Sonoda, T., Hirano, T., and Kishimoto, T. 1989. Interleukin-6 (IL-6) functions as an in vitro autocrine growth factor in renal cell carcinomas. *FEBS Lett* 250 (2):607-10.

Mishina, T., Scholer, D. W., and Edelman, I. S. 1981. Glucocorticoid receptors in rat kidney cortical tubules enriched in proximal and distal segments. *Am J Physiol* 240 (1):F38-45.

Moasser, M. M., DeBlasio, A., and Dmitrovsky, E. 1994. Response and resistance to retinoic acid are mediated through the retinoic acid nuclear receptor gamma in human teratocarcinomas. *Oncogene* 9 (3):833-40.

Moasser, M. M., Reuter, V. E., and Dmitrovsky, E. 1995. Overexpression of the retinoic acid receptor gamma directly induces terminal differentiation of human embryonal carcinoma cells. *Oncogene* 10 (8):1537-43.

Mongan, N. P., and Gudas, L. J. 2007. Diverse actions of retinoid receptors in cancer prevention and treatment. *Differentiation* 75 (9):853-70.

Morris, D. J., and Souness, G. W. 1992. Protective and specificity-conferring mechanisms of mineralocorticoid action. *Am J Physiol* 263 (5 Pt 2):F759-68.

Motzer, R. J., Hudes, G. R., Curti, B. D., McDermott, D. F., Escudier, B. J., Negrier, S., Duclos, B., Moore, L., O'Toole, T., Boni, J. P., and Dutcher, J. P. 2007. Phase I/II trial of temsirolimus combined with interferon alfa for advanced renal cell carcinoma. *J Clin Oncol* 25 (25):3958-64.

Motzer, R. J., Michaelson, M. D., Redman, B. G., Hudes, G. R., Wilding, G., Figlin, R. A., Ginsberg, M. S., Kim, S. T., Baum, C. M., DePrimo, S. E., Li, J. Z., Bello, C. L., Theuer, C. P., George, D. J., and Rini, B. I. 2006. Activity of SU11248, a multitargeted inhibitor of vascular endothelial growth factor receptor and platelet-derived growth factor receptor, in patients with metastatic renal cell carcinoma. *J Clin Oncol* 24 (1):16-24.

Motzer, R. J., Murphy, B. A., Bacik, J., Schwartz, L. H., Nanus, D. M., Mariani, T., Loehrer, P., Wilding, G., Fairclough, D. L., Cella, D., and Mazumdar, M. 2000. Phase III trial of interferon alfa-2a with or without 13-cis-retinoic acid for patients with advanced renal cell carcinoma. *J Clin Oncol* 18 (16):2972-80.

Muindi, J. R., Johnson, C. S., Trump, D. L., Christy, R., Engler, K. L., and Fakih, M. G. 2009. A phase I and pharmacokinetics study of intravenous calcitriol in combination with oral dexamethasone and gefitinib in patients with advanced solid tumors. *Cancer Chemother Pharmacol* 65 (1):33-40.

Muramatsu, M., and Inoue, S. 2000. Estrogen receptors: how do they control reproductive and nonreproductive functions? *Biochem Biophys Res Commun* 270 (1):1-10.

Nagakura, K., Abe, E., Suda, T., Hayakawa, M., Nakamura, H., and Tazaki, H. 1986. Inhibitory effect of 1 alpha,25-dihydroxyvitamin D3 on the growth of the renal carcinoma cell line. *Kidney Int* 29 (4):834-40.

Nakano, E., Tada, Y., Fujioka, H., Matsuda, M., Osafune, M., Kotake, T., Sato, B., Takaha, M., and Sonoda, T. 1984. Hormone receptor in renal cell carcinoma and correlation with clinical response to endocrine therapy. *J Urol* 132 (2):240-5.

Nakayama, T., Watanabe, M., Yamanaka, M., Hirokawa, Y., Suzuki, H., Ito, H., Yatani, R., and Shiraishi, T. 2001. The role of epigenetic modifications in retinoic acid receptor beta2 gene expression in human prostate cancers. *Lab Invest* 81 (7):1049-57.

Naray-Fejes-Toth, A., and Fejes-Toth, G. 1990. Glucocorticoid receptors mediate mineralocorticoid-like effects in cultured collecting duct cells. *Am J Physiol* 259 (4 Pt 2):F672-8.

Noronha, R. F., and Rao, B. R. 1985. Increased dihydrotestosterone receptor levels in high-stage renal adenocarcinoma. *Cancer* 56 (1):134-7.

Nykjaer, A., Dragun, D., Walther, D., Vorum, H., Jacobsen, C., Herz, J., Melsen, F., Christensen, E. I., and Willnow, T. E. 1999. An endocytic pathway essential for renal uptake and activation of the steroid 25-(OH) vitamin D3. *Cell* 96 (4):507-15.

Obara, W., Konda, R., Akasaka, S., Nakamura, S., Sugawara, A., and Fujioka, T. 2007. Prognostic significance of vitamin D receptor and retinoid X receptor expression in renal cell carcinoma. *J Urol* 178 (4 Pt 1):1497-503.

Obara, W., Suzuki, Y., Kato, K., Tanji, S., Konda, R., and Fujioka, T. 2007. Vitamin D receptor gene polymorphisms are associated with increased risk and progression of renal cell carcinoma in a Japanese population. *Int J Urol* 14 (6):483-7.

Omland, H., and Fossa, S. D. 1989. Spontaneous regression of cerebral and pulmonary metastases in renal cell carcinoma. *Scand J Urol Nephrol* 23 (2):159-60.

Pearson, J., Friedman, M. A., and Hoffman, P. G., Jr. 1981. Hormone receptors in renal cell carcinoma. Their utility as predictors of response to endocrine therapy. *Cancer Chemother Pharmacol* 6 (2):151-4.

Pemrick, S. M., Lucas, D. A., and Grippo, J. F. 1994. The retinoid receptors. *Leukemia* 8 Suppl 3:S1-10.

Porta, C., Tortora, G., Linassier, C., Papazisis, K., Awada, A., Berthold, D., Maroto, J. P., Powles, T., and De Santis, M. 2011. Maximising the duration of disease control in metastatic renal cell carcinoma with targeted agents: an expert agreement. *Med Oncol*.

Prufer, K., and Barsony, J. 2002. Retinoid X receptor dominates the nuclear import and export of the unliganded vitamin D receptor. *Mol Endocrinol* 16 (8):1738-51.

Pujols, L., Mullol, J., Roca-Ferrer, J., Torrego, A., Xaubet, A., Cidlowski, J. A., and Picado, C. 2002. Expression of glucocorticoid receptor alpha- and beta-isoforms in human cells and tissues. *Am J Physiol Cell Physiol* 283 (4):C1324-31.

Rafestin-Oblin, M. E., Roth-Meyer, C., Claire, M., Michaud, A., Baviera, E., Brisset, J. M., and Corvol, P. 1979. Are mineralocorticoid receptors present in human renal adenocarcinoma? *Clin Sci (Lond)* 57 (5):421-5.

Rashid, S. F., Moore, J. S., Walker, E., Driver, P. M., Engel, J., Edwards, C. E., Brown, G., Uskokovic, M. R., and Campbell, M. J. 2001. Synergistic growth inhibition of prostate cancer cells by 1 alpha,25 Dihydroxyvitamin D(3) and its 19-nor-hexafluoride analogs in combination with either sodium butyrate or trichostatin A. *Oncogene* 20 (15):1860-72.

Reichel, H., Koeffler, H. P., and Norman, A. W. 1989. The role of the vitamin D endocrine system in health and disease. *N Engl J Med* 320 (15):980-91.

Revollo, J. R., and Cidlowski, J. A. 2009. Mechanisms generating diversity in glucocorticoid receptor signaling. *Ann N Y Acad Sci* 1179:167-78.

Roland, B. L., Krozowski, Z. S., and Funder, J. W. 1995. Glucocorticoid receptor, mineralocorticoid receptors, 11 beta-hydroxysteroid dehydrogenase-1 and -2 expression in rat brain and kidney: in situ studies. *Mol Cell Endocrinol* 111 (1):R1-7.

Ruizeveld de Winter, J. A., Trapman, J., Vermey, M., Mulder, E., Zegers, N. D., and van der Kwast, T. H. 1991. Androgen receptor expression in human tissues: an immunohistochemical study. *J Histochem Cytochem* 39 (7):927-36.

Sabichi, A. L., Hendricks, D. T., Bober, M. A., and Birrer, M. J. 1998. Retinoic acid receptor beta expression and growth inhibition of gynecologic cancer cells by the synthetic retinoid N-(4-hydroxyphenyl) retinamide. *J Natl Cancer Inst* 90 (8):597-605.

Sasano, H., Fukushima, K., Sasaki, I., Matsuno, S., Nagura, H., and Krozowski, Z. S. 1992. Immunolocalization of mineralocorticoid receptor in human kidney, pancreas, salivary, mammary and sweat glands: a light and electron microscopic immunohistochemical study. *J Endocrinol* 132 (2):305-10.

Schug, T. T., Berry, D. C., Shaw, N. S., Travis, S. N., and Noy, N. 2007. Opposing effects of retinoic acid on cell growth result from alternate activation of two different nuclear receptors. *Cell* 129 (4):723-33.

Sheikh, M. S., Shao, Z. M., Li, X. S., Dawson, M., Jetten, A. M., Wu, S., Conley, B. A., Garcia, M., Rochefort, H., and Fontana, J. A. 1994. Retinoid-resistant estrogen receptor-negative human breast carcinoma cells transfected with retinoic acid receptor-alpha acquire sensitivity to growth inhibition by retinoids. *J Biol Chem* 269 (34):21440-7.

Siegel, R., Ward, E., Brawley, O., and Jemal, A. 2011. Cancer statistics, 2011: The impact of eliminating socioeconomic and racial disparities on premature cancer deaths. *CA Cancer J Clin* 61 (4):212-36.

Speirs, V., Parkes, A. T., Kerin, M. J., Walton, D. S., Carleton, P. J., Fox, J. N., and Atkin, S. L. 1999. Coexpression of estrogen receptor alpha and beta: poor prognostic factors in human breast cancer? *Cancer Res* 59 (3):525-8.

Storlie, J. A., Buckner, J. C., Wiseman, G. A., Burch, P. A., Hartmann, L. C., and Richardson, R. L. 1995. Prostate specific antigen levels and clinical response to low dose dexamethasone for hormone-refractory metastatic prostate carcinoma. *Cancer* 76 (1):96-100.

Suh, Y. A., Lee, H. Y., Virmani, A., Wong, J., Mann, K. K., Miller, W. H., Jr., Gazdar, A., and Kurie, J. M. 2002. Loss of retinoic acid receptor beta gene expression is linked to aberrant histone H3 acetylation in lung cancer cell lines. *Cancer Res* 62 (14):3945-9.

Swisshelm, K., Ryan, K., Lee, X., Tsou, H. C., Peacocke, M., and Sager, R. 1994. Down-regulation of retinoic acid receptor beta in mammary carcinoma cell lines and its up-regulation in senescing normal mammary epithelial cells. *Cell Growth Differ* 5 (2):133-41.

Takahashi, M., Yang, X. J., Sugimura, J., Backdahl, J., Tretiakova, M., Qian, C. N., Gray, S. G., Knapp, R., Anema, J., Kahnoski, R., Nicol, D., Vogelzang, N. J., Furge, K. A., Kanayama, H., Kagawa, S., and Teh, B. T. 2003. Molecular subclassification of kidney tumors and the discovery of new diagnostic markers. *Oncogene* 22 (43):6810-8.

Takeda, H., Chodak, G., Mutchnik, S., Nakamoto, T., and Chang, C. 1990. Immunohistochemical localization of androgen receptors with mono- and polyclonal antibodies to androgen receptor. *J Endocrinol* 126 (1):17-25.

Takenawa, J., Kaneko, Y., Okumura, K., Yoshida, O., Nakayama, H., and Fujita, J. 1995. Inhibitory effect of dexamethasone and progesterone in vitro on proliferation of human renal cell carcinomas and effects on expression of interleukin-6 or interleukin-6 receptor. *J Urol* 153 (3 Pt 1):858-62.

Tanaka, M., Fukuda, H., and Higashi, Y. 2003. [A case of complete regression of metastatic renal cell carcinoma following corticosteroid treatment]. *Hinyokika Kiyo* 49 (4):225-8.

Tang, X. H., and Gudas, L. J. 2011. Retinoids, retinoic acid receptors, and cancer. *Annu Rev Pathol* 6:345-64.

Thacher, T. D., and Clarke, B. L. 2011. Vitamin D insufficiency. *Mayo Clin Proc* 86 (1):50-60.

Thomas, C. P., Liu, K. Z., and Vats, H. S. 2006. Medroxyprogesterone acetate binds the glucocorticoid receptor to stimulate alpha-ENaC and sgk1 expression in renal collecting duct epithelia. *Am J Physiol Renal Physiol* 290 (2):F306-12.

Tickoo, S. K., Gopalan, A., Tu, J. J., Harik, L. R., Al-Ahmadie, H. A., Fine, S. W., Olgac, S., and Reuter, V. E. 2008. Estrogen and progesterone-receptor-positive stroma as a non-tumorous proliferation in kidneys: a possible metaplastic response to obstruction. *Mod Pathol* 21 (1):60-5.

Todd-Turla, K. M., Schnermann, J., Fejes-Toth, G., Naray-Fejes-Toth, A., Smart, A., Killen, P. D., and Briggs, J. P. 1993. Distribution of mineralocorticoid and glucocorticoid receptor mRNA along the nephron. *Am J Physiol* 264 (5 Pt 2):F781-91.

Trump, D. L., Hershberger, P. A., Bernardi, R. J., Ahmed, S., Muindi, J., Fakih, M., Yu, W. D., and Johnson, C. S. 2004. Anti-tumor activity of calcitriol: pre-clinical and clinical studies. *J Steroid Biochem Mol Biol* 89-90 (1-5):519-26.

Trump, D. L., Muindi, J., Fakih, M., Yu, W. D., and Johnson, C. S. 2006. Vitamin D compounds: clinical development as cancer therapy and prevention agents. *Anticancer Res* 26 (4A):2551-6.

Trydal, T., Bakke, A., Aksnes, L., and Aarskog, D. 1988. 1,25-Dihydroxyvitamin D3 receptor measurement in primary renal cell carcinomas and autologous normal kidney tissue. *Cancer Res* 48 (9):2458-61.

Turbiner, J., Amin, M. B., Humphrey, P. A., Srigley, J. R., De Leval, L., Radhakrishnan, A., and Oliva, E. 2007. Cystic nephroma and mixed epithelial and stromal tumor of kidney: a detailed clinicopathologic analysis of 34 cases and proposal for renal epithelial and stromal tumor (REST) as a unifying term. *Am J Surg Pathol* 31 (4):489-500.

Vanderleede, B., Opdenoordt, T., Vandenbrink, C., Ebert, T., and Vandersaag, P. 1995. Implication of retinoic Acid receptor-Beta in renal-cell carcinoma. *Int J Oncol* 6 (2):391-400.

Xu, X. C., Ro, J. Y., Lee, J. S., Shin, D. M., Hong, W. K., and Lotan, R. 1994. Differential expression of nuclear retinoid receptors in normal, premalignant, and malignant head and neck tissues. *Cancer Res* 54 (13):3580-7.

Yakirevich, E., Matoso, A., Sabo, E., Wang, L. J., Tavares, R., Meitner, P., Morris, D. J., Pareek, G., Delellis, R. A., and Resnick, M. B. 2011. Expression of the glucocorticoid receptor in renal cell neoplasms: an immunohistochemical and quantitative reverse transcriptase polymerase chain reaction study. *Hum Pathol.* 42 (11):1684-92.

Yakirevich, E., Morris, D. J., Tavares, R., Meitner, P. A., Lechpammer, M., Noble, L., de Rodriguez, A. F., Gomez-Sanchez, C. E., Wang, L. J., Sabo, E., Delellis, R. A., and Resnick, M. B. 2008. Mineralocorticoid receptor and 11beta-hydroxysteroid dehydrogenase type II expression in renal cell neoplasms: a tissue microarray and quantitative RT-PCR study. *Am J Surg Pathol* 32 (6):874-83.

Yang, J. C., Sherry, R. M., Steinberg, S. M., Topalian, S. L., Schwartzentruber, D. J., Hwu, P., Seipp, C. A., Rogers-Freezer, L., Morton, K. E., White, D. E., Liewehr, D. J., Merino, M. J., and Rosenberg, S. A. 2003. Randomized study of high-dose and low-dose interleukin-2 in patients with metastatic renal cancer. *J Clin Oncol* 21 (16):3127-32.

Yang, J. C., Haworth, L., Sherry, R. M., Hwu, P., Schwartzentruber, D. J., Topalian, S. L., Steinberg, S. M., Chen, H. X., Rosenberg, S. A. 2003. A randomized trial of bevacizumab, an anti-vascular endothelial growth factor antibody, for metastatic renal cancer. *N Engl J Med* 349 (5):427-34.

Young, A. N., Amin, M. B., Moreno, C. S., Lim, S. D., Cohen, C., Petros, J. A., Marshall, F. F., and Neish, A. S. 2001. Expression profiling of renal epithelial neoplasms: a method for tumor classification and discovery of diagnostic molecular markers. *Am J Pathol* 158 (5):1639-51.

Zhang, X. K., Liu, Y., Lee, M. O., and Pfahl, M. 1994. A specific defect in the retinoic acid response associated with human lung cancer cell lines. *Cancer Res* 54 (21):5663-9.

Zhuang, S. H., and Burnstein, K. L. 1998. Antiproliferative effect of 1alpha,25-dihydroxyvitamin D3 in human prostate cancer cell line LNCaP involves reduction of cyclin-dependent kinase 2 activity and persistent G1 accumulation. *Endocrinology* 139 (3):1197-207.

6

Anticancer Target Molecules Against the SCF Ubiquitin E3 Ligase in RCC: Potential Approaches to the NEDD8 Pathway

Tomoaki Tanaka and Tatsuya Nakatani
Osaka City University Graduate School of Medicine, Department of Urology
Japan

1. Introduction

Several alternative treatments have recently been developed for metastatic renal cell carcinoma (RCC). Vascular endothelial growth factor (VEGF) is a potent pro-angiogenic protein, which is responsible for increased vasculature and tumor-growth in RCC. Fundamentally, a mutation in the von Hippel-Lindau (VHL) tumor suppressor gene induces overexpression of VEGF via accumulation of hypoxia-inducible factor (HIF)-1 in RCC. Several agents inhibiting the VEGF signaling cascade, such as sorafenib, sunitinib and bevacizumab, have been found to exert significant anti-tumor effects and provide meaningful clinical benefits. Furthermore, temsirolimus and everolimus, inhibitors of the mammalian target of rapamycin (mTOR), which block the phosphoinositide 3-kinase (PI3K)/AKT signaling pathway involved in numerous cellular functions including cell proliferation, survival and angiogenesis, have been found to be effective agents against advanced RCC in the clinical setting. Although molecular targeting therapies against the VEGF or mTOR signaling pathway have revolutionized the treatment of advanced RCC, no curative therapy has yet been established.

In this chapter, we focus on potent molecules and agents possibly suppressing the tumor growth of RCC via regulation of the ubiquitination-proteasome system. NEDD8, one of the ubiquitin-like proteins, reportedly forms conjugates with cullin family proteins and thereby activates the Skp1-Cullin-F-box (SCF) ubiquitin protein ligase complex that catalyzes the ubiquitination of many cell-cycle regulators, e.g. cyclin E, p21, p73 and p27. It is possible that negative regulation of NEDD8 and its conjugation system induces an antiproliferative action on RCC, secondary to inhibition of ubiqitin-proteasome activity. We previously showed that these negative regulator proteins, such as NEDD8 ultimate buster 1 (NUB1) and a dominant negative form (Ubc12 C111S) of NEDD8 E2 ligase, exhibited remarkable antitumor effects against some tumors, including RCC. Moreover, MLN4924, a potent and selective inhibitor of NEDD8-activating enzyme (NAE), was recently reported to disrupt SCF ubiquitin E3 ligase-induced protein turnover leading to apoptosis in tumor cells via deregulation of the cell cycle. This compound has already been applied in the clinical setting, e.g., malignant lymphoma. Thus, negative regulation of NEDD8 and its conjugation is an attractive anti-cancer strategy based on evidence obtained by basic research. We have developed a hypoxia-inducible factor-1 (HIF-1)-triggered expression vector for the purpose of selective gene therapy using NEDD8 negative regulator molecules, including NUB1 and the Ubc12 dominant negative form.

In this chapter, we summarize the data on potent molecules associated with the ubiquitin-proteasome system as anti-cancer targets on the basis of our reseach and discuss future perspectives in the treatment of RCC.

2. Mechanisms of ubiquitination pathway

Programmed destruction of regulatory proteins is crucial for homeostasis of cellular biological functions. The ubiquitination-proteasome pathway is a major scavenger system associated with regulated proteolysis inside cells. The pathway of protein destruction begins by conjugating a chain of polyubiquitin to a target molecule (Hershko & Ciechanover, 1998). The first step in the production of this chain is to connect a monoubiquitin molecule to E1(ubiquitin-activating enzyme) through a thioester bond in an ATP-dependent manner. Next, E2 (ubiquitin-conjugating enzyme) receives an activated ubiquitin from E1 and transfers a ubiquitin to a lysine residue in a target protein with the assistance of an E3 ubiquitin ligase. Repeated cycles via the E1-E2-E3 cascade generate a polyubiquitin chain, namely a death signal, which is subsequently recognized by the regulatory subunit of the 26S proteasome machinery (Fig. 1).

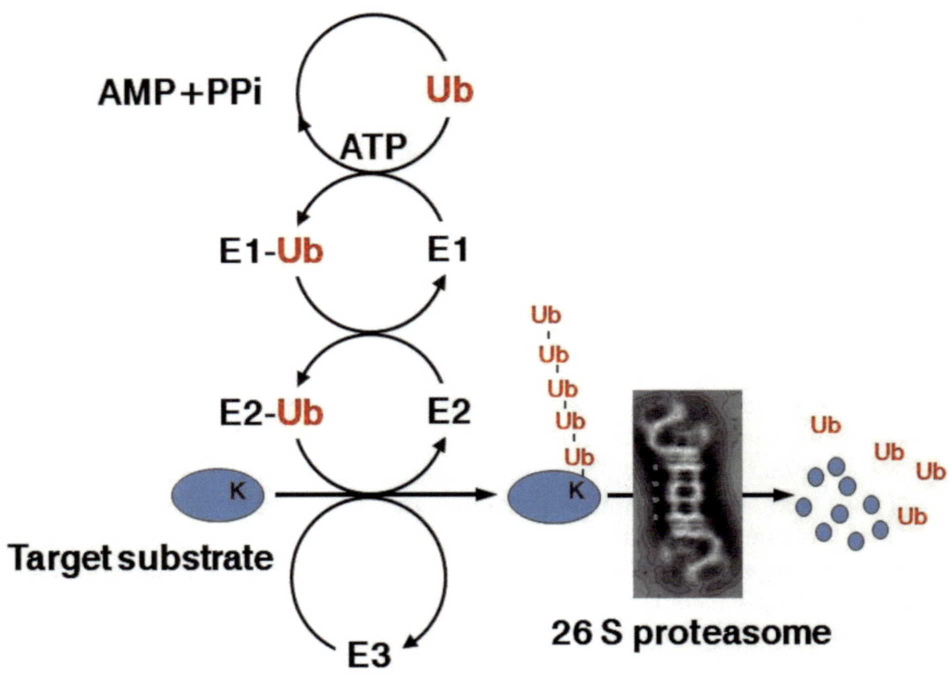

Fig. 1. Overview of the ubiquitination-proteasome pathway. Lysine residue (K) of the substrate is conjugated to ubiquitin (Ub).

2.1 Multiplicity of SCF (Skp-1, Cullins, F-box proteins) complex E3 ubiquitin ligases and their target proteins

The SCF complex E3 ligases or CRLs (Cullin-RING ubiquitin ligases), which are mainly comprised of Skp-1, Cullins, F-box proteins and Rbx/Roc RING finger proteins, are predominate among members of the E3 ubiquitin ligase family that promotes the ubiquitination of target proteins regulating various biological processes, including cell-cycle progression, signal transduction, and differentiation. The substrate specificity of SCF ligase depends on the combination pattern of its components, particularly the F-box binding domain. Numerous regulatory proteins targeted by SCF ligases have just recently been reported, as shown in Table 1. Therefore, deregulation of SCF E3 ligases may reinforce the instability of cellular functions; cell-cycle arrest, apoptosis, tumorigenesis, etc.

2.2 NEDD8, one of the ubiquitin-like proteins (UBLs), conjugation pathway

Several ubiquitin-like proteins (UBLs), including NEDD8, Sentrin/SUMO, ISG15, FAT10, Atg8 and Atg12, have been demonstrated to conjugate to a target molecule in a manner similar to ubiquitin. NEDD8 (neural precursor cell-expressed developmentally downregulated) was originally reported as a novel gene highly enriched in fetal mouse brain (Kumar et al., 1992). NEDD8 encodes a small protein of 81 amino acids, which is 60% identical and 80% homologous to ubiquitin, and equivalently conjugates to substrates (Kamitani et al., 1997). The crystal structure of NEDD8 is quite analogous to that of ubiquitin with the exception of two surface regions which are different (Fig. 2).

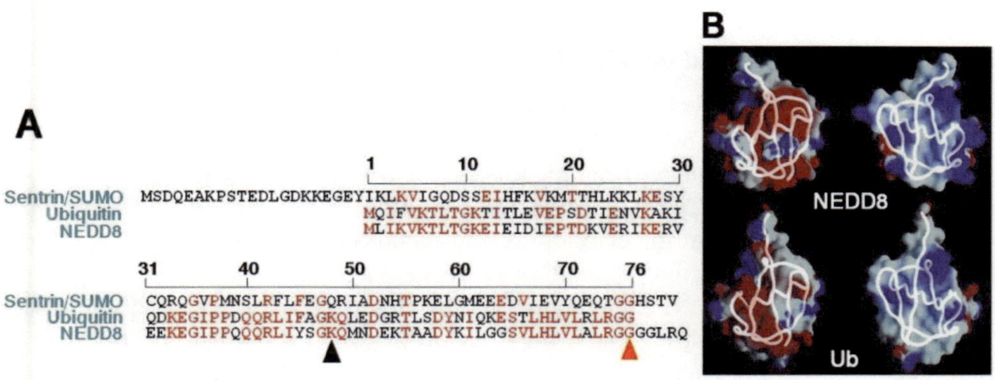

Fig. 2. (A) Alignment of amino acid sequences of human SUMO/Sentrin, Ubiquitin, and NEDD8. Black triangle; site of conjugation with lysine. Red triangle; active cleavage site for glycine. (B). 3D-structures of Ubiquitin and NEDD8.

The NEDD8 conjugation cascade, also known as neddylation, is mediated by E1 NEDD8-activating enzyme (NAE), E2 NEDD8 conjugating enzyme (Ubc12), and E3 NEDD8 ligase, which successively activate and transfer NEDD8 to a target molecule. First, the C-terminal glycine of NEDD8 is adenylated by an E1 NAE, which is composed of APP-BP1 and Uba3 heterodimer, in an ATP-dependent manner and transferred to E1 via a thiolester linkage. Second, activated NEDD8 is consecutively transferred to an E2 NEDD8 conjugation enzyme (Ubc12, Ube2f). Third, an E3 NEDD8 ligase transfers NEDD8 to a substrate lysine residue via an isopeptide bond. On the contrary, covalent neddylation of a substrate is reversibly deconjugated by the action of proteins (e.g. COP9 signalosome, NEDP1/DEN1, USP21) involved in deneddylation (Gong et al., 2000; Lyapina et al., 2001; Rabut & Peter, 2008) or inhibited by Cullin binding to CAND1 (Cullin-associated and neddylation-dissociate 1)(Goldenberg et al., 2004), or negatively down-regulated by NUB1 (NEDD8 ultimate buster 1) linked to the 26S proteasome (Kamitani et al., 2001; Kito et al., 2001) (Fig. 3).

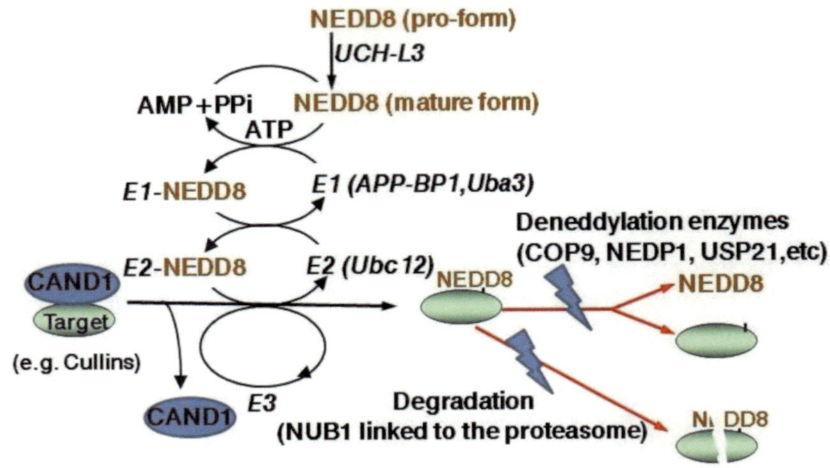

Fig. 3. Overview of the NEDD8 conjugation and deconjugation pathway.

2.2.1 Substrates conjugated by NEDD8; Cullins and other target molecules

Cullins, scaffold proteins assembling other components of an E3 SCF complex, are the substrates usually targeted by NEDD8 (Table 1). To date, seven Cullin family members (Cul-1, -2, -3, -4A, -4B, -5, -7) have been identified. Cul-1-based SCF complexes (CRL1), such as SCF^{Skp2}, $SCF^{\beta\text{-}Trcp}$ and SCF^{Fbw7}, are the most studied in terms of their cancer-related actions. SCF^{Skp2} is involved in the degradation of several cell-cycle regulators (e.g. cyclin D, $p27^{Kip1}$, $p21^{Cip1}$, p73, p130, etc) (Guardavaccaro & Pagano, 2004). $SCF^{\beta\text{-}Trcp}$ promotes degradation of Iκβα of the NFκB inhibitor and β-catenin (Skaar et al., 2009). Moreover, SCF^{Fbw7} has been reported to promote degradation of cyclin E, c-myc oncoproteins and Notch (Guardavaccaro & Pagano, 2004). A recent study identified more than 350 possible CRL1 substrates by employing global protein stability profiling (Yen & Elledge, 2008). Cul-2 properly generates a CRL2 complex (also known as VBC) with the von Hippel-Lindau gene product (pVHL) through elongin B and elongin C. This complex induces degradation of the hypoxia-inducible factor-1 α subunit (HIF-1α), of which proline residues are hydroxylated by prolyl hydroxylase in an oxygen-dependent manner and then targeted to pVHL for ubiquitination (Kaelin & Ratcliffe, 2008). Bialleic deletion of the VHL gene mainly results in the stability of HIF-1α and thereby ultimately contributes to tumorigenesis of sporadic clear-cell type RCC. The Cul-3-based SCF complex (CRL3), which is produced with Rbx1 and BTB-domain protein, promotes degradation of cyclin E, Mei-1 (a component of mitotic spindle), Dsh (a regulator of Wnt-β-catenin pathway) and NRF2 (a transcriptional factor associated with an anti-oxidant response) (Angers et al., 2006; Furukawa et al., 2003; Furukawa & Xiong, 2005). The CRL4 complex, including Cul-4 (A or B), a damaged DNA binding (DDB1) protein, and a DDB1 and Cul-4-associated factor (DCAF), controls DNA replication and nucleotide excision repair through ubiquitination of CDT1, p21, Histone H2A/H3/H4, XPC, etc (Hu et al., 2004; Jackson & Xiong, 2009; Kapetanaki et al., 2006). Interestingly, knockdown or a specific inhibitor of Cul-4A has attracted research attention as a strategy for treating Cul-4-amplified breast cancer (Chen et al., 1998) and UV-induced skin cancer (Liu et al., 2009). The CRL5 complex, comprised of Cul-5, a suppressor of cytokine signaling (SOCS) family proteins, Elongin B and C, and Rbx1, suppresses JAK-STAT signaling via degradation of JAK family proteins (Hilton, 1999). On the contrary, Cul-5 has been identified as a possible tumor suppressor, overexpression of which induces growth-inhibition of breast cancer cells (Johnson et al., 2007). As regards Cul-7, to date, there have been no reported observations indicating that it is neddylated in the formation of a CRL7 complex.

Scaffold	Adaptor	Receptor	Ring box	Substrates
Cul-1	Skp1	Skp2	Rbx1	p21, p27, p73, p130, Cyclin A/ D
Cul-1	Skp1	β-TrCP	Rbx1	IκBα, β-catenin, BimEL, Weel, p53
Cul-1	Skp1	Fbxw7	Rbx1	Cyclin E, c-Myc, c-Jun, Notch
Cul-2	Elongin BC	VHL	Rbx1	HIF1α
Cul-3		BTB-domain proteins	Rbx1	Cyclin E, Mei-1, Dsh, NRF2
Cul-4	DDB1	DCAF	Rbx1	CDT1, p21, Histone H2A/H3/H4, XPC
Cul-5	Elongin BC	SOCS	Rbx1	TEL-JAK2, JAK-STAT family proteins
Cul-7	Skp1	Fbxw8	Rbx1	IRS-1, Cyclin D

Table 1. SCF E3 ligases and their substrates.

As to NEDD8-target molecules other than Cullins, p53 is modified with NEDD8 via the function of MDM2, a RING finger E3 ligase, to facilitate its transactivation activity (Xirodimas et al., 2004). MDM2 also neddylates the proapoptotic protein, TAp73, and thereby enhances the localization of NEDD8-conjugated TAp73 in the cytoplasm to suppress its transactivation action (Watson et al., 2006). Moreover, MDM2 itself is also involved in NEDD8 modification, which contributes to its protein stability (Watson et al., 2010; Xirodimas et al., 2004). In addition, breast cancer-associated protein 3 (BCA3), which is highly expressed in breast and prostate cancers, was identified as a NEDD8 substrate (Gao et al., 2006). BCA3 inhibits NFκB-dependent transcription through its ability to bind to NFκB subunit p65 and the cyclin D1 promoter in a neddylation-dependent manner.

3. Focusing on the SCF E3 ligases for anticancer strategy

The SCF ubiquitin E3 ligases have been found to be dysregulated in a wide range of cancers, resulting in unlimited cell-proliferation and carcinogenesis via accumulation of their target-substrates. Consequently, the control of these E3 ligases is attracting attention as a possible strategy for treating cancers. The components (e.g. cullins, Skp-1/2, F-box proteins, Rbx1/2) and the molecules associated with modification by a SCF-activator protein, NEDD8, are potential candidates to be targeted in this approach.

3.1 Potent molecules involved in inhibition of SCF E3 ligases through deneddylation

As mentioned in section **2.2**, neddylation, i.e. conjugation of NEDD8 to target substrates, is catalyzed by certain known enzymes (E1, E2, E3) in a multistep fashion. Recently, MLN4924, a specific inhibitor of E1 NAE, was identified as an adenosine sulfamate derivative based on the results of a high throughput screen (HTS) study designed to identify NAE inhibitors (Soucy et al., 2009). Pharmaceutically, MLN4924 irreversibly forms a covalent adduct with NEDD8 via the NAE involved in the first NEDD8 adenylation step. MLN4924 is a potent ATP-competitive inhibitor that disrupts the thiolester bond between NEDD8 and Uba3, a subunit of NAE. Fundamentally, MLN4924-mediated suppression of cullin neddylation has been shown to increase expression levels of CRL-targeting substrates (Fig. 4). Moreover, MLN4924 was revealed to have antitumor effects against acute myeloid leukemia (AML) cells both in vitro and in xenograft models, simultaneously leading to increases in the amounts of CRL-specific substrates including Iκβα (Milhollen et al., 2010; Swords et al., 2010). Clinical trials using this agent are currently ongoing in AML patients.

Ubc12, an E2 NEDD8-conjugation enzyme, is also a key molecule in the neddylation cascade. Activated NEDD8 is transferred to the active site cystein residue of Ubc12 via a thiolester bond. Finally, Ubc12 conjugates NEDD8 to a single lysine residue of target substrates. Artificial Ubc12-C111S with mutant substitution of Cys-to-Ser in the active site (cys-111) was shown to have a dominant negative effect on the internal function of wild-type Ubc12, attributable to its covalent binding to NEDD8 (Wada et al., 2000) (Fig. 4). This mutant Ubc12-C111S has a forceful anti-proliferative action on cancer cells, concomitant with the instability of cellular morphology due to an actin cytoskeleton irregularity (Leck et al., 2010; Wada et al., 2000).

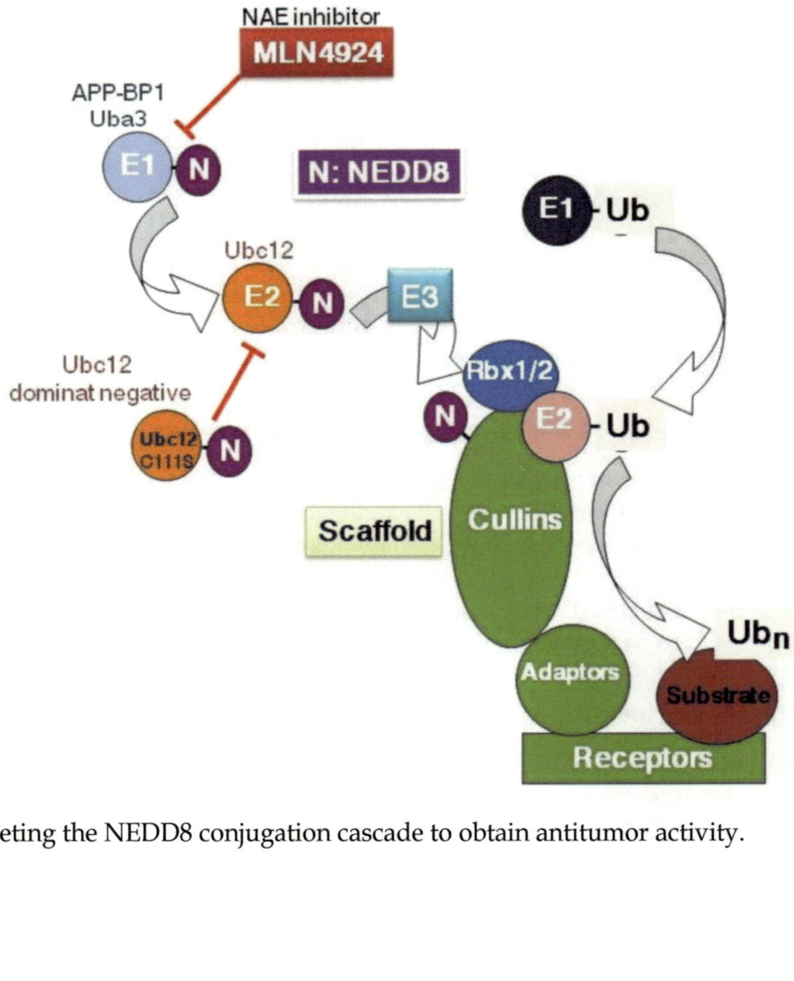

Fig. 4. Targeting the NEDD8 conjugation cascade to obtain antitumor activity.

3.1.1 Potent tumor-suppressor proteins of RCC, NUB1 (NEDD8 ultimate buster 1)/NUB1L

NUB1 is a NEDD8-interacting protein composed of 601 amino acid residues with a calculated molecular mass of 69.1 kDa. It is an interferon (IFN)-inducible protein and predominantly localizes in the nucleus. Moreover, NUB1L, a splicing variant of NUB1, possesses an insertion of 14 amino acids that codes for an additional ubiquitin-associated (UBA) domain, corresponding to a NEDD8-binding site (Fig. 5). Biologically, NUB1/NUB1L recruits NEDD8 and its conjugates to the proteasome for degradation and negatively regulates the NEDD8 conjugation system (Kamitani et al., 2001; Kito et al., 2001; Tanaka et al., 2003).

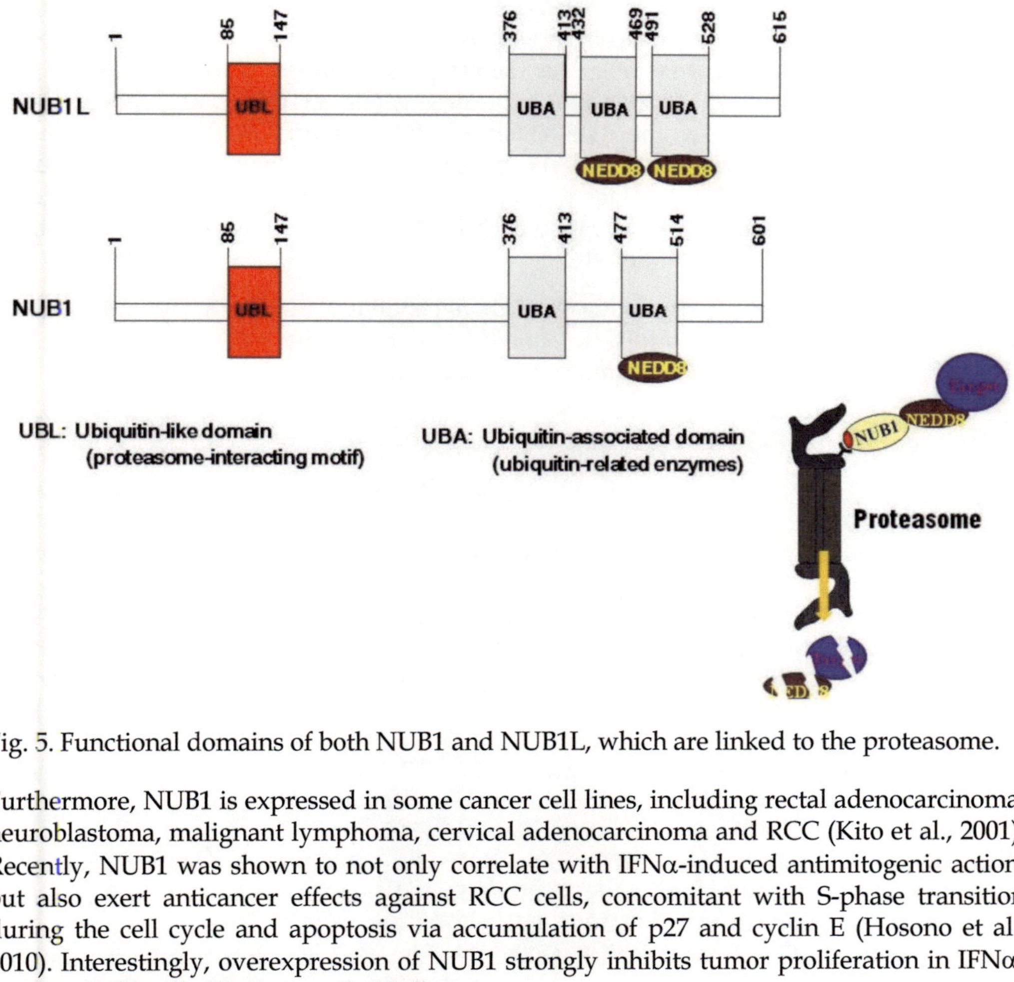

Fig. 5. Functional domains of both NUB1 and NUB1L, which are linked to the proteasome.

Furthermore, NUB1 is expressed in some cancer cell lines, including rectal adenocarcinoma, neuroblastoma, malignant lymphoma, cervical adenocarcinoma and RCC (Kito et al., 2001). Recently, NUB1 was shown to not only correlate with IFNα-induced antimitogenic action, but also exert anticancer effects against RCC cells, concomitant with S-phase transition during the cell cycle and apoptosis via accumulation of p27 and cyclin E (Hosono et al., 2010). Interestingly, overexpression of NUB1 strongly inhibits tumor proliferation in IFNα-resistant RCC cells (Hosono et al., 2010).

In general, tumorigenesis of RCCs, particularly clear cell carcinoma, is mainly attributed to HIF-1α-VEGF-mediated angiogenesis. HIF-1α is stabilized by loss of the function of a CRL2 complex via inactivation of VHL protein and of the hydroxylated oxygen-dependent degradation (ODD) domain of HIF-1α in a state of hypoxia inside RCC cells. For the purpose of developing tumor-specific gene therapy for RCCs, our laboratory constructed a potent delivery plasmid, composed of HIF-1-dependent reporter genes, in which 5 copies of the hypoxia-response element (5HRE) enhanced expression of the ODD domain and target gene under hypoxic conditions. Thus, these novel vectors including 5HRE-ODD-NUB1 or 5HRE-ODD-Ubc12 C111S may be useful for targeting advanced RCCs, even RCCs resistant to IFN, tyrosine kinase inhibitors, or mTOR inhibitors.

4. Conclusion

Potent agents (tyrosine kinase inhibitors, mTOR inhibitors), targeting VEGF and mTOR signal cascades, have recently been used worldwide for the purpose of treating metastatic RCC (mRCC) patients. Although these drugs have produced significant benefits in terms of overall survival and progression-free survival, as compared to traditional immunotherapy with IFN, there is no definitive strategy for the progressive-disease state of mRCC resistant to these target therapies. Alternative molecular targets (e.g. mTORC2, angiopoetin family proteins) complementary to the HIF-VEGF or PI3K-Akt-mTOR signal cascade are anticipated from future research. However, another approach distinct from conventional molecular targeting therapies is needed to prolong the survival of mRCC patients. Targeting neddylation as a procedure for inactivation of SCF E3 ligases was revealed to have a strong potential to suppress cancer cell growth.

Thus, a novel strategy for regulating NEDD8-dependent signal pathways may yield a breakthrough in the field of mRCC treatments, if it meets the criteria of showing high selectivity for cancer cells and being minimally toxic to normal cells.

5. References

Angers, S.; Thorpe, C.J.; Biechele, T.L.; Goldenberg, S.J.; Zheng, N.; MacCoss, M.J. & Moon, R.T. (2006). The KLHL12-Cullin-3 ubiquitin ligase negatively regulates the Wnt-beta-catenin pathway by targeting Dishevelled for degradation. *Nature Cell Biology,* Vol.8, No.4, (April 2006), pp. 348-357, ISSN 1465-7392

Chen, L.C.; Manjeshwar, S.; Lu, Y.; Moore, D.; Ljung, B.M.; Kuo, W.L.; Dairkee, S.H.; Wernick, M.; Collins, C. & Smith, H.S. (1998). The human homologue for the Caenorhabditis elegans cul-4 gene is amplified and overexpressed in primary breast cancers. *Cancer Research,* Vol.58, No.16, (August 1998), pp. 3677-3683, ISSN 0008-5472

Furukawa, M.; He, Y.J.; Borchers, C. & Xiong, Y. (2003). Targeting of protein ubiquitination by BTB-Cullin 3-Roc1 ubiquitin ligases. *Nature Cell Biology,* Vol.5, No.11, (November 2003), pp. 1001-1007, ISSN 1465-7392

Furukawa, M. & Xiong, Y. (2005). BTB protein Keap1 targets antioxidant transcription factor Nrf2 for ubiquitination by the Cullin 3-Roc1 ligase. *Molecular Cell Biology,* Vol.25, No.1, (January 2005), pp. 162-171, ISSN 0270-7306

Gao, F.; Cheng, J.; Shi, T. & Yeh, E.T. (2006). Neddylation of a breast cancer-associated protein recruits a class III histone deacetylase that represses NFkappaB-dependent transcription. *Nature Cell Biology,* Vol.8, No.10, (October 2006), pp. 1171-1177, ISSN 1465-7392

Goldenberg, S.J.; Cascio, T.C.; Shumway, S.D.; Garbutt, K.C.; Liu, J.; Xiong, Y. & Zheng, N. (2004). Structure of the Cand1-Cul1-Roc1 complex reveals regulatory mechanisms for the assembly of the multisubunit cullin-dependent ubiquitin ligases. *Cell,* Vol.119, No.4, (November 2004), pp. 517-528, ISSN 0092-8674

Gong, L.; Kamitani, T.; Millas, S. & Yeh, E.T. (2000). Identification of a novel isopeptidase with dual specificity for ubiquitin- and NEDD8-conjugated proteins. *The Journal Biological Chemistry,* Vol.275, No.19, (November 2000), pp 14212-14216, ISSN 0021-9258

Guardavaccaro, D. & Pagano, M. (2004). Oncogenic aberrations of cullin-dependent ubiquitin ligases. *Oncogene,* Vol.23, No.11, (March 2004), pp. 2037-2049, ISSN 0021-9258

Hershko, A. & Ciechanover, A. (1998). The ubiquitin system. *Annual Review of Biochemistry,* Vol.67, (July 1998), pp. 425-479, ISSN 0066-4154

Hilton, D.J. (1999). Negative regulators of cytokine signal transduction. *Cellular and Molecular Life Science,*Vol.55, No.12, (September 1999), pp. 1568-1577, ISSN 1420-682X

Hosono, T.; Tanaka, T.; Tanji, K.; Nakatani, T. & Kamitani, T. (2010). NUB1, an interferon-inducible protein, mediates anti-proliferative actions and apoptosis in renal cell carcinoma cells through cell-cycle regulation. *British Journal of Cancer,* Vol.102, No.5, (March 2010), pp. 873-882, ISSN 1532-1827

Hu, J.; McCall, C.M.; Ohta, T. & Xiong, Y. (2004). Targeted ubiquitination of CDT1 by the DDB1-CUL4A-ROC1 ligase in response to DNA damage. *Nature Cell Biology,* Vol.6, No.10, (October 2004), pp. 1003-1009, ISSN 1465-7392

Jackson, S. & Xiong, Y. (2009). CRL4s: the CUL4-RING E3 ubiquitin ligases. *Trends in Biochemical Sciences,* Vol.34, No.11, (November 2009), pp. 562-570, ISSN 0968-0004

Johnson, A.E.; Le, I.P.; Buchwalter, A. & Burnatowska-Hledin, M.A. (2007). Estrogen-dependent growth and estrogen receptor (ER)-alpha concentration in T47D breast cancer cells are inhibited by VACM-1, a cul 5 gene. *Molecular and Cellular Biochemistry,* Vol.301, No.1-2, (July 2007), pp. 13-20, ISSN 0300-8177

Kaelin, W.G., Jr.; Ratcliffe, P.J. (2008). Oxygen sensing by metazoans: the central role of the HIF hydroxylase pathway. *Molecular Cell,* Vol.30, No.4, (May 2008), pp. 393-402, ISSN 1097-4164

Kamitani, T.; Kito, K.; Fukuda-Kamitani, T. & Yeh, E.T. (2001). Targeting of NEDD8 and its conjugates for proteasomal degradation by NUB1. *The Journal of Biological Chemistry,* Vol.276, No.49, (December 2001), pp. 46655-46660, ISSN 0021-9258

Kamitani, T.; Kito, K.; Nguyen, H.P. & Yeh, E.T. (1997). Characterization of NEDD8, a developmentally down-regulated ubiquitin-like protein. *The Journal of Biological Chemistry,* Vol.272, No.45, (November 1997), pp. 28557-28562, ISSN 0021-9258

Kapetanaki, M.G.; Guerrero-Santoro, J.; Bisi, D.C.; Hsieh, C.L.; Rapic-Otrin, V. & Levine, A.S. (2006). The DDB1-CUL4ADDB2 ubiquitin ligase is deficient in xeroderma pigmentosum group E and targets histone H2A at UV-damaged DNA sites. *Proceedings of the National Academy of Sciences of the United States of America,* Vol.103, No.8, (February 2006), pp. 2588-2593, ISSN 0027-8424

Kito, K.; Yeh, E.T. & Kamitani, T. (2001). NUB1, a NEDD8-interacting protein, is induced by interferon and down-regulates the NEDD8 expression. *The Journal of Biological Chemistry,* Vol.276, No.23, (March 2001), pp. 20603-20609, ISSN 0021-9258

Kumar, S.; Tomooka, Y. & Noda, M. (1992). Identification of a set of genes with developmentally down-regulated expression in the mouse brain. *Biochemical and Biophysical Research Communications,* Vol.185, No.3, (June 1992), pp. 1155-1161, ISSN 0006-291X

Leck, Y.C.; Choo, Y.Y.; Tan, C.Y.; Smith, P.G. & Hagen, T. (2010). Biochemical and cellular effects of inhibiting Nedd8 conjugation. *Biochemical and Biophysical Research Communications,* Vol.398, No.3, (July 2010), pp. 588-593, ISSN 1090-2104

Liu, L.; Lee, S.; Zhang, J.; Peters, S.B.; Hannah, J.; Zhang, Y.; Yin, Y.; Koff, A.; Ma, L. & Zhou, P. (2009). CUL4A abrogation augments DNA damage response and protection against skin carcinogenesis. *Molecular Cell,* Vol.34, No.4, (May 2009), pp. 451-460, ISSN 1097-4164

Lyapina, S.; Cope, G.; Shevchenko, A.; Serino, G.; Tsuge, T.; Zhou, C.; Wolf, D.A.; Wei, N. & Deshaies, R.J. (2001). Promotion of NEDD-CUL1 conjugate cleavage by COP9 signalosome. *Science,* Vol.292, No.5520, (May 2001), pp. 1382-1385, ISSN 0036-8075

Milhollen, M.A.; Traore, T.; Adams-Duffy, J.; Thomas, M.P.; Berger, A.J.; Dang, L.; Dick, L.R.; Garnsey, J.J.; Koenig, E.; Langston, S.P.; Manfredi, M.; Narayanan, U.; Rolfe, M.; Staudt, L.M.; Soucy, T.A.; Yu, J.; Zhang, J.; Bolen, J.B. & Smith, P.G. (2010). MLN4924, a NEDD8-activating enzyme inhibitor, is active in diffuse large B-cell lymphoma models: rationale for treatment of NF-{kappa}B-dependent lymphoma. *Blood,* Vol.116, No.9, (September 2010), pp. 1515-1523, ISSN 1528-0020

Rabut, G. & Peter, M. (2008). Function and regulation of protein neddylation. 'Protein modifications: beyond the usual suspects' review series. *EMBO Reports,* Vol.9, No.10, (October 2008), pp. 969-976, ISSN 1469-3178

Skaar, J.R.; D'Angiolella, V.; Pagan, J.K. & Pagano, M. (2009). SnapShot: F Box Proteins II. *Cell,* Vol.137, No.7, (June 2009), pp. 1358, 1358 e1, ISSN 1097-4172

Soucy, T.A.; Smith, P.G.; Milhollen, M.A.; Berger, A.J.; Gavin, J.M.; Adhikari, S.; Brownell, J.E.; Burke, K.E.; Cardin, D.P.; Critchley, S.; Cullis, C.A.; Doucette, A.; Garnsey, J.J.; Gaulin, J.L.; Gershman, R.E.; Lublinsky, A.R.; McDonald, A.; Mizutani, H.; Narayanan, U.; Olhava, E.J.; Peluso, S.; Rezaei, M.; Sintchak, M.D.; Talreja, T.; Thomas, M.P.; Traore, T.; Vyskocil, S.; Weatherhead, G.S.; Yu, J.; Zhang, J.; Dick, L.R.; Claiborne, C.F.; Rolfe, M.; Bolen. J.B. & Langston, S.P. (2009). An inhibitor of NEDD8-activating enzyme as a new approach to treat cancer. *Nature,* vol.458, No.7239, (April 2009), pp. 732-736, ISSN 1476-4687

Swords, R.T.; Kelly, K.R.; Smith, P.G.; Garnsey, J.J.; Mahalingam, D.; Medina, E.; Oberheu, K.; Padmanabhan, S.; O'Dwyer, M.; Nawrocki, S.T.; Giles, F.J. & Carew, J.S. (2010). Inhibition of NEDD8-activating enzyme: a novel approach for the treatment of acute myeloid leukemia. *Blood,* Vol.115, No.18, (May 2010), pp. 3796-3800, ISSN 1528-0020

Tanaka, T.; Kawashima, H.; Yeh, E.T. & Kamitani, T. (2003). Regulation of the NEDD8 conjugation system by a splicing variant, NUB1L.*The Journal of Biological Chemistry,* Vol.278, No.35, (August 2003), pp. 32905-32913, ISSN 0021-9258

Wada, H.; Yeh, E.T. & Kamitani, T. (2000). A dominant-negative UBC12 mutant sequesters NEDD8 and inhibits NEDD8 conjugation in vivo. *The Journal of Biological Chemistry,* Vol.275, No.22, (June 2000), pp. 17008-17015, ISSN 0021-9258

Watson, I.R.; Blanch, A.; Lin, D.C.; Ohh, M. & Irwin, M.S. (2006). Mdm2-mediated NEDD8 modification of TAp73 regulates its transactivation function. *The Journal of Biological Chemistry,* Vol.281, No.45, (November 2006), pp. 34096-34103, ISSN 0021-9258

Watson, I.R.; Li, B.K.; Roche, O.; Blanch, A.; Ohh, M. & Irwin, M.S. (2010). Chemotherapy induces NEDP1-mediated destabilization of MDM2. *Oncogene,* Vol.29, No.2, (January 2010), pp. 297-304, ISSN 1476-5594

Xirodimas, D.P.; Saville, M.K.; Bourdon, J.C.; Hay, R.T. & Lane, D.P. (2004). Mdm2-mediated NEDD8 conjugation of p53 inhibits its transcriptional activity. *Cell,* Vol.118, No.1, (July 2004), pp. 83-97, ISSN 0092-8674

Yen, H.C. & Elledge, S.J. (2008). Identification of SCF ubiquitin ligase substrates by global protein stability profiling. *Science,* Vol.322, No.5903, (November 2008), pp. 923-929, ISSN 1095-9203

7

Oxidative Stress and Redox-Signaling in Renal Cell Cancer

Karen Block
The Veterans Health Care System, ALMD and
The University of Texas Health Science Center at San Antonio
USA

1. Introduction

Worldwide, approximately 150,000 people are diagnosed with Renal Cell Carcinoma (RCC) and 78,000 deaths are reported each year with the incidence on the rise (Jemel et al, 2010). Renal tumors are classified according to the "Heidelberg classification" where the tumors are separated based on their location within the nephron and linked to morphologic and genetic abnormalities (Schullerus et al, 1997). While most cases of RCC occur sporadically, inherited predisposition to renal cancer accounts for ~5% of cases. Hereditary and sporadic gene mutations associated with renal carcinoma include, von Hippel-Lindau *(VHL)* (Maher & Kaelin, 1997; Tory et al, 1989; Latif et al, 1993), tuberous sclerosis 2 *(TSC2),* (Washecka & Hanna, 1991), fumarate hydratase *(FH)* (Pfaffenroth & Linehan, 2008), succinate dehydrogenase *(SDH)* (Vanharanta et al, 2004; Henderson et al, 2009; Ricketts et al, 2008), MET (Schmidt et al, 1997; Lubensky et al, 1999), and Birt-Hogg-Dube' *(BHD)* (Pavlovich et al, 2002; Khoo et al, 2001, Schmidt et al, 2001). The diverse nature of these genes and the histologically distinct tumors they give rise to implicates various mechanisms and biological pathways in renal tumorigenesis. On the cellular level, inactivation of common pathogenic pathways and mechanisms involve oxidative stress. Oxidative stress is caused by an imbalance between the production of reactive oxygen species and the cells ability to neutralize the reactive intermediates. Adverse effects occur when the excess reactive oxygen species damage a cell's lipids, protein or DNA; together contributing to genomic instability and tumorigenesis. Additionally, reactive oxygen species can serve as important upstream regulators as well as downstream mediators of action through redox-signaling. Two major sources of oxidative stress in the kidney include the Mitochondria and NAD(P)H oxidases of the Nox family. Unlike natural byproducts of mitochondrial metabolism or mitochondrial dysfunction, reactive oxygen species generated by Nox oxidases function as signaling molecules that initiate and/or modulate different regulatory pathways involved in tumorigenesis and metastasis. Clinically, efforts to target specific enzymatic sources of reactive oxygen species production, that result in alterations of signaling and metabolism, represents novel therapeutic approaches to treat renal cancer. This chapter will review the links between genes inactivated in RCC that lead to enhanced oxidative stress, mediated by different enzymatic sources, and the biological pathways activated by redox-sensitive signaling molecules involved in cell growth, cell survival, and metastasis in RCC.

2. Sources of oxidative stress in renal cancer

Renal cell carcinoma, as is the case in many cancers, demonstrate oxidative stress (Szatrowski et al, 1991). Oxidative stress is defined as an imbalance between the production of reactive oxygen species and a biological system's ability to readily detoxify the reactive intermediates (Fridovich, 1978). Oxidative stress not only causes direct and irreversible oxidative damage to macromolecules but also disrupts key redox-dependent signaling processes. Reactive oxygen species include hydrogen peroxide (H_2O_2), hydroxyl radical (OH^-), peroxynitrite ($ONOO^-$), and superoxide (O_2-), many of which have been detected in renal cell carcinoma (Wickramasinghe, 1975; Block et al, 2007, 2010). Intracellular generation of the superoxide anion $O_2^{\bullet -}$ occurs, in part, by the semi-ubiquinone compound of the mitochondrial electron transport chain (Cadenas & Davies, 2000; Evans & Halliwell, 1999) and through NADPH-oxidases of the Nox family (Nox) (Babior, 1999; Vignais, 2002). Superoxide can interact with nitric oxide (NO) to produce peroxynitrite ($OONO^-$), a very reactive intermediate. Superoxide is converted into hydrogen peroxide enzymatically by the cytosolic antioxidant, superoxide-dismutase-1 (SOD1) or the mitochondrial superoxide-dismutase-2 (SOD2) and is then converted to water by glutathione peroxidase (GPX); however, this conversion is not 100% efficient and expression and activity of SOD1 is reduced in conventional renal cell carcinoma (Sarto et al, 1999; Fukai & Ushio-Fukai, 2011). Superoxide poorly crosses biological membranes (Evans & Halliwell, 1999); however, hydrogen peroxide can easily diffuse across biological membranes and is then removed by the antioxidant, catalase. Superoxide (O_2^-) and hydrogen peroxide (H_2O_2) can react to form a highly reactive and damaging hydroxyl (•OH) radical, which can not diffuse from the site of generation and quickly damages surrounding macromolecules such as amino acids, carbohydrates, lipids, and nucleic acids. Oxidative damage on nuclei acids form adducts such as deoxyguanidine (8-OH-dG), which if not cleared can potentially generate mutations (Novo & Parola, 2008). 8-OH-dG is often used an intracellular marker of oxidative stress. Together, overproduction of reactive oxygen species and/or alterations of the antioxidant system are key pathological triggers of cancer. Major sources of reactive oxygen species in renal cell carcinoma are NADPH oxidases of the Nox family and mitochondria. Unlike the mitochondria, which generate reactive oxygen species as a byproduct of cellular metabolism, NADPH oxidases of the Nox family generate reactive oxygen species that modulate redox-sensitive cellular responses and are essential mediators of normal cell physiology. However, as discussed below, excessive reactive oxygen species production by an overactive NADPH oxidase system, likely mediates constitutive activation of signaling pathways involved in the initiation and progression of renal carcinogenesis. This occurs through the selective oxidation of specific signaling enzymes/proteins that are linked to processes such as activation of transcription factors, secretion of cytokines or altering signaling proteins such as protein kinases and phosphatases. Redox research is providing evidence that increased and/or sustained levels of oxidative stress play a large role in the genesis of human cancers, including renal cancer.

2.1 NAD(P)H Oxidases of the Nox family as a source of oxidative stress in renal cell carcinoma

Figure 1. NAD(P)H oxidases of the Nox family are major sources of reactive oxygen species in renal cancer. Nox oxidases have six N-terminal transmembrane regions which contain four heme-binding histidines and in the C-terminal cytosolic region, they have an FAD and a NADPH-binding domain which together catalyse the reduction of molecular oxygen, using NADPH as an electron donor, to generate superoxide, (O_2^-) which is dismutated to hydrogen peroxide (H_2O_2) by superoxide dismutase (SOD). Although these oxidases are proposed to play a role in a variety of signaling events, such as cell growth, cell survival, oxygen sensing and inflammatory processes, their *bona fide* functions and regulation, as well as molecular composition, are largely unknown. Early studies on NAD(P)H oxidases were performed in neutrophils and phagocytic cells, investigating the respiratory burst NAD(P)H oxidase system. The molecular composition of the phagocyte respiratory burst oxidase or phagocyte NAD(P)H oxidase consists of two plasma membrane-associated proteins, gp91phox (the catalytic Nox subunit, now called Nox2) and the small regulatory subunit, p22phox, which comprise flavocytochrome b558. In addition to the membrane bound components, cytosolic factors, p47phox p67phox p40phox, and the small GTPase Rac are also necessary to activate the phagocyte NAD(P)H oxidase. Upon activation, the pg91phox phagocyte Nox oxidase generates a "burst" of reactive oxygen species, which functions in immunity. Homologs of Nox2, termed Nox (for NAD(P)H oxidase) proteins have been identified in somatic cells and generate reactive oxygen species at a much lower concentration than the phagocyte Nox oxidase. To date, the Nox family comprises seven members: Nox1-5 and the dual oxidases Duox-1 and -2 (Suh et al, 1999; Royer-Pokora et al, 1986; Cheng et al, 2001; Geiszt et al, 2000; Banfi et al, 2001; Dupuy et al, 1999; Deken et al, 2000). For the purpose of this chapter, Nox isoforms will only be considered. Nox1, Nox2, and Nox4, are the NAD(P)H oxidase isoforms that are predominantly expressed in the various renal cells (Bondi et al, 2010; Gorin et al, 2003, 2005; Block et al, 2007, 2009; Eid et al, 2009). The isoform Nox4/Renox was cloned from the kidney (Geiszt et al, 2000; Shiose et al, 2001). It is a 578-amino-acid protein that exhibits 39% identity to the phagocyte Nox2 with special conservation in the six membrane-spanning regions and binding sites for NAD(P)H, flavin adenine dinucleotide (FAD), and heme, the electron transfer centers that are required to pass electrons from NAD(P)H to oxygen to form superoxide and hydrogen peroxide (Lassegue & Griendling, 2010; Bedard & Krause, 2007; Brown & Griendling 2009; Geiszt, 2006; Selemidis et al, 2008; Geiszt et al, 2000; Shiose et al, 2001). The dehydrogenase domain of Nox4 exists in a conformation that allows spontaneous transfer of electrons from NAD(P)H to FAD, suggesting the enzyme has constitutive activity that is regulated primarily at the level of its expression in response to various stimuli (Nisimoto et al, 2010). Additional evidence suggests that in the presence of certain stimuli, Nox4 activity is enhanced when bound to p22phox, but does not require cytosolic subunits that are essential to activate other Nox isoforms (Bedard et al, 2007; Geiszt, 2006; Selemidis et al, 2008; Ambasta et al, 2004; Martyn et al, 2006). The localization of Nox4 may be cell type specific and has been documented to localize to intracellular membranes of the endoplasmic reticulum, focal adhesions and nucleus (Lassegue & Griendling, 2010; Bedard et al, 2007; Brown et al, 2009; Martyn et al, 2006; Pedruzzi et al, 2004; Hilenski et al, 2004). Nox4 harbors internal sequences that are predictive of a mitochondrial targeting sequence. Indeed, in the kidney, Nox4, unlike other Nox isoforms Nox4 localizes to the mitochondria (Block et al, 2009; Kuroda et al, 2010). This finding may suggest novel cross talk of the Nox oxidases and mitochondria in renal cancer. Nox1 is expressed in renal proximal tubular cells, glomerular mesangial cells, and podocytes. Activation mechanisms for Nox1 are similar to those of Nox2 and involve complex formation with regulatory cytosolic subunits upon agonist stimulation. However, in contrast to Nox2, Nox1 primarily interacts with the p47phox homolog, NoxO1 (Nox organizer 1), the p67phox homolog, NoxA1 (Nox activator 1), and

Rac upon activation (Lassegue & Griendling, 2010; Lambeth, 2007; Bedard & Krause, 2007; Brandes & Schroder, 2008; Geiszt, 2006; Selemidis et al, 2008). The expression of Nox regulatory subunits, p22phox, p47phox and p67phox are also expressed in renal cells (Jones et al, 1995). While Nox4 and p22phox over-expression seems to be a feature of renal cancer cells, ongoing studies are addressing the mechanisms by which Nox enzymes play a causal role in the renal cancer phenotype. Nox-dependent effects on cell division, angiogenesis, cell survival, mitogen, and cytokine signaling in a subset of human cancers provide putative mechanisms by which Nox enzymes may be linked to cancer development. For example, Nox1 over-expression transforms normal fibroblasts and creates a cell that is tumorigenic in athymic mice (Suh et al, 1999). Furthermore, Nox1 triggers an angiogenic switch and converts tumors from dormant to aggressive growth (Arbiser et al, 2002). Nox4 was found to regulate growth of malignant melanoma cells and to inhibit apoptosis of pancreatic cancer cells (Mochizuki et al, 2006; Vaquero et al, 2004). Nox5 mediates growth of prostate cancer cells (Brar et al, 2003). Overexpression of p22phox in normal proximal tubular epithelial cells can activate signaling pathways known to be constitutively active in the majority of renal cancers (Block et al, 2010). Nox activity is higher in renal cell carcinoma

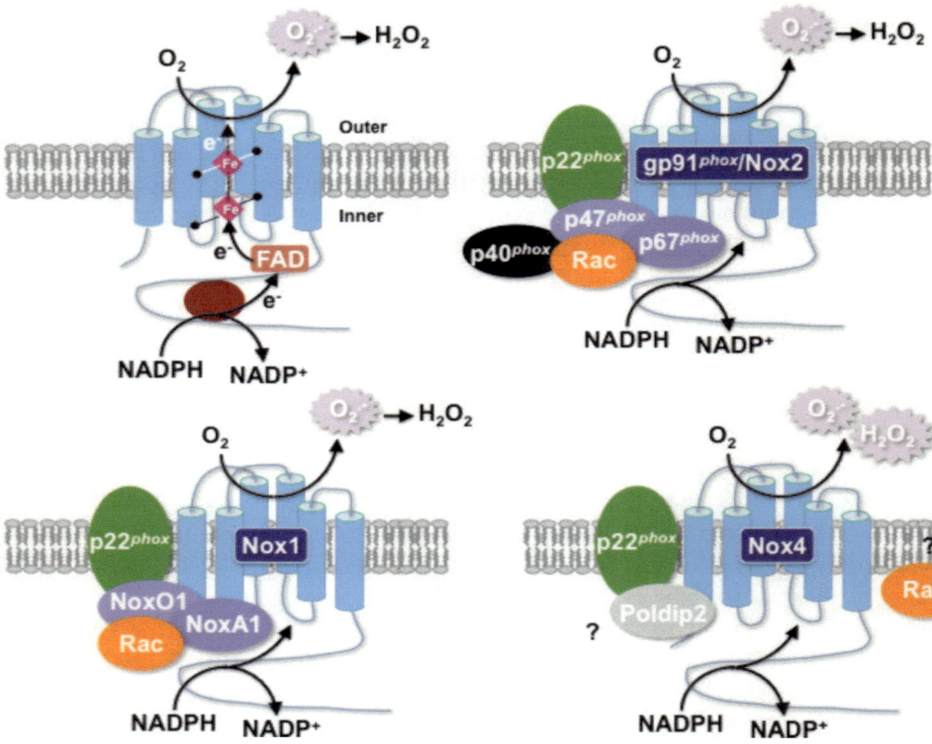

Fig. 1. Structure and molecular organization of the nicotinamide adenine dinucleotide phosphate, NAD(P)H oxidases of the Nox family. The top left panel illustrates the topology and the enzymatic reaction catalyzed by the Nox enzymes. The other panels represent the molecular structure of the different isoforms of Nox oxidases predominantly expressed in renal carcinoma cells, gp91phox/Nox2, Nox1, and Nox4. All Nox proteins can form a complex with p22phox, but the cytosolic subunits differ from the Nox oxidase isoforms. FAD, flavin adenine dinucleotide; H2O2, hydrogen peroxide; O_2^-, superoxide.

compared to normal proximal tubular epithelial cells and the expression of cytosolic SOD1 is reduced (Block et al, 2010). It has been demonstrated that superoxide is the main reactive oxygen species necessary for maintaining the expression of a critical protein involved in renal carcinogenesis, HIF-2alpha (Block et al, 2010).

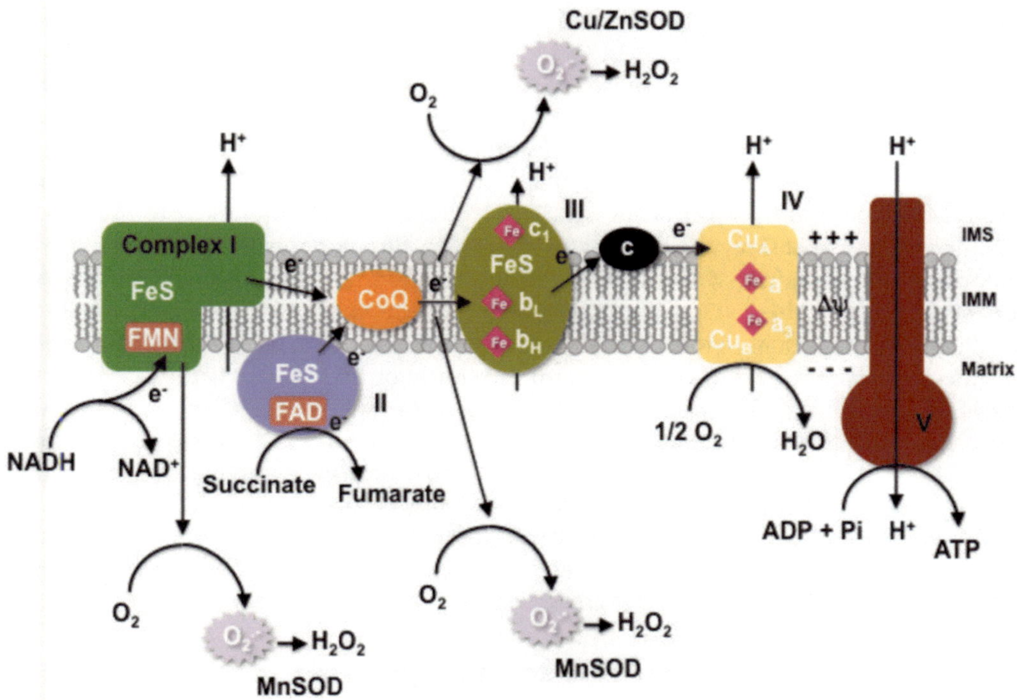

Fig. 2. Production of ROS by the mitochondrial electron-transport chain. IMS, intermembrane space; IMM, inner mitochondrial membrane; $\Delta\psi$m, mitochondrial membrane potential.

2.2 Mitochondria as a source of oxidative stress in renal cell carcinoma

Mitochondria play a central role in the generation of reactive oxygen species in cells and tissues. Aerobic energy metabolism relies on oxidative phosphorylation, a crucial process by which the oxidoreduction energy of mitochondrial electron transport is converted to the high-energy phosphate bond of ATP. During mitochondrial oxidative phosphorylation, superoxide anion and hydrogen peroxide can be formed. In normal respiratory cells, approximately 5% of electrons flowing through the electron transport chain can be diverted to form $O_2^{\bullet-}$ at the levels of complex I (NADH/ubiquinone oxidoreductase) and complex III (ubiquinol/cytochrome c oxidoreductase) (Cadenas & Davies, 2000; Halliwell et al, 1999) (**Figure 2**). $O_2^{\bullet-}$ is then converted by mitochondrial SOD (SOD2) into hydrogen peroxide (H_2O_2). Mitochondrial dysfunction, enhanced metabolism, or genetic alterations in mitochondrial DNA are potential mechanisms by which mitochondria-dependent reactive oxygen species generation is enhanced in cancer cells. Within the mitochondria, elements that are particularly vulnerable to free radicals include lipids, proteins, and mitochondrial DNA (mtDNA). Mitochondrial DNA is highly susceptible to damage because it is not protected by histones and is directly exposed to reactive oxygen species generated by the respiratory chain and DNA repair capacity is less efficient in the mitochondria. Free radical damage to mitochondrial proteins decrease their affinity for substrates or coenzymes resulting in reduced function and thus the production of more free radicals, which cause additional mitochondrial damage. Mitochondrial dysfunction is determined by a decrease in mitochondrial membrane potential and reduction of mitochondrial respiration with decreased ETC complex I and III activity while increasing mitochondrial-produced hydrogen peroxide. Tumor cells shown to exhibit mitochondrial dysfunction are those that have mutations in the tricarboxylic acid (TCA) cycle enzymes succinate dehydrogenase (SDH) or fumarate hydratase (FH). Electron microscopy of renal tumors has also demonstrated changes in the number, shape and function of mitochondria (Tickoo et al, 2000). Mitochondrial dysfunction in renal oncocytomas (BHD) are linked to mutations in subunits of complex I (Mayr et al, 2008). Additionally, chromophobe renal carcinoma exhibit abnormal mitochondria with altered cristae suggesting compromised mitochondrial function (Moreno et al, 2005). Alternatively, the production of reactive oxygen species may be altered by changes in mitochondrial metabolism. Cancer cells have enhanced expression of glucose transporters allowing increased consumption of glucose with high detectable levels of secreted lactate. This phenomenon, known as the "Warburg" effect, occurs when glucose is processed to pyruvate (via glycolysis) and pyruvate is converted into lactate in lieu of acetyl CoA (the primary intermediate of citric acid cycle) giving rise to glycolytic ATP production in the presence of oxygen (Warburg et al, 1924; Bui & Thompson, 2006; Brahimi-Horn et al, 2007). Overall, this altered metabolism, known as "tumor metabolism", mediates mitochondrial dysfunction and enhanced mitochondrial-dependent reactive oxygen species generation leading to enhanced cell growth and cell survival.

3. Gene inactivation and cellular factors that give rise to oxidative stress in RCC

Gene inactivation associated with oxidative stress

3.1 Loss of VHL

The von Hippel-Lindau gene (*VHL*) is inactivated in ~80% of renal cell carcinomas due to inherited or sporadic point mutations, deletions or promoter hypermethylation (Gnarra et al, 1994; Pfaffenroth & Linehan, 2008). Histologically, VHL-deficient tumors present as clear cell as the cytoplasm of these tumors are rich in lipids and glycogen, which provide the characteristic clear cytoplasm. Clear cell renal carcinoma is histologically the most common form of renal cancer and is likely derived from the renal tubular epithelium. The importance of VHL inactivation in renal carcinogenesis is underscored by the finding that restoration of VHL function in VHL-defective renal carcinoma cells suppresses tumor formation in nude mice (Gnarra et al, 1996; Iliopoulos et al, 1995). VHL is the substrate recognition module of an E3 ubiquitin ligase complex that contains elongin B, elongin C, Cul2, and Rbx1 (Kibel et al, 1995; Kamura et al, 1999). This complex targets the alpha subunits of the heterodimeric transcription factor HIF (hypoxia-inducible factor) for polyubiquitination and proteasomal degradation. Cells lacking wild-type VHL fail to degrade HIF-alpha subunits, thus hypoxia-inducible gene products are constitutively overproduced. Loss of VHL, and clear cell renal carcinoma in general, are associated with enhanced oxidative stress, mediated in large part by Nox oxidases. Nox-dependent superoxide generation is higher in cultured VHL-deficient

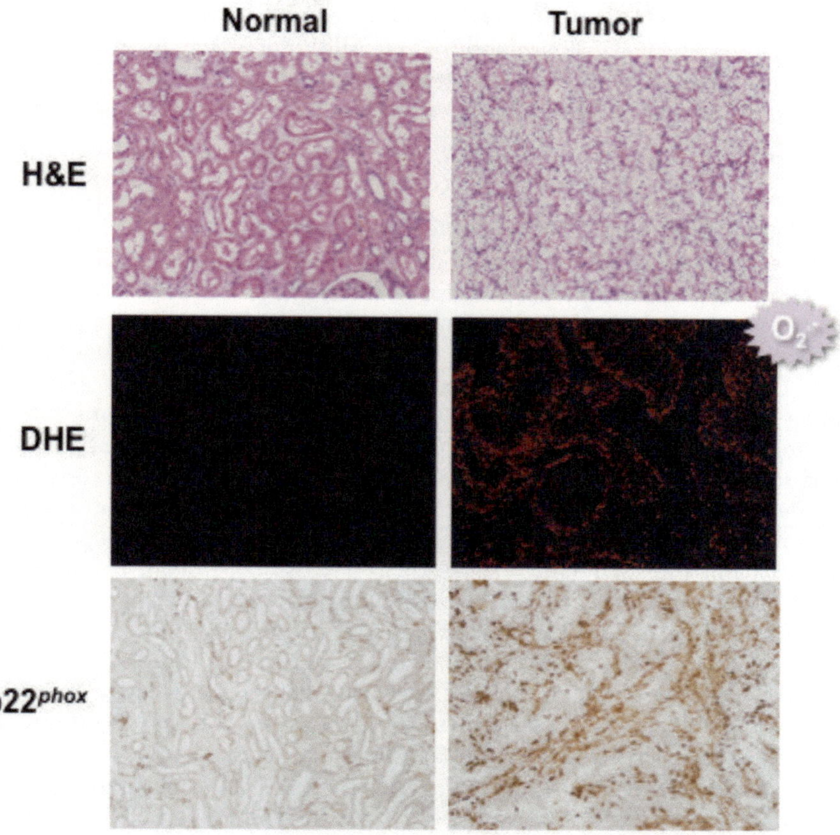

Fig. 3. p22*phox* protein expression and superoxide production is elevated in RCC tumors compared to normal adjacent renal tissue. Adapted from Block et al, 2010. *Top panel*, H&E staining. *Middle panel*, Detection of superoxide (O_2^-) in frozen 30-um-thick RCC sections, with dihydroethidium (DHE). *Bottom panel*, p22phox was detected by immunoperoxidase staining.

RCC cells compared to normal epithelial cells, mediated through p22phox-based Nox oxidases, **Figure 3**, (Block et al, 2007, 2010). p22phox protein expression, the Nox regulatory subunit necessary for Nox4 and Nox1 activation, is higher in VHL-deficient cultured renal cancer cells and in human renal tumors compared to normal controls (Block et al, 2007, 2010). Although the mechanism has not been fully defined, p22phox is an ubiquitinated protein and can associate with the von Hippel-Lindau protein *in vivo*, suggesting that p22phox-based Nox oxidase complexes may be stabilized upon the loss of the tumor suppressor protein, von Hippel-Lindau (pVHL). The Nox catalytic subunit, Nox4 is also overexpressed in VHL-deficient cells and in a subset of human RCCs at the mRNA and protein level (Maranchie & Zhan, 2005; Block et al, 2007, 2010). Although the mechanisms remain unclear, the Nox4 promoter harbors hypoxia responsive elements (HRE) known to be transcriptionally activated by HIFs (Diebold et al, 2010). Nox1 is expressed in renal tubular epithelial cells and is overexpressed in a subset of human RCC tumors compared to normal adjacent tissue (Block, 2010). Nox1 play a role in Nox-dependent reactive oxygen species and the genesis of RCC. Finally, it is clear in other cell types that Nox subunits and

Nox-derived ROS can be upregulated/activated by growth factors (Gorin et al, 2005; Bondi et al, 2010; Meng et al, 2008; Michaeloudes et al, 2011; Sturrock et al, 2006). Although the role of growth factor-induced Nox expression has not been explored, it is likely an alternative mechanism for enhanced Nox-derived reactive oxygen species in RCC.

3.2 TSC2

Tuberous sclerosis complex (TSC) is a multi-system genetic disease that causes tumors to form in several different organs, primarily in the kidney, brain, eyes, heart, skin and lungs. Tuberous sclerosis complex, like von Hippel–Lindau disease, are autosomal dominant tumor suppressor syndromes that can exhibit similar renal phenotypes and seem to share some signaling pathway components. TSC is caused by mutations in either the *TSC1* gene, located on chromosome 9 (Slegtenhorst et al, 1997) or the *TSC2* gene, located on chromosome 16 (European Chromosome 16 Tuberous Sclerosis Consortium, 1993). The TSC complex integrates cellular signaling inputs such as growth factors and cellular energy supply and regulates cell growth, proliferation, and survival. *TSC1* encodes hamartin and *TSC2* encodes tuberin, which form a heterodimer that inhibit mammalian target of rapamycin (mTOR) activity. mTOR is a key upstream regulator of protein synthesis activated in the majority of renal cancers and is discussed in detail below. Mutations in *TSC1* or *TSC2* genes give rise to tumors exhibiting increased phosphorylation of mTOR substrates and readouts of active mRNA translation, p70S6 kinase and 4E-BP1. Inactivation of TSC1/2 results in HIF accumulation through increased HIF mRNA translation by activated mTOR signaling. Rodent models harboring heterozygous mutations in the TSC2 gene develop spontaneous RCC, due to loss of heterozygosity (LOH). Kidneys of TSC2-/- rats demonstrate higher levels of the oxidative stress marker, 8-oxo-dG. In humans, between 60 and 80% of TSC patients have benign renal tumors called angiomyolipomas (AML) (Crino et al, 2006). These tumors are composed of vascular tissue (angio–), smooth muscle (–myo–), and fat (–lipoma). The discrepancy of benign and malignant TSC2-deficient tumors in the human and rodent disease respectively is unclear. In human AMLs, upregulation of the tumor suppressor phosphatase and tensin homolog (PTEN) by HIF-1 alpha was demonstrated to reduce Akt activation suggesting that PTEN may safeguard against developing malignant tumors in patients with TSC deficiency (Mahimainathan et al, 2009). A minority of TSC patients progress to renal cell carcinoma. Although the mechanisms remain unclear, oxidative stress may play a role. The DNA lesion caused by oxidative stress, 8-oxoguanine (8-oxy-dG), is normally excised and repaired by 8-oxoguanine DNA glycosylase 1 (hOGG1), which localizes in the nucleus and the mitochondria. Down regulation of OGG1 has also been linked to TSC-deficiency (Habib et al, 2008, 2009). Alternatively, *OGG1* is located on a chromosome region often demonstrating LOH, 3p25-26 in renal cell carcinoma (Gokden et al, 2008). Although genetic mutations in *TSC2* have not been detected in conventional clear cell renal carcinoma, Nox-dependent reactive oxygen species generation has been identified to post-translationally inactivate tuberin (Block et al, 2010). Taken together, reactive oxygen species may play a role in TSC inactivation, downregulation of OGG and DNA and lipid damage.

3.3 Tricarboxylic acid (Krebs) cycle genes, fumarate hydratase (FH)/succinate dehyrdogenase (SDH)

The tricarboxylic acid (TCA)/Krebs cycle is part of a metabolic pathway coupled to mitochondrial oxidative phosphorylation that converts nutrients to energy in aerobic cells.

The fumarate hydratase (*FH*) and succinate dehydrogenase (*SDH*) genes encode mitochondrial TCA cycle enzymes that play an essential role in energy production by catalyzing the conversion of fumarate to malate and succinate to fumarate respectively. Individuals who harbor germline mutations in either of these TCA cycle enzymes have an increased risk for developing renal tumors. Mutations in fumarate hydratase *(FH)* gene give rise to a rare form of hereditary leiomyomatosis and renal cell carcinoma (HLRCC). Renal tumors arising from genetic loss of FH range from type 2 papillary to tubulo-papillary to collecting-duct carcinomas. These tumors have significantly impaired oxidative phosphorylation and thus demonstrate aerobic glycolysis (Warburg effect) and are aggressive (Warburg et al, 1924). Positron emission tomography (PET) imaging demonstrates high glucose uptake in FH-deficient renal tumors lead to enhanced reactive oxygen species, mediated by a p47phox-based Nox oxidase, suggesting a role for the Nox oxidase isoform, Nox1 or Nox2 (Sudarshan, 2009). There is no evidence of genetic mutations in *FH* in sporadic conventional renal cell carcinoma; however, it has been demonstrated that mRNA and protein levels of FH are reduced in clear cell renal carcinoma (Sudarshan et al, 2011). Reduced levels of fumarate hydratase in clear cell renal carcinoma is associated with stabilized HIF-2alpha levels, likely mediated through an Akt-dependent mRNA translational pathway (Sudarshan et al, 2011). Additionally, overexpression of FH in VHL-deficient cells reduced cell invasion, suggesting that reduced levels of FH play a role in metastasis in clear cell renal carcinoma. Succinate dehydrogenase, SDH (complex II) is a functional member of both the Krebs cycle and the aerobic respiratory chain. Complex II couples the oxidation of succinate to fumarate in the mitochondrial matrix with the reduction of ubiquinone in the membrane (Cecchini et al, 2002). Mutations of the nuclear encoded genes of the mitochondrial oxidative phosphorylation complex, succinate dehyrdogenase B gene (SDHB) are associated with renal cell carcinoma (Vanharanta et al, 2004; Henderson et al, 2009; Ricketts et al, 2008). There is no detectable enhanced reactive oxygen species production in SDH mutated cells (Pollard & Tomlinson, 2005; King et al, 2006).

Cellular factors associated with oxidative stress

3.4 Hypoxia

Solid tumors exhibit intratumor hypoxic states, where regions of low oxygen (hypoxia) and necrosis is common Semenza, 2002; Maxwell et al, 1997). Hypoxia sensing and related signaling events, including activation of hypoxia-inducible factor 1 (HIF-1) now suggest that NAD(P)H oxidases, Nox1 and Nox4 serve as oxygen sensors. The human Nox4 promoter harbors putative hypoxia responsive element (HRE), which binds hypoxia-inducible factor-1 alpha (HIF-1a) (Diebold et al, 2010). Similarly, Nox1 mRNA and protein expression is enhanced in lung cells exposed to hypoxia (Goyal et al, 2004). Hypoxia-induced activation of Nox1-dependent reactive oxygen species generation was necessary for activation of HIF-1-dependent gene expression, which was blocked by the anti-oxidant, catalase (Goyal et al, 2004). In support of these conclusions, Nox1 and Nox4 are increased by chronic exposure of mice to hypoxia (Mittal et al, 2007). In RCC, the biological significance of hypoxia-induced Nox4 and Nox1 is unclear but may mediate HIF- and NF-kB-dependent signaling. In endothelial cells exposed to hypoxic conditions, superoxide is formed at the ubisemiquinone site of complex III in the mitochondria (Chandel et al, 2000). However, it is unclear if mitochondria participate in hypoxia-induced reactive oxygen species generation in renal cell carcinoma.

3.5 Growth factors

Stabilization of HIF-alpha binds to the HIF-beta subunit (ARNT) and the dimer translocates to the nucleus and binds to HIF-responsive elements, HREs (core sequence of 5′-RCGTG-3′ in the enhancer elements of target genes) which drives the transcriptional activation of over a hundred genes that support renal carcinogenesis including, but limited to, vascular endothelial growth factor (VEGF) and platelet-derived growth factor-beta (PDGF-b), implicated in angiogenesis and transforming growth factor alpha (TGF-a), which can establish a mitogenic autocrine loop with the epidermal growth factor (EGF) receptor (EGFR) (Knebelmann et al, 1998; Maxwell & van den Berg, 1999; de Paulsen et al, 2001) in renal epithelial cells. The growth factors bind to their respective receptors (VEGF-R, PDGF-R and EGF-R), which are each tyrosine kinase receptors. Growth factor-induced redox signaling by Nox oxidases is well established and involves several redox-sensitive steps. Activation of signaling pathways, mediated by the aforementioned tyrosine kinases, requires inactivation of a large family of enzymes that dephosphorylate tyrosine residues, protein tyrosine phosphatases (PTPs). All PTPs contain an essential cysteine residue, which is highly susceptible to oxidation by reactive oxygen species, especially by hydrogen peroxide, leading to reversible inhibition (Rhee et al, 2003; Chiarugi & Cirri, 2003; Lee et al, 1998). By inhibiting the activity of PTPs, NADPH oxidase derived reactive oxygen species can affect the activity of tyrosine kinase signaling pathways. For example, Nox4 has been implicated in modulating PDGF-induced cell growth, VEGF-induced angiogenic responses, insulin induced glucose uptake, and insulin-like growth factor-1-induced antiapoptotic effects, although in different types of cells (Mahadev et al, 2004; Datla et al, 2007; Wagner et al, 2007). Another kinase activated in the majority of RCCs is the phosphatidylinositol 3-kinase (PI3K). PI3K signaling is regulated by the tumor suppressor phosphatase and tensin

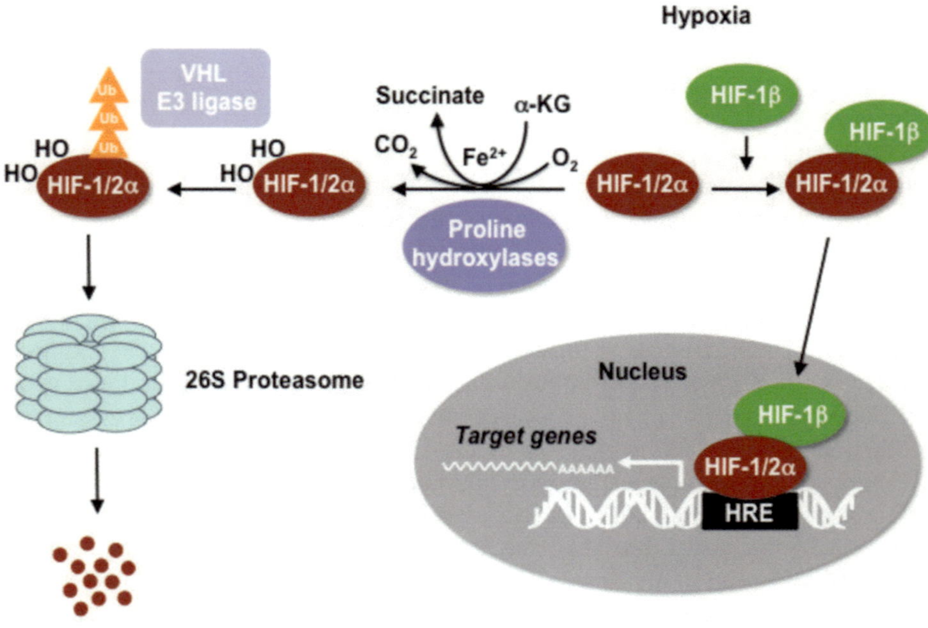

Fig. 4. Regulation of Hypoxia Inducible Factors (HIFs).

homolog (PTEN). PTEN dephosphorylates phosphatidylinositol 3,4,5-triphosphate, a product of the PI3 kinase (PI3K) reaction. In various cell types, overexpression of the Nox catalytic subunit, Nox1, potentiates PIP3 generation and activation of the protein kinase Akt induced by EGF, PDGF, and insulin as a result of hydrogen peroxide-dependent oxidation of essential cysteine residue of PTEN (Cho et al, 2004; Mahadev et al, 2004). Mutations in PTEN, although common in a number of cancers, are not commonly detected in RCC. However, reactive oxygen species -induced inactivation of PTEN has not been examined in RCC.

4. Redox-signaling in renal cancer

4.1 Redox regulation of hypoxia inducible factors (HIFs)

A common endpoint in the majority of RCC, independent of histological type, is the stabilization of HIF-alpha subunits through multi-step processes regulated at several levels by redox-sensitive pathways. HIF-alpha contains two highly conserved proline residues, located at the NH2-terminus in the oxygen-dependent degradation domains (ODDs), which are modified by a family of 4-prolyl hydroxylases (Epstein et al, 2001; Bruick & McKnight, 2001). Proline hydroxylases (PHDs) catalyze the hydroxylation reaction, which requires oxygen and 2-oxoglutarate (2-OG) as substrates and iron and ascorbate as cofactors. Proline hydroxylation promotes HIF-alpha binding to the multimeric VHL E3 ubiquitin ligase complex (Kamura et al, 1999). When hydroxylated and bound to VHL, HIF-alpha is polyubiquitinated and targeted for regulated protein degradation through the 26S proteasome (Jaakkola et al, 2001; Maxwell et al, 1999). HIF-alpha can also be hydroxylated at the COOH-terminus by asparaginyl hydroxylases which are Fe(II)- and 2-oxoglutarate (2-OG)-dependent family of dioxygenases (Masson & Ratcliffe 2003; Lando et al, 2002). Asparagine hydroxylation silences the COOH-terminal transactivation domains of HIF-alpha by preventing their interaction with the p300/CBP coactivator (Mahon et al, 2001). Reactive oxygen species inhibit PHD activity by oxidizing the PHD cofactors ferrous iron (Fe2+) to Fe3+ (Gerald et al, 2004). In solid VHL-competent tumors (hypoxic conditions), where mTOR is inactivated, reactive oxygen species are enhanced, likely stabilizing HIF-alpha subunits by inactivation of PHDs. Inactivation or loss of Fumarate Hydratase (FH) or Succinate dehydrogenase (SDH) can also lead to the inactivation of PHDs through different mechanisms. In FH-deficient cells, fumarate can competitively inhibit 2-OG-dependent HIF-hydroxylation resulting in the escape of VHL-dependent degradation (O'Flaherty et al, 2010), providing a VHL independent mechanism for dysregulation of HIF expression. Mutations in the Succinate dehydrogenase *(SHD)* gene promote the accumulation of succinate. Succinate is one of the end products of prolyl hydroxylase activity. Thus, succinate accumulation can block proly hydroxylase function and cause an accumulation of HIF-alpha (Pollard et al, 2005). In summary, loss of FH or SDH plays a role in HIF-alpha stabilization through inhibition of PHDs through metabolites and likely not through reactive oxygen species. Whereas, when VHL is mutated, expression of HIF-alpha subunits is maintained through Nox-dependent redox-sensitive pathways that mediate ongoing mRNA translation, discussed below (Block et al, 2007).

4.2 Redox regulation of PI3K-Akt signaling

The PI3K/Akt/mTOR signaling pathway is activated in the majority of renal cell carcinomas and mediates biological outputs such as cell growth, cell proliferation, metabolism, and cell survival (Manning & Cantley, 2007; Porta & Figlin, 2009). The PtdIns(3,4,5)P3 phosphatase PTEN that blocks PI3-kinase signaling is mutated in ~30% of renal cell carcinomas. Reactive oxygen species -dependent inactivation of PTEN in renal cell carcinoma has not been studied, but likely to occur. When PI3-kinase is activated, protein kinase B (Akt) and phosphoinositide-dependent protein kinase 1 (PDK1) translocate to the membrane and binds to PtdIns(3,4,5)P3 and PtdIns(3,4)P2 through the pleckstrin domain (Franke et al, 1997). The colocalization of activated PDK1 and Akt allows Akt to be phosphorylated by PDK1 on threonine 308, leading to partial activation of Akt. Full activation of Akt occurs upon phosphorylation of serine 473 by a Rictor-associated mTORC2 complex (see below). There are three isoforms of serine/threonine Akt in humans; Akt1, Akt2, and Akt3. In renal cell carcinoma, the Akt2 isoform maintains HIF-alpha expression in the absence of VHL (Toschi et al, 2008). The PI3K/Akt signaling pathway is regulated by reactive oxygen species produced by p22phox-based Nox oxidases (Block et al, 2007). Furthermore, the catalytic subunit implicated in reactive oxygen species-dependent Akt activation appears to be Nox1 and Nox4 (Block et al, 2007). Treatment of renal carcinoma cells with the PI3K inhibitor, LY29002 or wortmannin has no effect on Nox activity, suggesting Nox-derived reactive oxygen species act as an upstream regulator of PI3K/Akt signaling cascade (Block et al, 2007).

4.3 Redox regulation of mTOR signaling

Translational control of existing mRNAs allows for quick changes in cellular concentrations of encoded proteins. Regulation of the rate of translation is complex and occurs at several steps. One major step of translational regulation occurs at the cap-recognition stage. This is controlled by the formation of the eIF4F complex, which include the cap-binding factor eukaryotic translation initiation factor 4E, eIF4E, and its binding partners, eIF4G and the RNA helicase, eIF4A. Binding of eIF4F complex to the mRNA cap structure is inhibited by eIF4E- binding protein 1, 4E-BP1 (Gingras et al, 2004). 4E-BP1 competes with eIF4G for a common binding site within eIF4E (Marcotrigiano et al, 1999). Therefore, when eIF4E is bound to 4E-BP1, cap-dependent translation is inhibited. Release of 4E-BP1 from heterdimerization with eIF4E is regulated by mammalian target of rapamycin (mTOR)-dependent phosphorylation of 4E-BP1. Activation of mTOR is controlled by upstream kinases known to be constitutively active in most renal cancers, the PI3K/Akt- and the RAS/MAPK-signaling pathways. The regulation of the PI3K/Akt/mTOR signaling is redox-sensitive and is regulated by p22phox-based Nox oxidases (Block et al, 2007, 2009). The Nox catalytic isoforms, Nox1 and Nox4 play an important role in stabilizing/maintaining HIF-alpha protein expression in the absence of VHL through an Akt-mTOR signaling mRNA translational pathway. As previously discussed, activation of Akt signaling is likely mediated, in part, through inactivation of the PI3K-dependent phosphatase, PTEN. The hamartin/tuberin (TSC1/TSC2) complex is an upstream negative regulator of mammalian target of rapamycin complex 1 (mTORC1). Activation of Akt leads to Akt-mediated phosphorylation of TSC2 at amino acid, T1462, which leads to TSC2 dissociation from TSC1 and is targeted for regulated protein degradation through the 26S proteasome (Plas & Thompson, 2003). Post-translational inactivation of tuberin/TCS2 has been identified in conventional clear cell renal carcinoma, which exhibits hyperactive Akt signaling (Block et al, 2010). In cultured and human RCC where p22phox and Nox-derived reactive oxygen species are high, protein expression of TSC2 is significantly reduced due to

Akt-dependent phosphorylation and degradation. Activation of mTOR, in turn, phosphorylates, several substrates necessary to activate mRNA translation. Phosphorylation of 4E-BP1 results in its dissociation from eIF4E. mTOR-dependent phosphorylation of S6K leads to its activation and downstream phosphorylation of other proteins, which collectively affect translation initiation and elongation (Holz et al, 2005; Yang et al, 2003). The RAS/MAPK pathway mediates translation by phosphorylation of translational elongation factors, including eIF4E. eIF4E is a bonafide oncogene, that when activated, through phosphorylation, inhibits its binding to the translational repressor 4E-BP1 leading to aberrant and unregulated ongoing mRNA translation of oncogenes (Mamane et al, 2004). Therefore, eIF4E is considered an oncogene involved in cell cycle progression, cell transformation, and cell survival. Misregulation of mRNA translation and constitutive activation of mTOR contributes to renal cancer. mTOR is the catalytic subunit of two distinct complexes, mTOR complex 1 (mTORC1) and mTORC2. mTORC1 and mTORC2 are part of a multimeric complex commonly referred to as the Raptor-associated mTORC1 (Rapamycin sensitive), and Rictor-associated mTORC2 (rapamycin-insensitive). Raptor and Rictor are scaffolding proteins within each complex allowing the assembly of other proteins. mTORC1 complex consists of mTOR, Raptor, mammalian LST8/G-protein β-subunit like protein (mLST8/GβL), PRAS40 and Deptor (Kim et al, 2002, 2003; Harris & Lawrence, 2003). mTORC2 complex consists of mTOR, Rictor, GβL, and mammalian stress-activated protein kinase interacting protein 1 (mSIN1) (Sarbassov et al, 2004, 2005; Frias et al, 2006), Protor and Deptor. Unlike mTORC1, the regulation and downstream substrates of mTORC2 are less understood. mTORC2 phosphorylates AGC kinases such as the serine/threonine protein kinase Akt, at the hydrophobic motif (HM) site, Ser473 in the presence of growth factors, which is enhanced by PI3K activity. Rapamycin, a natural inhibitor of mTOR signaling, binds the FK506-binding protein (FKBP12) and, in turn, rapamycin–FKBP12 binds mTOR inhibiting phosphorylation of raptor-associated mTOR (mTORC1) substrates, but not rictor-associated mTOR (mTORC2) substrates. Prolonged treatment and higher dosage of rapamycin has been reported to inhibit mTORC2 in a subset of cell lines. Rapamycin analogues (mTORC1 inhibitors) have been utilized for the treatment for RCC. Despite initial excitement, objective response rates to these drugs remain low. One reason for rapamycin resistance of RCC may be due to absent and/or incomplete mTORC2 inhibition. In support of these clinical findings, *in vitro* studies have demonstrated that shRNA-mediated knockdown of Rictor (TORC2 complex) but not Raptor (TORC1 complex) reduces HIF-2alpha protein expression, suggesting TORC2 signals through yet unidentified pathways involved in mRNA translation to maintain HIF-2alpha protein expression (Toschi et al, 2008). A role for mTORC2 in mRNA translation is now becoming evident. mTORC2 complex has been found to associate with ribosomes in a PI3K-dependent manner and phosphorylates nascent Akt at the turn motif (TM; Thr450) site, which is not inducible by growth factors (Oh et al, 2010). In cancer cells, including renal cancer, where PI3K is constitutively active, mTORC2 binding to the ribosomes is enhanced. Additionally, it has been demonstrated that treatment of some cancer cell lines with rapamycin and rapalogs increase Akt and eIF4E phosphorylation involving PI3K and Mnk kinases (Wang et al, 2007, 2008). Importantly, cultured VHL-deficient cell lines and RCC cell lines cultured from patient tumors exhibit this phenomenon. Together, this provides an alternative mechanism for rapamycin resistance of RCC and may explain why so few patients respond to rapalog therapy.

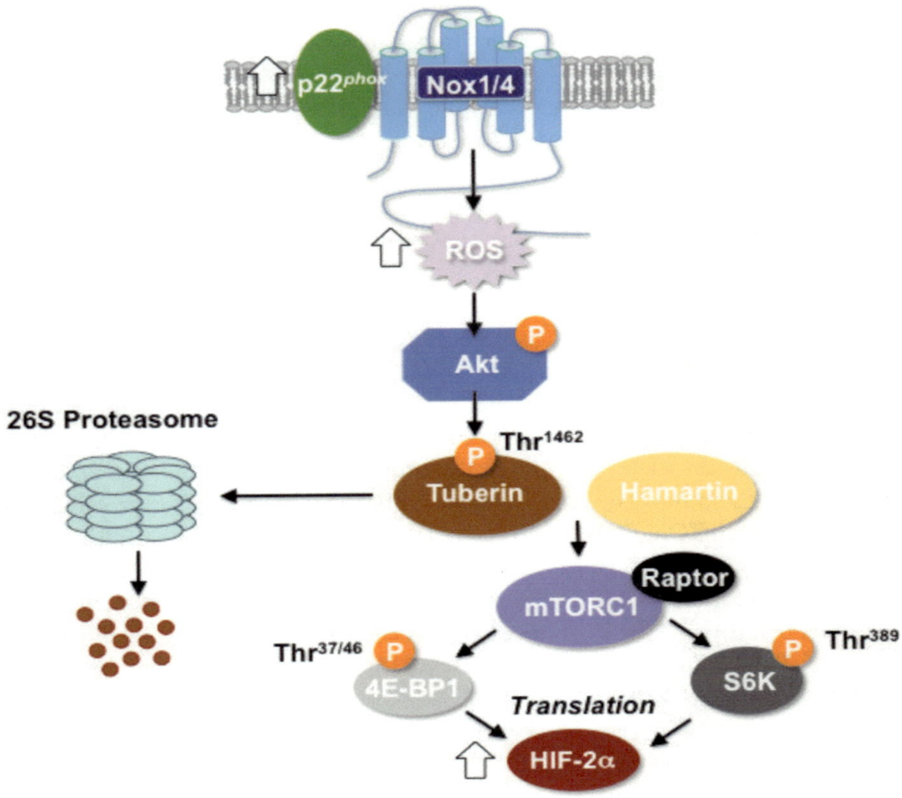

Fig. 5. Proposed mechanism of reactive oxygen species derived from p22phox-dependent Nox oxidases in the regulation of HIF-2alpha mRNA translation in RCC.

4.4 Redox regulation of nuclear factor kappa B (NF-kB) signaling

Nuclear factor kappa B (NF-κB) is a family of redox-sensitive dimeric transcription factors that regulate hundreds of genes involved in inflammation, proliferation, angiogenesis, and cell survival (Pande & Ramos, 2005). NFkB is constitutively expressed in a number of cancers, including renal cancer. It has been proposed that the resistance of RCC to chemotherapy and radiotherapy is due to increased levels of the nuclear factor kB activity and resistance to apoptosis (Oya et al, 2001; Qi & Ohh, 2003). In an unstimulated state, NF-kB binds a member of the inhibitory (IkB) family in the cytoplasm. Activation of NF-kB occurs in response to a wide variety of extracellular stimuli resulting in IkB phosphorylation and subsequent regulated protein degradation. The dissociation of IkB unmasks the NF-kB nuclear localization sequence allowing NF-kB to localize to into the nucleus where it heterodimerizes with a member of the NF-kB/Rel/Dorsal (NRD) family of proteins (Pande & Ramos, 2005). Although there are five known NRD members, RelA, cRel, RelB, p50 and p65, the classical dimer is composed of p50 and RelA. Reactive oxygen species have been implicated as second messengers involved in the activation of NF-kB as several studies have demonstrated that activation of NF-kB by nearly all stimuli can be blocked by antioxidants (Schulze-Osthoff et al, 1997, 1998; Giri & Aggarwal, 1998). Reactive oxygen species on NF-kB activation is further supported by studies demonstrating that hydrogen peroxide induces

NF-κB-dependent interleukin-8 expression in endothelial cells, which contributes to the angiogenic phenotype (Shono et al, 1996). Nox oxidase catalytic subunits, Nox1 and Nox4 have been implicated in the activation of NF-kB. Although the mechanisms remain to be determined, it is likely through regulation of IkK phosphorylation and degradation (Dröge, 2002). More recent studies suggest that NF-kB upregulates Nox oxidase expression and production of Nox-dependent reactive oxygen species. Here, overexpression of p65/RelA or IKKβ up-regulated Nox1, Nox4, and p22phox, mRNA, and protein expression through direct binding of the respective promoters (Manea, et al 2007, 2010). In contrast, NADPH-dependent superoxide production (Nox activity) was reduced in the presence of NF-kB inhibitors. Together, this suggests that NF-kB acts upstream to mediate Nox-dependent reactive oxygen species production and downstream NF-kB activity is positively regulated by Nox-generated reactive oxygen species.

5. Cell growth, survival and metastatic pathways regulated by redox-signaling in renal cancer

5.1 Mitochondrial-derived reactive oxygen species as a mediator of cell proliferation

Cancer cells utilize aerobic glycolysis and glutamine metabolism to generate the necessary resources for rapid cell proliferation and anchorage-independent cell growth. Altered glucose metabolism in cancer cells is termed the Warburg effect, which describes the propensity for most cancer cells to take up glucose avidly and convert it primarily to lactate, despite available oxygen (aerobic glycolysis) (Warburg et al, 1924). In addition to enhanced glucose metabolism, cancer cells also depend on continued mitochondrial function for metabolism, specifically glutaminolysis or glutamine metabolism. Glutamine's importance in tumor cell metabolism derives from characteristics it shares with glucose. The glutamine-fueled TCA cycle leads to the generation of reactive oxygen species by mitochondrial complexes of the electron transport chain and results in generation of ATP, NADPH, amino acids, nucleotides, and lipids (Wise et al, 2008; DeBerardinis, 2008). Mitochondrial metabolism of glutamine is elevated in cancer cells and the type of oncogenes activated in the tumor cells influences glutamine metabolism. For example, tumor cells that exhibit K-ras activation results in enhanced glutamine metabolism, fueling mitochondrial metabolism and mitochondrial derived reactive oxygen species-generation through complex III, independent of OXPHOS, which is necessary for cellular proliferation and anchorage-independent cell growth (Chandel et al, 2000). Additionally, c-Myc enhances glutamine metabolism in cancer cells by enhancing glutaminase (GLS), an amidohydrolase enzyme, which generates glutamate from glutamine. In prostate cancer cells, GLS is important for Myc-induced cell proliferation. K-ras and c-Myc amplification has been detected in RCC. Deciphering the pathways that fuel the TCA cycle differentially in renal cancer cells of various histologies will be important to elucidate the role of mitochondria in RCC cell proliferation and anchorage-independent growth.

5.2 Nox oxidase-derived reactive oxygen species as a mediator of cell proliferation

In renal cell carcinoma, inhibition of Nox oxidases using the NAD(P)H oxidase flavoprotein inhibitor diphenylene iodonium, DPI, reduces cell number and tumor growth in a xenograft nude mouse model; however, the mechanisms by which Nox-derived reactive oxygen species mediate cell proliferation remain unclear (Block et al, 2007). Kidney cancers demonstrate enhanced activation of redox-sensitive signaling pathways involved in cell proliferation. Notably, HIF-2alpha, rather than HIF-1alpha, has been shown to play a critical role in renal tumorigenesis due to HIF-2alpha driven TGF-alpha expression, the mitogen for proximal tubular epithelial cells. Up-regulation of TGF-alpha leads to its binding to the epidermal growth factor receptor (EGFR) with subsequent activation of the PI3K/Akt signaling pathway. As discussed earlier, growing evidence suggest that Nox-derived reactive oxygen species can stimulate signal transduction cascades through the EGFR likely through protein tyrosine phosphatase (PTP) inhibition. A role for Nox oxidases in agonist-induced cell proliferation has been demonstrated in a variety of other cell types; for example, proliferating keratinocytes showed higher reactive oxygen species generation and Nox1 expression than quiescent cells (Chamulitrat et al, 2003). Over-expression of Nox1 in several cell types is associated with increased cell division (Suh et al, 1999; Ranjan et al, 2006; Kamata et al, 2005). In addition, Nox overexpression has been seen in human renal, colon, prostate cancers and melanomas. In the case of Nox4 in melanoma cells and Nox5 in prostate cancer cells, inhibition of reactive oxygen species resulted in inhibition of cell proliferation, supporting a role for reactive oxygen species in mitogenic signaling (Lassegue & Clempus, 2003).

5.3 Reactive oxygen species as a mediator of cell survival

Increased reactive oxygen species is normally linked to cell death. However, in a subset of cancers, Nox-dependent reactive oxygen species has been associated with cell survival. For example, Nox4- and Nox1-derived reactive oxygen species inhibits apoptosis in pancreatic cancer cells and colon cancer cells respectively in a NF kappa-B- (Fukuyama et al, 2005) and Akt-dependent manner (Mochizuki et al, 2006). It is still unknown what role Nox oxidases and/or mitochondrial-derived reactive oxygen species play in RCC cell survival.

5.4 Reactive oxygen species as a mediator of angiogenesis

Renal tumors are known to be a highly vascular due to enhanced angiogenesis. Angiogenesis is the process in which tissue recruits blood vessels to form a neovasculature to vascularize the tissue. In most cases, the intratumor tissue experiences physiologic hypoxia and generates the angiogenic growth factor vascular endothelial growth factor (VEGF). VEGF induces angiogenesis by stimulating endothelial cell proliferation and migration primarily through the receptor tyrosine kinase VEGF receptor-2. VEGF binding initiates tyrosine phosphorylation of KDR, which results in activation of downstream signaling enzymes including ERK, Akt and eNOS, which contribute to angiogenic-related responses in endothelial cells (Colavitti et al, 2002; Matsumoto & Claesson-Welsh, 2001). Although NADPH oxidases are important for maintaining HIF-alpha expression in RCC, it is likely that Nox oxidases play a broader role in angiogenesis. Nox-derived reactive oxygen species function as signaling molecules to mediate various angiogenic-related responses such as cell proliferation, migration and angiogenic gene expression in endothelial cells (Ushio-Fukai et al, 2002, 2004, 2006). In endothelial cells, NADPH oxidase is activated by numerous stimuli including VEGF, EGF, cytokines, and hypoxia. Downregulation of Nox4 inhibits VEGF-induced endothelial cell migration and proliferation (Datla et al, 2007). Nox4 expression is upregulated in new capillaries in brain ischemia-induced angiogenesis of mice (Vallet et al, 2005). In animals of prostate cancer, Nox1 over-expression markedly increased angiogenesis by inducing the angiogenic factor VEGF correlating with an aggressive tumor phenotype (Lim et al, 2005). Nox1-induced hydrogen peroxide increases VEGF and VEGF receptor expression and MMP activity, markers of the angiogenic switch, thereby promoting vascularization and rapid expansion of melanoma tumors (Arbiser et al, 2002). Nox2 generates reactive oxygen species in endothelial cells by a number of agonists including VEGF and Ang 1, which are involved in angiogenesis (Ushio-Fukai et al, 2002; Gorlach et al, 2000; Li & Shah, 2002; Frey et al, 2002; Fürst et al., 2005; Harfouche et al, 2005). Neovascularization in response to ischemia or VEGF is inhibited in Nox2−/− mice and in wild-type mice treated with a NADPH oxidase inhibitor (Ushio-Fukai et al, 2002; Tojo et al, 2005; Al-Shabrawey et al, 2005). Taken together, accumulating evidence suggest that reactive oxygen species derived from NADPH oxidases play an important role in physiological and pathological angiogenesis; however, the enzymatic sources and role of reactive oxygen species involved in renal cancer angiogenesis remain undetermined.

6. Oxidative stress as potential novel biomarkers or therapeutic treatments in renal cancer

6.1 Novel biomarkers

Metabolites are the intermediates and products of metabolism. Whether its mitochondrial dysfunction, mutation in TCA cycle genes, or abnormal oxygen consumption, metabolic profiling can provide a metabolite fingerprint of intracellular physiology within a tumor. As the kidney is an organ, which secretes the water and waste drain from each kidney to the bladder and are eliminated from the body as urine, small-molecule metabolites are likely to be found in the urine. Metabolic profiling may be used for the establishment of non-invasive urinary biomarkers for the prediction of renal cancer, prognostic indicator, or responsiveness to therapy. A comprehensive metabolomics-driven approach is needed for the identification of biomarkers in various histologies of RCC. The most representative product that may reflect oxidative damage induced by reactive oxygen species detectable in the urine is 8-hydroxy-2'-deoxyguanosine (8-OHdG) (Sakano et al, 2009). F2-Isoprostanes and malondialdehyde (MDA) are considered reliable markers of lipid peroxidation *in vivo* and can also be detected in the urine. However, the use of oxidative stress markers as biomarkers for RCC may be challenging as many co-morbidities such as diabetes and hypertension induce oxidative stress that may be detected in the urine.

6.2 Antioxidants

The use of antioxidants to prevent disease is controversial. Antioxidants are manufactured within the body and are naturally found in fruits and vegetable food sources. As this chapter has just revealed a broad role for reactive oxygen species in renal tumorigenesis, it would be rational to think that antioxidants will slow or prevent activation of oncogene signaling in tumor cells. Indeed, *in vitro* studies demonstrate some beneficial effects of antioxidants on tumor cells and observational studies suggested a diet high in fruits and vegetables, both of which are rich with antioxidants, may prevent cancer development. However, many randomized trials have indicated that there is no benefit in preventing cancer or affecting mortality with antioxidant supplementation using vitamin C, vitamin E, or beta carotene in human patients (Lin et al, 2009). Supplementation with vitamin C, along with vitamins A, E, and beta-carotene did not prevent gastrointestinal cancer (Bjelakovic et al, 2004) did not lower the risk of prostate cancer (Kirsh et al, 2006) however, one study did find an association between the intake of vitamins A, C, or E and a reduced risk for cervical cancer (Kim et al, 2010). Are the successes or failure of antioxidants organ or genetic specific? All cells have intracellular antioxidant defense systems. However, as discussed, neutralization of free radicals are not 100% efficient and some proteins that function to neutralize the antioxidants are significantly reduced or inactivated in cancers, including renal cancer. Moreover, the enzymatic sources that generate reactive oxygen species are overactive and are not "turned off" by antioxidants. Here, it is likely that co-morbidities such as diabetes and hypertension play a systemic biological role in antioxidant failures, as diabetes and hypertension are known to induce oxidative stress alone, without the compounding issues of a tumor and tumor environment. Taken together, it is evident that a successful approach for antioxidant therapy will be to target the enzymatic sources that produce the reactive oxygen species such as NADPH oxidases or the mitochondria. Targeting Nox enzymes in an isoform-selective manner is likely to offer therapeutic advantages.

6.3 Novel therapeutic targets

Hypoxia inducible factors are master transcriptional regulators that activate over 100 genes involved in renal tumorigenesis. Therefore, targeting HIF-alpha subunits is an attractive therapeutic clinical goal. To date, agents with anti-angiogenic activity that inhibit VEGFR and PDGFR signaling (e.g. sorafenib, sunitinib), the VEGF ligand (bevacizumab), and the EGF ligand (cetuximab) have demonstrated some effectiveness in the management of renal cell cancer to different degrees (Patel et al, 2006; Sosman et al, 2007). However, these agents target only a small portion of the downstream genes regulated by HIF. As outlined here, the majority of renal cancer exhibits stabilization of HIF-alpha through the loss of VHL function or inhibition of proline hydroxylation activity together resulting in HIF-alpha overexpression. In the absence of VHL, maintaining HIF-alpha expression is dependent on ongoing mRNA translation, regulated by mTOR signaling. However, clinical trials using approved mTOR inhibitors such as temsirolimus (CCI-779) and everolimus (RAD001) do not exhibit beneficial outcomes long term. Importantly, renal carcinoma cells express HIF-2alpha or HIF-1alpha/HIF-2alpha and knockout and molecular studies have revealed that HIF-1alpha translation is dependent on mTORC1 signaling, whereas HIF-2alpha is downstream of the mTORC2 pathway; therefore, rapalogs have little to no effect on reducing HIF-2alpha expression in renal cell carcinoma (Toschi et al, 2008). Because Nox-dependent reactive oxygen species production maintain HIF-2alpha in the absence of proteasomal degradation by VHL and the broader role Nox oxidases play in other signaling pathways that mediate the genesis of RCC, suggest that novel development of specific inhibitors of NADPH oxidases may provide a novel approach for therapeutic targeting. For now, based on the literature and molecular mechanisms of mTOR signaling, new agents that target both the mTORC1 and mTORC2 pathways have the potential to downregulate both HIF-1alpha and HIF-2alpha in clear cell kidney cancers and could provide more antitumor activity than temsirolimus and everolimus, which again primarily target the mTORC1 pathway. Agents, which inhibit mTORC1, mTORC2 and PI3K pathways, such as AZD8055, demonstrates potent anti-tumor activity in *in vitro* and *in vivo* model systems (Chresta et al, 2010). It is unclear, if these inhibitors have indirect antioxidant effects.

7. Acknowledgement

I would like to thank my colleague, Dr. Yves Gorin for the creative design of the figures and critical reading of this chapter. KB is supported by Veterans Career Development Award & NIH/NCI CA131272.

8. References

Al-Shabrawey, M; Bartoli, M; El-Remessy, AB; Platt, DH; Matragoon, S; Behzadian, MA; Caldwell, RW; & Caldwell, RB. Inhibition of NAD(P)H oxidase activity blocks vascular endothelial growth factor overexpression and neovascularization during ischemic retinopathy. *Am J Pathol.* 167, (2005), 599-607.

Ambasta, RK; Kumar, P; Griendling, KK; Schmidt, HH; Busse, R; & Brandes, RP. Direct interaction of the novel Nox proteins with p22phox is required for the formation of a functionally active NADPH oxidase. *J Biol Chem* 279, (2004), 45935–45941.

Arbiser, JL; Petros, J; Klafter, R; Govindajaran, B; McLaughlin, ER; Brown, LF; Cohen, C; Moses, M; Kilroy, S; Arnold, RS; & Lambeth, JD. Reactive oxygen generated by Nox1 triggers the angiogenic switch. *Proc Natl Acad Sci U S A.* 99, (2002), 715-720.

Babior, BM. NADPH oxidase: an update. *Blood.* 93, (1999) 464-476.

Bánfi, B; Malgrange, B; Knisz, J; Steger, K; Dubois-Dauphin, M; & Krause, KH. NOX3, a superoxide-generating NADPH oxidase of the inner ear. *J Biol Chem.* 279, (2004), 46065-46072.

Bedard, K; & Krause, KH. The NOX family of ROS-generating NADPH oxidases: physiology and pathophysiology. *Physiol Rev* 87, (2007), 245–313.

Bjelakovic, G; Nikolova, D; Simonetti, RG; & Gluud, C. Antioxidant supplements for prevention of gastrointestinal cancers: a systematic review and meta-analysis. *Lancet.* 364, (2004), 1219-1228.

Block, K; Gorin; Hoover, P, Williams, P; Chelmicki, T; Clark, RA; Yoneda, T; & Abboud, HE. NAD(P)H oxidases regulate HIF-2alpha protein expression. *J Biol Chem.* 282, (2007), 8019-8026.

Block, K; Gorin, Y; & Abboud, HE. Subcellular localization of Nox4 and regulation in diabetes. *Proc Natl Acad Sci USA* 106, (2009), 14385–14390.

Block, K; Gorin, Y; New, DD; Eid, A; Chelmicki; T, Reed, A; Choudhury, GG; Parekh, DJ; & Abboud HE. The NADPH oxidase subunit p22phox inhibits the function of the tumor suppressor protein tuberin. *Am J Pathol.* 176, (2010), 2447-5245.

Bondi, CD; Manickam, N; Lee, DY; Block, K; Gorin, Y; Abboud, HE; & Barnes JL. NAD(P)H oxidase mediates TGF-beta1-induced activation of kidney myofibroblasts. *J Am Soc Nephrol.* 21, (2010), 93-102.

Brahimi-Horn, MC; Chiche, J; & Pouysségur, J. Hypoxia signalling controls metabolic demand. *Curr Opin Cell Biol.* 19, (2007), 223-239.

Brandes, RP; & Schroder, K. Composition and functions of vascular nicotinamide adenine dinucleotide phosphate oxidases. *Trends Cardiovasc Med.* 18, (2008), 15–19.

Brar, SS; Corbin, Z; Kennedy, TP; Hemendinger, R; Thornton, L; Bommarius, B; Arnold, RS; Whorton, AR; Sturrock, AB; Hueckstеadt, TP; Quinn, MT; Krenitsky, K; Ardie, KG; Lambeth, JD; & Hoidal, JR. NOX5 NAD(P)H oxidase regulates growth and apoptosis in DU 145 prostate cancer cells. *Am J Physiol Cell Physiol.* 285, (2003) C353-C369.

Bruick, RK; & McKnight, SL. *Science.* 294, (2001), 1337-1340. A conserved family of prolyl-4-hydroxylases that modify HIF.

Brown, DI; & Griendling, KK. Nox proteins in signal transduction. *Free Radic Biol Med* 47, (2009), 1239–1253.

Bui, T; & Thompson, CB. Cancer's sweet tooth. *Cancer Cell.* 9 (2006) 419-420.

Cadenas, E; & Davies, KJ. Mitochondrial free radical generation, oxidative stress, and aging. *Free Radic Biol Med.* 29, (2000), 222-230.

Cecchini, G; Schröder, I; Gunsalus, RP; & Maklashina, E. Succinate dehydrogenase and fumarate reductase from Escherichia coli. *Biochim Biophys Acta.* 1553, (2002), 140-157.

Chamulitrat, W; Schmidt, R; Tomakidi, P; Stremmel, W; Chunglok, W; Kawahara, T; & Rokutan, K. Association of gp91phox homolog Nox1 with anchorage-independent growth and MAP kinase-activation of transformed human keratinocytes. *Oncogene.* 22, (2003), 6045-6053.

Chandel, NS; McClintock, DS; Feliciano, CE; Wood, TM; Melendez, JA; Rodriguez, AM; & Schumacker, PT. Reactive oxygen species generated at mitochondrial complex III stabilize hypoxia-inducible factor-1alpha during hypoxia: a mechanism of O2 sensing. *J Biol Chem.* 275, (2000) 25130-15138.

Cheng, G; Cao, Z; Xu, X; van Meir, EG; & Lambeth, JD. Homologs of gp91phox: cloning and tissue expression of Nox3, Nox4, and Nox5. *Gene.* 269, (2001) 131-140.

Chiarugi, P; & Cirri, P. Redox regulation of protein tyrosine phosphatases during receptor tyrosine kinase signal transduction. *Trends Biochem Sci.* 28, (2003), 509-514

Cho, SH; Lee, CH; Ahn, Y; Kim, H; Kim, H; Ahn, CY; Yang, KS; & Lee, SR. Redox regulation of PTEN and protein tyrosine phosphatases in H(2)O(2) mediated cell signaling. *FEBS Lett.* 560, (2004), 7-13.

Chresta, CM; Davies, BR; Hickson, I; Harding, T; Cosulich, S; Critchlow, SE; Vincent, JP; Ellston, R; Jones, D; Sini, P; James, D; Howard, Z; Dudley, P; Hughes, G; Smith, L; Maguire, S; Hummersone, M; Malagu, K; Menear, K; Jenkins, R; Jacobsen, M; Smith, GC; Guichard, S; & Pass, M. AZD8055 is a potent, selective, and orally bioavailable ATP-competitive mammalian target of rapamycin kinase inhibitor with in vitro and in vivo antitumor activity. *Cancer Res.* 70, (2010), 288-298.

Colavitti, R; Pani, G; Bedogni, B; Anzevino, R; Borrello, S; Waltenberger, J; & Galeotti, T. Reactive oxygen species as downstream mediators of angiogenic signaling by vascular endothelial growth factor receptor-2/KDR. *J Biol Chem.* 277, (2002), 3101-3108.

Crino, PB; Nathanson, KL; & Henske, EP. The tuberous sclerosis complex. *N Engl J Med.* 355, (2006), 1345-1356.

Dang, CV; Resar, LM,; Emison, E; Kim, S; Li, Q; Prescott, JE; Wonsey, D; & Zeller, K. Function of the c-Myc oncogenic transcription factor. *Exp Cell Res.* 253, (1999), 63-77.

Datla, SR; Peshavariya, H; Dusting, GJ; Mahadev, K; Goldstein, BJ; & Jiang, F. Important role of Nox4 type NADPH oxidase in angiogenic responses in human microvascular endothelial cells in vitro. *Arterioscler Thromb Vasc Biol.* 27, (2007), 2319-2324.

DeBerardinis, RJ. Is cancer a disease of abnormal cellular metabolism? New angles on an old idea. *Genet Med.* 10, (2008), 767-777.

Deken, X; Wang, D; Many, MC; Costagliola, S; Libert, F; Vassart, G; Dumont, JE; & Miot, F. Cloning of two human thyroid cDNAs encoding new members of the NADPH oxidase family. *J Biol Chem.* 275, (2000), 23227-23233. de Paulsen, N; Brychzy, A; Fournier, MC; Klausner, RD; Gnarra, JR; Pause, A; & Lee, S. Role of transforming growth factor-alpha in von Hippel--Lindau (VHL)(-/-) clear cell renal carcinoma cell proliferation: a possible mechanism coupling VHL tumor suppressor inactivation and tumorigenesis. *Proc. Natl. Acad. Sci. U. S. A.* 98, (2001), 1387-1392.

Diebold, I, Petry, A, Hess, J, & Görlach, A. The NADPH oxidase subunit NOX4 is a new target gene of the hypoxia-inducible factor-1. *Mol Biol Cell.* 21, (2010), 2087-2096.

Dröge, W. Free radicals in the physiological control of cell function. *Physiol Rev.* 82, (2002) 47-95.

Dupuy, C, Ohayon, R, Valent, A, Noël-Hudson, MS, Dème, D, & Virion, A. Purification of a novel flavoprotein involved in the thyroid NADPH oxidase. Cloning of the porcine and human cdnas. *J Biol Chem.* 274, (1999), 37265-37269.

Eid, AA; Gorin, Y; Fagg, BM; Kasinath, BS; Gorin, Y; Ghosh-Choudhury, G; Barnes, JL; & Abboud, HE. Mechanisms of podocyte injury in diabetes: role of cytochrome P450 and NADPH oxidases. *Diabetes* 58, (2009), 1201–1211.

Epstein, AC; Gleadle, JM; McNeill, LA; Hewitson, KS; O'Rourke, J; Mole, DR; Mukherji, M; Metzen, E; Wilson, MI; Dhanda, A; Tian, YM; Masson, N; Hamilton, DL; Jaakkola, P; Barstead, R; Hodgkin, J; Maxwell, PH; Pugh, CW; Schofield, CJ; & Ratcliffe, PJ; C. elegans EGL-9 and mammalian homologs define a family of dioxygenases that regulate HIF by prolyl hydroxylation. *Cell.* 107, (2001), 43-54.

European Chromosome 16 Tuberous Sclerosis Consortium. Identification and characterization of the tuberous sclerosis gene on chromosome 16. *Cell.* 75, (1993), 1305-1315.

Evans, P; & Halliwell, B. Free radicals and hearing. Cause, consequence, and criteria. *Ann N Y Acad Sci.* 884, (1999), 19-40.

Franke, TF; Kaplan, DR; Cantley, LC; & Toker, A. Direct regulation of the Akt proto-oncogene product by phosphatidylinositol-3,4-bisphosphate. *Science.* 275, (1997), 665-668.

Frey, RS; Rahman, A; Kefer, JC; Minshall, RD; & Malik, AB. PKCzeta regulates TNF-alpha-induced activation of NADPH oxidase in endothelial cells. *Circ Res.* 90, (2002), 1012-1019.

Frias, MA; Thoreen, CC; Jaffe, JD; Schroder, W; Sculley, T; Carr, SA; & Sabatini, DM. mSin1 is necessary for Akt/PKB phosphorylation, and its isoforms define three distinct mTORC2s. *Curr Biol.* 16, (2006), 1865-1870.

Fridovich I. The biology of oxygen radicals. *Science.* 201,(1978), 875-880.

Fürst, R; Brueckl, C; Kuebler, WM; Zahler, S; Krötz, F; Görlach, A; Vollmar, AM; & Kiemer, AK. Atrial natriuretic peptide induces mitogen-activated protein kinase phosphatase-1 in human endothelial cells via Rac1 and NAD(P)H oxidase/Nox2-activation. *Circ Res.* 96, (2005), 43-53.

Fukai, T, & Ushio-Fukai, M. Superoxide Dismutases: Role in Redox Signaling, Vascular Function, and Diseases. *Antioxid Redox Signal.* (2011).

Fukuyama, M; Rokutan, K; Sano, T; Miyake, H; Shimada, M; & Tashiro, S. Overexpression of a novel superoxide-producing enzyme, NADPH oxidase 1, in adenoma and well differentiated adenocarcinoma of the human colon. *Cancer Lett.* 221, (2005), 97-104.

Geiszt, M; Kopp, JB; Várnai, P; & Leto, TL. Identification of renox, an NAD(P)H oxidase in kidney. *Proc Natl Acad Sci U S A.* 97, (2000), 8010-8014.

Geiszt, M. NADPH oxidases: new kids on the block. *Cardiovasc Res* 71, (2006), 289–299.

Gerald, D; Berra, E; Frapart, YM; Chan, DA; Giaccia, AJ; Mansuy, D; Pouysségur, J; Yaniv, M; & Mechta-Grigoriou, F. JunD reduces tumor angiogenesis by protecting cells from oxidative stress. *Cell.* 118, (2004), 781-794.

Gingras, AC, Raught, B, & Sonenberg, N. mTOR signaling to translation. *Curr Top Microbiol Immunol.* 279, (2004), 169-97.

Giri, DK; & Aggarwal, BB. Constitutive activation of NF-kappaB causes resistance to apoptosis in human cutaneous T cell lymphoma HuT-78 cells. Autocrine role of tumor necrosis factor and reactive oxygen intermediates. J Biol Chem. 273, (1998), 14008-14014.

Gnarra, JR; Tory, K; Weng ,Y; Schmidt, L; Wei, MH; Li, H; Latif, F; Liu, S; Chen, F; Duh, FM; et al. Mutations of the VHL tumour suppressor gene in renal carcinoma. *Nat Genet.* 7, (1994), 85-90.

Gnarra, JR; Duan, DR; Weng, Y; Humphrey, JS; Chen, DY; Lee, S; Pause, A; Dudley, CF; Latif, F; Kuzmin, I; Schmidt, L; Duh, FM; Stackhouse, T; Chen, F; Kishida, T; Wei, MH; Lerman, MI; Zbar, B; Klausner, RD; & Linehan, WM. Molecular cloning of the von Hippel-Lindau tumor suppressor gene and its role in renal carcinoma. *Biochim Biophys Acta.* 1242, (1996), 201-210.

Gokden, N; Li, L; Zhang, H; Schafer, RF; Schichman, S; Scott, MA; Smoller, BR; & Fan, CY. Loss of heterozygosity of DNA repair gene, hOGG1, in renal cell carcinoma but not in renal papillary adenoma. *Pathol Int.* 58, (2008), 339-343.

Gorin, Y; Ricono, JM; Kim, NH; Bhandari, B, Choudhury, GG; & Abboud, HE. Nox4 mediates angiotensin II-induced activation of Akt/protein kinase B in mesangial cells. *Am J Physiol Renal Physiol.* 285, (2003), F219–F229.

Gorin, Y; Block, K; Hernandez, J; Bhandari, B; Wagner, B; Barnes, JL; & Abboud, HE. Nox4 NAD(P)H oxidase mediates hypertrophy and fibronectin expression in the diabetic kidney. *J Biol Chem* 280, (2005), 39616–39626.

Goyal, P; Weissmann, N; Grimminger, F; Hegel, C; Bader, L; Rose, F; Fink, L; Ghofrani, HA;, Schermuly, RT; Schmidt, HH; Seeger, W; & Hänze, J. Upregulation of NAD(P)H oxidase 1 in hypoxia activates hypoxia-inducible factor 1 via increase in reactive oxygen species. *Free Radic Biol Med.* 36, (2004), 1279-1288.

Habib SL. Molecular mechanism of regulation of OGG1: tuberin deficiency results in cytoplasmic redistribution of transcriptional factor NF-YA. *J Mol Signal.* 4, (2009), 8.

Habib, SL, Simone, S, Barnes, JJ, & Abboud, HE. Tuberin haploinsufficiency is associated with the loss of OGG1 in rat kidney tumors. *Mol Cancer.* 24, 7, (2008), 10.

Harfouche, R; Malak, NA; Brandes, RP; Karsan, A; Irani, K; & Hussain, SN. Roles of reactive oxygen species in angiopoietin-1/tie-2 receptor signaling. FASEB J. 12, (2005), 1728-1730.

Harris ,TE; & Lawrence, JC Jr. TOR signaling. *Sci STKE*. 212, (2003), 15.

Henderson, A; Douglas, F; Perros, P; Morgan, C; & Maher, ER. SDHB-associated renal oncocytoma suggests a broadening of the renal phenotype in hereditary paragangliomatosis. Fam Cancer. 8, (2009), 257-260.

Hilenski, LL; Clempus, RE; Quinn, MT; Lambeth, JD; Griendling, KK. Distinct subcellular localizations of Nox1 and Nox4 in vascular smooth muscle cells. *Arterioscler Thromb Vasc Biol* 24, (2004), 677–683.

Holz, MK; Ballif, BA; Gygi, SP; & Blenis, J. mTOR and S6K1 mediate assembly of the translation preinitiation complex through dynamic protein interchange and ordered phosphorylation events. *Cell*. 123, (2005), 569-580.

Iliopoulos, O; Kibel, A; Gray, S; & Kaelin, WG Jr. Tumour suppression by the human von Hippel-Lindau gene product. *Nat Med*. 1, (1995), 822-826.

Jaakkola, P; Mole, DR; Tian, YM; Wilson, MI; Gielbert, J; Gaskell, SJ; Kriegsheim, Av; Hebestreit, HF; Mukherji, M; Schofield, CJ; Maxwell, PH; Pugh, CW; & Ratcliffe, PJ. Targeting of HIF-alpha to the von Hippel-Lindau ubiquitylation complex by O2-regulated prolyl hydroxylation. *Science*. 292, (2001), 468-472.

Jemal, A; Murray, T; Ward, E; Samuels, A; Tiwari, RC; Ghafoor, A; Feuer, EJ; & Thun, MJ. *Cancer statistics. CA. Cancer J. Clin*. 55, (2005), 10-30.

Jones, SA, Hancock, JT, Jones, OT, Neubauer, A, & Topley, N. The expression of NADPH oxidase components in human glomerular mesangial cells: detection of protein and mRNA for p47phox, p67phox, and p22phox. *J Am Soc Nephrol*. 5, (1995), 1483-1491.

Kamata, H; Honda, S; Maeda, S; Chang, L; Hirata, H; & Karin, M. Reactive oxygen species promote TNFalpha-induced death and sustained JNK activation by inhibiting MAP kinase phosphatases. *Cell*. 120, (2005), 649-661.

Kamura, T; Koepp, DM; Conrad, MN; Skowyra, D; Moreland, RJ; Iliopoulos, O; Lane, WS; Kaelin, WG Jr; Elledge, SJ; Conaway, RC; Harper, JW; & Conaway, JW. Rbx1, a component of the VHL tumor suppressor complex and SCF ubiquitin ligase. *Science*. 284, (1999), 657-661.

Khoo, SK; Bradley, M; Wong, FK; Hedblad, MA; Nordenskjöld, M; & Teh, BT. Birt-Hogg-Dubé syndrome: mapping of a novel hereditary neoplasia gene to chromosome 17p12-q11.2. Oncogene. 20, (2001), 5239-5242.

Kibel, A; Iliopoulos, O; DeCaprio, JA; & Kaelin, WG Jr. Binding of the von Hippel-Lindau tumor suppressor protein to Elongin B and C. *Science*. 269, (1995), 1444-1446.

Kim, DH; Sarbassov, DD; Ali, SM; King, JE; Latek, RR, Erdjument-Bromage, H; Tempst, P; & Sabatini, DM. mTOR interacts with raptor to form a nutrient-sensitive complex that signals to the cell growth machinery. *Cell*. 110, (2002), 163-175.

Kim, J; Kim, MK; Lee, JK; Kim, JH; Son, SK; Song, ES; Lee, KB; Lee, JP, Lee, JM; & Yun, YM. Intakes of vitamin A, C, and E, and beta-carotene are associated with risk of cervical cancer: a case-control study in Korea. Nutr Cancer. 62, (2010), 181-189.

King, A; Selak, MA; & Gottlieb, E. Succinate dehydrogenase and fumarate hydratase: linking mitochondrial dysfunction and cancer. *Oncogene*. 25, (2006), 4675-4682.

Kirsh, VA; Hayes, RB; Mayne, ST; Chatterjee, N; Subar, AF; Dixon, LB; Albanes, D; Andriole, GL; Urban, DA; & Peters U. PLCO Trial. Supplemental and dietary vitamin E, beta-carotene, and vitamin C intakes and prostate cancer risk. *J Natl Cancer Inst*. 98, (2006), 245-254.

Knebelmann, B; Ananth, S; Cohen, HT; & Sukhatme, VP. Transforming growth factor alpha is a target for the von Hippel-Lindau tumor suppressor. *Cancer Res*. 58, (1998), 226-231.

Kuroda, J; Ago, T; Matsushima, S; Zhai, P; Schneider, MD; & Sadoshima, J. NADPH oxidase 4 (Nox4) is a major source of oxidative stress in the failing heart. *Proc Natl Acad Sci U S A*. 107, (2010), 15565-15570.

Lambeth, JD. Nox enzymes, ROS, and chronic disease: an example of antagonistic pleiotropy. *Free Radic Biol Med* 43, (2007), 332–347.

Lassegue, B; & Clempus, RE. Vascular NAD(P)H oxidases: specific features, expression, and regulation. *Am J Physiol Reg Integr Compar Physiol* 285, (2003), R277–R297.

Lassègue, B; & Griendling, KK. NADPH oxidases: functions and pathologies in the vasculature. *Arterioscler Thromb Vasc Biol*. 30, (2010), 653-661.

Latif, F; Tory, K; Gnarra, J; Yao, M; Duh, FM; Orcutt, ML; Stackhouse, T; Kuzmin, I; Modi, W; Geil, L, et al. Identification of the von Hippel-Lindau disease tumor suppressor gene. *Science*. 260, (1993), 1317-1320.

Lee, SR; Kwon, KS; Kim, SR; & Rhee, SG. Reversible inactivation of protein-tyrosine phosphatase 1B in A431 cells stimulated with epidermal growth factor. *J Biol Chem*. 273, (1998), 15366-15372.

Li, JM; & Shah, AM. Intracellular localization and preassembly of the NADPH oxidase complex in cultured endothelial cells. *J Biol Chem*. 277, (2002), 19952-19960.

Lim, SD; Sun, C; Lambeth, JD; Marshall, F; Amin, M; Chung, L; Petros, JA; Arnold, RS. Increased Nox1 and hydrogen peroxide in prostate cancer. *Prostate*. 62, (2005), 200-207.

Lin, J; Cook, NR; Albert, C; Zaharris, E; Gaziano, JM; Van Denburgh, M; Buring, JE; & Manson, JE. Vitamins C and E and beta carotene supplementation and cancer risk: a randomized controlled trial. *J Natl Cancer Inst*. 101, (2009), 14-23.

Lubensky, IA; Schmidt, L; Zhuang, Z; Weirich, G; Pack, S, Zambrano, N; Walther, MM; Choyke, P; Linehan, WM; & Zbar, B. Hereditary and sporadic papillary renal carcinomas with c-met mutations share a distinct morphological phenotype. *Am J Pathol*. 155, (1999), 517-526.

Mahadev, K; Motoshima, H; Wu, X; Ruddy, JM; Arnold, RS; Cheng, G; Lambeth, JD; & Goldstein, BJ. The NAD(P)H oxidase homolog Nox4 modulates insulin-stimulated generation of H2O2 and plays an integral role in insulin signal transduction. *Mol Cell Biol*. 24, (2004), 1844-1854.

Maher, ER; & Kaelin, WG Jr. von Hippel-Lindau disease. *Medicine (Baltimore*). 76, (1997), 381-391.

Mahimainathan, L; Ghosh-Choudhury, N; Venkatesan, B; Das, F; Mandal, CC; Dey, N; Habib, SL; Kasinath, BS; Abboud, HE; & Ghosh Choudhury, G. TSC2 deficiency increases PTEN via HIF1alpha. *J Biol Chem*. 284, (2009), 27790-27798.

Mahon, PC; Hirota, K; & Semenza, GL. FIH-1: a novel protein that interacts with HIF-1alpha and VHL to mediate repression of HIF-1 transcriptional activity. *Genes Dev*. 15, (2001), 2675-2686.

Mamane, Y; Petroulakis, E; Rong, L; Yoshida, K; Ler, LW; Sonenberg, N. eIF4E--from translation to transformation. *Oncogene*. 23, (2004), 3172-3179.

Manea, A; Manea, SA; Gafencu, AV; & Raicu, M. Regulation of NADPH oxidase subunit p22(phox) by NF-kB in human aortic smooth muscle cells. *Arch Physiol Biochem.* 113, (2007), 163-172.

Manea, A; Tanase, LI; Raicu, M; & Simionescu, M. Transcriptional regulation of NADPH oxidase isoforms, Nox1 and Nox4, by nuclear factor-kappaB in human aortic smooth muscle cells. *Biochem Biophys Res Commun.* 396, (2010), 901-907.

Manning, BD; & Cantley, LC. AKT/PKB signaling: navigating downstream. *Cell.* 129, (2007), 1261-1274.

Maranchie, JK; & Zhan, Y. Nox4 is critical for hypoxia-inducible factor 2-alpha transcriptional activity in von Hippel-Lindau-deficient renal cell carcinoma. *Cancer Res.* 65, (2005), 9190-9193.

Marcotrigiano, J, Gingras, AC, Sonenberg, N, & Burley, SK. Cap-dependent translation initiation in eukaryotes is regulated by a molecular mimic of eIF4G. *Mol Cell.* 3, (1999), 707-716.

Martyn, KD; Frederick, LM; von Loehneysen, K; Dinauer, MC; & Knaus, UG. Functional analysis of Nox4 reveals unique characteristics compared to other NADPH oxidases. *Cell Signal* 18, (2006), 69–82.

Masson, N; & Ratcliffe, PJ. HIF prolyl and asparaginyl hydroxylases in the biological response to intracellular O(2) levels. *J Cell Sci.* 116, (2003), 3041-3049.

Matsumoto, T; & Claesson-Welsh, L. VEGF receptor signal transduction. *Sci STKE.* 112, (2001), re21.

Maxwell, PH, Dachs, GU; Gleadle, JM; Nicholls, LG; Harris, AL; Stratford, IJ; Hankinson, O; Pugh, CW; & Ratcliffe, PJ. Hypoxia-inducible factor-1 modulates gene expression in solid tumors and influences both angiogenesis and tumor growth. *Proc Natl Acad Sci U S A.* 94, (1997), 8104-8109.

Maxwell, PH; Wiesener, MS; Chang, GW; Clifford, SC; Vaux, EC; Cockman, ME; Wykoff, CC; Pugh, CW; Maher, ER; & Ratcliffe, PJ. The tumour suppressor protein VHL targets hypoxia-inducible factors for oxygen-dependent proteolysis. *Nature.* 399, (1999), 271-275.

Maxwell, P; & van den Berg, HW. Changes in the secretion of insulin-like growth factor binding proteins -2 and -4 associated with the development of tamoxifen resistance and estrogen independence in human breast cancer cell lines. *Cancer Lett.* 139, (1999), 121-127.

Mayr, JA; Meierhofer, D; Zimmermann, F; Feichtinger, R; Kögler, C; Ratschek, M; Schmeller, N; Sperl, W; & Kofler, B. Loss of complex I due to mitochondrial DNA mutations in renal oncocytoma. *Clin Cancer Res.* 14, (2008), 2270-2275.

Meng, D; Lv, DD; & Fang, J. Insulin-like growth factor-I induces reactive oxygen species production and cell migration through Nox4 and Rac1 in vascular smooth muscle cells. *Cardiovasc Res.* 80, (2008), 299-308.

Michaeloudes, C; Sukkar, MB; Khorasani, NM; Bhavsar, PK; & Chung, KF. TGF-β regulates Nox4, MnSOD and catalase expression, and IL-6 release in airway smooth muscle cells. *Am J Physiol Lung Cell Mol Physiol.* (2011).

Mochizuki, T; Furuta, S; Mitsushita J; Shang, WH; Ito, M; Yokoo, Y; Yamaura, M; Ishizone, S, Nakayama, J; Konagai, A; Hirose, K; Kiyosawa, K; & Kamata, T. Inhibition of NADPH oxidase 4 activates apoptosis via the AKT/apoptosis signal-regulating kinase 1 pathway in pancreatic cancer PANC-1 cells. *Oncogene*. 25, (2006), 3699-36707.

Moreno, SM; Benítez, IA; & Martínez González, MA. Ultrastructural studies in a series of 18 cases of chromophobe renal cell carcinoma. *Ultrastruct Pathol*. 29, (2005), 377-387.

Nisimoto, Y; Jackson, HM; Ogawa, H; Kawahara, T; & Lambeth, JD. Constitutive NADPH-dependent electron transferase activity of the Nox4 dehydrogenase domain. *Biochemistry*. 49, (2010), 2433–2442.

Novo, E; & Parola, M. Redox mechanisms in hepatic chronic wound healing and fibrogenesis. *Fibrogenesis Tissue Repair*. (2008).

O'Flaherty, L; Adam, J; Heather, LC; Zhdanov, AV; Chung, YL; Miranda, MX; Croft, J; Olpin, S; Clarke, K; Pugh, CW,; Griffiths, J; Papkovsky, D; Ashrafian, H; Ratcliffe, PJ; & Pollard, PJ. Dysregulation of hypoxia pathways in fumarate hydratase-deficient cells is independent of defective mitochondrial metabolism. *Hum Mol Genet*. 19, (2010), 3844-3851.

Oya, M; Ohtsubo, M; Takayanagi, A; Tachibana, M;Shimizu, N; & Murai, M. Constitutive activation of nuclear factor-kappaB prevents TRAIL-induced apoptosis in renal cancer cells. *Oncogene*. 20, (2001), 3888-3896.

Pande, V; & Ramos, MJ. NF-kappaB in human disease: current inhibitors and prospects for de novo structure based design of inhibitors. *Curr Med Chem*. 12, (2005), 357-374.

Patel, PH, Chaganti, RS, & Motzer, RJ. Targeted therapy for metastatic renal cell carcinoma. *Br J Cancer*. 94, (2006), 614-619.

Plas, DR, & Thompson, CB. Akt activation promotes degradation of tuberin and FOXO3a via the proteasome. *J Biol Chem*. 278, (2003), 12361-12366.

Pavlovich, CP; Walther, MM; Eyler, RA; Hewitt, SM; Zbar, B; Linehan, WM; & Merino, MJ. Renal tumors in the Birt-Hogg-Dubé syndrome. *Am J Surg Pathol*. 26, (2002), 1542-1552.

Pedruzzi, E; Guichard, C; Ollivier, V; Driss, F; Fay, M; Prunet, C; Marie. JC; Pouzet, C; Samadi, M; Elbim, C; O'dowd, Y; Bens, M; Vandewalle, A; Gougerot-Pocidalo, MA; Lizard, G; & Ogier-Denis, E. NAD(P)H oxidase Nox-4 mediates 7-ketocholesterol-induced endoplasmic reticulum stress and apoptosis in human aortic smooth muscle cells. *Mol Cell Biol* 24, (2004), 10703–10717.

Pfaffenroth, EC: & Linehan, WM. Genetic basis for kidney cancer: opportunity for disease-specific approaches to therapy. *Expert Opin Biol Ther*. 8, (2008), 779-790.

Pollard, PJ; Brière, JJ; Alam, NA; Barwell, J; Barclay, E; Wortham, NC; Hunt, T; Mitchell, M; Olpin, S; Moat, SJ; Hargreaves, IP; Heales, SJ; Chung, YL; Griffiths, JR; Dalgleish, A; McGrath, JA; Gleeson, MJ; Hodgson, SV; Poulsom, R; Rustin, P; Tomlinson, IP. Accumulation of Krebs cycle intermediates and over-expression of HIF1alpha in tumours which result from germline FH and SDH mutations. *Hum Mol Genet*. 14, (2005), 2231-2239.

Porta, C; & Figlin, RA. Phosphatidylinositol-3-kinase/Akt signaling pathway and kidney cancer, and the therapeutic potential of phosphatidylinositol-3-kinase/Akt inhibitors. *J Urol*. 182, (2009), 2569-2577.

Oh, WJ; Wu, CC; Kim, SJ; Facchinetti, V; Julien, LA; Finlan, M; Roux, PP; Su, B; & Jacinto, E. mTORC2 can associate with ribosomes to promote cotranslational phosphorylation and stability of nascent Akt polypeptide. *EMBO J*. 29, (2010), 3939-3951.

Qi, H; & Ohh, M. The von Hippel-Lindau tumor suppressor protein sensitizes renal cell carcinoma cells to tumor necrosis factor-induced cytotoxicity by suppressing the nuclear factor-kappaB-dependent antiapoptotic pathway. *Cancer Res.* 63, (2003), 7076-7080.

Ranjan, P; Anathy, V; Burch, PM; Weirather, K; Lambeth, JD; Heintz, NH. Redox-dependent expression of cyclin D1 and cell proliferation by Nox1 in mouse lung epithelial cells. *Antioxid Redox Signal.* 8, (2006), 1447-1459.

Rhee, SG; Chang, TS; Bae, YS; Lee, SR; Kang, SW. Cellular regulation by hydrogen peroxide. J Am Soc Nephrol. 14, (2003), S211-S215.

Ricketts, C; Woodward, ER; Killick, P; Morris, MR; Astuti, D; Latif, F; & Maher, ER. Germline SDHB mutations and familial renal cell carcinoma. *J Natl Cancer Inst.* 100, (2008), 1260-1262.

Royer-Pokora, B; Kunkel, LM; Monaco, AP; Goff, SC; Newburger, PE; Baehner, RL; Cole, FS; Curnutte, JT; & Orkin, SH. Cloning the gene for an inherited human disorder--chronic granulomatous disease--on the basis of its chromosomal location. Nature. 322, (1986), 32-38.

Sakano, N; Wang, DH; Takahashi, N; Wang, B; Sauriasari, R; Kanbara, S; Sato, Y; Takigawa, T; Takaki, J; & Ogino, K. Oxidative stress biomarkers and lifestyles in Japanese healthy people. *J Clin Biochem Nutr.* 44, (2009), 185-195.

Sarbassov DD, Guertin DA, Ali SM, Sabatini DM. Phosphorylation and regulation of Akt/PKB by the rictor-mTOR complex. Science. 2005 Feb 18;307(5712):1098-101.

Sarbassov, DD; Ali, SM; Kim, DH; Guertin, DA; Latek, RR; Erdjument-Bromage, H; Tempst, P; & Sabatini, DM. Rictor, a novel binding partner of mTOR, defines a rapamycin-insensitive and raptor-independent pathway that regulates the cytoskeleton. *Curr Biol.* 14, (2004), 1296-1302.

Sarto, C; Frutiger, S; Cappellano, F; Sanchez, JC; Doro, G; Catanzaro, F; Hughes, GJ; Hochstrasser, DF; & Mocarelli, P. Modified expression of plasma glutathione peroxidase and manganese superoxide dismutase in human renal cell carcinoma. *Electrophoresis.* 20, (1999), 3458-3466.

Schmidt, L; Duh, FM; Chen, F; Kishida, T; Glenn, G; Choyke, P; Scherer, SW; Zhuang, Z; Lubensky, I; Dean, M; Allikmets, R; Chidambaram, A; Bergerheim, UR; Feltis, JT; Casadevall, C; Zamarron, A; Bernues, M; Richard, S; Lips, CJ; Walther, MM; Tsui, LC; Geil, L; Orcutt, ML; Stackhouse, T; Lipan, J; Slife, L; Brauch, H; Decker, J; Niehans, G; Hughson, MD; Moch, H; Storkel S; Lerman, MI; Linehan, WM; Zbar, B. Germline and somatic mutations in the tyrosine kinase domain of the MET proto-oncogene in papillary renal carcinomas. *Nat Genet.* 16, (1997), 68-73.

Schmidt, LS; Warren, MB; Nickerson, ML; Weirich, G; Matrosova, V; Toro, JR; Turner, ML; Duray, P; Merino, M; Hewitt, S; Pavlovich, CP; Glenn, G; Greenberg, CR; Linehan, WM; & Zbar B. Birt-Hogg-Dubé syndrome, a genodermatosis associated with spontaneous pneumothorax and kidney neoplasia, maps to chromosome 17p11.2. Am J Hum Genet. 69, (2001), 876-882.

Schullerus, D; Herbers, J; Chudek, J; Kanamaru, H; & Kovacs, G. Loss of heterozygosity at chromosomes 8p, 9p, and 14q is associated with stage and grade of non-papillary renal cell carcinomas. *J Pathol.* 183, (1997), 151-155.

Schulze-Osthoff, K; Ferrari, D; Riehemann, K; & Wesselborg, S. Regulation of NF-kappa B activation by MAP kinase cascades. Immunobiology. 198, (1997), 35-49.

Schulze-Osthoff, K; Ferrari, D; Los, M; Wesselborg, S; & Peter, ME. Apoptosis signaling by death receptors. *Eur J Biochem*. 254, (1998), 439-459.

Selemidis, S; Sobey, CG; Wingler, K; Schmidt, HH; Drummond, GR. NADPH oxidases in the vasculature: molecular features, roles in disease and pharmacological inhibition. *Pharmacol Ther*. 120, (2008), 254–291.

Semenza, GL. HIF-1 and tumor progression: pathophysiology and therapeutics. *Trends Mol Med*. 8, (2002), S62-S67.

Shiose, A; Kuroda, J; Tsuruya, K; Hirai, M; Hirakata, H; Naito, S; Hattori, M; Sakaki, Y; & Sumimoto, H. A novel superoxide-producing NAD(P)H oxidase in kidney. *J Biol Chem* 276, (2001), 1417–1423.

Shono, T; Ono, M; Izumi, H; Jimi, SI; Matsushima, K; Okamoto, T; Kohno, K; & Kuwano, M. Involvement of the transcription factor NF-kappaB in tubular morphogenesis of human microvascular endothelial cells by oxidative stress. *Mol Cell Biol*. 16, (1996), 4231-4239.

Sturrock, A; Cahill, B; Norman, K; Huecksteadt, TP; Hill, K; Sanders, K; Karwande, SV; Stringham, JC; Bull, DA; Gleich, M; Kennedy, TP; & Hoidal, JR. Transforming growth factor-beta1 induces Nox4 NAD(P)H oxidase and reactive oxygen species-dependent proliferation in human pulmonary artery smooth muscle cells. *Am J Physiol Lung Cell Mol Physiol*. 290, (2006), L661-L673.

Sudarshan, S; Sourbier, C; Kong, HS; Block, K; Valera, Romero, VA; Yang, Y; Galindo, C; Mollapour, M; Scroggins, B; Goode, N; Lee, MJ; Gourlay, CW; Trepel, J; Linehan, WM; & Neckers, L. Fumarate hydratase deficiency in renal cancer induces glycolytic addiction and hypoxia-inducible transcription factor 1alpha stabilization by glucose-dependent generation of reactive oxygen species. *Mol Cell Biol*. 29, (2009), 4080-4090.

Sudarshan, S; Shanmugasundaram, K; Naylor, SL; Lin, S; Livi, CB; O'Neill, CF; Parekh, DJ; Yeh, IT;Sun, LZ; & Block, K. Reduced Expression of Fumarate Hydratase in Clear Cell Renal Cancer Mediates HIF-2α Accumulation and Promotes Migration and Invasion. *PLoS One*. 6, (2011), e21037.

Suh, YA; Arnold, RS; Lassegue, B; Shi, J; Xu, X; Sorescu, D; Chung, AB; Griendling, KK; & Lambeth, JD. Cell transformation by the superoxide-generating oxidase Mox1. *Nature*. 401, (1999), 79-82.

Sosman, JA; Puzanov, I; & Atkins, MB. Opportunities and obstacles to combination targeted therapy in renal cell cancer. *Clin Cancer Res*. 13, (2007), 764s-769s.

Szatrowski, TP; & Nathan, CF. Production of large amounts of hydrogen peroxide by human tumor cells. *Cancer Res*. 51, (1991), 794-798.

Tickoo, SK; Lee, MW; Eble, JN; Amin, M; Christopherson, T; Zarbo, RJ; & Amin, MB. Ultrastructural observations on mitochondria and microvesicles in renal oncocytoma, chromophobe renal cell carcinoma, and eosinophilic variant of conventional (clear cell) renal cell carcinoma. *Am J Surg Pathol*. 24, (2000), 1247-1256.

Tojo, T; Ushio-Fukai, M; Yamaoka-Tojo, M; Ikeda, S; Patrushev, N; & Alexander, RW. Role of gp91phox (Nox2)-containing NAD(P)H oxidase in angiogenesis in response to hindlimb ischemia. *Circulation*. 111, (2005), 2347-2355.

Tory, K; Brauch, H; Linehan, M; Barba, D; Oldfield, E; Filling-Katz; M, Seizinger, B; Nakamura, Y; White, R; Marshall, FF, et al. Specific genetic change in tumors associated with von Hippel-Lindau disease. *J Natl Cancer Inst.* 81, (1989), 1097-1101.

Toschi, A; Lee, E; Gadir, N; Ohh, M; & Foster, DA. Differential dependence of hypoxia-inducible factors 1 alpha and 2 alpha on mTORC1 and mTORC2. *J Biol Chem.* 283, (2008), 34495-34499.

Ushio-Fukai, M; Tang, Y; Fukai, T; Dikalov, SI; Ma, Y; Fujimoto, M; Quinn, MT; Pagano, PJ; Johnson, C; & Alexander, RW. Novel role of gp91(phox)-containing NAD(P)H oxidase in vascular endothelial growth factor-induced signaling and angiogenesis. *Circ Res.* 91, (2002), 1160-1167.

Ushio-Fukai, M, & Alexander, RW. Reactive oxygen species as mediators of angiogenesis signaling: role of NAD(P)H oxidase. *Mol Cell Biochem.* 264, (2004), 85-97.

Ushio-Fukai M. Redox signaling in angiogenesis: role of NADPH oxidase. *Cardiovasc Res.* 71, (2006), 226-235.

Vallet, P; Charnay, Y; Steger, K; Ogier-Denis, E; Kovari, E; Herrmann, F; Michel, JP; & Szanto, I. Neuronal expression of the NADPH oxidase NOX4, and its regulation in mouse experimental brain ischemia. *Neuroscience.* 132, (2005), 233-238.

van Slegtenhorst, M; de Hoogt, R; Hermans, C; Nellist, M; Janssen, B; Verhoef, S; Lindhout, D; van den Ouweland, A; Halley, D; Young, J; Burley, M; Jeremiah, S; Woodward, K; Nahmias, J; Fox, M; Ekong, R; Osborne, J; Wolfe, J; Povey, S; Snell, RG; Cheadle, JP; Jones, AC; Tachataki, M; Ravine, D; Sampson, JR; Reeve, MP; Richardson, P; Wilmer, F; Munro, C; Hawkins, TL; Sepp, T; Ali, JB; Ward, S; Green, AJ; Yates, JR; Kwiatkowska, J; Henske, EP; Short, MP; Haines, JH; Jozwiak, S; & Kwiatkowski, DJ. Identification of the tuberous sclerosis gene TSC1 on chromosome 9q34. *Science.* 277, (1997), 805-808.

Vaquero, EC; Edderkaoui, M; Pandol, SJ; Gukovsky, I; & Gukovskaya, AS. Reactive oxygen species produced by NAD(P)H oxidase inhibit apoptosis in pancreatic cancer cells. *J Biol Chem.* 279, (2004), 34643-34654.

Vanharanta, S; Buchta, M; McWhinney, SR; Virta, SK; Peçzkowska, M; Morrison, CD; Lehtonen, R; Januszewicz, A; Järvinen, H; Juhola, M; Mecklin, JP; Pukkala, E; Herva, R; Kiuru, M; Nupponen, NN; Aaltonen, LA; Neumann, HP; & Eng, C. Early-onset renal cell carcinoma as a novel extraparaganglial component of SDHB-associated heritable paraganglioma. *Am J Hum Genet.* 74, (2004), 153-159.

Vignais, PV. The superoxide-generating NADPH oxidase: structural aspects and activation mechanism. *Cell Mol Life Sci.* 59, (2002), 1428-1459.

Wagner, B; Ricono, JM; Gorin, Y; Block, K; Arar, M; Riley, D; Choudhury, GG; & Abboud, HE. Mitogenic signaling via platelet-derived growth factor beta in metanephric mesenchymal cells. *J Am Soc Nephrol.* 18, (2007), 2903-2911.

Wang, X; Hawk, N; Yue, P; Kauh, J; Ramalingam, SS; Fu, H; Khuri, FR; & Sun, SY. Overcoming mTOR inhibition-induced paradoxical activation of survival signaling pathways enhances mTOR inhibitors' anticancer efficacy. *Cancer Biol Ther.* 7, (2008), 1952-1958.

Wang, X; Yue, P; Chan, CB; Ye, K; Ueda, T; Watanabe-Fukunaga, R; Fukunaga, R; Fu, H, Khuri; FR, & Sun, SY. Inhibition of mammalian target of rapamycin induces phosphatidylinositol 3-kinase-dependent and Mnk-mediated eukaryotic translation initiation factor 4E phosphorylation. *Mol Cell Biol.* 27, (2007), 7405-7413.

Warburg, O; Posener, K; & Negelein, E. Über den Stoffwechsel der Tumoren. *Biochem. Z.* 152,319-344, (1924).

Washecka, R; & Hanna, M. Malignant renal tumors in tuberous sclerosis. *Urology*. 37, (1991), 340-343.

Wickramasinghe, RH. Biological aspects of cytochrome P450 and associated hydroxylation reactions. *Enzyme*. 19, (1975), 348-376.

Wise, DR; DeBerardinis, RJ; Mancuso, A; Sayed, N; Zhang, XY; Pfeiffer, HK; Nissim, I; Daikhin, E; Yudkoff, M; McMahon, SB, & Thompson, CB. Myc regulates a transcriptional program that stimulates mitochondrial glutaminolysis and leads to glutamine addiction. *Proc Natl Acad Sci U S A*. 105, (2008), 18782-18787.

Yang, HS; Jansen, AP; Komar, AA; Zheng, X; Merrick, WC; Costes, S; Lockett, SJ; Sonenberg, N; & Colburn, NH. The transformation suppressor Pdcd4 is a novel eukaryotic translation initiation factor 4A binding protein that inhibits translation. *Mol Cell Biol*. 23, (2003), 26-37.

8

Biological Aspects in Renal Cell Carcinoma

Vanessa Medina Villaamil[1], Guadalupe Aparicio Gallego[1]
and Luis Miguel Antón Aparicio[2,3]
[1]*INIBIC, A Coruña University Hospital, A Coruña,*
[2]*Medical Oncology Service, A Coruña University Hospital, A Coruña,*
[3]*Medicine Department, University of A Coruña, A Coruña*
Spain

1. Introduction

A growing understanding of the underlying molecular biology of renal cell carcinoma (RCC) has identified several pathways pertinent to its pathophysiology. Cellular hypoxia and metabolic stress have been observed in many cancer types. Hypoxia-induced factor (HIF) is considered a central regulator of oxygen homeostasis. The HIF transcription factor complex has been demonstrated to transcriptionally induce the expression of genes involved in angiogenesis, anaerobic glucose metabolism, cell motility and metastasis, growth and survival, apoptosis, and telomere maintenance. Notable genes induced by HIF that are involved in angiogenesis include vascular endothelial growth factor (VEGF) and platelet-derived growth factor (PDGF), as well as other proangiogenic factors, such as angiopoietin-4 (Ang4). These factors promote the proliferation, migration, and maturation of endothelial cells and pericytes supporting the recruitment of vessels or neoangiogenesis necessary to restore blood supply to an ischemic region. In the case of RCC, this process leads to the rampant, disorganised proliferation of vessels in this highly vascular tumour type. Additional factors include proteins involved in promoting the cellular switch to anaerobic glycolysis, such as the glucose transporter Glut1; enzymes of glucose metabolism, such as hexokinase (HK) and lactate dehydrogenase (LDH), the antigen carbonic anhydrase IX (CAIX, also called G250) and the lactate transporter MCT-4. This hypoxic repertoire of gene upregulation likely contributes to the highly glycolytic phenotype of RCC, even in the presence of abundant oxygen with which to perform oxidative phosphorylation for energy generation. Like other processes that integrate endothelial cell vascular network expansion, tumour angiogenesis is dependent on secreted VEGF to promote existing vessel in growth into the tumour and the expansion of vascular networks by neovascularisation. Inappropriate activation of the hypoxia response pathway is a major mechanism of VEGF transcriptional regulation in RCC. A variety of mechanisms account for the increase in VEGF, with activation of the hypoxic response pathway via the transcription factors HIF1-α and HIF2-α as the classic mechanism of induction.

RCC presents a unique clinical setting, in which a tumour type nearly universally usurps a proangiogenic cellular homeostatic mechanism.

Knowledge of the genetic basis of RCC has important implications for diagnosis and management of this disease. Study of the genes for RCC has revealed that kidney cancer is fundamentally a metabolic disorder. The seven RCC genes (*VHL, MET, BHD, TSC1, TSC2, fumarate hydratase* (*FH*) and *succinate dehydrogenase* (*SDH*)) represent disorders of energy, nutrient, iron and oxygen sensing.

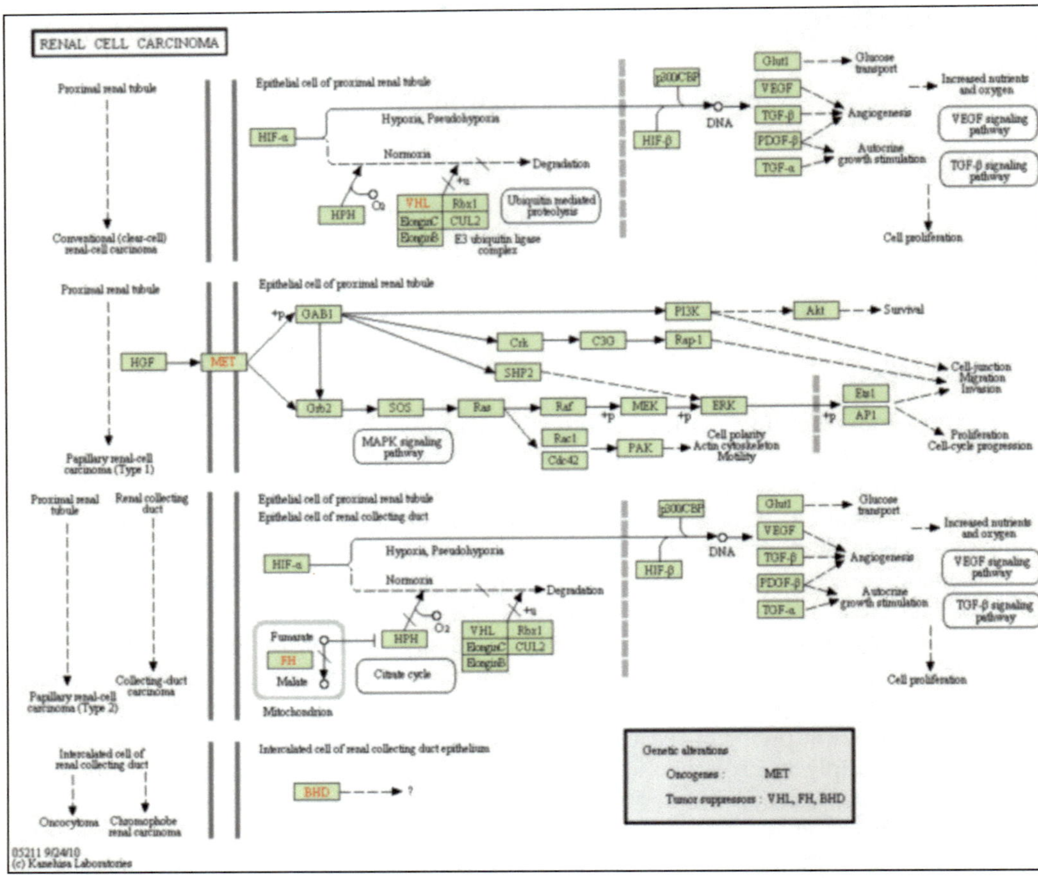

Fig. 1. Renal Cell Carcinoma Pathway (Kanehisa et al., 2010). Renal cell cancer (RCC) accounts for ~3% of human malignancies and its incidence appears to be rising. Although most cases of RCC seem to occur sporadically, an inherited predisposition to renal cancer accounts for 1-4% of cases. RCC is not a single disease, it has several morphological subtypes. Conventional RCC (clear cell RCC) accounts for ~80% of cases, followed by papillary RCC (10-15%), chromophobe RCC (5%), and collecting duct RCC (<1%). Genes potentially involved in sporadic neoplasms of each particular type are VHL, MET, BHD, and FH respectively. In the absence of VHL, hypoxia-inducible factor alpha (HIF- α) accumulates, leading to production of several growth factors, including vascular endothelial growth factor and platelet-derived growth factor. Activated MET mediates a number of biological effects including motility, invasion of extracellular matrix, cellular transformation, prevention of apoptosis and metastasis formation. Loss of functional FH leads to accumulation of fumarate in the cell, triggering inhibition of HPH and preventing targeted pVHL-mediated degradation of HIF- α. BHD mutations cause the Birt-Hogg-Dube syndrome and its associated chromophobe, hybrid oncocytic, and conventional (clear cell) RCC.

Targeting the basic metabolic alterations in RCC has the potential to provide a more durable and effective approach to therapy.

2. Overview of hypoxia-inducible signalling

Over the last decade, major advances have been made in deciphering the molecular mechanisms that allow cells to respond and adapt to low PO2. As key mediators in cellular oxygen homeostasis, hypoxia-inducible factor-1 and -2 (HIF-1 and HIF-2) facilitate both oxygen delivery and adaptation to oxygen deprivation by regulating the expression of gene products that are involved in cellular energy metabolism and glucose transport, angiogenesis, erythropoiesis and iron metabolism, pH regulation, apoptosis, and cell proliferation, as well as cell-cell and cell-matrix interactions (Schofield et al., 2004). Examples of classic HIF target genes are phosphoglycerate kinase-1 (PGK), glucose transporter-1 (GLUT1), vascular endothelial growth factor (VEGF), and erythropoietin (EPO).

HIF-1 and HIF-2 (collectively referred to here as HIF) are members of the Per-ARNT-Sim (PAS) family of heterodimeric basic helix-loop-helix (bHLH) transcription factors and consist of an oxygen-sensitive α-subunit and a constitutively expressed β-unit, also known as the aryl hydrocarbon receptor nuclear translocator (ARNT) or simply HIF-β.

Direct transcriptional regulation occurs through the binding of HIF heterodimers to hypoxia-response elements (HREs), which are present in the regulatory regions of hypoxia-sensitive genes. With regard to their ability to transcriptionally regulate specific hypoxia-responsive genes, HIF-1 and HIF-2 have distinct functions and only partially overlap. For example, glycolytic genes appear to be predominantly regulated by HIF-1 (Hu et al., 2003), whereas HIF-2 has been suggested as the main regulator of hypoxic VEGF and EPO induction in tissues that express both HIF-1 and HIF-2 (Rankin et al., 2005).

In addition to heterodimerisation with HIF-β resulting in the formation of a bHLH transcription factor that mediates the canonical hypoxia response, HIF-α subunits also regulate biological processes through direct protein-protein interaction with other factors. These include, among others, the tumour suppressor protein p53 and the c-Myc proto-oncogene (Koshiji et al., 2004). A more recent example is the ability of HIF-1α to biochemically associate with the intracellular domain of Notch (Notch ICD), thereby increasing Notch signalling through upregulation of Notch target genes such as Hey and Hes (Gustafsson et al., 2005). The observation that HIF-1α modulates Notch signalling through a direct protein-protein interaction underscores the importance of HIF-α as a regulator of important intracellular pathways, independent of its role in HRE-mediated transcription.

HIF activation is dependent on the stabilisation of the oxygen-sensitive α-subunit and its subsequent translocation to the nucleus, where it dimerises with HIF-β and recruits transcriptional cofactors such as CBP and p300 (Schofield et al., 2004). Normally, under conditions of adequate oxygen supply, hydroxylated HIF-α binds to the von Hippel-Lindau tumour suppressor protein (pVHL), which is part of an E3-ubiquitin ligase complex that targets HIF-α for proteasomal degradation. The pVHL/HIF-α interaction is highly conserved between species and requires iron- and oxygen-dependent hydroxylation of specific proline residues within the oxygen-dependent degradation domain (ODD) of HIF-α. Prolyl-hydroxylation by prolyl-4-hydroxylases and binding to pVHL are absolutely required for the execution of HIF proteolysis under normoxia. During hypoxia, prolyl-hydroxylases are inactive, and HIF-α degradation is inhibited. Three major mammalian HIF prolyl-hydroxylases have been identified, all of which are expressed in renal epithelial cells (Soilleux et al., 2005).

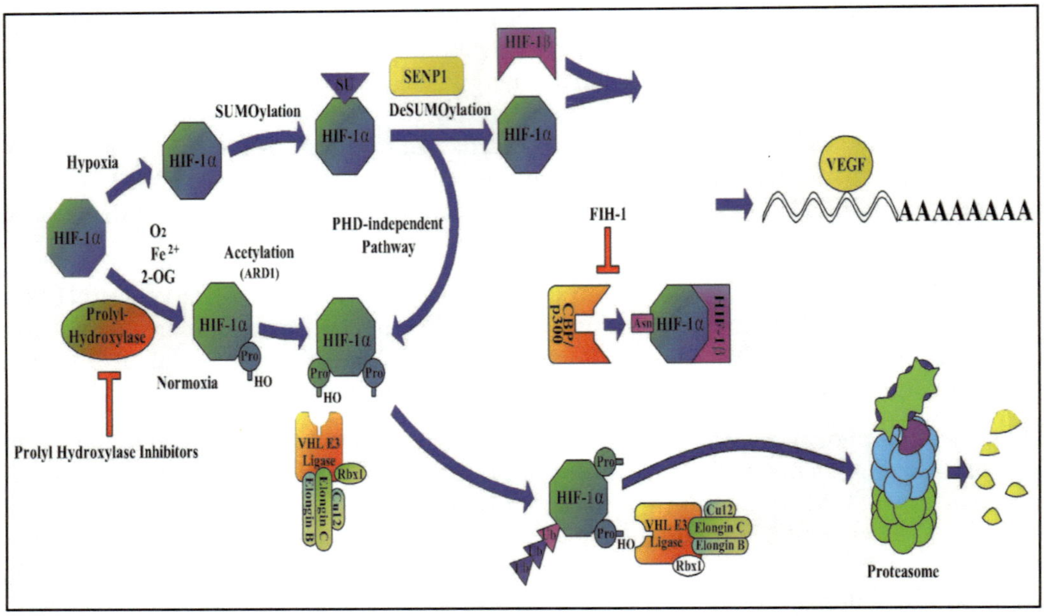

Fig. 2. Regulatory pathway of HIF. HIF-α is hydroxylated in the oxygen dependent destruction domain and at an asparagine residue in the C terminal transactivation domain. Prolyl hydroxylation by PHD is required for binding to the pVHL-E3-ubiquitin ligase complex, whereas asparaginyl hydroxylation prevents the interaction of HIF-α with CBP/p300 transcriptional co-activator. Upon binding to the E3-ligase complex, HIF-α is polyubiquitinated and then degraded by the proteasome. Acetylation of HIF-α by ARD1 enhances binding to pVHL and subsequent ubiquitination. During hypoxia when prolyl-hydroxylases are inactive, HIF-α is stabilized and translocates to the nucleus, where it is SUMOylated by SUMO conjugases. Failure to deSUMOylate HIF-α targets HIF-α for VHL/proteasome-dependent degradation by providing an alternate signal (prolyl hydroxylation-independent) for pVHL binding. DeSUMOylated HIF-α escapes degradation, heterodimerizes with HIF-1β, binds to the hypoxia response elements (consensus binding site), and increases transcription of HIF target genes such as VEGF. Oxygen-dependent asparagine hydroxylation of HIF-α by factor-inhibiting HIF-1 (FIH 1) blocks recruitment of the CBP/p300 co-factor to the HIF transcriptional complex.

A second hypoxic switch operates in the COOH-terminal transactivation domain of HIF-α upon the hydroxylation of a specific asparagine residue. During hypoxia, asparagine hydroxylation is blocked, and CBP/p300 recruitment is facilitated, enabling increased levels of transcription. Factor-inhibiting-HIF (FIH) hydroxylates the asparagine residue. FIH is expressed in renal tubular epithelial cells and glomeruli (Soilleux et al., 2005).

In addition to hypoxic activation, a nonhypoxic increase in HIF transcriptional activity has been shown to be mediated by nitric oxide and TNF-α (Sandau et al., 2001), interleukin 1 (Stiehl et al., 2002), angiotensin II (Richard et al., 2000), and a variety of growth factors, including epidermal growth factor, insulin, and insulin-like growth factors (Jiang et al., 2001; Stiehl et al., 2002; Treins et al., 2002). Nitric oxide, ROS, and certain oncogenes such as v-Src and activated Ras have been shown to inhibit HIF prolyl-hydroxylation (Kaelin 2005). In contrast, HIF activation induced through the phosphoinositide 3-kinase/Akt-1/mammalian target of rapamycin pathway appears to be mediated through increased HIF-α protein translation (Fukuda et al., 2002). Thus, HIF activation is likely to occur in a variety of different renal disease settings even in the absence of significant hypoxia.

Whereas HIF-1α is ubiquitously expressed, HIF-2α expression is more restricted. HIF-2α has been found in hepatocytes, cardiomyocytes, glial cells, type II pneumocytes, and endothelial cells (Wiesener et al., 2003).

The list of HIF-regulated genes (either directly or indirectly regulated by HIF) has grown rapidly. HIF is involved in the regulation of a multitude of biological processes that are relevant to kidney function under physiological and pathological conditions.

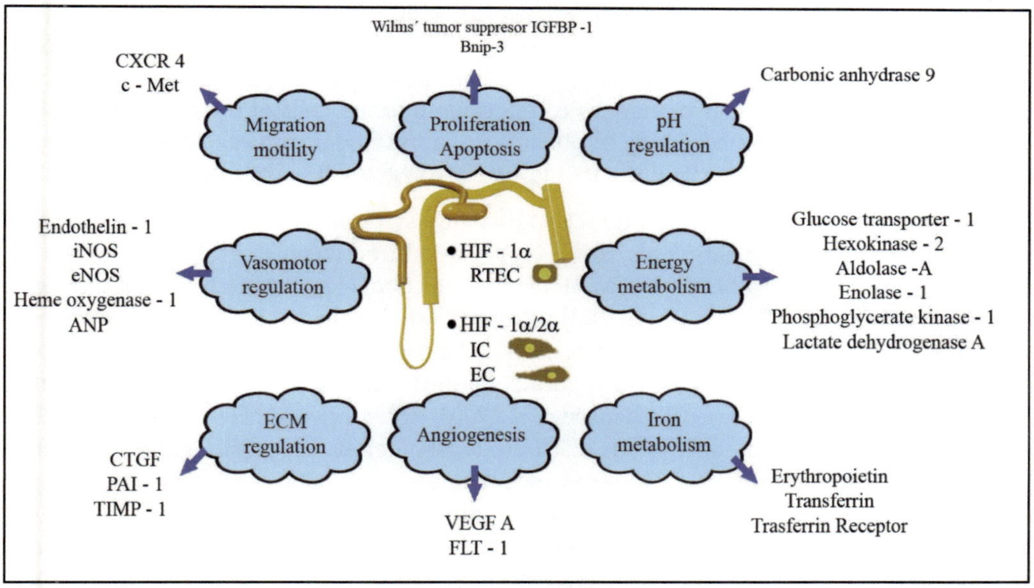

Fig. 3. Overview of selected hypoxia/HIF-regulated biological processes that have been shown or have been proposed to play important roles in the pathogenesis of renal cancer. RTEC (renal tubular epithelial cell), IC (intersticial cell), EC (endothelial cell).

3. Renal injury in cancer patients: Hypoxia and Inflammation

Whereas acutely injured kidneys appear to benefit from the protective effects of HIF-regulated biological processes, chronic hypoxia, mediated in part through HIF-1, can contribute to increased extracellular matrix production and the epithelial-to-mesenchymal transition (EMT), thereby potentially promoting renal fibrosis and the progression of renal disease. HIF may impact the pathogenesis of tubulointerstitial disease through the regulation of inflammatory responses. Microenvironmental changes, such as hypoxia, strongly impact inflammatory cell recruitment (Kong et al., 2004) and function (Cramer et al., 2003). HIF-1 is essential for myeloid cell-mediated inflammation mainly through its effects on cellular ATP generation. Inactivation of HIF-1 results in a profound impairment of myeloid cell aggregation, motility, and invasiveness, whereas forced expression of HIF-1 has the opposite effect (Kong et al., 2004). Alterations in HIF signalling in inflammatory cells may also play a significant role in renal inflammation, subsequent fibrosis and, thus, the progression of chronic renal disease.

Patients with neoplasia are subject to a variety of different types of renal, fluid and electrolyte disorders, either from direct effects such as urinary tract obstruction or infiltration or from indirect effects such as hyperkalaemia. Glomerulonephritis and nephrotic syndrome are due to immunologic reactions associated with neoplasia.

Just as hypoxia can induce inflammation, inflamed lesions often become severely hypoxic. Because of the steep oxygen gradient between the anaerobic intestinal lumen and the metabolically active lamina propria mucosae, intestinal epithelial cells are normally hypoxic (Karhausen et al., 2004).

Contributors to tissue hypoxia during inflammation include an increase in the metabolic demands of cells and a reduction in metabolic substrates caused by thrombosis, trauma, compression (interstitial hypertension), or atelectasis (airway plugging). Moreover, multiplication of intracellular pathogens can deprive infected cells of oxygen (Kempf et al., 2005). In the case of inflamed tissue, hypoxia is not a bystander; rather, it can influence the environment of the tissue, particularly by regulating oxygen-dependent gene expression.

Activation of the prolyl hydroxylase (PHDs)–HIF pathway promotes the resolution of mucosal inflammation in mice (Colgan et al., 2010). Hypoxia-induced changes in gene expression by epithelial cells help to promote mucosal barrier function (e.g., through the activation of intestinal trefoil factor) (Furuta et al., 2001) or to increase the production by the epithelium of anti-inflammatory signalling molecules such as adenosine (Eltzschig 2009). These adaptive responses to hypoxia are activated during mucosal inflammation and promote the resolution of inflammatory bowel disease (Karhausen et al., 2004; Robinson et al., 2008; Eckle et al., 2008) and acute lung injury (Rosenberg et al., 2009; Reutershan et al., 2009; Schingnitz et al., 2010). Several studies have shown that hypoxia enhances the enzymatic conversion of precursor nucleotides, such as ATP, adenosine diphosphate, or AMP, to adenosine (Eltzschig et al., 2003), thereby elevating extracellular levels of adenosine, an anti-inflammatory signalling molecule involved in restraining innate immune responses.

HIF stimulates the production of extracellular adenosine and suppresses both its uptake into the intracellular compartment and its intracellular metabolism (Morote-García et al., 2008). HIF also enhances adenosine receptor signalling by increasing the expression on the cell surface of adenosine receptors (Eckle et al., 2008), an effect that attenuates immune responses, vascular fluid leakage, and neutrophil accumulation in the presence of myocardial, renal, hepatic, or intestinal ischemia or acute lung injury.

Concentrations of oxygen in solid tumors, as compared with those in normal tissues, are frequently lower (Semenza 2003). Solid tumours contain increased levels of HIF-1α and HIF-2α. Hypoxia in a solid tumour stabilises HIF through hypoxia-dependent inhibition of PHDs. Similarly, the activation of oncogenes, or the loss of function of tumour-suppressor genes, results in the stabilisation of HIF, as happens in the case of the VHL tumour-suppressor gene. Hypoxia and inflammation meet at several points in the setting of cancer. In tumour cells oncogenes, inflammatory signals (mediated in part through Toll-like receptors [TLRs]), and hypoxia-activated nuclear factor κB (NF-κB) and hypoxia-inducible factor (HIF) 1α (which activate one another). These factors induce a gene program that recruits and activates leukocytes (through the release of chemokines and cytokines), stimulates angiogenesis and the formation of an abnormal vasculature and endothelium (through release of angiogenic signals), and increases tumour-cell invasion, metastasis, epithelial-to-mesenchymal transition (EMT), survival, proliferation, and metabolic reprogramming. In leukocytes, hypoxia also activates NF-κB and HIF-1α; endogenous ligands, released from necrotic cancer cells, activate TLRs upstream of NF-κB and HIF-1α, and HIF-1α up-regulates TLR expression. The resultant gene-expression profile leads to the production of cytokines and angiogenic signals and skews their polarisation phenotype. Tumour vessels with two PHDs-domain 2 (PHD2) alleles have an abnormal endothelium, are hypo-perfused, and cause tumour hypoxia, which fuels tumour-cell invasiveness and metastasis. In contrast, tumour vessels lacking one PHD2 allele have increased HIF-2α levels, which results in an up-regulation of factors that counteract the development of tumour endothelial abnormalities; this, in turn, results in improved tumour-vessel perfusion and oxygenation and, secondarily, reduced metastasis.

Experimental evidence indicates that inhibition of HIF within the inflamed tumour core attenuates the growth and vascularisation of tumours and enhances the sensitivity of tumours to radiation (Semenza et al., 2010). In contrast, inhibition of PHD2 and stabilisation of HIF within the tumour vasculature may play an important role in tumour therapy, if the means can be found to selectively direct inhibitors of PHD to the tumour vasculature and inhibitors of HIF to the hypoxic core.

4. Hypoxia inducible factor and renal cancer

The most common form of kidney cancer is renal cell cancer of the clear cell type (CC-RCC). A molecular hallmark of sporadic CC-RCC and hereditary CC-RCC associated with the von Hippel-Lindau familial tumour syndrome are mutations in the VHL tumour suppressor pVHL. Loss of pVHL function results in oxygen-independent HIF-α stabilisation, increased HIF transcriptional activity, and constitutive upregulation of HIF target genes. While patients with sporadic CC-RCC are characterised by somatic inactivation of both VHL gene copies in renal epithelial cells, patients with the VHL tumour syndrome transmit germ line mutations of the VHL gene. Although the highly vascular nature of VHL-deficient tumours is easily explained by increased VEGF production as a result of increased HIF transcriptional activity, VHL-associated renal carcinogenesis is more difficult to understand and most likely requires multiple other genetic events beyond the loss of pVHL function. In addition to regulating the degradation of HIF-α-subunits, pVHL has been shown to have additional biological functions, which may or may not be critical for renal tumourigenesis (Haase 2005).

Aside from a regulatory role in tumour angiogenesis, HIF plays a key role in the regulation of factors that are important for the development and invasiveness of CC-RCC. These include, among others, TGF-α, a potent renal epithelial mitogen, cell cycle regulator cyclin D1 (CCND1), and chemokine receptor CXCR4 (Bindra et al., 2002; Raval et al., 2005; Smith et al., 2005; Staller et al., 2003; Wykoff et al., 2004; Zatyka et al., 2002). With regard to the individual contribution of HIF-1 and HIF-2 to renal tumour development, a substantial number of VHL-defective CC-RCC cell lines do not express HIF-1α but do express HIF-2α (Maxwell et al., 1999). This is in contrast to normal, nontransformed renal epithelial cells, in which HIF-2α is not detectable during ischemia (Rosenberger et al., 2002).

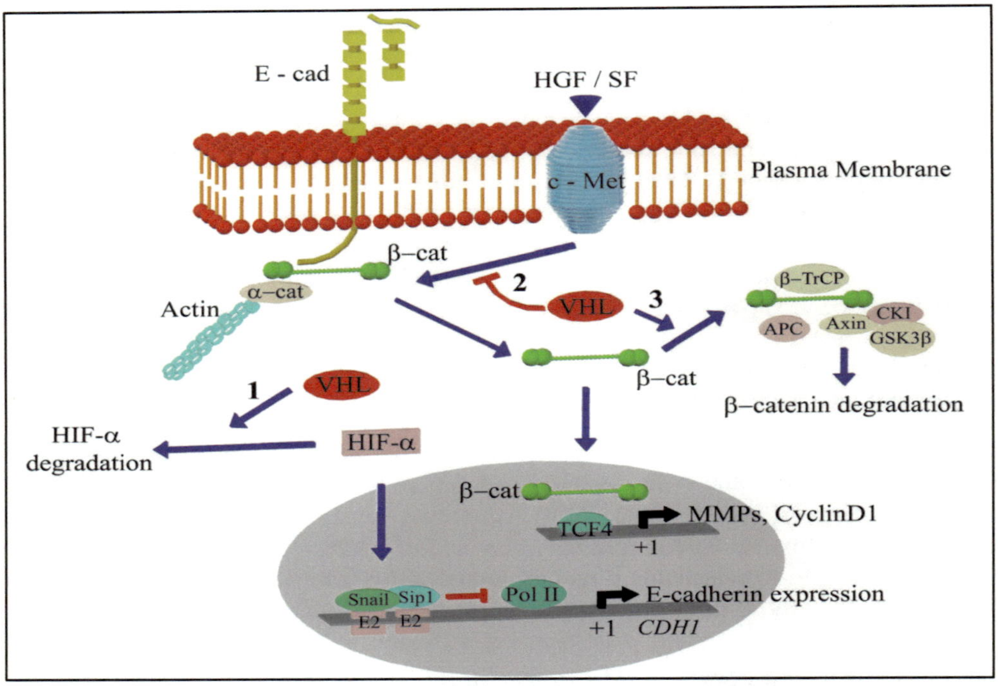

Fig. 4. Role of VHL in the regulation of E-cadherin and β-catenin. Loss of VHL leads to the stabilization of HIFα (1), which promotes the transactivation of E-cadherin-specific repressors, reducing E-caherin expression. Loss of VHL also causes constitutive phosphorylation of c-Met (2) and subsequent release, activation and stabilization of β-catenin (3).

HIF-1 and HIF-2 have diverse functions with regard to VHL renal tumourigenesis. HIF-2 has been proposed to preferentially regulate signalling pathways critical for renal cell growth, such as signalling through the TGF-α/epidermal growth factor receptor pathway and through the cell cycle regulator cyclin D1 (Bindra et al., 2002; Raval et al., 2005; Smith et al., 2005; Staller et al., 2003; Wykoff et al., 2004; Zatyka et al., 2002).

In addition to VHL-associated CC-RCC, HIF-α stabilisation can be found in renal cell cancers that are associated with mutations of the tuberous sclerosis tumour suppressor TSC-2 (Liu et al., 2003) and in rare leiomyomatosis-associated renal cancers. The latter form of renal cancer is characterised by fumarate hydratase deficiency, the inability to convert fumarate to malate, which results in HIF prolyl-hydroxylase inhibition; fumarate acts as a competitive inhibitor of HIF prolyl-hydroxylation (Isaacs et al., 2005). It is unclear whether an increase in HIF-1 and HIF-2 activity in these rare forms of renal cancer has the same biological effects as in VHL-negative CC-RCC, and further investigation is required.

5. Energy disorders in RCC

Tumours are characterised by specific metabolic alterations providing a metabolic signature in malignant transformation at different stages; end stage carcinomas are most dependent on anaerobic glucose degradation (aerobic glycolysis, fermentation) and least dependent on mitochondrial energy supplies. The metabolic endpoint of this transformation is the anaerobic degradation of glucose even in the presence of oxygen (Koppenol et al., 2011).Concomitant with this metabolic switch, high lactate concentrations occur and result in the immune protection of cancer cells, acid-mediated matrix degradation, invasiveness and metastasis (Hutterer et al., 2007).

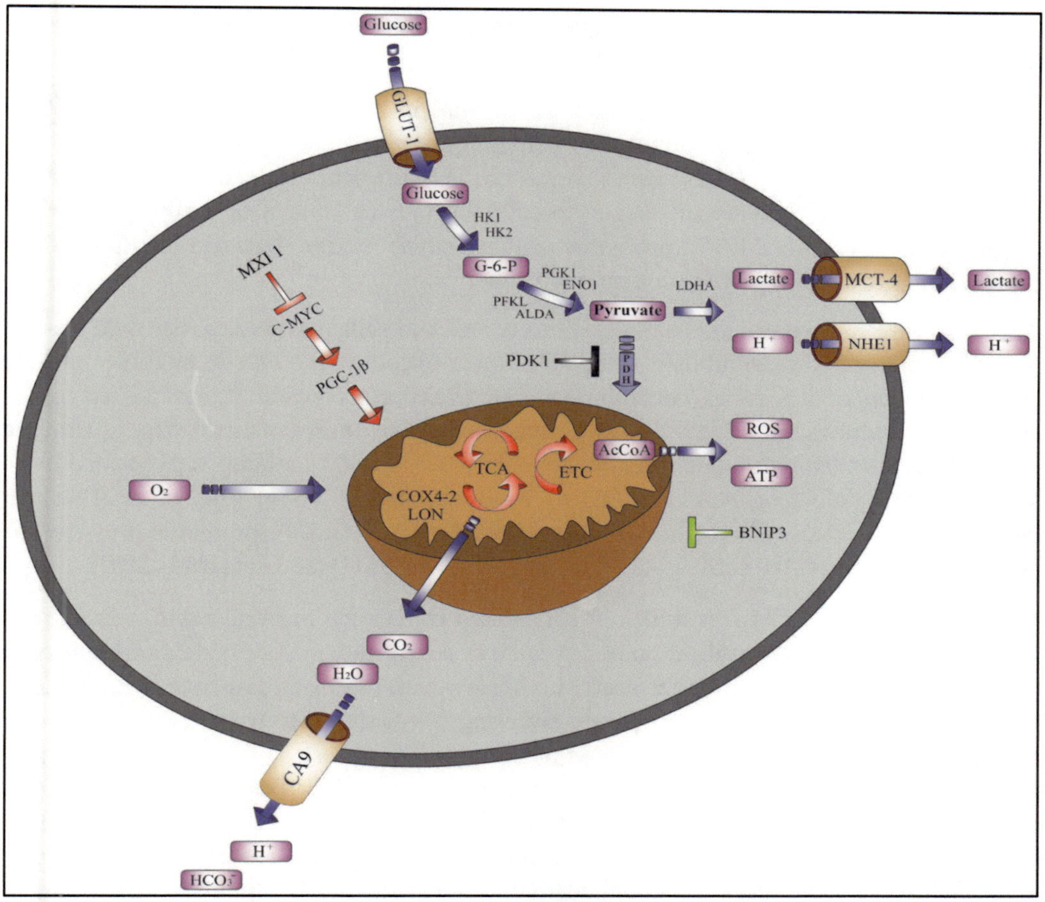

Fig. 5. Regulation of proteins required for glucose uptake and energy metabolism by HIF-1. Metabolic substrates and products are shown in purple and HIF-1-regulated gene products are shown in brown. Red arrows, mitochondrial biogenesis mediated by C-MYC (in renal carcinoma cells). Green blocked arrow, mitochondrial autophagy mediated by BNIP3 (in mouse embryo fibroblasts). AcCoA, acetyl coenzyme A; ALD, aldolase; CA9, carbonic anhydrase; COX, cytochrome c oxidase; ENO, enolase; G-6-P, glucose-6-phosphate; GLUT, glucose transporter; HK, hexokinase; LDH, lactate dehydrogenase; MCT, monocarboxylate transporter; NHE, sodium-hydrogen exchanger; PDH, pyruvate dehydrogenase; PDK, PDH kinase; PFK, phosphofructokinase; PGC, PPAR-γ co-activator; PGK, phosphoglycerate kinase.

Increased total activity of the transketolase-dependent, nonoxidative branch of the pentose phosphate pathway (PPP) in cancer cells is due to the overexpression of the transketolase-like-1 (TKTL1) protein (Hu et al., 2007).

The complex regulation of tumour metabolism switches from mitochondrial oxidative to nonoxidative energy production, which is dependent on the PPP. Both the oxidative and nonoxidative branches of the PPP have been described as activated in carcinogenesis (Ramos-Montoya et al., 2006). It is assumed that the enzymes of the oxidative branch of the PPP [glucose-6-phosphate-dehydrogenase (G6PD) and 6-phosphogluconate dehydrogenase] are triggered by an increased need for NADPH, whereas the enzymes of the nonoxidative branch (TKTL1, transaldolases) are triggered by an increased need for ribose and energy (Ramos-Montoya et al., 2006).

HIF-1 regulates the expression of hundreds of genes in human cells (Manalo et al., 2005; Elvidge et al., 2006) and is essential for embryonic development in mice (Iyer et al., 1998; Ryan et al., 1998). Many of these genes contribute to two essential functions of HIF-1. First, HIF-1 promotes the delivery of oxygen to cells through its control of erythropoiesis and angiogenesis. Second, HIF-1 promotes cell survival under hypoxic conditions by reprogramming cellular glucose and energy metabolism.

Analysis of mRNA expression in mouse embryonic stem cells that were either wild type or homozygous for a knockout allele at the *Hif1a* locus encoding the HIF-1α subunit revealed that expression of the genes encoding glucose transporters 1 and 3 and the glycolytic enzymes hexokinase 1 and 2, glucose phosphate isomerase, phosphofructokinase L, aldolase A and C, triosephosphate isomerase, phosphoglycerate kinase 1, enolase 1, pyruvate kinase M, and lactate dehydrogenase A (LDH-A) was regulated by HIF-1 (Iyer et al., 1998). In human VHL-deficient renal cell carcinoma, upregulation of GLUT1 protein expression has been demonstrated at the earliest stages of tumour formation (Mandriota et al., 2002).

The upregulation of LDH-A results in the increased conversion of pyruvate to lactate at the expense of mitochondrial utilisation of pyruvate as a substrate for pyruvate dehydrogenase (PDH), which converts pyruvate to acetyl CoA. However, recent studies have demonstrated that HIF-1 plays a direct role in actively shunting pyruvate away from the mitochondria through its regulation of the PDK1 gene (encoding PDH kinase 1) in multiple cell types, including VHL deficient renal carcinoma cells (Kim et al., 2006; Papandreou et al., 2006). Phosphorylation of the catalytic subunit of PDH by PDK1 inactivates the enzyme. In mouse embryo fibroblasts cultured from HIF-1α-null embryos, prolonged hypoxic incubation induces ROS production leading to cell death that can be rescued by the forced expression of PDK1 (Kim et al., 2006). HIF-1α-null mouse embryo fibroblasts also manifest increased cell death (relative to wild-type cells) when incubated under hypoxic conditions in the presence of the hypoxic cytotoxin tirapazamine (Papandreou et al., 2006). These results suggest that HIF-1 actively inhibits the oxidative metabolism of glucose under hypoxic conditions.

The decrease in oxygen consumption under moderate hypoxia is likely to be an adaptive mechanism to avoid the development of anoxia. During hypoxia, cells that fail to decrease their oxygen consumption are likely to become anoxic faster than cells that can suppress their rate of oxygen consumption (Denko 2008).

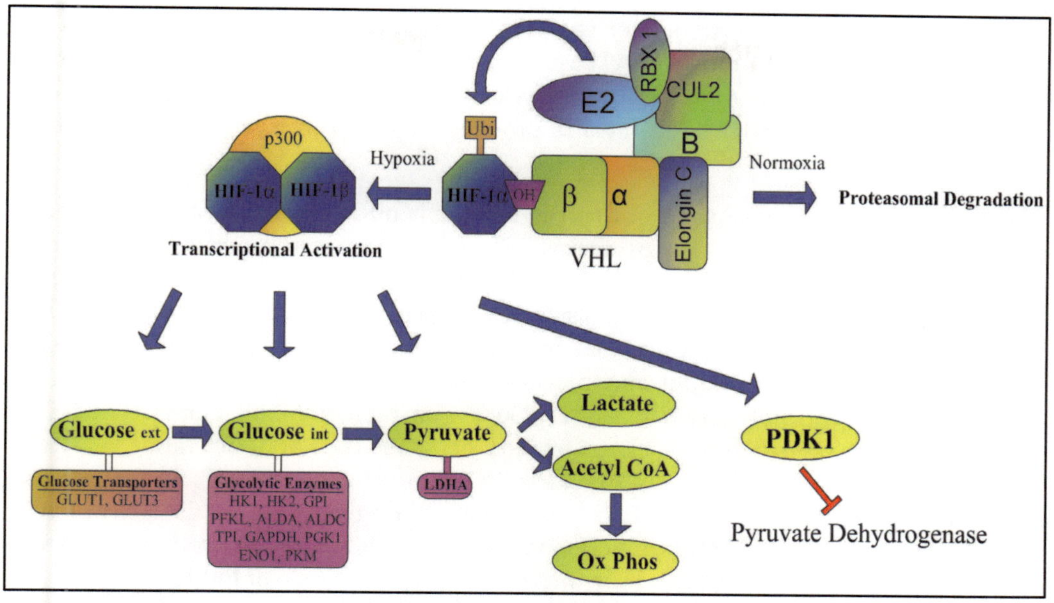

Fig. 6. Regulation of glucose metabolism by HIF-1. Under normoxic conditions, HIF-1α (or HIF-2α) is hydroxylated by PHD2, bound by VHL, ubiquitinated by an E3 ligase complex containing elongin B, elongin C, cullin 2, and Rbx1, and degraded by the proteasome. VHL loss-of-function (in clear cell renal carcinoma) or hypoxic conditions leads to the accumulation of non-hydroxylated, non-ubiquitinated HIF-1α (or HIF-2α), which dimerizes with HIF-1β, recruits the coactivator p300 (or CBP) and activates the transcription of genes encoding glucose transporter (GLUT) 1 and 3, hexokinase (HK) 1 and 2, glucosephosphate isomerase (GPI), phosphofructokinase (PFK) L, aldolase (ALD) A and C, triosephosphate isomerase (TPI), glyceraldephosphate dehydrogenase (GAPDH), phosphoglycerate kinase (PGK) 1, enolase (ENO) 1, pyruvate kinase (PK) M, lactate dehydrogenase (LDH) A, and pyruvate dehydrogenase kinase (PDK) 1.

Mitochondrial respiration in cells is controlled by cellular ATP utilisation. One model suggests that increased cytoplasmic ATP utilisation decreases cytosolic ATP levels and increases cytosolic ADP and Pi levels (Chance et al., 1955). The rise in cytosolic ADP levels leads to a rise in mitochondrial ADP via the increased activity of the adenine nucleotide carrier. The increased mitochondrial ADP concentration stimulates ATP synthase to augment the rate of ATP synthesis. The increased ATP synthesis results in a decrease in the mitochondrial membrane potential, which stimulates the respiratory chain to consume oxygen. Aside from cellular ATP utilisation, the other factors that control mitochondrial respiration are the NADH supply, the respiratory chain, and the degree of proton leak (Jones et al., 1993). The major reason for the decrease in respiration during hypoxia is the decrease in cellular ATP utilisation.

A major ATP consumer that hypoxia inhibits is Na/K-ATPase. The activity of Na/K-ATPase alone can account for 20–70% of the oxygen expenditure of mammalian cells (Milligan et al., 1985). Na/K-ATPase is a transmembrane protein found in higher eukaryotes that transports Na^+ and K^+ across the plasma membrane to maintain ionic gradients (Skou

1957). Na/K-ATPase is a heterodimer composed of α and β subunits (Kaplan 2002). The hypoxia-induced decrease of Na/K-ATPase activity is due to endocytosis of the α subunit from the plasma membrane by PKC zeta. Hypoxia stimulates the AMPK alpha-1 isoform, which directly phosphorylates PKC zeta to promote Na/K-ATPase endocytosis (Gusarova et al., 2009).

The other major ATP consumer that hypoxia inhibits is mRNA translation (Wouters et al., 2005). The mammalian target rapamycin (mTOR) and pancreatic eIF2α kinase(PERK) are the key regulators of translation during hypoxia (Arsham et al., 2003; Koumenis et al., 2002). In growth-promoting conditions, mTOR sustains translation by phosphorylating eIF4E-binding proteins (4EBPs) and ribosomal protein S6 kinases (S6Ks) (Gingras et al., 2001). Hypoxia (1.5% O_2) causes rapid and reversible hypophosphorylation of mTOR and its effectors 4E-BP1 and S6K (Arsham et al., 2003). The rapid inhibition of mTOR is HIF independent and occurs through the activation of AMPK76. Rapid activation of AMPK during hypoxia is dependent on mitochondrial ROS (Emerling et al., 2009). The other major contributor to the decrease in mRNA translation during hypoxia is the activation of PERK73, resulting in eIF2α phosphorylation and the inhibition of mRNA translation initiation. Mitochondrial ROS have been implicated in the activation of PERK.

Mitochondrial respiration is regulated by the availability of oxygen, ADP and reducing equivalents (NADH and $FADH_2$ from the TCA cycle). Oxygen is limiting for respiration under severely hypoxic conditions (<0.5% O_2). Thus, under physiological hypoxia (1–3% O_2), oxygen is not limiting for maximal respiration. The major controller of mitochondrial respiration is ADP availability from cellular ATP utilisation. Hypoxia through mitochondrial ROS also diminishes the activity of Na/K-ATPase and mRNA translation. This results in a decrease in cellular ATP utilisation and a decrease in ADP availability to mitochondria. Hypoxia also stimulates the release of mitochondrial ROS from complex III to activate HIF-1, which induces the transcription of PDK1. PDK1 negatively regulates PDH, an enzyme that converts pyruvate to acetyl-CoA. Thus, an increase in HIF-1 dependent PDK1 expression results in diminished availability of acetyl-CoA. This also contributes to diminished respiration during hypoxia by decreasing TCA cycle activity.

Although HIF-1 and HIF-2 are activated by similar mechanisms by hypoxia, they have both overlapping and distinct gene targets. HIF-1 regulates metabolic genes, whereas HIF-2 regulates EPO and the mitochondrial matrix protein superoxide dismutase 2 (SOD2). Depending on the genetic background, the loss of HIF-2 in adult mice results in profound anaemia (Gruber et al., 2007) or multiple organ pathology due to increased oxidative stress (Scortegagna M., 2003). The role of HIF-2 regulation of oxidative stress is further supported by the observation that SOD2 levels are markedly increased in VHL-null renal cell carcinoma cells (Hervouet et al., 2008). It will be interesting to determine whether activation of HIF-2 prevents oxidative stress-induced injury in other organs, such as brain, lung and heart.

6. Nutrient disorders in RCC

Diets rich in fruits and vegetables have typically been shown to decrease RCC risk, possibly through antioxidant effects, while consumption of fried foods has commonly been shown to increase risk, possibly due to the potential carcinogenic effects of acrylamides (Chow et al., 2008). Recently, epidemiological studies suggest that vitamin D, which is found in food (vitamin D2 and D3) and produced in the body after exposure to ultraviolet (UV) rays from the sun (vitamin D3), may be inversely associated with RCC risk (Karami et al., 2008). Both vitamin D2 and D3 are hydroxylated in the liver and subsequently in the kidney to form active vitamin D (1,25(OH)2D3). Dietary intake of vitamin D accounts for a small (approximately 10%) proportion of vitamin D levels (Holick 2006). However, dietary intake of vitamin D and vitamin D rich foods may play a role in determining RCC risk, given that vitamin D has been associated with anticarcinogenic properties and is primarily metabolised within the kidneys (Holick 2006). Vitamin D and its metabolites are thought to impede carcinogenesis by stimulating cell differentiation, inhibiting cell proliferation, inducing apoptosis, and suppressing invasiveness, angiogenesis, and metastasis (Valdivielso et al., 2006). Vitamin D activation is mediated by binding to vitamin D receptors (VDRs), transcription factors that are part of the nuclear hormone receptor family. Forming a heterodimer complex with the retinoid-X-receptor (RXR) gene, VDR can regulate the transcription of other genes involved in cell regulation, growth, and immunity (Valdivielso et al., 2006; Thibault et al., 2006). Most epidemiological studies have focused on the VDR gene; however, a recent evaluation of 139 single nucleotide polymorphisms (SNPs) across eight genes in the vitamin D pathway found a significant association between RCC risk and certain VDR and RXRA genetic variants (Karami et al., 2009).

The kidney is the most important organ for vitamin D metabolism and activity as well as calcium homeostasis. Within the kidneys, calcium has been shown to influence active vitamin D levels (Holick et al., 2006). Thus, investigations of dietary vitamin D and calcium in RCC aetiology are highly relevant. A Canadian RCC case-control study showed no association for the intake of individual foods rich in vitamin D (i.e., fish and eggs) or calcium (i.e., milk, dairy, and cheese) (Hu et al., 2003). In contrast, calcium supplement intakes were shown to significantly reduce RCC risk as the number of years of intake increased. Different polymorphisms in the VDR gene have been speculated to result in variations of VDR expression and changes to circulating levels of active vitamin D (Ikuyama et al., 2002). For this reason, epidemiological studies suggest that tissue specific expression of vitamin D pathway genes function as the primary mechanism involved in linking vitamin D status with the anticarcinogenic effects of 1,25(OH)2D3. Therefore, a lower renal cancer risk may be associated with higher circulating levels of 25(OH)D, the storage form of vitamin D, by providing substrates for renal tissue-specific synthesis of 1,25(OH)2D3 (McCullough et al., 2008). RXRA, on the other hand, may play a critical role in vitamin D activity, particularly from dietary sources, since this gene has been shown to regulate cholesterol (Hegele et al., 2001), which is abundant in eggs and yogurt, the food groups that were statistically associated with renal cancer risk in this study. RXRA regulated fatty acid and cholesterol metabolism through intestinal cholesterol absorption and bile acid synthesis (Hegele et al., 2001). Cholesterol metabolism has been associated with atherosclerosis, which is associated with hypertension and cardiovascular risk, known risk factors of RCC.

Antioxidant-rich foods have several preventive effects against different diseases, such as cancer, coronary disease, inflammatory disorders, and neurologic degeneration. Honey has been used as a traditional food source since ancient times. It is made when the nectar and sweet deposits from plants are gathered, modified, and stored in the honeycomb by honeybees. The major components of honey are fructose and glucose; honey also contains carbohydrates, proteins, amino acids, vitamins, water, minerals, and enzymes. In general, honey is also rich in antioxidants and has antibacterial properties (Brudzynski 2006). Honey not only promotes growth of new skin tissue by creating a moist environment but also prevents infection by way of its antimicrobial properties. Moreover, honey is harmless; in fact, it enables faster healing of the wounds by forming new tissues. Honey is thought to exhibit a broad spectrum of therapeutic properties, including antibacterial, antifungal, cytostatic, and anti-inflammatory activity (Jeddar et al., 1985). Honey potentiated the antitumour activity of chemotherapeutic drugs, such as 5-fluorouracil and cyclophosphamide, and contains many biologically active compounds, including caffeic acid, caffeic acid phenethyl ester, and flavonoid glycones. These compounds have been shown to have an inhibitory effect on tumour cell proliferation and transformation by the downregulation of many cellular enzymatic pathways, including protein tyrosine kinase, cyclooxygenase, and ornithine decarboxylase pathways (Chinthalapally et al., 1993).

Honey is also a dietary source for flavonoids, which have been demonstrated to have anticarcinogenic and anti-inflammatory activities. Although crude honey was reported by some authors to be a proliferative agent that enhances the proliferation of both normal and malignant cells (Rady 2005), it was also reported to be a promising antitumour agent with pronounced antimetastatic effects (Orsolic et al., 2005). The proliferative effect of honey on tumour cells was suggested to be a nutritional effect rather than a carcinogenic effect, and the antitumour effect was reported to result from many activities, such as the inhibition of DNA synthesis with no signs of cytotoxicity and the downregulation of MMP-2 and MMP-9, which have been implicated in the induction of the angiogenic switch in different model systems (Egeblad et al., 2002). Honey has cytotoxic activity against carcinomic human kidney cells, indicating that honey possesses antitumour and anticarcinogenic activities (Abdel Aziz et al., 2009).

Leptin is an adipocyte-derived hormone/cytokine that links nutritional status with neuroendocrine and immune functions. Leptin was the first adipocyte-derived hormone described, and the amount of leptin produced is directly proportional to the amount of adipose tissue. Leptin activates the anorexigenic axis in the hypothalamus. Leptin is a key intermediary between energy homeostasis and the immune system, and it may play roles in inflammation and obesity-related diseases, including atherosclerosis and cancer. The characterisation of leptin functions and signalling pathways in regulating lipid metabolism, inflammatory mediator production and lipid body biogenesis in macrophages and other cells are important for understanding the roles of leptin in the pathogenesis of inflammatory diseases.

The mTOR kinase pathway is a well-studied and evolutionarily conserved intracellular nutrient-sensing pathway (Lindsley et al., 2004). This pathway integrates nutrient- and growth factor-derived signals to set overall growth rates, and interfaces with the cell cycle machinery to coordinate cell growth and division (Richardson et al., 2004).

New findings are starting to unveil an important role for mTOR in leptin signalling, in the hypothalamic centres as well as in peripheral cells (Cota et al., 2006).

The activation of mTOR complex 1 in the hypothalamus is important for the effects of leptin on the hypothalamic axis, which modulates food intake (Cota et al., 2006). These authors showed that the activation of the mTOR pathway occurs in response to leptin stimulation and that rapamycin inhibits the anorexigenic signal of leptin. Moreover, the amino acid leucine directly activates mTOR in the hypothalamus, functioning as a redundant signal with leptin. Several nutrient sensing mediators that activate mTOR in adipose tissue, including insulin, leucine and UDP-N-acetylglucosamine, also induce leptin synthesis (Lindsley et al., 2004). The role of leptin in regulating lipid accumulation and foam cell formation in macrophages is beginning to be characterised and involves key steps mediated by mTOR-dependent signalling. Typically, increases in the size and numbers of lipid bodies are accompanied by accumulation of triacylglycerides and cholesterol esters in their hydrophobic core. In different cell systems, including adipocytes and macrophages, intracellular lipids are stored and metabolised in hydrophobic organelles called lipid bodies or lipid droplets. Although lipid bodies were long considered inert fat depots, lipid bodies are now viewed as dynamic organelles with roles in integrating lipid metabolism, inflammatory mediator production, membrane trafficking and intracellular signalling (Wang et al., 2007). Accordingly, the regulatory mechanisms of lipid body biogenesis and functions are of major interest for the study of atherosclerosis, obesity, cancer and other inflammatory diseases. In addition, the mTOR inhibitor rapamycin upregulates the expression of genes that promote fatty acid oxidation, while downregulating genes that participate in fatty acid synthesis (Peng et al., 2002). However, it should be noted that depending on the cell type and model system used, leptin might have opposite effects on intracellular lipid storage and metabolism (O´Rourke et al., 2002). In fact, leptin diminishes lipid accumulation in the liver, kidney and adipose tissue (Motomura et al., 2006). These data point to different roles and possibly different signalling pathways for leptin, depending on the tissue.

Numerous studies have established a link between diet and cancer risk or progression; as a result, the World Cancer Research Fund has recently acknowledged that after smoking, diet may be the second most important contributor to the global burden of cancer (http://www.wcrf-uk.org/preventing cancer/index.php.).

7. Iron disorders in RCC

Iron metabolism is crucial in all aspects of energy production in the body (Anderson et al., 2009) and is particularly important for cells that are characterised by high-energy demands, such as tumourous cells. Iron has the ability to shuttle between two oxidative states (ferric and ferrous iron), which makes it an efficient cofactor for several enzymes and the catalyst of numerous biochemical reactions (Anderson et al., 2009). The ferrous form Fe(II) can donate electrons, while the Fe(III) form can accept electrons. Iron plays a crucial role in oxygen transport (as a component of hemoglobin (Hb)), oxygen storage (as a component of myoglobin), and oxidative metabolism (as a component of oxidative enzymes and respiratory chain processes).

Ion is also involved in the synthesis and degradation of lipids, carbohydrates, DNA, and RNA as well as in the metabolism of collagen, tyrosine, and catecholamines.

Therefore, iron deficiency can impair oxidative metabolism, cellular energetics, and cellular immune mechanisms.

Experimental studies in animals have shown that severe iron deficiency can cause diastolic dysfunction and heart failure with pulmonary congestion, left ventricular hypertrophy and dilation, cardiac fibrosis, a reduction in erythropoietin levels and a worsening of the molecular signalling pathways (as measured by cardiac STAT3 phosphorylation), an increase in the inflammatory cytokine TNFα, and proteinuria (Dong et al., 2005). Iron may have anti-inflammatory effects. Compared to haemodialysis patients taking EPO alone, those taking EPO and IV iron had lower proinflammatory TNFα levels and higher anti-inflammatory cytokine IL-4 levels as well as lower levels of total peroxide (a marker of free radical concentration) (Weiss et al., 2003).

The biology of iron and oxygen is closely related, and known regulatory pathways involving HIF and iron-regulatory proteins (IRPs) are responsive to both these stimuli.

In humans, iron is absorbed only in the small intestine, stored in the liver and the reticuloendothelial (RE) system, and is mainly used in bone marrow. Intestinal absorption of iron depends on four types of proteins of iron metabolism: duodenal cytochrome b (Dcytb), divalent metal transporter 1 (DMT1), ferroportin 1 (FP1) and hephaestin (Hp).

Many proteins of iron metabolism show a high degree of expression in tumour cells, indicating that iron plays an important role in tumourigenesis and development. However, regulatory factors of iron metabolism and their mechanisms remain to be studied. New treatment strategies may be developed by combining imaging agents or targeted drugs with proteins related to iron metabolism. Recently, magnetic nanoparticles carrying chemotherapeutic drugs provide a new thinking for solid tumour targeted therapy. For example, the combination of the magnetic nanoparticle Fe_3O_4 with cisplatin (DDP) is used to reverse DDP resistance in the human ovarian cancer cell line SKOV3/DDP through increasing intracellular drug concentrations and promoting cell apoptosis by reducing mRNA expression of the antiapoptosis genes *bcl2* and *survivin* (Jiang et al., 2009).

8. Oxygen sensing and RCC

Tumours are characterised by specific metabolic alterations providing a metabolic signature in malignant transformation at different stages; end stage carcinomas are most dependent on anaerobic glucose degradation (aerobic glycolysis, fermentation) and least dependent on mitochondrial energy supplies (Ramanathan et al., 2005). The metabolic endpoint of this transformation, the anaerobic degradation of glucose even in the presence of oxygen, was first described by Nobel laureate Otto Warburg (Warburg et al., 1924). Concomitant with this metabolic switch, high lactate concentrations occur and result in immune protection of cancer cells, acid-mediated matrix degradation, invasiveness and metastasis. Furthermore, transformation to a more malignant phenotype is associated with resistance to chemo- and radiation-therapy (Cao et al., 2007).

Increased total activity of the transketolase-dependent, nonoxidative branch of the pentose phosphate pathway (PPP) in cancer cells is due to the overexpression of the transketolase-like-1 (TKTL1) protein (Hu et al., 2007).

The complex regulation of tumour metabolism switches from mitochondrial oxidative to nonoxidative energy production, which is dependent on the PPP. Both the oxidative and nonoxidative branches of the PPP have been described as activated in carcinogenesis. It is assumed that the enzymes of the oxidative branch of the PPP [glucose-6-phosphate-dehydrogenase (G6PD) and 6-phosphogluconate dehydrogenase] are triggered by an increased need for NADPH, whereas the enzymes of the nonoxidative branch (TKTL1, transaldolases) are triggered by an increased need for ribose and energy (Ramos-Montoya et al., 2006).

During malignant transformation of cancer cells, a metabolic switch from mitochondrially based, oxygen-dependent ATP production (oxidative phosphorylation) to anaerobic glucose degradation (aerobic glycolysis, fermentation) leading to oxygen- and mitochondria-independent ATP generation takes place, even in the presence of oxygen (Ramanathan et al., 2005).

Activation of HIF-1, a key transcription factor that upregulates genes involved in glycolytic energy metabolism, is a common feature of RCC and has been linked to malignant transformation, metastasis and treatment resistance. In the absence of a functional von Hippel-Lindau tumour suppressor protein (70% of sporadic RCCs), irrespective of oxygen concentration, HIF-1α is not degraded and translocates to the nucleus where it dimerises with HIF-1β to form transcriptionally active HIF. HIF-1α is increased by hypoxia, insulin, insulin-like growth factor, epidermal growth factor and angiotensin II. The glycolysis-activated accumulation of HIF-1 protein once again stresses the crucial role of aerobic glycolysis in carcinogenesis and has been demonstrated to be a potent target in anticancer therapy (Oh et al., 2008).

Increased lactic-acid production and excretion by fermenting tumour cells results in suppression of cytokine production, T-cell inactivation, acid-mediated matrix degradation and apoptosis of surrounding healthy cells, leading to invasion and metastasis. Thus, high lactate production results in an exceptional growth advantage for tumour cells. The correlation between mitochondrial dysfunction and increased aerobic glycolysis in carcinogenesis has been investigated, but the competitive advantage for tumour cells is still under discussion (Ramanathan et al., 2005; Brandon et al., 2006). Mitochondrial energy production is correlated with release of reactive oxygen species (ROS) that damage proteins and macromolecules such as DNA. During proliferation, DNA is exposed to ROS that leads to severe DNA damage and mutations. Fermentative cancer cells do not produce mitochondrial ROS, thus preventing ROS-induced DNA alterations.

Anaerobic glucose metabolism is believed to have a poorer energy output in relation to the energy stored in the glucose molecule. Therefore, the elevated demand for glucose is compensated by the upregulation of glucose transporters and the onset of aerobic glycolysis in a PI-3K-dependent manner, resulting in high lactate concentrations (Walenta et al., 2004). The switch to anaerobic energy production by the TKTL1-dependent, nonoxidative branch of the PPP supports the enormous demand for (ROS-free) energy and anabolic substrates, such as ribose, NADPH and acetyl-CoA. The modified, TKTL1-dependent PPP seems a general biochemical program suitable for safe and enhanced energy release, and the anabolic substrate production necessary for rapid cell proliferation.

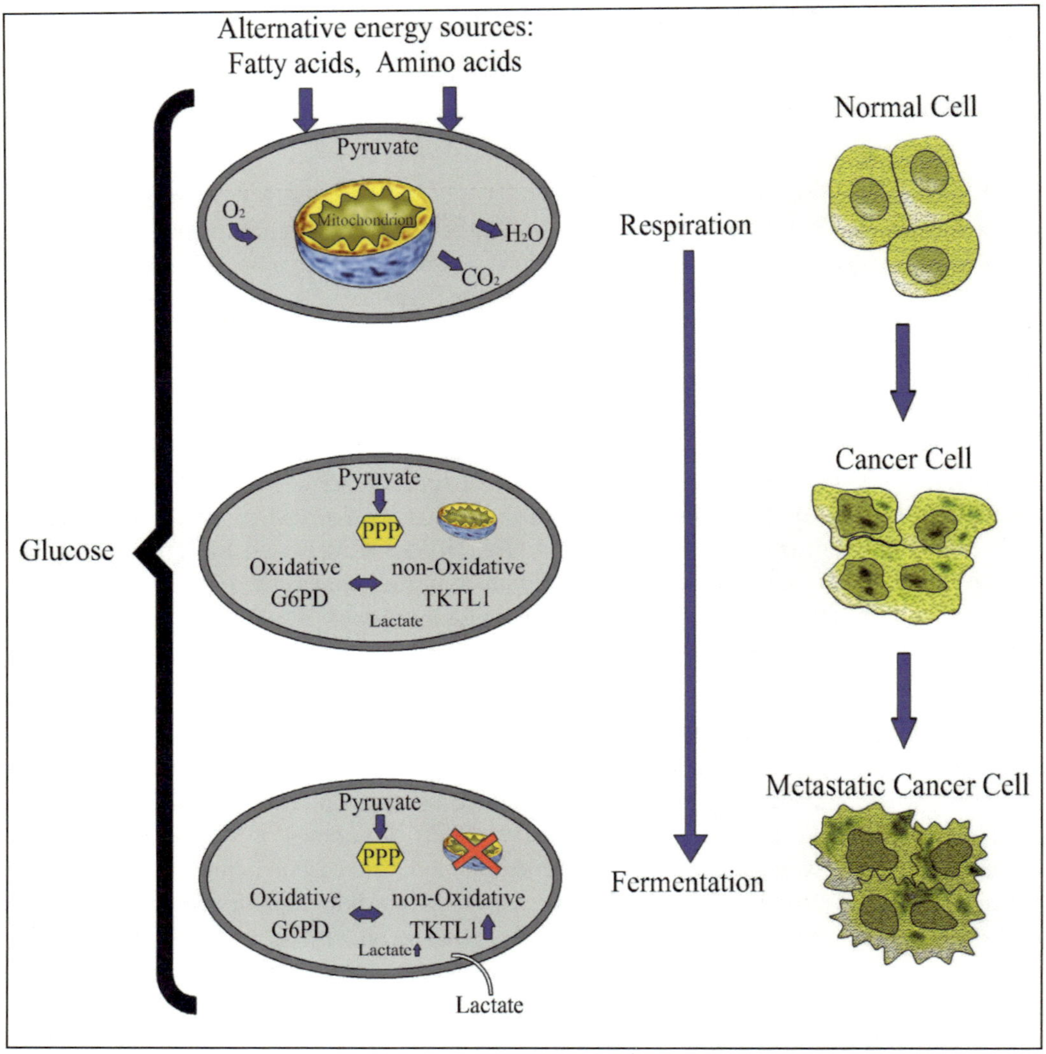

Fig. 7. Malignant transformation of cancer cells: renal tumors are present with an altered glucose metabolism. Enhanced glycolysis leads to increased activity of the enzymes in the oxidative (G6PD) and nonoxidative branches (TKTL1) of the PPP. Progressing tumors are characterized by specific upregulation of the nonoxidative branch of the PPP, ensuring ribose and energy, and supporting acidification of the tumor microenvironment. Acidification is a major step in invasive tumor growth, metastasis and immune escape. Additionally, upregulation of the anaerobic energy supply without ROS production, and G6PD activity for increased reducing equivalents, protects cancer cells from oxidative stress.

9. Conclusions

The oxygen-dependent regulation of HIF activity involves very complex pathways that involve prolyl hydroxylases and the VHL tumour suppressor protein, both of which are highly modulated by environmental and physiologic cues. The exact roles of the different HIF-α isoforms in these processes are still under intense investigation.

In the past decade, studying the regulation of HIFs has led to an appreciation that mitochondrial metabolism and ROS are essential regulators of HIFs. Conversely, HIFs have also been shown to regulate mitochondrial metabolism and ROS levels. Because mitochondria are the major consumers of oxygen, it is not surprising that HIFs and mitochondria are inter-connected.

The evidence accumulated from ecologic and case control studies show that diet has an important role in the development of RCC. Energy intake and several dietary factors should be considered as potentially involved in the development of renal cell cancer at different stages of tumourigenesis.

In this chapter, we have summarised the most recent findings in HIF signalling and have attempted to provide a perspective on how recent advances in HIF biology may affect our understanding of renal cancer.

10. References

Abdel Aziz A, Rady H, Amer MA, and Kiwan HS. (2009) Effect of Some Honey Bee Extracts on the Proliferation, Proteolytic and Gelatinolytic Activities of the Hepatocellular Carcinoma Hepg2 Cell Line. *Aus J Basic App Sci* 3, 2754–69

Anderson GJ and Vulpe CD (2009) Mammalian iron transport. *Cellular and Molecular Life Sciences* 66, 3241–3261

Arsham AM, Howell JJ, and Simon MC. (2003) A novel hypoxia-inducible factor-independent hypoxic response regulating mammalian target of rapamycin and its targets. *J Biol Chem* 278, 29655–29660

Bindra RS, Vasselli JR, Stearman R, Linehan WM, and Klausner RD. (2002) VHL-mediated hypoxia regulation of cyclin D1 in renal carcinoma cells. *Cancer Res* 62, 3014–3019

Brandon M, Baldi P, and Wallace DC. (2006) Mitochondrial mutations in cancer. *Oncogene* 25, 4647–62

Brudzynski K. (2006) Effect of hydrogen peroxide on antibacterial activities of Canadian honeys. *Can J Microbiol.* 52, 1228–37

Cao X, Fang L, Gibbs S, Huang Y, Dai Z, Wen P, Zheng X, Sadee W, and Sun D. (2007) Glucose uptake inhibitor sensitizes cancer cells to daunorubicin and overcomes drug resistance in hypoxia. *Cancer Chemother Pharmacol* 59:495–505

Chance B and Williams GR. (1955) Respiratory enzymes in oxidative phosphorylation. I. Kinetics of oxygen utilization. *J Biol Chem* 217, 383–393

Chinthalapally V, Dhimant D, Barbara S, Nalini K, Shantu A, and Bandaru R. (1993) Inhibitory effect of caffeic acid esters on azoxymethane-induced biochemical changes and aberrant crypt foci formation in rat colon. *Cancer Res* 53, 4182–8

Chow WH and Devesa SS. (2008) Contemporary epidemiology of renal cell cancer *Cancer Journal* 14, 288–301

Colgan SP, and Taylor CT. (2010) Hypoxia: an alarm signal during intestinal inflammation. *Nat Rev Gastroenterol Hepatol* 7, 281-7

Cota D, Proulx K, Smith KA, Kozma SC, Thomas G, Woods SC, and Seeley RJ.(2006) Hypothalamic mTOR signaling regulates food intake. *Science* 312, 927-30

Cramer T, Yamanishi Y, Clausen BE, Forster I, Pawlinski R, Mackman N, Haase VH, Jaenisch R, Corr M, Nizet V, Firestein GS, Gerber HP, Ferrara N, and Johnson RS.(2003) HIF-1α is essential for myeloid cell-mediated inflammation. *Cell* 112, 645–657

Denko NC. (2008) Hypoxia, HIF1 and glucose metabolism in the solid tumour. *Nat Rev Cancer* 8, 705–713

Dong F, Zhang X, Culver B, Chew HG, Kelley RO, and Ren J (2005) Dietary iron deficiency induces ventricular dilation, mitochondrial ultrastructural aberrations and cytochrome c release: involvement of nitric oxide synthase and protein tyrosine nitration. *Clinical Science* 109, 277–286

Eckle T, Grenz A, Laucher S, and Eltzschig HK. A2B adenosine receptor signaling attenuates acute lung injury by enhancing alveolar fluid clearance in mice. *J Clin Invest* 118, 3301-15

Eckle T, Köler D, Lehmann R, El Kasmi KC, and Eltzschig HK. (2008) Hypoxia-inducible factor-1 is central to cardioprotection: a new paradigm for ischemic preconditioning. *Circulation* 118, 166-75

Egeblad M, and Werb Z. (2002) New functions for the matrix metalloproteinases in cancer progression. *Nat Rev Cancer* 2, 161–74

Eltzschig HK, Ibla JC, Furuta GT, Leonard MO, Jacobson KA, Enjyoji K, Robson SC, and Colgan SP. (2003) Coordinated adenine nucleotide phosphohydrolysis and nucleoside signaling in posthypoxic endothelium: role of ectonucleotidases and adenosine A2B receptors. *J Exp Med* 198, 783-96

Eltzschig HK. (2009) Adenosine: an old drug newly discovered. *Anesthesiology* 111, 904-15

Elvidge GP, Glenny L, Appelhoff RJ, Ratcliffe PJ, Ragoussis J, and Gleadle JM (2006) Concordant regulation of gene expression by hypoxia and 2-oxoglutarate-dependent dioxygenase inhibition: the role of HIF-1alpha, HIF-2alpha, and other pathways. *J Biol Chem* 281, 15215–15226

Emerling BM, Weinberg F, Snyder C, Burgess Z, Mutlu GM, Viollet B, Budinger GR, and Chandel NS. (2009) Hypoxic activation of AMPK is dependent on mitochondrial ROS but independent of an increase in AMP/ATP ratio. *Free Radic Biol Med* 46, 1386–1391

Fukuda R, Hirota K, Fan F, Jung YD, Ellis LM, and Semenza GL. (2002) Insulin-like growth factor 1 induces hypoxia-inducible factor 1-mediated vascular endothelial growth factor expression, which is dependent on MAP kinase and phosphatidylinositol 3-kinase signaling in colon cancer cells. *J Biol Chem* 277, 38205–38211

Furuta GT, Turner JR, Taylor CT, Hershberg RM, Comerford K, Narravula S, Podolsky DK, and Colgan SP. (2001) Hypoxia-inducible factor 1-dependent induction of intestinal trefoil factor protects barrier function during hypoxia. *J Exp Med* 193, 1027-34

Gingras AC, Raught B, Gygi SP, Niedzwiecka A, Miron M, Burley SK, Polakiewicz RD, Wyslouch-Cieszynska A, Aebersold R, and Sonenberg N. (2001) Hierarchical phosphorylation of the translation inhibitor 4EBP1.*Genes Dev* 15, 2852–2864

Gruber M, Hu CJ, Johnson RS, Brown EJ, Keith B, and Simon MC. (2007) Acute postnatal ablation of Hif-2alpha results in anemia. *Proc Natl Acad Sci U S A.* 104, 2301–2306

Gusarova GA, Dada LA, Kelly AM, Brodie C, Witters LA, Chandel NS, and Sznajder JI. (2009) Alpha1-AMP-activated protein kinase regulates hypoxia-induced Na,K-ATPase endocytosis via direct phosphorylation of protein kinase C zeta. *Mol Cell Biol* 29, 3455–3464

Gustafsson MV, Zheng X, Pereira T, Gradin K, Jin S, Lundkvist J, Ruas JL, Poellinger L, Lendahl U, and Bondesson M. (2005) Hypoxia requires notch signaling to maintain the undifferentiated cell state. *Dev Cell* 9, 617–628

Haase VH. (2005) The VHL tumor suppressor in development and disease: functional studies in mice by conditional gene targeting. *Semin Cell Dev Biol* 16, 564–574

Hegele RA and Cao H. (2001) Single nucleotide polymorphisms of RXRA encoding retinoid X receptor alpha. *Journal of Human Genetics* 46, 423–425

Hervouet E, Cízková A, Demont J, Vojtísková A, Pecina P, Franssen-van Hal NL, Keijer J, Simonnet H, Ivánek R, Kmoch S, Godinot C, and Houstek J. (2008) HIF and reactive oxygen species regulate oxidative phosphorylation in cancer. Carcinogenesis 29, 1528–1537

Holick MF (2006) Vitamin D: its role in cancer prevention and treatment *Progress in Biophysics and Molecular Biology* 92, 49–59

Hu CJ, Wang LY, Chodosh LA, Keith B, and Simon MC. (2003) Differential roles of hypoxia-inducible factor 1α (HIF-1α) and HIF-2α in hypoxic gene regulation. *Mol Cell Biol* 23, 9361–9374

Hu J, Mao Y, and White K. (2003) Diet and vitamin or mineral supplements and risk of renal cell carcinoma in Canada. *Cancer Causes Control* 14, 705–714

Hu LH, Yang JH, Zhang DT, Zhang S, Wang L, Cai PC, Zheng JF, and Huang JS. (2007) The TKTL1 gene influences total transketolase activity and cell proliferation in human colon cancer LoVo cells. *Anticancer Drugs* 18, 427–33

Hu LH, Yang JH, Zhang DT, Zhang S, Wang L, Cai PC, Zheng JF, and Huang JS. (2007) The TKTL1 gene influences total transketolase activity and cell proliferation in human colon cancer LoVo cells. *Anticancer Drugs* 18, 427–33

Hutterer GC, Patard JJ, Perrotte P, Ionescu C, de La Taille A, Salomon L, Verhoest G, Tostain J, Cindolo L, Ficarra V, Artibani W, Schips L, Zigeuner R, Mulders PF, Valeri A, Chautard D, Descotes JL, Rambeaud JJ, Mejean A, and Karakiewicz PI. (2007) Patients with renal cell carcinoma nodal metastases can be accurately identified: external validation of a new nomogram. *Int J Cancer* 121, 2556–61

Ikuyama T, Hamasaki T, Inatomi H, Katoh T, Muratani T, and Matsumoto T. (2002) Association of vitamin D receptor gene polymorphism with renal cell carcinoma in Japanese *Endocrine Journal* 49, 433–438

Isaacs JS, Jung YJ, Mole DR, Lee S, Torres-Cabala C, Chung YL, Merino M, Trepel J, Zbar B, Toro J, Ratcliffe PJ, Linehan WM, and Neckers L. (2005) HIF overexpression correlates with biallelic loss of fumarate hydratase in renal cancer: novel role of fumarate in regulation of HIF stability. *Cancer Cell* 8, 143–153

Iyer NV, Kotch LE, Agani F, Leung SW, Laughner E, Wenger RH, Gassmann M, Gearhart JD, Lawler AM, Yu AY, and Semenza GL (1998) Cellular and developmental control of O2 homeostasis by hypoxia-inducible factor 1 alpha. *Genes Dev* 12, 149–162

Jeddar A, Khassany A, Ramsaroop VG, Bhamjei IE, Moosa A. (1985) The antibacterial action of honey: an in vitro study. *S Afr Med J* 67, 257–9

Jiang BH, Jiang G, Zheng JZ, Lu Z, Hunter T, and Vogt PK. (2001) Phosphatidylinositol 3-kinase signaling controls levels of hypoxia-inducible factor 1. *Cell Growth Differ* 12, 363–369

Jiang Z, Chen BA, Wu Q, Xia GH, Zhang Y, Gao F, Hong TY, Xu CR, Cheng J, Li GH, Chen WJ, Liu LJ, Li XM, and Wang XM. (2009) Reversal effect of Fe3O4-magnetic nanoparticles on multi-drug resistance of ovarian carcinoma cells and its correlation with apoptosis-associated genes *J Chin J Cancer* 28, 1158-1162

Jones DP, Shan X and Park Y. (1993) Coordinated multisite regulation of cellular energy metabolism. *Annu Rev Nutr* 12, 327–343

Kaelin WG. Proline hydroxylation and gene expression. (2005) *Annu Rev Biochem* 74, 115–128

Kanehisa M, Goto S, Furumichi M, Tanabe M, and Hirakawa M. (2010) KEGG for representation and analysis of molecular networks involving diseases and drugs. *Nucleic Acids Res.* 38, D355-D360

Kaplan JH. (2002) Biochemistry of Na,K-ATPase. *Annu Rev Biochem* 71, 511–535

Karami S, Brennan P, Hung RJ, Boffetta P, Toro J, Wilson RT, Zaridze D, Navratilova M, Chatterjee N, Mates D, Janout V, Kollarova H, Bencko V, Szeszenia-Dabrowska N, Holcatova I, Moukeria A, Welch R, Chanock S, Rothman N, Chow WH, and Moore LE. (2008)Vitamin D receptor polymorphisms and renal cancer risk in Central and Eastern Europe *Journal of Toxicology and Environmental Health A* 6, 367–372

Karami S, Brennan P, Rosenberg PS, Navratilova M, Mates D, Zaridze D, Janout V, Kollarova H, Bencko V, Matveev V, Szeszenia-Dabrowska N, Holcatova I, Yeager M, Chanock S, Menashe I, Rothman N, Chow WH, Boffetta P, and Moore LE. (2009) Analysis of SNPs and haplotypes in vitamin D pathway genes and renal cancer risk. PLoS ONE 4, e7013

Karhausen J, Furuta GT, Tomaszewski JE, Johnson RS, Colgan SP, Haase VH. (2004) Epithelial hypoxia-inducible factor-1 is protective in murine experimental colitis. *J Clin Invest* 114, 1098-106

Kempf VA, Lebiedziejewski M, Alitalo K, Wälzlein JH, Ehehalt U, Fiebig J, Huber S, Schütt B, Sander CA, Müller S, Grassl G, Yazdi AS, Brehm B, and Autenrieth IB. (2005) Activation of hypoxia-inducible factor-1 in bacillary angiomatosis: evidence for a role of hypoxia-inducible factor- 1 in bacterial infections. *Circulation* 111, 1054-62

Kim J-W, Tchernyshyov I, Semenza GL, and Dang CV (2006) HIF-1-mediated expression of pyruvate dehydrogenase kinase: a metabolic switch required for cellular adaptation to hypoxia. *Cell Metab* 3, 177–185

Kong T, Eltzschig HK, Karhausen J, Colgan SP, and Shelley CS. (2004) Leukocyte adhesion during hypoxia is mediated by HIF-1-dependent induction of β2 integrin gene expression. *Proc Natl Acad Sci USA* 101, 10440–10445

Koppenol WH, Bounds PL, and Dang CV. (2011) Otto Warburg's contributions to current concepts of cancer metabolism. *Nat Rev Cancer* 11, 325-37

Koshiji M, Kageyama Y, Pete EA, Horikawa I, Barrett JC, and Huang LE. (2004) HIF-1α induces cell cycle arrest by functionally counteracting Myc. *EMBO J* 23, 1949–1956

Koumenis C, Naczki C, Koritzinsky M, Rastani S, Diehl A, Sonenberg N, Koromilas A, and Wouters BG. (2002) Regulation of protein synthesis by hypoxia via activation of the endoplasmic reticulum kinase PERK and phosphorylation of the translation initiation factor eIF2alpha. *Mol Cell Biol* 22, 7405–7416

Lindsley JE, and Rutter J. (2004) Nutrient sensing and metabolic decisions. *Comp Biochem Physiol B Biochem Mol Biol* 139, 543-59

Liu MY, Poellinger L, and Walker CL. (2003) Up-regulation of hypoxiainducible factor 2α in renal cell carcinoma associated with loss of Tsc-2 tumor suppressor gene. *Cancer Res* 63, 2675–2680

Manalo DJ, Rowan A, Lavoie T, Natarajan L, Kelly BD, Ye SQ, Garcia JG, and Semenza GL (2005) Transcriptional regulation of vascular endothelial cell responses to hypoxia by HIF-1. *Blood* 105, 659–669

Mandriota SJ, Turner KJ, Davies DR, Murray PG, Morgan NV, Sowter HM, Wykoff CC, Maher ER, Harris AL, Ratcliffe PJ, and Maxwell PH (2002) HIF activation identifies early lesions in VHL kidneys: evidence for site-specific tumor suppressor function in the nephron. *Cancer Cell* 1, 459–468

McCullough ML, Bandera EV, Moore DF, and Kushi LH. (2008) Vitamin D and calcium intake in relation to risk of endometrial cancer: a systematic review of the literature. *Prev Med* 46, 298-302

Morote-Garcia JC, Rosenberger P, Kuhlicke J, and Eltzschig HK. (2008) HIF-1-dependent repression of adenosine kinase attenuates hypoxia-induced vascular leak. *Blood* 111, 5571-80

Motomura W, Inoue M, Ohtake T, Takahashi N, Nagamine M, Tanno S, Kohgo Y, and Okumura T. (2006) Upregulation of ADRP in fatty liver in human and liver steatosis in mice fed with high fat diet. *Biochem Biophys Res Commun* 340, 1111-8

Multiple organ pathology, metabolic abnormalities and impaired homeostasis of reactive oxygen species in Epas1-/- mice. (2003) Multiple organ pathology, metabolic abnormalities and impaired homeostasis of reactive oxygen species in Epas1−/− mice. *Nat Genet* 35, 331–340

O'Rourke L, Gronning LM, Yeaman SJ, and Shepherd PR. (2002) Glucose-dependent regulation of cholesterol ester metabolism in macrophages by insulin and leptin. *J Biol Chem* 277, 42557-62

Oh SH, Woo JK, Jin Q, Kang HJ, Jeong JW, Kim KW, Hong WK, and Lee HY. (2008) Identification of novel antiangiogenic anticancer activities of deguelin targeting hypoxia-inducible factor-1a. *Int J Cancer* 122, 5–14

Orsolic N, Terzic S, Sver L, and Basic I. (2005) Honey-bee products in prevention and/or therapy of murine transplantable tumours. *J Sci Food Agri* 85, 363–70

Papandreou I, Cairns RA, Fontana L, Lim AL, and Denko NC (2006) HIF-1 mediates adaptation to hypoxia by actively downregulating mitochondrial oxygen consumption. *Cell Metab* 3, 187-197

Peng T, Golub TR, and Sabatini DM. (2002) The immunosuppressant rapamycin mimics a starvation-like signal distinct from amino acid and glucose deprivation. *Mol Cell Biol* 22, 5575-84

Rady H. (2005) Faculty of Science. Cairo University; Phytochemical and biological study of an antitumor agent of plant origin mixed withhoney on malignant human cells in vitro.

Ramanathan A, Wang C, and Schreiber SL. (2005) Perturbational profiling of a cell-line model of tumorigenesis by using metabolic measurements. *Proc Natl Acad Sci USA* 102, 5992–7

Ramos-Montoya A, Lee WN, Bassilian S, Lim S, Trebukhina RV, Kazhyna MV, Ciudad CJ, Noe V, Centelles JJ, and Cascante M. (2006) Pentose phosphate cycle oxidative and nonoxidative balance: a new vulnerable target for overcoming drug resistance in cancer. *Int J Cancer* 119, 2733–41

Ramos-Montoya A, Lee WN, Bassilian S, Lim S, Trebukhina RV, Kazhyna MV, Ciudad CJ, Noe V, Centelles JJ, and Cascante M. (2006) Pentose phosphate cycle oxidative and nonoxidative balance: a new vulnerable target for overcoming drug resistance in cancer. *Int J Cancer* 119, 2733–41

Rankin EB, Higgins DF, Walisser JA, Johnson RS, Bradfield CA, and Haase VH. (2005) Inactivation of the arylhydrocarbon receptor nuclear translocator (Arnt) suppresses von Hippel-Lindau disease-associated vascular tumors in mice. *Mol Cell Biol* 25, 3163–3172

- Raval RR, Lau KW, Tran MG, Sowter HM, Mandriota SJ, Li JL, Pugh CW, Maxwell PH, Harris AL, and Ratcliffe PJ. (2005) Contrasting properties of hypoxia-inducible factor 1 (HIF-1) and HIF-2 in von Hippel-Lindau-associated renal cell carcinoma. *Mol Cell Biol* 25, 5675–5686

Reutershan J, Vollmer I, Stark S, Wagner R, Ngamsri KC, and Eltzschig HK. (2009) Adenosine and inflammation: CD39 and CD73 are critical mediators in LPS-induced PMN trafficking into the lungs. *FASEB J* 23, 473-82

Richard DE, Berra E, and Pouyssegur J. (2000) Nonhypoxic pathway mediates the induction of hypoxia-inducible factor 1α in vascular smooth muscle cells. *J Biol Chem* 275, 26765–26771

Richardson CJ, Schalm SS, and Blenis J. (2004) PI3-kinase and TOR: PIKTORing cell growth. *Semin Cell Dev Biol* 15, 147-59

Robinson A, Keely S, Karhausen J, Gerich ME, Furuta GT, and Colgan SP. (2008) Mucosal protection by hypoxia-inducible factor prolyl hydroxylase inhibition. *Gastroenterology* 134, 145-55

Rosenberger C, Mandriota S, Jurgensen JS, Wiesener MS, Horstrup JH, Frei U, Ratcliffe PJ, Maxwell PH, Bachmann S, and Eckardt KU. (2002) Expression of hypoxia-inducible factor-1α and -2α in hypoxic and ischemic rat kidneys. *J Am Soc Nephrol* 13, 1721–1732

Rosenberger P, Schwab JM, Mirakaj V, Masekowsky E, Mager A, Morote-Garcia JC, Unertl K, and Eltzschig HK. (2009) Hypoxia-inducible factor-dependent induction of netrin-1 dampens inflammation caused by hypoxia. *Nat Immunol* 10, 195-202

Ryan HE, Lo J, and Johnson RS (1998) HIF-1 alpha is required for solid tumor formation and embryonic vascularization. *EMBO J* 17, 3005–3015

Sandau KB, Zhou J, Kietzmann T, and Brune B. (2001) Regulation of the hypoxia-inducible factor 1α by the inflammatory mediators nitric oxide and tumor necrosis factor-α in contrast to desferroxamine and phenylarsine oxide. *J Biol Chem* 276, 39805–39811

Schingnitz U, Hartmann K, Macmanus CF, Eckle T, Zug S, Colgan SP, Eltzschig HK. (2010) Signaling through the A2B adenosine receptor dampens endotoxininduced acute lung injury. *J Immunol* 184, 5271-9

Schofield CJ and Ratcliffe PJ. (2004) Oxygen sensing by HIF hydroxylases. *Nat Rev Mol Cell Biol* 5, 343–354

Semenza GL. (2003) Targeting HIF-1 for cancer therapy. *Nat Rev Cancer* 3, 721-32

Skou JC. (1957) The influence of some cations on an adenosine triphosphatase from peripheral nerves. *Biochim Biophys Acta* 23, 394–401

Smith K, Gunaratnam L, Morley M, Franovic A, Mekhail K, and Lee S. (2005) Silencing of epidermal growth factor receptor suppresses hypoxiainducible factor-2-driven VHL-/- renal cancer. *Cancer Res* 65: 5221–5230

Soilleux EJ, Turley H, Tian YM, Pugh CW, Gatter KC, and Harris AL. (2005) Use of novel monoclonal antibodies to determine the expression and distribution of the hypoxia regulatory factors PHD-1, PHD-2, PHD-3 and FIH in normal and neoplastic human tissues. *Histopathology* 47, 602–610

Staller P, Sulitkova J, Lisztwan J, Moch H, Oakeley EJ, and Krek W. (2003) Chemokine receptor CXCR4 downregulated by von Hippel-Lindau tumour suppressor pVHL. *Nature* 425, 307–311

The Word Cancer Resarch Fund, June 2009, http://www.wcrf-uk.org/preventing cancer/index.php.

Thibault F, Cancel-Tassin G, and Cussenot O. (2006) Low penetrance genetic susceptibility to kidney cancer *BJU International* 98, 735–738

Treins C, Giorgetti-Peraldi S, Murdaca J, Semenza GL, and Van Obberghen E. (2002) Insulin stimulates hypoxia-inducible factor 1 through a phosphatidylinositol 3-kinase/target of rapamycin-dependent signalling pathway. *J Biol Chem* 277: 27975–27981

Valdivielso JM and Fernandez E. (2006) Vitamin D receptor polymorphisms and diseases *Clinica Chimica Acta* 371, 1–12

Walenta S, and Mueller-Klieser WF. (2004) Lactate: mirror and motor of tumor malignancy. *Semin Radiat Oncol* 14, 267–74

Warburg O, Posener K, and Negelein E. (1924) Über den Stoffwechsel der Carcinomcelle. *Biochem* 152, 309–44

Weiss G, Meusburger E, Radacher G, Garimorth K, Neyer U, and Mayer G. (2003) Effect of iron treatment on circulating cytokine levels in ESRD patients receiving recombinant human erythropoietin. *Kidney International* 64, 572–578

Wouters BG, van den Beucken T, Magagnin MG, Koritzinsky M, Fels D, and Koumenis C. (2005) Control of the hypoxic response through regulation of mRNA translation. *Semin Cell Dev Biol* 16, 487–501

Wykoff CC, Sotiriou C, Cockman ME, Ratcliffe PJ, Maxwell P, Liu E, and Harris AL. (2004) Gene array of VHL mutation and hypoxia shows novel hypoxia-induced genes and that cyclin D1 is a VHL target gene. *Br J Cancer* 90, 1235–1243

Zatyka M, da Silva NF, Clifford SC, Morris MR, Wiesener MS, Eckardt KU, Houlston RS, Richards FM, Latif F, and Maher ER. (2002) Identification of cyclin D1 and other novel targets for the von Hippel-Lindau tumor suppressor gene by expression array analysis and investigation of cyclin D1 genotype as a modifier in von Hippel-Lindau disease. *Cancer Res* 62, 3803–3811

9

Immunotherapy of Renal Cell Carcinoma – From Antigen Identification to Patient Treatment

Heiko Schuster[1], Mathias Walzer[1,2] and Stefan Stevanović[1]
[1]Department of Immunology, Institute for Cell Biology, University of Tübingen
[2]Applied Bioinformatics Group, Center for Bioinformatics, University of Tübingen
Germany

1. Introduction

Renal cell carcinoma (RCC) ist the 3rd most common urologic cancer leading to an estimated 271 000 new cancer cases worldwide each year (Ferlay *et al.* 2010). RCC is generally associated with poor prognosis because of late diagnosis and bad responsiveness to classical radio- and chemotherapy. For a long period of time immunotherapy with IL-2 or Interferon alpha (IFNα) have been the only therapeutic options to treat advanced stage RCCs. In recent years targeted therapy with tyrosine kinase inhibitors (TKIs; Sunitinib, Sorafenib) or mTor inhibitors (Everolimus, Temsirolimus) has replaced cytokine based immunotherapy as a first line treatment in the management of metastatic RCCs (mRCC). IFNα is nevertheless still playing an important role in the treatment of mRCC not as a monotherapy, but rather in combination with the antibody Bevacizumab which is directed against proangiogenic vascular endothelial growth factor (VEGF).

Despite these recent improvements resistance to this new class of drugs frequently occurs and curative treatment of RCC is still only possible by surgical resection of the tumor mass at an early non-metastatic stage (Rini & Atkins 2009). A lot of effort has therefore been put into the development of a targeted immunotherapeutic approach that aims at the *in vivo* induction or reinforcement of an anti tumor immune response.

2. Cancer immunotherapy in the course of history

The underlying idea that the immune system is able to recognise and kill transformed cells is actually not new (Parish 2003). As early as the 19th century William Coley and others noticed that cancer patients suffering from a bacterial infection sometimes experienced tumor regression. William Coley was also the first to translate this observation into clinical practice by treating cancer patients with a bacterial preparation of Streptococcus pyogenes known as Coley's toxin (Coley 1893). In 1909 Paul Ehrlich evaluated the role of the immune system in tumor control and suggested that without the immune system cancers would occur in much higher frequency (Ehrlich 1909). Unfortunately it took more than half a century before Ehrlich's idea regained attention. First experimental evidence during the 1950s could show that syngenic animals could be immunized against transplantable tumors. In the early 1960s Lewis Thomas argued that long-lived organisms must have developed mechanisms that resemble homograft rejection in order to counter neoplastic diseases

(Lawrence 1959). Based on Thomas' views Frank M. Burnet formulated in 1967 his revolutionary „Immunosurveillance Theory" in which he stated that immune cells were constantly surveying host tissues for the presence of transformed cells that could be recognized by neo-antigens acquired during the transformation process (Burnet 1967). However Burnet's idea remained controversial simply because many people could not believe that the immune system could properly differentiate between healthy tissue and transformed cancer cells. Experiments with athymic nude mice also argued against Burnets idea (Stutman 1979). Despite their supposed lack of mature T cells (which was later shown to be not completely true (Maleckar & Sherman 1987)) these mice had no higher incidence in tumor development as originally predicted by Ehrlich. Since the late 80s, more and more evidence accumulated that revived the immunosurveillance theory. The discovery of tumor associated antigens (TAA) in mice and humans as well as the observation that truly immunodeficient knockout mice (*e.g.* RAG2$^{-/-}$, STAT1$^{-/-}$) really showed a higher incidence in cancer development finally proved Burnets idea.

3. Immunotherapeutical studies in RCC

RCC, along with melanoma, are considered to be the most immunogenic tumor in humans. This is based on the occurence of spontaneous regressions even in metastatic disease (Lokich 1997), the high amount of lymphocytic infiltrates found in tumor tissue (Van den Hove *et al.* 1997) and the comparably good response to nonspecific immunotherapy with cytokines like IL-2 or IFNα, at least in some part of the patients (10-20%) (Negrier *et al.* 1998). First clinical trials using a specific immunotherapy for RCC were therefore conducted during the mid - 90s already. Table 1 provides a comprehensive summary of published results regarding anti-tumor vaccination approaches from that time until today. Many different strategies involving lysate from autologous tumor tissue, allogenic tumor cell lines, whole tumor cell RNA as well as defined antigens (*e.g.* peptides derived from TAAs CAIX or MUC1) have been used. In most cases these antigens were applied in combination with an adjuvant (*e.g.* GM-CSF, BCG or incomplete Freunds adjuvant) or after loading onto dendritic cells (DCs) usually from the same patient. Dendritic cells are professional antigen presenting cells that have the capacity to take up tumor derived products spontaneously (in some trials also inforced by electrofusion with tumor cells) and to present antigen derived peptides *via* HLA class I and II molecules to cytotoxic- and also T helper cells. In most trials dendritic cells were generated from autologous peripheral blood derived monocytes or CD34^{+} bone marrow cells that can both develop *ex vivo* into immature dendritic cells (iDCs). More recent studies almost uniformly apply a cytokine maturation step to generate mature dendritic cells (mDCs) as iDCs have been shown to posess tolerogenic rather than immune stimulatory functionality (Figdor *et al.* 2004). Keyhole limpet hemocyanin has been also applied in many trials as an immunostimulant because it was previously shown to improve dendritic cell based vaccinations by inducing a potent CD4^{+} T helper cell response at least in mouse models (Shimizu *et al.* 2001). Other approaches to enhance the immunogenicity of the vaccine have been tried by virally transducing autologous tumor cells and allogenic cell lines with cytokines (GM-CSF, IL2) or T-cell costimulatory molecule CD80 (B7.1).

Vaccination with all these different approaches has proven to be well tolerated and side effects have been rare and were usually limited to allergic reactions at the site of injection as well as induration or erythema. In trials in which additional cytokine treatment (IL-2, IFNα) was employed, further side effects like fatigue, fever, vomiting and hypotension could be observed.

In some cases systemic application of high dose cytokines can however also lead to serious and life-threatening side effects. These symptoms have been known for a long time to also occur under cytokine monotherapy and are therefore not directly associated with the vaccine.

Author	Setting	Antigen	Adjuvant	N*	Results
Inactivated tumor cells and gene modified tumor vaccines:					
(Galligioni *et al.* 1996)	Adjuvant after nephrectomy	Autol. Irradiated tumor cells	BCG	60 (60)	5-year DFS 63% vs. control 72%; 5-year OS 69% vs. control 78%
(Simons & Mikhak 1998)	mRCC	Autol. Irradiated tumor cells transduced with GM-CSF	None	16	1 PR
(Schwaab *et al.* 2000)	metastatic RCC	Autol. Irradiated tumor cells	BCG IFNg+ IFNa	14	3 MR, 5 SD, 1 PD
Dillman(Dillman *et al.* 2004)	8 primary RCC, 17 mRCC	Autol. Irradiated tumor cells	BCG, GM-CSF, IFNa, IFNg, IL2, CP	25	median PFS 2.4 months, median OS 10,2 months
(Jocham *et al.* 2004)	Adjuvant after nephrectomy	Autol. tumor lysate vaccine (Reniale)	None	177 (202)	5 year PFS 77.4% vs control 67.8%
(Dudek *et al.* 2008)	stage IV RCC	Autol. large multivalent immunogen vaccine	none, CP, IL-2 + CP	31	median PFS 12.2, 1 PR, 12 SD
(May *et al.* 2009)	Adjuvant after nephrectomy	Autol. tumor lysate vaccine (Reniale)	None	495 (495)	5-year OS 80.6% vs. control 79,2%, 10-year OS 79,2% vs. control 62,1%
(Antonia *et al.* 2002)	mRCC	Autol. Irradiated tumor cells transduced with B7-1	IL-2	15	2 PR, 2SD
(Tani *et al.* 2004)	stage IV RCC	Autol. Irradiated tumor cells transduced with GM-CSF	none, low dose IL-2	4	1 SD, 1MR
(Pizza *et al.* 2004)	mRCC	Autol. fixed tumor cells + allog. ACHN cell line transduced with IL-2	None	30 (131)	1 CR, 4 PR, 9 SD
(Moiseyenko *et al.* 2005)	mRCC after cytoreductive surgery	Autol. Irradiated tumor cells transfected with tag7/PGRP-S	None	4	1 SD
(Fishman *et al.* 2008)	stage IV RCC	Autol. Irradiated tumor cells transduced with B7-1	IL-2	39	1 CR, 24 SD
(Buchner *et al.* 2010)	mRCC	Allog.RCC-26 tumor cell line transduced with CD80 and IL 2	None	15	median PFS 5.3 months, median OS 15.6 months
Peptide based vaccines					
Authors	**Setting**	**Antigen**	**Adjuvant**	**N***	**Results**
(Uemura *et al.* 2006)	mRCC, HLA-A*24 pos.	CA9 derived peptides (p219-227, p288-296, p323-331)	IFA	23	3 PR, 6SD, median OS 21 months
(Iiyama *et al.* 2007)	mRCC, HLA-A*24 pos.	WT1 anchor modified peptide	IFA	3	2 SD
(Suekane *et al.* 2007)	mRCC, HLA-A*24 pos or HLA-A*2 pos.	Personalized cocktail of 4 peptides based on presence of Anti Peptide IgG or CTLs	IFA	10	6 SD
(Wood *et al.* 2008)	Adjuvant after nephrectomy	Autol. tumor derived heat-shock protein-peptide complex (Vitespen)	None	367 (361)	No difference in RFS
(Jonasch *et al.* 2008)	mRCC	Autol. tumor derived heat-shock protein-peptide complex (Vitespen)	None, IL2	60	2 CR, 2PR, 7SD
(Reinhardt *et al.* 2010)	mRCC, HLA-A*02 pos.	IMA901, 9 HLA-A*02 + 1 panDR restricted peptides	GMCSF, single dose CP before vaccination	64	OS after 18 months 63% and 80% with CP pretreament

Dendritic cell based vaccines					
Authors	**Setting**	**DC + Antigen**	**Adjuvant/ Additional Treatment**	**N***	**Results**
(Oosterwijk-Wakka *et al.* 2002)	mRCC	Autol. iDCs loaded with autol. tumor cell lysate	IL-2;/ DC pulsed with KLH,none	12	8 SD
(Marten *et al.* 2002)	mRCC	Autol. mDCs loaded with autol. tumor cell lysate	none;/ DC pulsed with KLH, none	15	1 PR, 7 SD
(Holtl *et al.* 2002)	mRCC	Autol. mDCs loaded with autol. tumor cell lysate or allog. A498 cell line lysate	none / DC pulsed with KLH	35	2 CR, 1 PR, 7 SD
(Azuma *et al.* 2002)	mRCC	Autol. iDCs loaded with autol. tumor cell lysate	none / DC pulsed with KLH	3	1 SD
(Marten *et al.* 2003)	mRCC	Allog. mDCs fused with autol. tumor cells	None	12	4 SD
(Marten *et al.* 2006)	mRCC, HLA matched	Autol. mDCs loaded with a telomerase derived peptide	none; DC pulsed with KLH	10	1 MR, 1 SD
(Gitlitz *et al.* 2003)	mRCC	Autol. iDCs loaded with autol. tumor cell lysate	None	12	1 PR, 3 SD
(Barbuto *et al.* 2004)	mRCC	Allog. mDCs fused with autol. tumor derived cells	None	19	3 OR, 14 SD
(Avigan *et al.* 2007)	stage IV RCC	Allog. mDCs fused with autol. tumor derived cells	None	20	2 PR, 8 SD
(Avigan *et al.* 2004)	mRCC	Allog. iDCs fused with autol. tumor derived cells	DC pulsed with KLH	13	5 SD
(Pandha *et al.* 2004)	mRCC	Autol. iDCs loaded with allog. lysate of tumor cell line JM-RCC	KLH	5	2 SD
(Arroyo *et al.* 2004)	mRCC	Autol. mDCs loaded with autol. tumor cell lysate	DC pulsed with KLH	5	3 SD
(Dannull *et al.* 2005)	mRCC	Autol. mDCs transfected with whole tumor RNA	Pretreatment with ONTAK (Treg depletion)	11	not evaluated
(Holtl *et al.* 2005)	mRCC	Allog. mDCs laded with autol. tumor cell lysate	none/ Cyclophosphamide; DC pulsed with KLH	20	2 MR, 3 SD
(Wierecky *et al.* 2006)	mRCC HLA-A*02	Autol. mDCs loaded with two HLA-A*02 MUC1 peptides	pan DR-peptide PADRE, IL-2 (post vaccination period)	20	1 CR, 2 PR, 2 MR, 5 SD
(Bleumer *et al.* 2007)	metastatic ccRCC HLA-A*02	Autol. mDCs loaded with an HLA-A*02 and HLA-DR restricted CA9 derived peptide	DC pulsed with KLH	6	all PD
(Wei *et al.* 2007)	mRCC	Autol. mDCs fused with autol. tumor derived cells (Dendritomas)	IL-2	10	1 PR, 3 SD
(Matsumoto *et al.* 2007)	mRCC	Autol. mDCs loaded with autol. Primary tumor derived cell lysate	DC pulsed with KLH	3	1 SD
(Kim *et al.* 2007)	mRCC	Autol. mDCs loaded with autol. Primary tumor derived cell lysate	DC pulsed with KLH	9	1 PR, 5 SD
(Berntsen *et al.* 2008)	mRCC, HLA-A*02 pos or neg	Autol. mDCs loaded with allog. cell line lysate (A*02 neg) or a mix of 9 different hTERT and 11 Survivin derived peptides (A*02 pos)	IL-2, pan DR-peptide PADRE, DC pulsed with KLH (only A*02 neg)	27	13 SD
(Tatsugami *et al.* 2008)	mRCC	Autol. mDCs loaded with autol. Primary tumor derived cell lysate	IFNa	7	5 SD
(Schwaab *et al.* 2009)	mRCC	Autol. mDCs loaded with autol. Primary tumor derived cell lysate	IL-2 and IFNa	18	3 CR, 6 PR, 6 SD

*Number of patients treated versus number of patients in control group in brackets. mRCC: metastatic renal cell carcinoma, ccRCC: clear cell renal cell carcinoma, autol.: autologous, allog.: allogenic, mDC: mature dendritic cells, iDC: immature dendritic cells, BCG: Bacille Calmette Guerin, IFA: Incomplete Freunds adjuvant CP: Cyclophosphamide, CR: complete response, PR: partial response, MR: mixed response, OR: objective response, SD: stable disease, PD: progressive disease, OS.: overall survival RFS.: regression free survival, PFS: progression free survival, DFS: disease free survival.

Table 1. Immunotherapeutical studies in RCC

Apart from the tumor vaccination studies mentioned above other approaches involving the transfer of leukocytes such as adoptive T-cell transfer and even stem cell transplantation have been applied in some cases. Allogenic stem cell transplantation has been used succesfully for several decades in hematological cancers. Lymphocytes, in particular T-cells of HLA identical donors, are thought to exert a graft-vs-leukaemia effect mainly by recognition of minor histocompatibility antigens on recipient tissues (Bleakley & Riddell 2004) but probably also tumor cell specific antigens (Tykodi *et al.* 2004). The curative or graft-vs-leukaemia effect (GvL) therefore often directly correlates with the appearance of graft vs host disease (GvHD). The use of stem cell transplantation in solid tumors has been shown to provide a similiar graft-vs-tumor (GvT) effect in renal cell carcinoma, but also in ovarian (Bay *et al.* 2002) and breast cancer patients (Bishop *et al.* 2004). In the context of solid tumors non-myeloablative regimens have been preferred to avoid the substantial side effects of myeloablation with high dose chemotherapy and irradiation. Engraftment thus does not lead to complete substitution of the host's immune system but rather to a chimeric state incorperationg both the recipient's and the donor's hematological system. First studies of non-myeloablative allogenic stem cell transplantation (NST) in 17 mRCC patients showed quite promising results (Childs *et al.* 2000) with partial regression in over 50% including three patients with prolonged complete response. Further studies have been conducted (for a comprehensive overview see (Demirer *et al.* 2008)) with small patient numbers and varying response rates ranging from 0% (Rini *et al.* 2006) to more than 50% (Bregni *et al.* 2002) . However, NST is also facing several other difficulties. Besides the need for an HLA matched donor, severe and sometimes fatal complications from transplantation and subsequent GvHD can occur. Furthermore the time from treatment to response can take several months and in order to avoid graft rejection, patients have to be kept in an immunosuppressive state which allows for and might even accelerate rapid disease progression.

Adoptive T cell transfer in RCC has played a rather minor role compared to trials in other immunogenic tumors, especially in melanoma. Initial studies with isolated and *ex vivo* expanded tumor infiltrating lymphocytes (TILs) that have been reinfused into the patient usually in combination with IL-2, showed only modest response (Topalian *et al.* 1988; Kradin *et al.* 1989). In a larger phase III trial involving 160 patients with metastatic RCC, treatment with *ex vivo* expanded TILs and IL-2 showed no benefit compared to IL-2 alone (Figlin *et al.* 1999). Because of these disappointing results and because of the lack of tumor specific T-cell epitopes further use of (antigen specific) adoptive T-cell transfer has been limited although recently the usage of gammadelta T cells in RCC patients has moved into the focus of ongoing research (Bennouna *et al.* 2008; Kobayashi *et al.* 2010). In order to complete the picture of current immunotherapeutic approaches, WX-G250 (Girentuximab) has to be mentioned. This is an antibody developed by Wilex that is specifically intended for adjuvant use in non-metastatic RCC patients and is currently undergoing Phase III clinical trials (Reichert 2011). The chimeric IgG1 antibody is directed against Carbonic anhydrase 9, which is a tumor associated antigen expressed by more than 90% of clear cell renal cell carcinoma. Data from a recent Phase I/II trial of Girentuximab in combination with IFNα for metastatic RCC patients have shown good tolerability, safety and also clinical benefit (Siebels *et al.* 2011).

Considering the diversity of different immunotherapeutic approaches, especially in tumor vaccination, the question remains why many of these studies failed or showed rather limited clinical success, with only a few trials progressing to clinical phase III. In order to answer this question we will first look at the main problem of all immunotherapeutic approaches, namely the ability of a tumor to escape a directed immune response by inducing an immunosuppresive environment. In this context we will also discuss methodological deficiencies and contradictions that have contributed to clinical failure and describe more promising directions for future immunotherapy.

4. Immunosuppression and tumor escape

As mentioned above, renal cell carcinomas, like other tumors, are highly infiltrated by leukocytes and especially T cells (> 60%) mainly of the $CD8^+$ rather than the $CD4^+$ phenotype. Natural killer cells have also been found to be enriched within the TIL population in some studies at least whereas B cells make up only a minor subset. (Van den Hove, Van Gool et al. 1997). Infiltrating T cells are predominantly of the antigen experienced effector memory type (T_{EM}), and $CD8^+$ cells also encompass highly differentiated T_{EMRA} effector cells (Attig *et al.* 2009). Expression of several lymphocyte activation markers such as CD69 or HLA-DR on TILs has been confirmed and oligoclonal expansion of certain TCR-Vβ regions indicates that a selection of potentially tumor specific T cells has taken place (Angevin *et al.* 1997). Furthermore, after isolation and ex vivo culture T cells are able to express cytokines and show normal cytotoxic activity. However if these TILs show functionality *ex vivo* then why are they not reactive within the tumor microenvironment? Indeed, freshly isolated uncultured TILs often show a reduced capacity of their cytotoxic function (Van den Hove, Van Gool et al. 1997) and also an impaired cytokine production or altered cytokine profile, demonstrating that some kind of immunosuppressive milieu must be present within the tumor microenvironment (Gouttefangeas *et al.* 2007). Defects in T-cell signalling and downregulation of the CD3 ζ-chain, which is necessary for TCR signal transduction into the cell, can be frequently found in T cells isolated from RCC patients (Frey & Monu 2008). Several mechanisms responsible for this locoregional immunosuppression have been discovered within the last decades and only the most important findings will be described here. Some of these mechanisms, such as the activation of T regulatory cells (T_{regs}), have been intentionally developed by evolution to counteract deleterious long term activation of an immune response in order to avoid autoimmune diseases. Others, such as the generation of inhibitory signals have been developed or rather selected within the heterogeneity of tumor cells to escape an existing immune response and thereby provide a selection advantage. Among the latter are immunosuppressive cytokines IL-10 or TGF-β, which are known to inhibit T-cell activation as well as proliferation and can also lead to downregulation of MHC class I molecules (Khong & Restifo 2002; Li *et al.* 2006). In renal cell carcinoma, proangiogenic vascular endothelial growth factor (VEGF), which acts also immunosuppressively by inhibiting DC maturation (Ohm & Carbone 2001) plays a major role because it is usually found highly overexpressed in clear cell RCCs (Rini 2005). Apart from the expression of immunosuppressive factors, tumor cells can also downregulate costimulatory molecules from their surface. Despite the fact that tumor cells are not professional APCs and therefore not supposed to prime T cells, the complete lack of costimulatory molecules such as CD80 (B7.1) or CD86 (B7.2) can lead to a decreased T-cell activation or even induction of T-cell anergy (Jung *et al.* 1999; Lang *et al.* 2000). In this context another B7 family member should be mentioned which, in contrast to the aforementioned, is often found highly upregulated in different types of cancer. B7-H1

(PDL1) is usually expressed on macrophages and provides costimulatiory function for T cells. However, due to its high abundance on tumor cells it has a predominantly negative regulatory activity. After binding to its receptor PD1 on activated T cells B7-H1 can downmodulate T cell activation and even induce apoptosis (Dong *et al.* 2002). B7-H1, and more recently another associate of the B7 family with a similiar function, B7-H4, have been shown to be expressed in RCC patients and their expression correlated with adverse clinical prognosis (Thompson *et al.* 2005).

In order to escape an already existing specific immune response, cancer cells can either escape by downregulating the antigen or even parts of the HLA presentation machinery. Indeed downregulation of HLA expression can be observed in several cancer types preferentially in late metastasized stages (Marincola *et al.* 2000; Campoli *et al.* 2002). Different mechanisms underlying this process of downregulation or even complete loss of HLA expression have been elucidated from several tumor cell lines and seem to affect nearly all parts of the antigen processing machinery (Seliger *et al.* 2002). To which extent HLA downregulation or loss plays a role in RCC is still controversial. Whereas some publications suggest that HLA downregulation is a frequent event (Romero *et al.* 2006) other more recent data could clearly show that HLA-expression is not diminished but rather upregulated in comparison to benign kidney tissue (Saenz-Lopez *et al.* 2010; Stickel *et al.* 2011).

Tumor cells can also indirectly inhibit an immune response by depriving proliferating immune cells of essential nutrients. Indoleamine-2,3-dioxygenase (IDO) is an enzyme that catalyzes the first and also rate-limiting step in the degradation of the essential amino acid tryptophane. IDO has been found to be nearly ubiquitously expressed in human tumors (Uyttenhove *et al.* 2003). By locally depleting tryptophane, IDO can inhibit the proliferation of TILs and also induce or recruit T_{regs} (Prendergast *et al.* 2009).

$CD4^{+}$ $CD25^{high}$ $FoxP3^{+}$ regulatory T cells have become a major field of investigation in immunotherapy because of their potential to induce tolerance by suppressing (tumor) antigen specific priming of T cells and also T cell effector functions (Zou 2006). T_{regs} are known to accumulate within the microenvironment of different tumors (Woo *et al.* 2001) and higher levels of T_{regs} in the peripheral blood of cancer patients have been detected. In RCC patients a higher frequency of T_{regs} within the tumor and periphery have been described and correlate with an adverse clinical outcome (Liotta *et al.* 2011). A plethora of different mechanisms have been described on how T_{regs} exert their immunosuppressive functions that range from the expression of immunosuppressive cytokines (IL 10, TGFβ)(Taylor *et al.* 2006), induction of IDO and B7-H4 in APCs (Fallarino *et al.* 2003; Sica *et al.* 2003), and consumption of IL-2 (von Boehmer 2005) to direct cell mediated cytotoxicity (Grossman *et al.* 2004). Antigen specific T_{regs} have been described (Wang *et al.* 2004) but after activation, the suppressive activity of CD4+ T_{regs} seems to be antigen non-specific affecting T cells of varying specificity (Thornton & Shevach 2000). Another type of immunosuppresive cells are the myeloid derived suppressor cells (MDSCs) which have recently acquired increasing attention (Kusmartsev & Vieweg 2009). MDSCs are a heterogeneous population of progenitor cells of the myeloid lineage. Under healthy conditions these cells rapidly differentiate into mature granulocytes, macrophages and also dendritic cells. However, in patients suffering from different types of cancer that include RCC (Rodriguez *et al.* 2009), these immature cells have been shown to strongly accumulate in peripheral blood and also

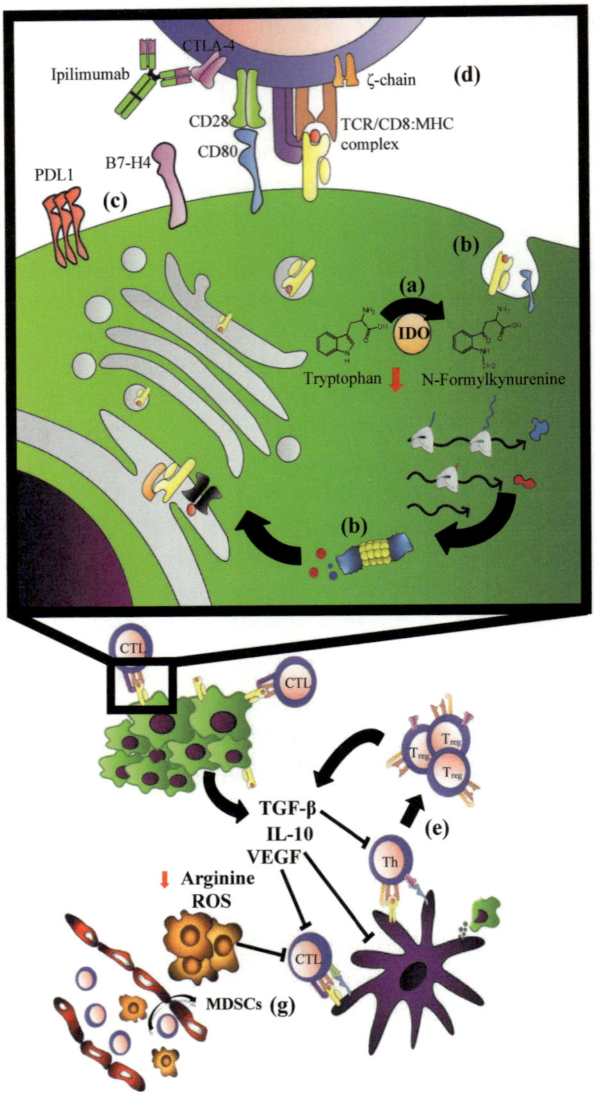

Fig. 1. Immunosuppressive Mechanisms: (a) Overexpression of Indoleamin-2.3-dioxyngenase (IDO) leads to reduced extracellular tryptophan levels thereby inhibiting T cell proliferation. (b) Defects in antigen presentation machinery or downregulation of MHC molecules prevent recognition by cytotoxic lymphocytes (CTLs). (c) Aberrant expression of PDL1 or upregulation of coinhibitory molecules B7-H4 decrease costimulation. (d) Downregulation of T-cell receptor (TCR) ζ-chain inhibits intracellular signalling. (e) Secretion of immunosuppressive cytokines by tumor cells or regulatory T cells (T_{regs}) inhibits activation of T cells (IL-10, TGF-β) and dendritic cells (VEGF). In addition induction of Tregs (f) from the CD4+ T helper cell (Th) population is inceased. (g) Infiltration of myeloid derived suppressor cells (MDSCs) from the blood lead to production of reactive oxygen species (ROS)) and enhanced arginine catabolism through arginase and iNOS thereby further hampering T cell proliferation.

within the tumor microenvironment (Young *et al.* 1997; Nagaraj & Gabrilovich 2010) where they exert potent immunosuppressive effects. Myeloid suppressor cells seem to highly express two enzymes involved in the arginine metabolism: Arginase and inducible nitric oxid synthase (iNOS). These enzymes drive the enhanced catabolism of arginine which subsequently leads to an arginine depletion from the tumor microenvironment thereby strongly inhibiting T-cell proliferation (Ochoa *et al.* 2007; Gabrilovich & Nagaraj 2009). Higher arginase activity in PBMCs from RCC patients could indeed be demonstrated (Zea *et al.* 2005). Other mechanisms of MDSC mediated immunosuppression, such as the production of reactive oxygen species (ROS) *e.g.* peroxynitrite (Kusmartsev *et al.* 2004), the secretion of immunosuppressive cytokine TGF-β (Filipazzi *et al.* 2007) and the induction of other immune suppressive cells such as T_{regs} (Serafini *et al.* 2008) could also be observed.

Despite all these different immunosuppressive cells and the mechanisms discussed (see Figure 1), the infiltration of cancer tissue by leukocytes still remains a reliable marker for patient outcome and correlates positively with clinical prognosis in RCC patients (Pages *et al.* 2010). Galon et. al have shown that the presence and composition of the immunological infiltrate is highly predictive for clinical outcome in colon cancer patients and can even be superior to classical TNM staging (Galon *et al.* 2006).

5. Counteracting immunosuppression

In view of all these sophisticated immunosuppresive mechanisms there are doubts that we will ever be able to overcome immunosuppression and tumor escape. In order to generate a long lasting immune response which keeps the immune system up and running, tumor associated antigens ant T-cell epitopes represent only a part of the whole picture. Adjuvants are therefore urgently needed to specifically address this difficult task. Adjuvants or„Immunologist's dirty little secrets" as Janeway termed them (Janeway 1989) are an active component of most protective vaccines against infectious diseases particularly intended to enhance or modulate a specific immune response. Most of the adjuvants approved for human treatment (Alumn, MPL) were actually developed for passive vaccination of healthy patients against infectious diseases - a setting in which an enormously high safety profile of the adjuvant is clearly necessary. However, considering the highly immunosuppressive environment of late stage tumors in particular, the need for stronger immunostimulatory adjuvants has emerged even if they reduce safety and bear the risk of provoking autoimmunity. In the majority of trials involving RCC patients (Table 1) cytokines such as GM-CSF, IL-2 or IFNα have been used to ensure effective priming of T cells and enhance the immune response. Regardless of toxicity problems considering the systemic application of IL-2 and Interferon α, new studies could show that IL-2 also leads to the induction and stimulation of regulatory T cells (Brandenburg *et al.* 2008). Similarly GM-CSF has been shown to stimulate the recruitment of myeloid derived suppressor cells (Serafini *et al.* 2004) and its beneficial effect in cancer vaccination has been challenged by two randomized vaccination trials in melanoma in which patients that additionally received GM-CSF had an inferior immunologic and patient outcome (Faries *et al.* 2009; Slingluff *et al.* 2009). The use of incomplete Freund's adjuvant and BCG as adjuvants in cancer immunotherapy appears rather outdated. Nevertheless, BCG is still approved for the treatment of superficial bladder cancer. Metabolizable squalene based emulsions (MF59, AF03) and saponins (Quil-A, ISCOM, QS-2) have replaced mineral oil based formulations like Freunds adjuvant. The use of live-attenuated bacteria like BCG has been discontinued in favor of molecularly defined

TLR agonists. The discovery that toll like receptors (TLRs) constitute part of the innate immune system and can act as pattern recognition receptors (PRRs) for different pathogen associated molecular patterns (PAMPs) has boosted the search for agonistic TLR ligands. Synthetic TLR ligands can, as their natural counterparts, bind to TLRs on different cell types and subsequently lead to the activation of the cell (*e.g.* maturation, release of proinflammatory cytokines, enhanced antigen presentation or effector function). In theory a combination of different TLR agonists can be used to tailor an immune response to fit individual needs (Adams 2009). For example, TLRs 3, 7/8 and 9 have been shown to lead to the preferential activation of a Th1 response which has been known for a long time to be a prognostic factor in cancer immunotherapy correlating with favourable outcome. Several of these synthetic TLR agonists such as PolyI:C (TLR3 agonist), Resimiquimod (TLR7/8 agonist) and CpG (TLR9 agonist) are currently being evaluated in clinical trials (Adams *et al.* 2008; Cheever 2008).

Only very few studies in RCC patients have attempted to address the specific requirements needed to overcome immune escape. Some groups have used cyclophosphamide prior to or during vaccination because it is known that low doses of this chemotherapeutic drug lead to improved immune responses potentially by depleting T_{regs}. (Ghiringhelli *et al.* 2004; Lutsiak *et al.* 2005). Denileukin (Diftitox, Ontak), a recombinant fusion protein of IL-2 and diphtheria toxin has been also used successfully for the same purpose (Atchison *et al.* 2010). However some studies have described severe side effects in conjunction with Denileukin like vision loss and vascular leak syndrome (Park *et al.* 2007; Avarbock *et al.* 2008), treatment failure has also been reported (Welters *et al.* 2009). Recent studies are suggesting that pretreatment with less toxic Sunitinib might have a similar effect on regulatory T cells (Finke *et al.* 2008).

The most promising agents that are currently being developed to overcome tumor induced immunosuppression are immune modulating antibodies that inhibit immune checkpoint controls (Fife & Bluestone 2008). The first antibody with this mode of action (Ipilimumab) has just recently been approved by regulatory authorities in the US and Europe as a monotherapy for the treatment of late stage melanoma. Ipilimumab is directed against cytotoxic T-lymphocyte antigen 4 (CTLA-4), a negative immunoregulatory receptor expressed by activated T cells, in particular T_{regs}. CTLA-4 binds to costimulatory molecules (*e.g.* CD80, CD86) on APCs or tumor cells and thereby directly competes with T cell coactivating molecule CD28. However whereas signalling through CD28 is leads to T cell activation CTLA-4 signalling is rather inhibitory and promotes T cell tolerization and anergy. Blocking of CTLA-4 by Ipilimumab consequently leads to an increase in T-cell activating signals resulting in a greatly sustained activation of an immune repsonse. Considering its unspecific mechanism of action it is not surprising that among the different side effects experienced after treatment with Ipilimumab, the induction of autoimmune phenomena was also quite frequent. Nevertheless, in most cases the treatment with corticosteroids was effective and did not interfere with clinical benefit.

Based on this very recent breakthrough, several trials are currently evaluating combinations of Ipilimumab with targeted immunotherapeutic approaches in order to highlight the direction to activated T cells. Another immunomodulating antibody directed against PD1 (MDX-1106) is currently being applied in late phase clinical trials. Interaction of PD1 with its ligand B7-H1, which is broadly overexpressed on tumor cells has already been discussed as an established tumor escape mechanism.

The advent of new immunotherapies has also clearly revealed another problem regarding the kinetics and study endpoints of clinical immunotherapeutic trials (Hoos *et al.* 2010). Evaluation of clinical benefit is usually based on world health organization (WHO) (World Health Organization. 1979) or response evaluation criteria in solid tumors (RECIST) (Therasse *et al.* 2000; Eisenhauer *et al.* 2009). These are criteria that were originally developed for treatment with cytotoxic agents. However, patterns of clinical response may greatly differ in immunotherapeutic trials. Compared to chemotherapeutics, the manifestation of clinical response is often delayed in immunotherapeutic trials and develops after an initial phase of stable disease or even tumor progression. This effect is frequently observed in immunotherapeutic trials and is expressed by a delayed separation of Kaplan-Meyer survival curves (Hoos *et al.* 2010). Furthermore, a well-known discrepancy of many immunotherapies that fail to achieve clinical benefit in progression-free survival but do show an objective effect on overall survival can be explained by this effect. In order to accommodate these observations, new immune related response criteria (irRC) have been proposed and are currently being tested for their significance and applicability in immunotherapeutical trials (Wolchok *et al.* 2009).

Another question that remains in this context is the appropriate general setting of an immunotherapeutic approach. Nearly all trials mentioned in Table 1 focus on late stage patients with metastatic RCC that have often not responded to previous therapies and have acquired a resistance to cytokine treatment and targeted therapy. Some authors have suggested that this might be a rather unfavourable setting for testing the efficiency of an immunotherapeutic approach because the immune system has probably lost the battle against the cancer at a much earlier stge and immune suppressive mechanisms may have progressed to an irreversible state. The use of immunotherapies should therefore be tested preferentially in an adjuvant or minimal residual disease setting (Morse *et al.* 2005; Hoos *et al.* 2007).

6. Tumor associated antigens: the good, the bad, and the ugly

The lack of defined tumor specific antigens in RCC can already be deduced from the list of studies undertaken so far. Only few invoke defined antigens, most make use of autologous tumor tissue alone, in combination with adjuvant or after loading on dendritic cells. The use of non-defined antigens has several inherent problems however. First, the quality of the vaccine is critically dependent on the purity of the antigen and tissue material received from surgery is undoubtedly of varying quality. Furthermore, some studies have shown that only apoptotic and not necrotic cell vaccines can induce a regular immune response (Scheffer *et al.* 2003). Second, a mixture of different unknown antigens always has the potential of partially or preferentially inducing tolerogenic T cells or, even worse, inducing autoimmunity against self-antigens. Last but not least, immunomonitoring of patients, which has become a powerful tool in recent immunotherapeutic studies, can only be carried out accurately if the antigen is known in advance. Compared with full length proteins, antigenic peptides have the advantage of simple chemically defined production in GMP quality. This allows for the combination of different antigenic peptides to a multi-epitope vaccine. Thereby the individuality of a patient's immune response is taken into account, indicating that not every patient will develop an equally strong immune response against one and the same antigen. The major disadvantage of defined T-cell epitopes is that they are usually restricted to for one HLA allotype requiring the patient to match to a certain HLA in order to benefit from the treatment. This further underlines the need for the identification of additional tumor-associated antigen-derived peptides for less common HLA alleles (Klug *et al.* 2009).

How can we now decide whether an identified antigen is also a good vaccination candidate and what are the hallmarks of these antigens? The most important but often carelessly neglected requirement of any good vaccination candidate is the presence of the antigen on the tumor cell. In terms of an immunotherapy this means that the antigen needs to be accessible in order to be recognized by immune cells, preferentially T cells. At first glance this sounds trivial but in fact most studies have made use of antigens that have actually never been found to be presented by MHC molecules and instead emanated from *in vitro* tested or *in silico* predicted T cell epitopes of previously known tumor associated antigens that were shown to be overexpressed within tumor tissue at the mRNA or protein level. In doing so basic principles of immunology are ignored since T cells are not given insight into tumor cells but have to rely on a showcase of peptide antigens presented by MHC molecules. Indeed it could be shown that the gene expression level of a certain protein and presentation of corresponding protein-derived peptides only reveal a very faint correlation (Weinzierl *et al.* 2007).

The second most important requirement is the immunogenicity of the antigen. This is indeed a crucial point, since many of the tumor antigens are derived from self proteins and hence show only weak immunogenicity if at all because of central or peripheral T-cell tolerance. One great exception are unique antigens that arise from gene mutations or fusion proteins which accumulate during the course of tumor development. These neo-antigens are therefore not affected by tolerance mechanisms, either in the thymus during lymphocyte maturation by clonal deletion or in the periphery by anergy induction. Because of the large set of distinct mutations acquired within each tumor not only within different genes, but also at a multitude of locations within the gene, the application of mutated antigens in tumor vaccination will be restricted to a patient individualized approach.

Other frequently examined antigens including cancer testis or differentiation antigens show a rather restricted expression pattern that can in some cases also be considered to be tumor specific. During the course of tumorigenesis cancer cells often acquire epigenetic alterations that lead to the expression of genes (MAGE, NY-ESO-1) which are usually only transcribed during embryonic development and hence remain silenced within adult tissue. Some of these cancer testis antigens (CTA) have, however, also been found to be expressed in thymic epithelium so that central tolerance by deletion of CTA-specific T cells cannot be excluded (Gotter *et al.* 2004). Differentiation antigens are commonly expressed in malignant and normal cells of the same lineage *e.g.* Melan-A, gp100 and TRP1 in melanoma tumor tissue and benign melanocytes. In cases in which the benign tissue expressing the differentiation antigen is dispensable as, for instance, in prostate cancer patients after prostatectomy, differentiation antigens like PSA become highly specific for the tumor. The great majority of potential vaccination antigens is, however, derived from tumor antigens that are rather ubquitously expressed but show a (high) overexpression on cancer tissue (CA9, Her2/neu, MUC1) (Kessler & Melief 2007). Differentiation and overexpressed antigens are usually subject to central and peripheral tolerance mechanisms. Self tolerance for many antigens, however is not always complete. The prior testing of T-cell immunogenicity for theses antigens is therefore absolutely essential.

Another aspect that should be considered before choosing a vaccination antigen is its impact on tumor oncogenicity. Preferentially, antigens should be targeted that are involved in the oncogenic process and hence indispensable for tumor growth and maintenance of the neoplastic state.

Based on similar but not identical criteria, a ranking of potentially suitable tumor associated antigens for clinical use has been published in an initiative from the National Cancer Institute involving different working groups in the US (Cheever *et al.* 2009). They used an analytical hierachy process generated ranking which further included objective criteria like therapeutic functionality, the expression of the antigen within stem cells, number of patients expressing the antigen, the number of known antigen derived T-cell epitopes and also the cellular localisation of the antigen.

7. Identification of new tumor associated antigens

Having described the hallmarks of optimal tumor associated and specific antigens in the context of an anti-tumor vaccine we would now like to present state-of-the-art technology for the identification of respective antigens with a clear focus on tumor associated HLA ligands. There are several strategies which can be divided into two basic sets: Top-down approaches carried out - by directly analysing the tumor antigens present within or presented by tumor cells, and bottom-up. The latter represent a reverse approach usually starting from the gene level *via* the protein level and subsequently to the HLA ligand level.

7.1 Bottom-up

One of the first approaches developed for the large scale identification of tumor associated antigens is the serological identification of antigens by recombinant expression cloning SEREX (Sahin *et al.* 1995). The method is based on cDNA expression libraries created from tumor cell lines or tissues which are subsequently packaged into lambda-phage vectors that can be used to infect *E. coli* bacteria. During the lytic phase the production of recombinant proteins is induced and clones can be screened for the presence of tumor reactive antibodies using cancer patient sera. Selection, cloning and sequencing of antibody reacting clones allows for the straightforward molecular description of the antigen, as the recombinant proteins are located in the same *E.coli* clone plaque as the respective cDNA (Tureci *et al.* 2005). The major advantage of cDNA expression libraries is that only genes that are actually expressed within the cell/tisue of origin are incorporated and that they can be generated from various sources that include patient derived autologous tumor tissue. SEREX is still a valued, commonly used tool for antigen identification (Wang *et al.* 2009; Kiyamova *et al.* 2010). Several modifications have been incoporated to overcome restrictions for instance regarding the prokaryotic expression system, which does not allow for posttranslational modifications (Kim *et al.* 2007). With the advent of the „omics" era a comparatively high throughput analysis of differences in the gene expression level could be done with relative ease. Now large databases summarizing these data are publicly available (Edgar *et al.* 2002). New approaches aim at gaining a deeper understanding of the tumor and its genetic basis by sequencing the complete tumor genome. The whole genome approach has profited from the rapid progress in next-generation sequencing techniques over the last few years which is fortunately accompanied by decreasing costs (Wong *et al.* 2011). The complete and differential sequencing of tumor tissue and corresponding normal tissue shows alterations directly on genomic level that the tumor has acquired during its development (see Fig. 2 blue section). The subset of potential tumor antigens can be assessed by the selection of non-silent mutational events. Further reconciliation with databases of known sequence polymorphisms (dbSNP, (Smigielski *et al.* 2000)) or known mutations in cancer (COSMIC, (Bamford *et al.* 2004)) can help to distinguish tumor driver from passenger mutations.

The bottom-up approach yields proteins without any post-translational modifications. A prerequisite for successful peptide vaccination therapy is the presentation on the tumor cell surface by MHC molecules. *In silico* digestion and HLA binding prediction (Feldhahn *et al.* 2009) of the respective parts can shed light on which of these are putative tumor antigens suitable for further evaluation of immunogenicity in T-cell arrays.

A major determinant for peptide:HLA binding is the steric configuration defined by the MHC molecule and the amino acid sequence of the peptide (Bjorkman *et al.* 1987). The HLA molecule forms a peptide binding groove with prominent binding pockets for individual amino acid side chains. The polymorphism of the HLA alleles results in different polypeptides and therefore different binding pocket properties. This yields characteristic peptide sequence motifs for ligands to bind the HLA molecule. The most conserved positions in these motifs form the anchor residues, whose side chains fit best in the binding pockets for strong interaction.

With sufficient ligandome analysis that takes sequence statistics for the given peptide:HLA molecule pairs into consideration one can generate Position Specific Scoring Matrices (PSSMs). Each position holds higher scores for more frequently occurring amino acids. Summing up the scores for each position, these matrices can be used to estimate the binding capability with an HLA molecule for any given peptide sequence. The SYFPEITHI method uses PSSMs generated from naturally processed HLA ligands from the SYFPEITHI database (Rammensee *et al.* 1999) in an expert system fashion also accounting for given chemical conditions. The assumption of independent contribution of each amino acid to the overall binding affinity is one drawback of PSSM approaches. Non-linear fashion machine learning methods can create prediction models that address this issue with different techniques (support vector machine (SVM) based SVMHC (Dönnes & Kohlbacher 2006), artificial neural network (ANN) training method based NetMHC (Buus *et al.* 2003). Prediction quality for all approaches is heavily dependent on the sampling coverage for an an allele-specific HLA ligandome available (discussion of efficiency is out of scope).

There also exist prediction methods for the steps preceding peptide presentation, the proteasomal cleavage of proteins (PAProC (Nussbaum *et al.* 2001), NetChop, (Kesmir *et al.* 2002)) and the TAP transport (TAPPred, (Bhasin & Raghava 2004)). As these steps are very complex and depend on a huge variety of parameters, the results may not adequately reflect the naturally occurring process. The framework for T-cell epitope detection FRED provides easy accession to most prediction methods for MHC binding as well as creating a general infrastructure for the handling of antigen sequence data. It includes the possibility for integrated analysis of protein polymorphisms influences and simultaneous accession of different prediction methods. Analysis pipelines intended for high throughput capability profit immensely from such frameworks. They integrate different algorithms with differing input and output types and therefore provide a flexible means to implement of accelerating the analysis process.

7.2 Top-down

Until now straightforward proteomics approaches have mainly focused on the identification of serum cancer biomarkers rather than target antigens for cancer therapy (Seliger *et al.* 2003). One exception is serological proteome analysis, SERPA, a modified SEREX approach translated to the protein level. In contrast to SEREX, screening with autologous patient sera is not carried out against cDNA expression libraries but against protein lysates separated by two dimensional polyacrylamide gel electrophoresis (2D-PAGE) or directly against protein arrays (Desmetz *et al.* 2009). The comparative full proteome analysis of tumor and benign tissue usually requires the pre-separation of proteins, for example by 2D-PAGE or multidimensional liquid chromatography, due to the overall complexity of the protein lysate. This approach has in the past suffered from low sensitivity and weak reproducibility (Baggerman *et al.* 2005). Identification of tumor associated target antigens has remained rare since standard proteomics approaches often fail to detect low abundant proteins (Joshi *et al.* 2011). Nevertheless proteomics is a rapidly developing field. Taking the steadily increasing mass spectrometric sensitivity (Yates *et al.* 2009), the use of *in vitro* (*e.g.* chemical modification) or *in vivo* (*e.g.* SILAC) differential labeling approaches for quantification (Schulze & Usadel 2010) and also MALDI imaging technology (Fournier *et al.* 2008) into account, proteomics will clearly contribute to a greater extent to TAA identification in the future.

In contrast to standard proteomics, HLA ligandomics is a well established, straightforward approach and perfectly suited for the identification of tumor associated HLA ligands (Schirle *et al.* 2000). HLA molecules can be directly isolated from dissected tumors and autologous normal tissue. The method of choice is immunoaffinity chromatography using antibodies specific for different HLA molecules (see table 2) immobilised on a sepharose matrix. Application of a crude tissue lysate leads to the binding of respective HLA molecules which can be subsequently eluted by acid treatment. At the same time, pH shift also leads to the release of bound peptides from the HLA binding grooves. Due to the narrow mass range of these peptide ligands, they can be easily separated from higher molecular weight substances (>10 kDa) by ultra-filtration. Lyophilisation of the filtrate yields a mixture of different HLA derived peptides ready for concomitant separation and analysis using liquid-chromatography coupled mass spectrometry (LC-MS, see Fig. 2a).

Clone	**∝HLA**	**Reference**
W6/32	A,B,C	(Barnstable *et al.* 1978)
B1.23.2	B,C	(Rebai & Malissen 1983)
BB7.2	A2	(Parham & Brodsky 1981)
GAP-A3	A3	(Berger *et al.* 1982)
Spv-L3	DQ	(Spits *et al.* 1983)
Tü-39	DR, DQ, DP	(Maeda & Hirata 1984)
L243	DR	(Lampson & Levy 1980)
IVD-12	DQ	(Kolstad *et al.* 1987)

Table 2. HLA directed antibodies

The greates benefit is that the described procedure yields natural ligands, so that neither the proteasomal cleavage nor intracellular transport and loading onto HLA molecules has to be determined for the respective peptide. The challenge is the molecular characterisation of the heterogenous mixture of isolated peptides.

Peptide and protein sequencing can be accomplished via tandem mass spectrometry. This is an advanced technique of proteomics analysis and offers a versatile, high-throughput procedure for investigation of protein samples, including sequence identification. The measurement is conducted by recording the mass-to-charge ratio (m/z) of peptide ions with high sensitivity down to the sub-femtomole level. For better identification a second mass analyzer can be added in tandem, where molecules of selected masses are further fragmented (Roepstorff & Fohlman 1984; Johnson *et al.* 1987) and the resulting mass-to-charge ratios measured (see Table 3). Fragmentation of peptides occurs most prominently at the backbone structure, *i.e.* the peptide bonds concatenating the amino acids. The result of a tandem mass spectrometric analysis is a spectrum of fragment m/z values. The fragments containing the N-terminus of the peptide are called „b-ions" whereas those containing the C-terminus are called „y-ions", each enumerated by the number of retained amino acids. *Via* the masses of the fragments the spectra can be annotated with the peptide's sequence.

	b-ions	Mass	y-ions	Mass	
1	(S)	-	YFPEITHI	1019.5197	8
2	SY	251.1026	FPEITHI	856.4563	7
3	SYF	398.1710	PEITHI	709.3879	6
4	SYFP	495.2238	EITHI	612.3352	5
5	SYFPE	624.2664	ITHI	483.2926	4
6	SYFPEI	737.3505	THI	370.2085	3
7	SYFPEIT	838.3981	HI	269.1608	2
8	SYFPEITH	975.4571	I	132.1019	1

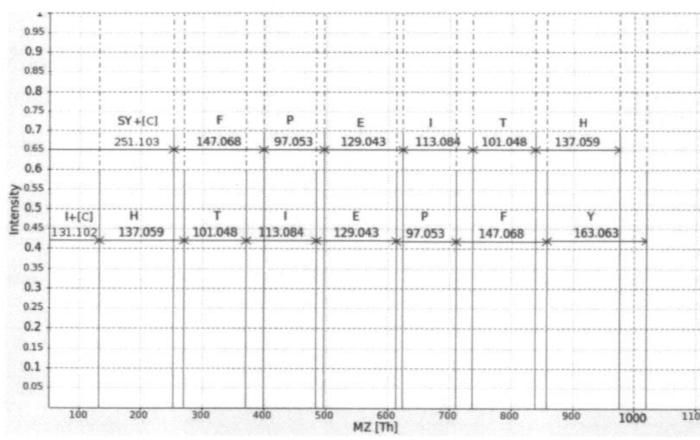

Table 3. Theoretical fragmentation spectrum of SYFPEITHI peptide.

Missing peaks make the spectrum annotation a complex problem. These are due to: technical detection thresholds, complex or incomplete fragmentation, contamination and measurement noise. This can be addressed by computational methods for mass spectrometry proteomics. Spectra can be identified by either algorithmic comparison to a database of known spectra (Eng *et al.* 1994), directly by de novo methods (Bertsch *et al.* 2009) that do not depend on databases or by comparison with a sequence database (Perkins *et al.* 1999).

The latter and in most cases very robust method infers theoretical spectra from a set of compatible sequences and matches the experimentally determined masses with those calculated. The method is robust because it is possible to infer a statistical significance evaluation, *i.e.* a score, from the size of the database as well as the number and quality of matches. Another technique to introduce robustness to the results is the use of a false discovery cut off. The introduction of a decoy database (most commonly the inverse input database) allows for calculation of a false discovery rate, defined as the number of false discoveries (from the decoy) over the number of false and correct discoveries (from both databases) given a score. A false discovery rate of 5% discerns a score within one experiment which guarantees that scores equal or better will be false discoveries only by the chance of p=0.05 (i.e. 5%).

Sophisticated methods for high throughput identification of natural HLA ligands are beginning to emerge. Established proteomics methods are specifically suited for this task. OpenMS (Sturm *et al.* 2008) is an open and flexible framework for proteomics data analysis. As explained, integrated analysis is a major advantage for high throughput oriented analysis. In the case of individualized cancer therapy, different disciplines with diverse methods come together which does not permit a comprehensive framework. One solution for maintaining high throughput capability is a tailored workflow development that integrates analysis tools of different trades. OpenMS/TOPP also comes with tools for workflow development (Kohlbacher *et al.* 2007) for virtually seamless integration of other computational aspects of immunology, such as the *in silico* prediction of HLA presented peptides or database connection and reconciliation containing very different types of data.

7.3 Validation and selection of peptide candidates

The final verification step of identified HLA ligands includes the chemical synthesis of peptides. The tandem mass spectrometric measurement of the synthesized peptide represents a crucial aspect of reliability. As fragmentation patterns define the sequence and are preserved throughout the measurements, the corresponding spectra as well as the retention time of the synthetic and identified peptide will be nearly identical. A putative T-cell epitope needs to be further validated in T-cell priming experiments. For this reason a plethora of protocols has been established to prime naive T cells usually from healthy donors with either natural (*e.g.* dendritic cells) or artificial APCs presenting the synthetic peptide. Proliferation and priming efficiency can subsequently be assayed by a variety of functional tests, *e.g.* enzyme linked immunospot technique (ELISPOT), intracellular cytokine staining (ICS) or tetramer staining.

In order to work reasonably well in a preferably diverse target group, the design of a vaccine also poses the challenge of combining several vaccination candidate peptides to a multi-epitope vaccine. Recently, Toussaint et al. (Toussaint & Kohlbacher 2009) proposed a mathematical framework for the selection of an optimal set of peptides for vaccination. Given a set of candidate epitopes, a target population, information on the respective T-cell reactivities to the peptides (or HLA binding affinities), along with other user-defined information to be incorporated in the selection process, the framework efficiently determines an optimal epitope set.

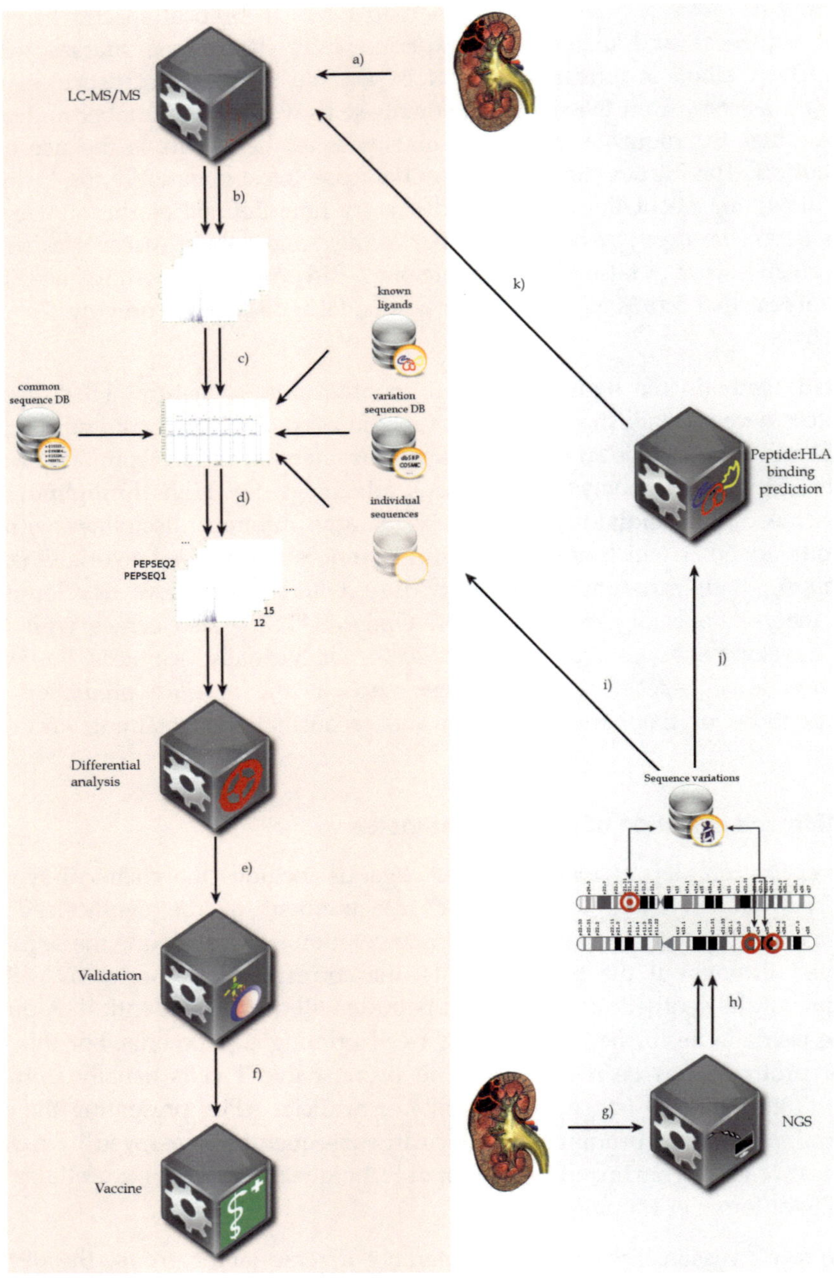

Fig. 2. The workflow for standard HLA ligandome analysis (red) and with mounted bottom-up approach methods (blue) for patient individualisation. a) sample preparation, b) MS analysis, c) peptide identification, d) FDR filter, e) differential analys f) HLA ligand validation, g) vaccine design and application, h) genome sequencing, i) variation detection, j) peptide:HLA binding prediction, k) identification of peptides with sequence variation, l) targeted search. Chromosome figures are modified from a screenshot at http://genome.ucsc.edu (Kent et al. 2002).

8. Outlook

The therapeutic situation in advanced stage renal cell carcinoma leaves much rome for improvement with frequent resistance development to TKIs and still no cure in sight. Despite the lack of convincing clinical succes, targeted immunotherapy remains a promising approach. We are only just beginning to understand the complex relationship between the tumor and the surrounding microenvironment. The sophisticated mechanisms of immune evasion that hamper an active immune response are still a major hindrance on the road to success. First steps to overcoming this are by specifically addressing immunosuppression presented through the advent of immune modulatory antibodies such as Ipilimumab. However improvement of targeted immunotherapy is also clearly dependent on the identification of new tumor associated and also specific antigens as well as HLA ligands (Stevanovic 2002). This stresses the need for concise epitope libraries comprising ligands from different tumor entities and benign tissue for various HLA alleles (Krüger *et al.* 2005).

8.1 Targeting the individual patient

The greatest leap forward in the struggle for a successful immunotherapy, at least from the authors' point of view are expected from a patient individualised approach. Tremendous progress in DNA sequencing during the last few years has enabled us to look at the genetic basis of each individual cancer. Comparison of somatic mutations within different tumors has shown that distinct mutational patterns are not only present between different tumor types but also between tumors of the same entity clearly underlining the need for an individualized approach (Ocana & Pandiella 2010).

Combination of whole genome sequencing with HLA ligandome analysis will in future lead to the identification of mutated tumor specific HLA ligands presented on tumor cells. The advanced utilisation of computer-aided high throughput methods enables fast and accurate identification of vaccine candidates. This demonstrates that individualised anti-tumor therapy is also feasible within a certain time frame (first vaccination estimated 5-7 weeks post surgery see Table 4).

Step	Approx. Duration	Section in Figure 2
Genome sequencing	> 2 Weeks	Blue
Ligandome analysis	1-2 weeks	Red
GMP grade peptide synthesis	>2 Weeks	Red
	$\sum$ ~ 6 Weeks	

Table 4. Current time limitations until vaccine availability

The use of mutated HLA ligands should also eliminate the need for time consuming *in vitro* T-cell immunogenicity testing since these antigens are tumor specific neoantigens and thus foreign to the immune system. Differences in the strength of an immune response towards a certain mutated peptide antigen can, however, not be excluded. Nevertheless, the probability of response failure can be greatly reduced by a combination of several mutated peptides to a multi-epitope vaccine.

Compared to other treatment strategies, immunotherapy aimed at mutated antigens does not necessarily need to target tumor driver mutations, which are usually key to oncogenic properties. Instead, any mutation specific for a certain tumor which is found to be expressed and presented by HLA molecules can be used. Thereby the amount of possible vaccination candidate peptides is greatly increased. The importance of this fact is obvious given that only 2-5 driver mutations among the 1000-10000 somatic mutations found can be unambiguously identified within each tumor (Stratton 2011).

8.2 Targeting the tumor microenvironment

Failure to eradicate cancer by targeting tumor cells exclusively has extended the focus in anticancer therapy during the last few years to include the tumor microenvironment (Kenny *et al.* 2007). Evidence is accumulating to confirm intense crosstalk between tumor cells and their surroundings. Tumor cells not just passively profit from nutritional factors but actively shape their own environment towards their specific needs in a process of coevolution (Polyak *et al.* 2009). Clear cell renal cell carcinoma are a prime example of this since they are usually hypervascularized. This is nearly always the result of a genetic defect in the hypoxia inducible factor 1 signalling cascade leading to secretion of large amounts of proangiogenic VEGF (Sufan *et al.* 2004). Other well established mechanisms of tumor-stroma interaction are the remodelling of the extracellular matrix by tumor-associated macrophages(Mantovani *et al.* 2006), the expression of stimulatory growth factors by tumor asociated fibroblasts (Bhowmick *et al.* 2004) and of course the attraction of immune suppressive cells (Baglole *et al.* 2006). The idea of targeting the cancer's „safe haven" might therefore not only deprive the tumor from its nutritional basis but hopefully also, at least in part reverse immunosuppression. Targeting the tumor stroma in RCC is already being done: tyrosine kinase inhibitors, which currently represent first line treatment for metastatic RCC, are thought to act primarily on endothelial cells, thereby inhibiting angiogenesis.

Combination therapy of TKIs together with cytokine treatment (Miller & Larkin 2009) as well as TKIs with targeted immunotherapy (Rini *et al.* 2011) are already being tested in clinical trials. But what about targeting the stroma directly with a specific immunotherapy? Stroma cells within tumor cells seem to differ in various aspects from their normal counterparts. Endothelial cells within the tumor show a highly fenestrated chaotic organization and often lack supportive smooth muscle cells as well as a regular basement membrane (Aird 2009). Cancer associated fibroblasts have an activated phenotype with high proliferative capacity, less growth requirements and show a high capacity to recruit endothelial progenitor cells (Orimo & Weinberg 2006; Li *et al.* 2007). Differences between normal and tumor stroma can also be observed on the level of gene expression (Ma *et al.* 2009) and are probably based on different epigenetic alterations (Hu *et al.* 2005). Some groups have reported that tumor associated stroma cells are also subject to clonally selected somatic mutations in tumor suppressor genes (TP53) (Kurose *et al.* 2002) and oncogenes (EGFR) (Weber *et al.* 2005) and further show a high degree of genomic instability (loss of chromosomal heterozygosity) (Moinfar *et al.* 2000). However these results are still controversial and might also be due to technical issues (Polyak, Haviv et al. 2009).

Nevertheless, considering the overall changes within tumor associated stroma might render these cells susceptible to an attack by different immune cells. In order to include the targeting of tumor stroma cells into an immunotherapeutic approach, immunological accessible antigens, especially HLA ligands which are exclusively expressed on tumor stroma need to be identified.

8.3 Targeting cancer stem cells

Another upcoming field in cancer therapy is based on the observation that tumor cells within some cancer types at least show a hierarchical organization which is closely resembling that of normal benign tissue. According to the cancer stem cell hypothesis only a rare population of tumor cells termed cancer stem cells (CSC) or tumor initiating cells (TIC) are ultimately responsible for initiating and driving tumor growth. CSCs share some characteristics with normal tissue stem cells including the potential of self renewal, indefinite division, slow replication rate, greatly increased DNA repair capacity and finally the ability to divide asymmetrically, thereby giving rise to new cancer stem cells and rapidly dividing more differentiated tumor cells that make up the bulk of the tumor (Wang & Dick 2005). Evidence for the existence of a tumor initiating cell population was first provided in acute myeloid leukaemia by John Dick and colleagues in the mid 90s (Lapidot *et al.* 1994; Bonnet & Dick 1997). They demonstrated that tumorigenicity of leukaemia cells was much higher in a subpopulation of $CD34^{+}CD38^{-}$ tumor cells. Less than 500 cells exhibiting this particular phenotype were sufficient to engraft immunodeficient mice, whereas even a 100-fold higher number of $CD34^{+}CD38^{+}$ tumor cells, which constitute the gross of leukaemic cells, could not initiate engraftment. Even more important engraftment of isolated $CD34^{+}CD38^{-}$ cells repeated the composition of the original tumor in that $CD34^{+}CD38^{-}$ cells also gave rise to the major leukaemic cell population of $CD34^{+}CD38^{+}$ cells.

Several years later, the presence of a cancer stem cell population in solid tumors was shown for breast cancer (Al-Hajj *et al.* 2003). Since then, the existence of a CSC-population has been shown for many different types of cancer including brain, prostate, liver, colon and lung (for a review see (Visvader & Lindeman 2008)). In renal cell carcinoma, the existence of a $CD105^{+}$ cancer stem cell population has also been postulated but final proof regarding its existence is still missing (Bussolati *et al.* 2008). The attraction of the cancer stem cell model is in part based on its ability to explain long known but still poorly understood clinical phenomena, the relapse of cancer patients after a period of tumor regression and even absence of detectable lesions. CSC are known to be highly resistant to chemo- and radiotherapy. They can remain quiescent for a prolonged period of time and then restart tumor growth at a distant site leading to metastasis. This bears a fundamental clinical impact for the treatment of cancer patients. As long as CSCs are not effectively killed by a treatment we won't be able to completely eradicate a certain tumor (Clevers 2011). Considering the resistance mechanisms to standard therapeutic approaches, immunotherapy may indeed be the only therapeutic option to directly target these cells. Therefore cancer stem cell specific antigens urgently need to be discovered and their potential for a targeted immunotherapy evaluated.

There is ample evidence that specific immunotherapy will play a very important role in the future not only in RCC but rather for the treatment of different cancer types. The first targeted immunotherapy Provenge (Sipuleucel-T) manufactured by Dendreon has just recently been approved by the FDA for the treatment of advanced prostate cancer. Provenge consists of an autologous dendritic cell vaccine loaded with a fusion protein of GM-CSF with the prostate specific antigen prostatic acid phosphatase (PAP). Although it is far too early to speak of a triumphal course of this new category of cancer treatment at least a start has been made.

9. Acknowledgements

We specially thank Lynne Yakes for expert proofreading.

10. References

Adams, S. (2009). Toll-like receptor agonists in cancer therapy. *Immunotherapy*, 1, 6, (Nov, 2009) pp. 949-964

Adams, S., *et al.* (2008). Immunization of malignant melanoma patients with full-length NY-ESO-1 protein using TLR7 agonist imiquimod as vaccine adjuvant. *J Immunol*, 181, 1, (Jul 1, 2008) pp. 776-784

Aird, W. C. (2009). Molecular heterogeneity of tumor endothelium. *Cell Tissue Res*, 335, 1, (Jan, 2009) pp. 271-281

Al-Hajj, M., *et al.* (2003). Prospective identification of tumorigenic breast cancer cells. *Proc Natl Acad Sci U S A*, 100, 7, (Apr 1, 2003) pp. 3983-3988

Angevin, E., *et al.* (1997). Analysis of T-cell immune response in renal cell carcinoma: polarization to type 1-like differentiation pattern, clonal T-cell expansion and tumor-specific cytotoxicity. *Int J Cancer*, 72, 3, (Jul 29, 1997) pp. 431-440

Antonia, S. J., *et al.* (2002). Phase I trial of a B7-1 (CD80) gene modified autologous tumor cell vaccine in combination with systemic interleukin-2 in patients with metastatic renal cell carcinoma. *J Urol*, 167, 5, (May, 2002) pp. 1995-2000

Arroyo, J. C., *et al.* (2004). Immune response induced in vitro by CD16- and CD16+ monocyte-derived dendritic cells in patients with metastatic renal cell carcinoma treated with dendritic cell vaccines. *J Clin Immunol*, 24, 1, (Jan, 2004) pp. 86-96

Atchison, E., *et al.* (2010). A pilot study of denileukin diftitox (DD) in combination with high-dose interleukin-2 (IL-2) for patients with metastatic renal cell carcinoma (RCC). *J Immunother*, 33, 7, (Sep, 2010) pp. 716-722

Attig, S., *et al.* (2009). Simultaneous infiltration of polyfunctional effector and suppressor T cells into renal cell carcinomas. *Cancer Res*, 69, 21, (Nov 1, 2009) pp. 8412-8419

Avarbock, A. B., *et al.* (2008). Lethal vascular leak syndrome after denileukin diftitox administration to a patient with cutaneous gamma/delta T-cell lymphoma and occult cirrhosis. *Am J Hematol*, 83, 7, (Jul, 2008) pp. 593-595

Avigan, D., *et al.* (2004). Fusion cell vaccination of patients with metastatic breast and renal cancer induces immunological and clinical responses. *Clin Cancer Res*, 10, 14, (Jul 15, 2004) pp. 4699-4708

Avigan, D. E., *et al.* (2007). Phase I/II study of vaccination with electrofused allogeneic dendritic cells/autologous tumor-derived cells in patients with stage IV renal cell carcinoma. *J Immunother*, 30, 7, (Oct, 2007) pp. 749-761

Azuma, T., *et al.* (2002). Dendritic cell immunotherapy for patients with metastatic renal cell carcinoma: University of Tokyo experience. *Int J Urol*, 9, 6, (Jun, 2002) pp. 340-346

Baggerman, G., *et al.* (2005). Gel-based versus gel-free proteomics: a review. *Comb Chem High Throughput Screen*, 8, 8, (Dec, 2005) pp. 669-677

Baglole, C. J., *et al.* (2006). More than structural cells, fibroblasts create and orchestrate the tumor microenvironment. *Immunol Invest*, 35, pp. 297-325

Bamford, S., *et al.* (2004). The COSMIC (Catalogue of Somatic Mutations in Cancer) database and website. *Br J Cancer*, 91, 2, (Jul, 2004) pp. 355--358

Barbuto, J. A., *et al.* (2004). Dendritic cell-tumor cell hybrid vaccination for metastatic cancer. *Cancer Immunol Immunother*, 53, 12, (Dec, 2004) pp. 1111-1118

Barnstable, C. J., *et al.* (1978). Production of monoclonal antibodies to group A erythrocytes, HLA and other human cell surface antigens-new tools for genetic analysis. *Cell*, 14, 1, (May, 1978) pp. 9-20

Bay, J. O., *et al.* (2002). Allogeneic hematopoietic stem cell transplantation in ovarian carcinoma: results of five patients. *Bone Marrow Transplant*, 30, 2, (Jul, 2002) pp. 95-102

Bennouna, J., *et al.* (2008). Phase-I study of Innacell gammadelta, an autologous cell-therapy product highly enriched in gamma9delta2 T lymphocytes, in combination with IL-2, in patients with metastatic renal cell carcinoma. *Cancer Immunol Immunother*, 57, 11, (Nov, 2008) pp. 1599-1609

Berger, A. E., *et al.* (1982). Monoclonal antibody to HLA-A3. *Hybridoma*, pp. 87-90

Berntsen, A., *et al.* (2008). Therapeutic dendritic cell vaccination of patients with metastatic renal cell carcinoma: a clinical phase 1/2 trial. *J Immunother*, 31, 8, (Oct, 2008) pp. 771-780

Bertsch, A., *et al.* (2009). De novo peptide sequencing by tandem MS using complementary CID and electron transfer dissociation. *Electrophoresis*, 30, 21, (Nov, 2009) pp. 3736--3747

Bhasin, M. & G. P. S. Raghava (2004). Analysis and prediction of affinity of TAP binding peptides using cascade SVM. *Protein Sci*, 13, 3, (Mar, 2004) pp. 596--607

Bhowmick, N. A., *et al.* (2004). Stromal fibroblasts in cancer initiation and progression. *Nature*, 432, 7015, (Nov 18, 2004) pp. 332-337

Bishop, M. R., *et al.* (2004). Allogeneic lymphocytes induce tumor regression of advanced metastatic breast cancer. *J Clin Oncol*, 22, 19, (Oct 1, 2004) pp. 3886-3892

Bjorkman, P. J., *et al.* (1987). Structure of the human class I histocompatibility antigen, HLA-A2. *Nature*, 329, 6139, (Oct, 1987) pp. 506-512

Bleakley, M. & S. R. Riddell (2004). Molecules and mechanisms of the graft-versus-leukaemia effect. *Nat Rev Cancer*, 4, 5, (May, 2004) pp. 371-380

Bleumer, I., *et al.* (2007). Preliminary analysis of patients with progressive renal cell carcinoma vaccinated with CA9-peptide-pulsed mature dendritic cells. *J Immunother*, 30, 1, (Jan, 2007) pp. 116-122

Bonnet, D. & J. E. Dick (1997). Human acute myeloid leukemia is organized as a hierarchy that originates from a primitive hematopoietic cell. *Nat Med*, 3, 7, (Jul, 1997) pp. 730-737

Brandenburg, S., *et al.* (2008). IL-2 induces in vivo suppression by CD4(+)CD25(+)Foxp3(+) regulatory T cells. *Eur J Immunol*, 38, 6, (Jun, 2008) pp. 1643-1653

Bregni, M., *et al.* (2002). Nonmyeloablative conditioning followed by hematopoietic cell allografting and donor lymphocyte infusions for patients with metastatic renal and breast cancer. *Blood*, 99, 11, (Jun 1, 2002) pp. 4234-4236

Buchner, A., *et al.* (2010). Phase 1 trial of allogeneic gene-modified tumor cell vaccine RCC-26/CD80/IL-2 in patients with metastatic renal cell carcinoma. *Hum Gene Ther*, 21, 3, (Mar, 2010) pp. 285-297

Burnet, F. M. (1967). Immunological aspects of malignant disease. *Lancet*, 1, 7501, (Jun 3, 1967) pp. 1171-1174

Bussolati, B., *et al.* (2008). Identification of a tumor-initiating stem cell population in human renal carcinomas. *FASEB J*, 22, 10, (Oct, 2008) pp. 3696-3705

Buus, S., *et al.* (2003). Sensitive quantitative predictions of peptide-MHC binding by a 'Query by Committee' artificial neural network approach. *Tissue Antigens*, 62, 5, (Nov, 2003) pp. 378--384

Campoli, M., *et al.* (2002). HLA class I antigen loss, tumor immune escape and immune selection. *Vaccine*, 20 Suppl 4, (Dec 19, 2002) pp. A40-45

Cheever, M. A. (2008). Twelve immunotherapy drugs that could cure cancers. *Immunol Rev*, 222, (Apr, 2008) pp. 357-368

Cheever, M. A., *et al.* (2009). The prioritization of cancer antigens: a national cancer institute pilot project for the acceleration of translational research. *Clin Cancer Res*, 15, 17, (Sep 1, 2009) pp. 5323-5337

Childs, R., *et al.* (2000). Regression of metastatic renal-cell carcinoma after nonmyeloablative allogeneic peripheral-blood stem-cell transplantation. *N Engl J Med*, 343, 11, (Sep 14, 2000) pp. 750-758

Clevers, H. (2011). The cancer stem cell: premises, promises and challenges. *Nat Med*, 17, 3, (Mar, 2011) pp. 313-319

Coley, W. B. (1893). The treatment of malignant tumors by repeated inoculations of erysipelas. With a report of ten original cases. *Am. J. Med. Sci.*, 105, (Jan, 1893) pp. 487-511

Dannull, J., *et al.* (2005). Enhancement of vaccine-mediated antitumor immunity in cancer patients after depletion of regulatory T cells. *J Clin Invest*, 115, 12, (Dec, 2005) pp. 3623-3633

Demirer, T., *et al.* (2008). Transplantation of allogeneic hematopoietic stem cells: an emerging treatment modality for solid tumors. *Nat Clin Pract Oncol*, 5, 5, (May, 2008) pp. 256-267

Desmetz, C., *et al.* (2009). Humoral response to cancer as a tool for biomarker discovery. *J Proteomics*, 72, 6, (Aug 20, 2009) pp. 982-988

Dillman, R., *et al.* (2004). Autologous tumor cell line-derived vaccine for patient-specific treatment of advanced renal cell carcinoma. *Cancer Biother Radiopharm*, 19, 5, (Oct, 2004) pp. 570-580

Dong, H., *et al.* (2002). Tumor-associated B7-H1 promotes T-cell apoptosis: a potential mechanism of immune evasion. *Nat Med*, 8, 8, (Aug, 2002) pp. 793-800

Dönnes, P. & O. Kohlbacher (2006). SVMHC: a server for prediction of MHC-binding peptides. *Nucleic Acids Res*, 34, Web Server issue, (Jul, 2006) pp. 194-197

Dudek, A. Z., *et al.* (2008). Autologous large multivalent immunogen vaccine in patients with metastatic melanoma and renal cell carcinoma. *Am J Clin Oncol*, 31, 2, (Apr, 2008) pp. 173-181

Edgar, R., *et al.* (2002). Gene Expression Omnibus: NCBI gene expression and hybridization array data repository. *Nucleic Acids Res*, 30, 1, (Jan 1, 2002) pp. 207-210

Ehrlich, P. (1909). Über den jetzigen Stand der Karzinomforschung. *Ned. Tijdschr. Geneeskd.*, 5, pp. 273-290

Eisenhauer, E. A., *et al.* (2009). New response evaluation criteria in solid tumours: revised RECIST guideline (version 1.1). *Eur J Cancer*, 45, 2, (Jan, 2009) pp. 228-247

Eng, J. K., *et al.* (1994). An approach to correlate tandem mass spectral data of peptides with amino acid sequences in a protein database. *Journal of the American Society for Mass Spectrometry*, 5, 11, (November, 1994) pp. 976--989

Fallarino, F., *et al.* (2003). Modulation of tryptophan catabolism by regulatory T cells. *Nat Immunol*, 4, 12, (Dec, 2003) pp. 1206-1212

Faries, M. B., *et al.* (2009). Effect of granulocyte/macrophage colony-stimulating factor on vaccination with an allogeneic whole-cell melanoma vaccine. *Clin Cancer Res*, 15, 22, (Nov 15, 2009) pp. 7029-7035

Feldhahn, M., *et al.* (2009). FRED--a framework for T-cell epitope detection. *Bioinformatics*, 25, 20, (Oct, 2009) pp. 2758--2759

Ferlay, J., *et al.* (2010). Estimates of worldwide burden of cancer in 2008: GLOBOCAN 2008. *Int J Cancer*, 127, 12, (Dec 15, 2010) pp. 2893-2917

Fife, B. T. & J. A. Bluestone (2008). Control of peripheral T-cell tolerance and autoimmunity via the CTLA-4 and PD-1 pathways. *Immunol Rev*, 224, (Aug, 2008) pp. 166-182

Figdor, C. G., *et al.* (2004). Dendritic cell immunotherapy: mapping the way. *Nat Med*, 10, 5, (May, 2004) pp. 475-480

Figlin, R. A., *et al.* (1999). Multicenter, randomized, phase III trial of CD8(+) tumor-infiltrating lymphocytes in combination with recombinant interleukin-2 in metastatic renal cell carcinoma. *J Clin Oncol*, 17, 8, (Aug, 1999) pp. 2521-2529

Filipazzi, P., *et al.* (2007). Identification of a new subset of myeloid suppressor cells in peripheral blood of melanoma patients with modulation by a granulocyte-macrophage colony-stimulation factor-based antitumor vaccine. *J Clin Oncol*, 25, 18, (Jun 20, 2007) pp. 2546-2553

Finke, J. H., *et al.* (2008). Sunitinib reverses type-1 immune suppression and decreases T-regulatory cells in renal cell carcinoma patients. *Clin Cancer Res*, 14, 20, (Oct 15, 2008) pp. 6674-6682

Fishman, M., *et al.* (2008). Phase II trial of B7-1 (CD-86) transduced, cultured autologous tumor cell vaccine plus subcutaneous interleukin-2 for treatment of stage IV renal cell carcinoma. *J Immunother*, 31, 1, (Jan, 2008) pp. 72-80

Fournier, I., *et al.* (2008). Tissue imaging using MALDI-MS: a new frontier of histopathology proteomics. *Expert Rev Proteomics*, 5, 3, (Jun, 2008) pp. 413-424

Frey, A. B. & N. Monu (2008). Signaling defects in anti-tumor T cells. *Immunol Rev*, 222, (Apr, 2008) pp. 192-205

Gabrilovich, D. I. & S. Nagaraj (2009). Myeloid-derived suppressor cells as regulators of the immune system. *Nat Rev Immunol*, 9, 3, (Mar, 2009) pp. 162-174

Galligioni, E., *et al.* (1996). Adjuvant immunotherapy treatment of renal carcinoma patients with autologous tumor cells and bacillus Calmette-Guerin: five-year results of a prospective randomized study. *Cancer*, 77, 12, (Jun 15, 1996) pp. 2560-2566

Galon, J., *et al.* (2006). Type, density, and location of immune cells within human colorectal tumors predict clinical outcome. *Science*, 313, 5795, (Sep 29, 2006) pp. 1960-1964

Ghiringhelli, F., *et al.* (2004). CD4+CD25+ regulatory T cells suppress tumor immunity but are sensitive to cyclophosphamide which allows immunotherapy of established tumors to be curative. *Eur J Immunol*, 34, 2, (Feb, 2004) pp. 336-344

Gitlitz, B. J., *et al.* (2003). A pilot trial of tumor lysate-loaded dendritic cells for the treatment of metastatic renal cell carcinoma. *J Immunother*, 26, 5, (Sep-Oct, 2003) pp. 412-419

Gotter, J., *et al.* (2004). Medullary epithelial cells of the human thymus express a highly diverse selection of tissue-specific genes colocalized in chromosomal clusters. *J Exp Med*, 199, 2, (Jan 19, 2004) pp. 155-166

Gouttefangeas, C., *et al.* (2007). Immunotherapy of renal cell carcinoma. *Cancer Immunol Immunother*, 56, 1, (Jan, 2007) pp. 117-128

Grossman, W. J., *et al.* (2004). Human T regulatory cells can use the perforin pathway to cause autologous target cell death. *Immunity*, 21, 4, (Oct, 2004) pp. 589-601

Holtl, L., *et al.* (2005). Allogeneic dendritic cell vaccination against metastatic renal cell carcinoma with or without cyclophosphamide. *Cancer Immunol Immunother*, 54, 7, (Jul, 2005) pp. 663-670

Holtl, L., *et al.* (2002). Immunotherapy of metastatic renal cell carcinoma with tumor lysate-pulsed autologous dendritic cells. *Clin Cancer Res*, 8, 11, (Nov, 2002) pp. 3369-3376

Hoos, A., *et al.* (2010). Improved endpoints for cancer immunotherapy trials. *J Natl Cancer Inst*, 102, 18, (Sep 22, 2010) pp. 1388-1397

Hoos, A., *et al.* (2010). Development of ipilimumab: contribution to a new paradigm for cancer immunotherapy. *Semin Oncol*, 37, 5, (Oct, 2010) pp. 533-546

Hoos, A., *et al.* (2007). A clinical development paradigm for cancer vaccines and related biologics. *J Immunother*, 30, 1, (Jan, 2007) pp. 1-15

Hu, M., *et al.* (2005). Distinct epigenetic changes in the stromal cells of breast cancers. *Nat Genet*, 37, 8, (Aug, 2005) pp. 899-905

Iiyama, T., *et al.* (2007). WT1 (Wilms' tumor 1) peptide immunotherapy for renal cell carcinoma. *Microbiol Immunol*, 51, 5, pp. 519-530

Janeway, C. A., Jr. (1989). Approaching the asymptote? Evolution and revolution in immunology. *Cold Spring Harb Symp Quant Biol*, 54 Pt 1, 1989) pp. 1-13

Jocham, D., *et al.* (2004). Adjuvant autologous renal tumour cell vaccine and risk of tumour progression in patients with renal-cell carcinoma after radical nephrectomy: phase III, randomised controlled trial. *Lancet*, 363, 9409, (Feb 21, 2004) pp. 594-599

Johnson, R. S., *et al.* (1987). Novel fragmentation process of peptides by collision-induced decomposition in a tandem mass spectrometer: differentiation of leucine and isoleucine. *Anal Chem*, 59, 21, (Nov, 1987) pp. 2621--2625

Jonasch, E., *et al.* (2008). Vaccination of metastatic renal cell carcinoma patients with autologous tumour-derived vitespen vaccine: clinical findings. *Br J Cancer*, 98, 8, (Apr 22, 2008) pp. 1336-1341

Joshi, S., *et al.* (2011). Oncoproteomics. *Clin Chim Acta*, 412, 3-4, (Jan 30, 2011) pp. 217-226

Jung, D., *et al.* (1999). Gene transfer of the Co-stimulatory molecules B7-1 and B7-2 enhances the immunogenicity of human renal cell carcinoma to a different extent. *Scand J Immunol*, 50, 3, (Sep, 1999) pp. 242-249

Kenny, P. A., *et al.* (2007). Targeting the tumor microenvironment. *Front Biosci*, 12, 2007) pp. 3468-3474

Kent, W. J., *et al.* (2002). The human genome browser at UCSC. *Genome Res*, 12, 6, (Jun, 2002) pp. 996--1006

Kesmir, C., *et al.* (2002). Prediction of proteasome cleavage motifs by neural networks. *Protein Eng*, 15, 4, (Apr, 2002) pp. 287-296

Kessler, J. H. & C. J. Melief (2007). Identification of T-cell epitopes for cancer immunotherapy. *Leukemia*, 21, 9, (Sep, 2007) pp. 1859-1874

Khong, H. T. & N. P. Restifo (2002). Natural selection of tumor variants in the generation of "tumor escape" phenotypes. *Nat Immunol*, 3, 11, (Nov, 2002) pp. 999-1005

Kim, J. H., *et al.* (2007). Phase I/II study of immunotherapy using autologous tumor lysate-pulsed dendritic cells in patients with metastatic renal cell carcinoma. *Clin Immunol*, 125, 3, (Dec, 2007) pp. 257-267

Kim, M. S., *et al.* (2007). Optimized serological isolation of lung-cancer-associated antigens from a yeast surface-expressed cDNA library. *J Microbiol Biotechnol*, 17, 6, (Jun, 2007) pp. 993-1001

Kiyamova, R., *et al.* (2010). Identification of tumor-associated antigens from medullary breast carcinoma by a modified SEREX approach. *Mol Biotechnol*, 46, 2, (Oct, 2010) pp. 105-112

Klug, F., *et al.* (2009). Characterization of MHC ligands for peptide based tumor vaccination. *Curr Pharm Des*, 15, 28, 2009) pp. 3221-3236

Kobayashi, H., *et al.* (2010). Complete remission of lung metastasis following adoptive immunotherapy using activated autologous gammadelta T-cells in a patient with renal cell carcinoma. *Anticancer Res*, 30, 2, (Feb, 2010) pp. 575-579

Kohlbacher, O., *et al.* (2007). TOPP--the OpenMS proteomics pipeline. *Bioinformatics*, 23, 2, (Jan, 2007) pp. e191--e197

Kolstad, A., *et al.* (1987). A human-human hybridoma antibody (TrB12) defining subgroups of HLA-DQw1 and -DQw3. *Hum Immunol*, 20, 3, (Nov, 1987) pp. 219-231

Kradin, R. L., *et al.* (1989). Tumour-infiltrating lymphocytes and interleukin-2 in treatment of advanced cancer. *Lancet*, 1, 8638, (Mar 18, 1989) pp. 577-580

Krüger, T., *et al.* (2005). Lessons to be learned from primary renal cell carcinomas: novel tumor antigens and HLA ligands for immunotherapy. *Cancer Immunol Immunother*, 54, 9, (Sep, 2005) pp. 826-836

Kurose, K., *et al.* (2002). Frequent somatic mutations in PTEN and TP53 are mutually exclusive in the stroma of breast carcinomas. *Nat Genet*, 32, 3, (Nov, 2002) pp. 355-357

Kusmartsev, S., *et al.* (2004). Antigen-specific inhibition of CD8+ T cell response by immature myeloid cells in cancer is mediated by reactive oxygen species. *J Immunol*, 172, 2, (Jan 15, 2004) pp. 989-999

Kusmartsev, S. & J. Vieweg (2009). Enhancing the efficacy of cancer vaccines in urologic oncology: new directions. *Nat Rev Urol*, 6, 10, (Oct, 2009) pp. 540-549

Lampson, L. A. & R. Levy (1980). Two populations of Ia-like molecules on a human B cell line. *J Immunol*, 125, 1, (Jul, 1980) pp. 293-299

Lang, S., *et al.* (2000). B7.1 on human carcinomas: costimulation of T cells and enhanced tumor-induced T-cell death. *Cell Immunol*, 201, 2, (May 1, 2000) pp. 132-143

Lapidot, T., *et al.* (1994). A cell initiating human acute myeloid leukaemia after transplantation into SCID mice. *Nature*, 367, 6464, (Feb 17, 1994) pp. 645-648

Lawrence, H. S., (1959). *Cellular and humoral aspects of the hypersensitive states*, P.B. Hoeber, ISBN, New York, USA

Li, H., *et al.* (2007). Tumor microenvironment: the role of the tumor stroma in cancer. *J Cell Biochem*, 101, 4, (Jul 1, 2007) pp. 805-815

Li, M. O., *et al.* (2006). Transforming growth factor-beta regulation of immune responses. *Annu Rev Immunol*, 24, pp. 99-146

Liotta, F., *et al.* (2011). Frequency of regulatory T cells in peripheral blood and in tumour-infiltrating lymphocytes correlates with poor prognosis in renal cell carcinoma. *BJU Int*, 107, 9, (May, 2011) pp. 1500-1506

Lokich, J. (1997). Spontaneous regression of metastatic renal cancer. Case report and literature review. *Am J Clin Oncol*, 20, 4, (Aug, 1997) pp. 416-418

Lutsiak, M. E., *et al.* (2005). Inhibition of CD4(+)25+ T regulatory cell function implicated in enhanced immune response by low-dose cyclophosphamide. *Blood*, 105, 7, (Apr 1, 2005) pp. 2862-2868

Ma, X. J., *et al.* (2009). Gene expression profiling of the tumor microenvironment during breast cancer progression. *Breast Cancer Res*, 11, 1, 2009) pp. R7

Maeda, H. & R. Hirata (1984). Separation of four class II molecules from DR2 and DRw6 homozygous B lymphoid cell lines. *Immunogenetics*, 20, 6, pp. 639-647

Maleckar, J. R. & L. A. Sherman (1987). The composition of the T cell receptor repertoire in nude mice. *J Immunol*, 138, 11, (Jun 1, 1987) pp. 3873-3876

Mantovani, A., *et al.* (2006). Role of tumor-associated macrophages in tumor progression and invasion. *Cancer Metastasis Rev*, 25, 3, (Sep, 2006) pp. 315-322

Marincola, F. M., *et al.* (2000). Escape of human solid tumors from T-cell recognition: molecular mechanisms and functional significance. *Adv Immunol*, 74, 2000) pp. 181-273

Marten, A., *et al.* (2002). Therapeutic vaccination against metastatic renal cell carcinoma by autologous dendritic cells: preclinical results and outcome of a first clinical phase I/II trial. *Cancer Immunol Immunother*, 51, 11-12, (Dec, 2002) pp. 637-644

Marten, A., *et al.* (2003). Allogeneic dendritic cells fused with tumor cells: preclinical results and outcome of a clinical phase I/II trial in patients with metastatic renal cell carcinoma. *Hum Gene Ther*, 14, 5, (Mar 20, 2003) pp. 483-494

Marten, A., *et al.* (2006). Telomerase-pulsed dendritic cells: preclinical results and outcome of a clinical phase I/II trial in patients with metastatic renal cell carcinoma. *Ger Med Sci*, 4, 2006) pp. Doc02

Matsumoto, A., *et al.* (2007). Immunotherapy against metastatic renal cell carcinoma with mature dendritic cells. *Int J Urol*, 14, 4, (Apr, 2007) pp. 277-283

May, M., *et al.* (2009). [Adjuvant autologous tumour cell vaccination in patients with renal cell carcinoma. Overall survival analysis with a follow-up period in excess of more than 10 years]. *Urologe A*, 48, 9, (Sep, 2009) pp. 1075-1083

Miller, R. E. & J. M. Larkin (2009). Combination systemic therapy for advanced renal cell carcinoma. *Oncologist*, 14, 12, (Dec, 2009) pp. 1218-1224

Moinfar, F., *et al.* (2000). Concurrent and independent genetic alterations in the stromal and epithelial cells of mammary carcinoma: implications for tumorigenesis. *Cancer Res*, 60, 9, (May 1, 2000) pp. 2562-2566

Moiseyenko, V. M., *et al.* (2005). Phase I/II trial of gene therapy with autologous tumor cells modified with tag7/PGRP-S gene in patients with disseminated solid tumors: miscellaneous tumors. *Ann Oncol*, 16, 1, (Jan, 2005) pp. 162-168

Morse, M. A., *et al.* (2005). Recent developments in therapeutic cancer vaccines. *Nat Clin Pract Oncol*, 2, 2, (Feb, 2005) pp. 108-113

Nagaraj, S. & D. I. Gabrilovich (2010). Myeloid-derived suppressor cells in human cancer. *Cancer J*, 16, 4, (Jul-Aug, 2010) pp. 348-353

Negrier, S., *et al.* (1998). Recombinant human interleukin-2, recombinant human interferon alfa-2a, or both in metastatic renal-cell carcinoma. Groupe Francais d'Immunotherapie. *N Engl J Med*, 338, 18, (Apr 30, 1998) pp. 1272-1278

Nussbaum, A. K., *et al.* (2001). PAProC: a prediction algorithm for proteasomal cleavages available on the WWW. *Immunogenetics*, 53, 2, (Mar, 2001) pp. 87-94

Ocana, A. & A. Pandiella (2010). Personalized therapies in the cancer "omics" era. *Mol Cancer*, 9, 2010) pp. 202

Ochoa, A. C., *et al.* (2007). Arginase, prostaglandins, and myeloid-derived suppressor cells in renal cell carcinoma. *Clin Cancer Res*, 13, 2 Pt 2, (Jan 15, 2007) pp. 721s-726s

Ohm, J. E. & D. P. Carbone (2001). VEGF as a mediator of tumor-associated immunodeficiency. *Immunol Res*, 23, 2-3, 2001) pp. 263-272

Oosterwijk-Wakka, J. C., *et al.* (2002). Vaccination of patients with metastatic renal cell carcinoma with autologous dendritic cells pulsed with autologous tumor antigens in combination with interleukin-2: a phase 1 study. *J Immunother*, 25, 6, (Nov-Dec, 2002) pp. 500-508

Orimo, A. & R. A. Weinberg (2006). Stromal fibroblasts in cancer: a novel tumor-promoting cell type. *Cell Cycle*, 5, 15, (Aug, 2006) pp. 1597-1601

Pages, F., *et al.* (2010). Immune infiltration in human tumors: a prognostic factor that should not be ignored. *Oncogene*, 29, 8, (Feb 25, 2010) pp. 1093-1102

Pandha, H. S., *et al.* (2004). Dendritic cell immunotherapy for urological cancers using cryopreserved allogeneic tumour lysate-pulsed cells: a phase I/II study. *BJU Int*, 94, 3, (Aug, 2004) pp. 412-418

Parham, P. & F. M. Brodsky (1981). Partial purification and some properties of BB7.2. A cytotoxic monoclonal antibody with specificity for HLA-A2 and a variant of HLA-A28. *Hum Immunol*, 3, 4, (Dec, 1981) pp. 277-299

Parish, C. R. (2003). Cancer immunotherapy: the past, the present and the future. *Immunol Cell Biol*, 81, 2, (Apr, 2003) pp. 106-113

Park, M., *et al.* (2007). Vision loss following denileukin diftitox treatment: a case report of possible posterior ischemic optic neuropathy. *Leuk Lymphoma*, 48, 4, (Apr, 2007) pp. 808-811

Perkins, D. N., *et al.* (1999). Probability-based protein identification by searching sequence databases using mass spectrometry data. *Electrophoresis*, 20, 18, (Dec, 1999) pp. 3551--3567

Pizza, G., *et al.* (2004). Allogeneic gene-modified tumour cells in metastatic kidney cancer. Report II. *Folia Biol (Praha)*, 50, 6, pp. 175-183

Polyak, K., *et al.* (2009). Co-evolution of tumor cells and their microenvironment. *Trends Genet*, 25, 1, (Jan, 2009) pp. 30-38

Prendergast, G. C., *et al.* (2009). IDO recruits Tregs in melanoma. *Cell Cycle*, 8, 12, (Jun 15, 2009) pp. 1818-1819

Rammensee, H., *et al.* (1999). SYFPEITHI: database for MHC ligands and peptide motifs. *Immunogenetics*, 50, 3-4, (Nov, 1999) pp. 213-219

Rebai, N. & B. Malissen (1983). Structural and genetic analyses of HLA class I molecules using monoclonal xenoantibodies. *Tissue Antigens*, 22, 2, (Aug, 1983) pp. 107-117

Reichert, J. M. (2011). Antibody-based therapeutics to watch in 2011. *MAbs*, 3, 1, (Jan-Feb, 2011) pp. 76-99

Reinhardt, C., *et al.* (2010). Results of a randomized Phase 2 study investigating multi-peptide vaccination with IMA901 in advanced renal cell carcinoma (RCC). *Proceedings of the American Society of Clinical Oncology (ASCO)*, Chicago, IL, USA, June 2010

Rini, B. I. (2005). VEGF-targeted therapy in metastatic renal cell carcinoma. *Oncologist*, 10, 3, (Mar, 2005) pp. 191-197

Rini, B. I. & M. B. Atkins (2009). Resistance to targeted therapy in renal-cell carcinoma. *Lancet Oncol*, 10, 10, (Oct, 2009) pp. 992-1000

Rini, B. I., *et al.* (2006). Adoptive immunotherapy by allogeneic stem cell transplantation for metastatic renal cell carcinoma: a CALGB intergroup phase II study. *Biol Blood Marrow Transplant*, 12, 7, (Jul, 2006) pp. 778-785

Rini, B. I., *et al.* (2011). IMA901 multi-peptide vaccine randomized INTernational phase III trial (IMPRINT): A randomized, controlled Phase III study investigating IMA901 multipeptide cancer vaccine in patients receiving sunitinib as first-line therapy for advanced/metastatic RCC, Retrieved 12 Jul 2011, Available from http://www.immatics.com/

Rodriguez, P. C., *et al.* (2009). Arginase I-producing myeloid-derived suppressor cells in renal cell carcinoma are a subpopulation of activated granulocytes. *Cancer Res*, 69, 4, (Feb 15, 2009) pp. 1553-1560

Roepstorff, P. & J. Fohlman (1984). Letter to the editors. *Biological Mass Spectrometry*, 11, 11, 1984) pp. 601--601

Romero, J. M., *et al.* (2006). Analysis of the expression of HLA class I, proinflammatory cytokines and chemokines in primary tumors from patients with localized and metastatic renal cell carcinoma. *Tissue Antigens*, 68, 4, (Oct, 2006) pp. 303-310

Saenz-Lopez, P., *et al.* (2010). Higher HLA class I expression in renal cell carcinoma than in autologous normal tissue. *Tissue Antigens*, 75, 2, (Feb, 2010) pp. 110-118

Sahin, U., *et al.* (1995). Human neoplasms elicit multiple specific immune responses in the autologous host. *Proc Natl Acad Sci U S A*, 92, 25, (Dec, 1995) pp. 11810--11813

Scheffer, S. R., *et al.* (2003). Apoptotic, but not necrotic, tumor cell vaccines induce a potent immune response in vivo. *Int J Cancer*, 103, 2, (Jan 10, 2003) pp. 205-211

Schirle, M., *et al.* (2000). Identification of tumor-associated MHC class I ligands by a novel T cell-independent approach. *Eur J Immunol*, 30, 8, (Aug, 2000) pp. 2216-2225

Schulze, W. X. & B. Usadel (2010). Quantitation in mass-spectrometry-based proteomics. *Annu Rev Plant Biol*, 61, 2010) pp. 491-516

Schwaab, T., *et al.* (2000). A randomized phase II trial comparing two different sequence combinations of autologous vaccine and human recombinant interferon gamma and human recombinant interferon alpha2B therapy in patients with metastatic renal cell carcinoma: clinical outcome and analysis of immunological parameters. *J Urol*, 163, 4, (Apr, 2000) pp. 1322-1327

Schwaab, T., *et al.* (2009). Clinical and immunologic effects of intranodal autologous tumor lysate-dendritic cell vaccine with Aldesleukin (Interleukin 2) and IFN-{alpha}2a therapy in metastatic renal cell carcinoma patients. *Clin Cancer Res*, 15, 15, (Aug 1, 2009) pp. 4986-4992

Seliger, B., *et al.* (2002). HLA class I antigen abnormalities and immune escape by malignant cells. *Semin Cancer Biol*, 12, 1, (Feb, 2002) pp. 3-13

Seliger, B., *et al.* (2003). Detection of renal cell carcinoma-associated markers via proteome- and other 'ome'-based analyses. *Brief Funct Genomic Proteomic*, 2, 3, (Oct, 2003) pp. 194-212

Serafini, P., *et al.* (2004). High-dose granulocyte-macrophage colony-stimulating factor-producing vaccines impair the immune response through the recruitment of myeloid suppressor cells. *Cancer Res*, 64, 17, (Sep 1, 2004) pp. 6337-6343

Serafini, P., *et al.* (2008). Myeloid-derived suppressor cells promote cross-tolerance in B-cell lymphoma by expanding regulatory T cells. *Cancer Res*, 68, 13, (Jul 1, 2008) pp. 5439-5449

Shimizu, K., *et al.* (2001). Enhancement of tumor lysate- and peptide-pulsed dendritic cell-based vaccines by the addition of foreign helper protein. *Cancer Res*, 61, 6, (Mar 15, 2001) pp. 2618-2624

Sica, G. L., *et al.* (2003). B7-H4, a molecule of the B7 family, negatively regulates T cell immunity. *Immunity*, 18, 6, (Jun, 2003) pp. 849-861

Siebels, M., *et al.* (2011). A clinical phase I/II trial with the monoclonal antibody cG250 (RENCAREX(R)) and interferon-alpha-2a in metastatic renal cell carcinoma patients. *World J Urol*, 29, 1, (Feb, 2011) pp. 121-126

Simons, J. W. & B. Mikhak (1998). Ex-vivo gene therapy using cytokine-transduced tumor vaccines: molecular and clinical pharmacology. *Semin Oncol*, 25, 6, (Dec, 1998) pp. 661-676

Slingluff, C. L., Jr., *et al.* (2009). Effect of granulocyte/macrophage colony-stimulating factor on circulating CD8+ and CD4+ T-cell responses to a multipeptide melanoma vaccine: outcome of a multicenter randomized trial. *Clin Cancer Res*, 15, 22, (Nov 15, 2009) pp. 7036-7044

Smigielski, E. M., *et al.* (2000). dbSNP: a database of single nucleotide polymorphisms. *Nucleic Acids Res*, 28, 1, (Jan, 2000) pp. 352--355

Spits, H., *et al.* (1983). Characterization of monoclonal antibodies against cell surface molecules associated with cytotoxic activity of natural and activated killer cells and cloned CTL lines. *Hybridoma*, 2, 4, 1983) pp. 423-437

Stevanovic, S. (2002). Identification of tumour-associated T-cell epitopes for vaccine development. *Nat Rev Cancer*, 2, 7, (Jul, 2002) pp. 514-520

Stickel, J. S., *et al.* (2011). Quantification of HLA class I molecules on renal cell carcinoma using Edman degradation. *BMC Urol*, 11, pp. 1

Stratton, M. R. (2011). Exploring the genomes of cancer cells: progress and promise. *Science*, 331, 6024, (Mar 25, 2011) pp. 1553-1558

Sturm, M., *et al.* (2008). OpenMS - an open-source software framework for mass spectrometry. *BMC Bioinformatics*, 9, 2008) pp. 163

Stutman, O. (1979). Spontaneous tumors in nude mice: effect of the viable yellow gene. *Exp Cell Biol*, 47, 2, 1979) pp. 129-135

Suekane, S., *et al.* (2007). Phase I trial of personalized peptide vaccination for cytokine-refractory metastatic renal cell carcinoma patients. *Cancer Sci*, 98, 12, (Dec, 2007) pp. 1965-1968

Sufan, R. I., *et al.* (2004). The role of von Hippel-Lindau tumor suppressor protein and hypoxia in renal clear cell carcinoma. *Am J Physiol Renal Physiol*, 287, 1, (Jul, 2004) pp. F1-6

Tani, K., *et al.* (2004). Phase I study of autologous tumor vaccines transduced with the GM-CSF gene in four patients with stage IV renal cell cancer in Japan: clinical and immunological findings. *Mol Ther*, 10, 4, (Oct, 2004) pp. 799-816

Tatsugami, K., *et al.* (2008). Dendritic cell therapy in combination with interferon-alpha for the treatment of metastatic renal cell carcinoma. *Int J Urol*, 15, 8, (Aug, 2008) pp. 694-698

Taylor, A., *et al.* (2006). Mechanisms of immune suppression by interleukin-10 and transforming growth factor-beta: the role of T regulatory cells. *Immunology*, 117, 4, (Apr, 2006) pp. 433-442

Therasse, P., *et al.* (2000). New guidelines to evaluate the response to treatment in solid tumors. European Organization for Research and Treatment of Cancer, National Cancer Institute of the United States, National Cancer Institute of Canada. *J Natl Cancer Inst*, 92, 3, (Feb 2, 2000) pp. 205-216

Thompson, R. H., *et al.* (2005). Costimulatory molecule B7-H1 in primary and metastatic clear cell renal cell carcinoma. *Cancer*, 104, 10, (Nov 15, 2005) pp. 2084-2091

Thornton, A. M. & E. M. Shevach (2000). Suppressor effector function of CD4+CD25+ immunoregulatory T cells is antigen nonspecific. *J Immunol*, 164, 1, (Jan 1, 2000) pp. 183-190

Topalian, S. L., *et al.* (1988). Immunotherapy of patients with advanced cancer using tumor-infiltrating lymphocytes and recombinant interleukin-2: a pilot study. *J Clin Oncol*, 6, 5, (May, 1988) pp. 839-853

Toussaint, N. C. & O. Kohlbacher (2009). OptiTope--a web server for the selection of an optimal set of peptides for epitope-based vaccines. *Nucleic Acids Res*, 37, Web Server issue, (Jul, 2009) pp. W617--W622

Tureci, O., *et al.* (2005). Identification of tumor-associated autoantigens with SEREX. *Methods Mol Med*, 109, pp. 137-154

Tykodi, S. S., *et al.* (2004). Allogeneic hematopoietic cell transplantation for metastatic renal cell carcinoma after nonmyeloablative conditioning: toxicity, clinical response, and immunological response to minor histocompatibility antigens. *Clin Cancer Res*, 10, 23, (Dec 1, 2004) pp. 7799-7811

Uemura, H., *et al.* (2006). A phase I trial of vaccination of CA9-derived peptides for HLA-A24-positive patients with cytokine-refractory metastatic renal cell carcinoma. *Clin Cancer Res*, 12, 6, (Mar 15, 2006) pp. 1768-1775

Uyttenhove, C., *et al.* (2003). Evidence for a tumoral immune resistance mechanism based on tryptophan degradation by indoleamine 2,3-dioxygenase. *Nat Med*, 9, 10, (Oct, 2003) pp. 1269-1274

Van den Hove, L. E., *et al.* (1997). Phenotype, cytokine production and cytolytic capacity of fresh (uncultured) tumour-infiltrating T lymphocytes in human renal cell carcinoma. *Clin Exp Immunol*, 109, 3, (Sep, 1997) pp. 501-509

Visvader, J. E. & G. J. Lindeman (2008). Cancer stem cells in solid tumours: accumulating evidence and unresolved questions. *Nat Rev Cancer*, 8, 10, (Oct, 2008) pp. 755-768

von Boehmer, H. (2005). Mechanisms of suppression by suppressor T cells. *Nat Immunol*, 6, 4, (Apr, 2005) pp. 338-344

Wang, H. Y., *et al.* (2004). Tumor-specific human CD4+ regulatory T cells and their ligands: implications for immunotherapy. *Immunity*, 20, 1, (Jan, 2004) pp. 107-118

Wang, J. C. & J. E. Dick (2005). Cancer stem cells: lessons from leukemia. *Trends Cell Biol*, 15, 9, (Sep, 2005) pp. 494-501

Wang, K., *et al.* (2009). Identification of tumor-associated antigens by using SEREX in hepatocellular carcinoma. *Cancer Lett*, 281, 2, (Aug 28, 2009) pp. 144-150

Weber, F., *et al.* (2005). Variability in organ-specific EGFR mutational spectra in tumour epithelium and stroma may be the biological basis for differential responses to tyrosine kinase inhibitors. *Br J Cancer*, 92, 10, (May 23, 2005) pp. 1922-1926

Wei, Y. C., *et al.* (2007). Combined treatment of dendritoma vaccine and low-dose interleukin-2 in stage IV renal cell carcinoma patients induced clinical response: A pilot study. *Oncol Rep*, 18, 3, (Sep, 2007) pp. 665-671

Weinzierl, A. O., *et al.* (2007). Distorted relation between mRNA copy number and corresponding major histocompatibility complex ligand density on the cell surface. *Mol Cell Proteomics*, 6, 1, (Jan, 2007) pp. 102-113

Welters, M. J., *et al.* (2009). Report on the sixth annual meeting of the Association for Immunotherapy of Cancer (CIMT), May 15 and 16, 2008 in Mainz, Germany. *Cancer Immunol Immunother*, 58, 5, (May, 2009) pp. 777-787

Wierecky, J., *et al.* (2006). Immunologic and clinical responses after vaccinations with peptide-pulsed dendritic cells in metastatic renal cancer patients. *Cancer Res*, 66, 11, (Jun 1, 2006) pp. 5910-5918

Wolchok, J. D., *et al.* (2009). Guidelines for the evaluation of immune therapy activity in solid tumors: immune-related response criteria. *Clin Cancer Res*, 15, 23, (Dec 1, 2009) pp. 7412-7420

Wong, K. M., *et al.* (2011). Unraveling the Genetics of Cancer: Genome Sequencing and Beyond. *Annu Rev Genomics Hum Genet*, (Jun 2, 2011)

Woo, E. Y., *et al.* (2001). Regulatory CD4(+)CD25(+) T cells in tumors from patients with early-stage non-small cell lung cancer and late-stage ovarian cancer. *Cancer Res*, 61, 12, (Jun 15, 2001) pp. 4766-4772

Wood, C., *et al.* (2008). An adjuvant autologous therapeutic vaccine (HSPPC-96; vitespen) versus observation alone for patients at high risk of recurrence after nephrectomy for renal cell carcinoma: a multicentre, open-label, randomised phase III trial. *Lancet*, 372, 9633, (Jul 12, 2008) pp. 145-154

World Health Organization., (1979). *WHO handbook for reporting results of cancer treatment*, World Health Organization, ISBN: 9241700483, Geneva, Albany, N.Y.

Yates, J. R., *et al.* (2009). Proteomics by mass spectrometry: approaches, advances, and applications. *Annu Rev Biomed Eng*, 11, 2009) pp. 49-79

Young, M. R., *et al.* (1997). Increased recurrence and metastasis in patients whose primary head and neck squamous cell carcinomas secreted granulocyte-macrophage colony-stimulating factor and contained CD34+ natural suppressor cells. *Int J Cancer*, 74, 1, (Feb 20, 1997) pp. 69-74

Zea, A. H., *et al.* (2005). Arginase-producing myeloid suppressor cells in renal cell carcinoma patients: a mechanism of tumor evasion. *Cancer Res*, 65, 8, (Apr 15, 2005) pp. 3044-3048

Zou, W. (2006). Regulatory T cells, tumour immunity and immunotherapy. *Nat Rev Immunol*, 6, 4, (Apr, 2006) pp. 295-307

Part 2

Surgery

10

Clinical Spectrum of Patients with Renal Cell Carcinoma

Mehrnaz Asadi Gharabaghi
Tehran University of Medical Sciences
Iran

1. Introduction

The classic triad of flank pain, palpable mass and hematuria exists in less than 20 percent of patients with renal cell carcinoma, and the tumor may become large in its origin before any local sign or symptom arises. Therefore, it is common to detect the tumor only after the metastasis develops.

Renal cell carcinoma (RCC) may present with diverse range of clinical manifestations. Many cases of renal cell carcinoma are unsuspected initially. The same is true for tumor recurrence even several years after primary tumor resection. For instance, it is not uncommon for a thyroid nodule to be the presenting feature of metastatic RCC. Renal cell carcinoma may masquerade any other illness so it is named tumor of internal medicine. Here the clinical presentations of the tumor within different body organs are discussed. In the followings, the clinical spectrum is arranged by each system in the body. The symptoms and signs of tumor in the urinary system are discussed separately. The systemic manifestations of cancer-related treatment are not discussed here.

2. Skin manifestations

Dermatological manifestations of renal cell carcinoma are not common. However, there are reports of coetaneous metastases as the primary clue to the tumor diagnosis (Mueller et al., 2004; Srinivasan, 2010). Skin nodules are more common. Scalp is the most prevalent site followed by chest and abdomen (Arrabal-Polo et al, 2009; Dorairajan et al., 1999).

Small vessel vasculitis limited to skin has been noted in renal cell carcinoma. It causes papules, nodules and even skin ulceration. Maynard et al reported a case of an adult male with renal cell carcinoma that initially presented with leukocytoclastic vasculitis involving skin, joints and gastrointestinal tracts (Maynard, 2010).

Palmar fibromatosis,acanthosis nigricans,hypertrichosis lanuginose,paraneoplastic erythroderma, bullous pemphigoid, and acquired ichthyosis are rare coetaneous manifestations of internal malignancies that are rarely reported in cases of renal cell carcinoma (Klein et al., 2009; Tebbe et al.,1991).

Hence, it cannot be over emphasized that an occult cancer such as renal cell carcinoma needs to be considered in evaluation of an elderly patient presenting with systemic vasculitis or certain dermatologic disorders.

3. Musculoskeletal manifestations

Renal cell carcinoma avidly involves the skeleton .After lung; the skeleton is the second most common site for metastases (Fottner et al., 2010). It ranks as the sixth solid tumor responsible for bone metastases that cause severe bone pain or debilitating skeletal complications such as pathologic fractures and spinal cord compression. Pelvis, ribs and vertebrae are the most prevalent sites for bone metastases. Patients with bone involvement portend a grave prognosis and most of them die within a year. Various therapeutic modalities such as chemo radiotherapy, surgery and bisphosphonates have been introduced with variable success (Lipton et al., 2004).

A 54 year-old man presented with multiple pathologic fractures of thoracic vertebrae to my department. He was finally diagnosed to suffer from advanced renal cell carcinoma. He was a truck driver and noticed the severe back pain while fixing his truck. The fractures occurred when he was tightening the screws forcefully. Therefore, it seems prudent to look for a kidney cancer while confronting bone metastasis with unknown origin.

Cancer and autoimmunity is a well-known inter-disciplinary entity .Tumor products behave as haptens triggering an overwhelming autoimmune response within the body. The autoimmune disorder may herald the presence of an occult cancer.

Inflammatory myopathies, myositis and inclusion body myositis are reported as paraneoplastic syndromes associated with renal cell carcinoma. Klausner et al reported a case of 45- year -old man presented with polymyosistis that finally diagnosed to have renal cell carcinoma (Klausner et al, 2002). Similarly, Respicio et al reported a case of concurrent renal cell carcinoma, interstitial lung disease and polymyositis in a 58 year-old man (Respicio et al., 2007).It is not exactly known whether it is possible to predict the type of solid tumor at the time of inflammatory mysoitis by means of tumor biologic markers. Amoura et al reported that markers as CA-125 and CA19-9 may predict developing the offending tumor in advance and need to be included in evaluation of patients with inflammatory myopathic syndromes(Amoura et al.,2005).

A syndrome resembling to polymyalgia rheumatica (PMR) has been described as a paraneoplastic manifestation of solid tumors. The syndrome is not steroid responsive. Yet, it is not clear whether it will be improved after nephrectomy (Sidhom et al., 1993). Hence, it is reasonable to look for an occult solid tumor such as renal cell carcinoma in a patient with PMR refractory to steroids. Niccoli et al reported three patients presenting with PMR mimicking syndrome heralding renal cell carcinoma. They suggested that besides inefficacy of steroids, absence of morning stiffness and characteristic sonographic findings of shoulder are features of PMR mimicking syndrome associated with RCC (Niccoli et al., 2002).

RS3PE (remitting symmetric sero negative synovitis with pitting edema) is a syndrome with symptoms similar to PMR; it occurs in patients older than 50 and may be associated with solid tumors or hematologic malignancies. It is mandatory to rule out an occult malignancy in the setting of RS3PE syndrome. Lung, breast, prostate and rarely kidney cancers have been reported as the underlying solid tumors in patients with this syndrome (Juncadella et al., 2003; Marto et al., 2010; Russel, 2005).

Other rare rheumatic manifestations of renal cell carcinoma include metastatic monoarthritis and multi centric reticulo histiocytosis (MR). The latter is a syndrome presenting with coetaneous nodules and severe destructive arthritis .It may be associated with an internal malignancy. Tan et al reported two cases of MR associated with urologic malignancies (Placed et al, 2010; Tan et al.2011).

4. Nervous system manifestations

Paraneoplastic neuropathy is a well-known autoimmune neuropathy associated with anti neuronal nuclear antibody. Roy et al (Roy et al., 2002) reported chronic sensory motor polyneuropathy in a 65-year-old man several months before the diagnosis of RCC. Allen et al also reported a case of acute demyelinating neuropathy in a case of papillary renal cell carcinoma that resolved following nephrectomy (Allen et al., 2011). Torvik et al reported three cases with necrotizing vasculitic involvement of peripheral nerves that were diagnosed to have renal cell carcinoma through postmortem follow up (Torvik & Berntzen, 1968).

Numb chin syndrome is numbness of lower lip, chine and gingiva of anterior lower teeth. It may be associated with a visceral malignancy such as lung, breast cancer or leukemia; however, it has been reported in renal cell carcinoma. Inferior alveolar/mental nerve is involved due to metastasis to mandible or nerve sheath infiltration by tumor (Divya et al., 2010; Lata & Kumar, 2010).

Opsoclonus is an ocular dyskinesia characterized by involuntary, repetitive, rapid conjugate saccades. It is most commonly seen in children. In an adult, it may herald an internal malignancy. Koukoulis A et al reported a case of paraneoplastic opsoclonus in a 64 year- old man. The patient was diagnosed to have papillary renal cell carcinoma 6 months after the diagnosis of opsoclonus (Koukoulis et al., 1998).

Antinueronal nuclear antibody type 1 (classically known as anti –Hu) is detected in cancer associated autoimmune neurologic disorders (lucchinetti et al., 1998) .Patients develop various forms of neurologic disease including Lambert-Eaton myasthenic syndrome, encephalitis, cerebellar ataxia and so forth. For instance, Ammar et al reported a case of 64-year- old woman who presented with acute cerebellar ataxia as the initial manifestation of renal cell carcinoma (Ammar et al., 2008). There is also a report of bilateral diaphragmatic paralysis as a paraneoplastic neurologic disease secondary to RCC that ameliorated after nephrectomy (Rijnders & Decramer, 2000).Therefore, it is appropriate to investigate for an occult cancer when confronting an idiopathic bilateral diaphragmatic paralysis.

Brain and spinal metastases are common in advanced stages of RCC. However, solitary brain metastasis and relevant clinical findings such as headache and focal neurologic deficit may be the presenting signs of the cancer (Candiano et al., 2010). Spinal metastases are usually extra dural but intradural involvement with resulting neurologic deficits, especially cauda equina syndrome were reported (Lin et al., 2011). Back pain and sciatica due to metastatic nerve root infiltration of lumbo sacral nerves have been reported in RCC patients (Shakeel et al., 2009). Intramedullary spinal metastasis that are the rarest type of spinal involvement have also been reported as the presenting sign in RCC (Asadi et al., 2009; Donovan& Freeman, 2006; Gómez de la Riva et al., 2005; Schijns et al., 2000). Although uncommon, an occult cancer such as renal cell carcinoma needs to be considered in differential diagnosis of the above-mentioned syndromes.

5. Vascular system manifestations

Renal vein and caval thromboses are among the well- known thrombotic events associated with renal cell carcinoma. Left-sided varicocele that does not decompress after taking the recumbent position is a well -known complication of the locally advanced RCC. It is due to tumor thrombus extending along the renal vein that blocks drainage of left spermatic vein into inferior vena cava (IVC).It is not just left spermatic vein that may become clogged .Right spermatic vein is at risk too. Shinsaka et al reported a case of right varicocele as a result of RCC thrombus in right spermatic vein without simultaneous caval thrombosis (Al-Taan et al., 2007;Shinsaka et al., 2006).Furthermore, prothrombotic state as a paraneoplastic feature of RCC may cause thrombosis in unusual sites such as subclavian veins(Hameed et al.,2011). Hence, it is worthwhile to consider RCC in evaluating patients with idiopathic venous thrombosis, especially in an unusual site.

6. Hematologic manifestations

Cytopenia, especially anemia is a common feature of the tumor. Polycythemia may also be seen, although less frequently (Mohammed Ilyas et al., 2008). Although, micro angiopathic hemolytic anemia, hemolytic uremic syndrome and disseminated intravascular coagulopathy may occur because of cancer chemotherapy in RCC, the tumor rarely presents with such a hematologic manifestation as thrombocytopenia .Yet, there are reports of metastatic RCC presenting with thrombocytopenia due to bone marrow carcinomatosis (Florcken et al., 2009).

Disturbation in fibrinolysis system is a well -known feature of hematologic and non-hematologic tumors such as prostate cancer. Plasminogen is converted to plasmin; tissue plasminogen activator (t PA) or urokinase- type plasminogen activator (uPA) promotes the conversion. Some tumors express high level of tPA activity. This feature not only brings some sort of bleeding diathesis but also seems to be vital for tumor survival. In fact, the variable expression of fibrinolysis system components in a given cancer may affect the prognosis. For instance, patients with greater expression of u-PA on breast cancer cells have shorter survival and increased chance of relapse (Bell, 1996).In renal cell carcinoma, it has been demonstrated that expression of plasminogen inhibitor-1 is an independent poor prognostic factor as it promotes tumor angiogenesis and metastasis (Choi et al.,2011;Zubcaet al.,2010). Therefore, changes in hematologic parameters are not only paraneoplstic features of RCC but also of prognostic value.

7. Pulmonary manifestations

Lung metastases are common in natural history of RCC. Single or multiple variable -sized pulmonary nodules are usually detected in patients with advanced RCC. Regarding large reserve volume of lung, tumor burden may become so huge before any respiratory symptom such as dyspnea or cough develops. Besides this common mode of presentation, lymphangitic carcinomatosis may develop in setting of metastatic RCC. It is an interstitial lung disorder caused by lymphangitic spread of tumors such as breast, lung and rarely kidney cancer. It usually manifests with obstinate cough and progressive dyspnea. Wallach et al reported a case of 68 year -old man who presented with respiratory symptoms 20 months after nephrectomy for stage III RCC. He had lymphangitic carcinomatosis.

According to their review of literature, there are less than 10 reports of such patients (Wallach et al., 2011).

RCC metastases are not confined to lung parenchyma. There are reports of endobronchial metastases from RCC .Therefore hemoptysis or a pulmonary atelectasis may result from endobronchial spread of RCC.As the tumor is a hyper vascular one, it is mandatory to take precaution while planning local therapeutic modalities for symptomatic metastases (Mathai et al., 2007; Suyama et al., 2011).

Malignant pleural effusion secondary to RCC is rare and usually seen with papillary and clear cell histological types. There are reports of special cases of malignant effusion secondary to RCC.As an example; Chetcuti K et al reported a case of massive spontaneous hemothorax in a 78 year- old man with a history of RCC. The culprit was a chest wall metastasis of RCC (Chetcuti et al., 2010; Teresa et al., 2011).

Mediastinal lymph adenopathy and masses are seen in advanced stages of renal cell carcinoma or as presenting features of primary tumor or tumor recurrence. They are closely correlated with poor prognosis (Mattana et al., 1996; Winter et al., 2010). Niikura S et al reported a case of 62 year- old man presented with mediastinal lymph node enlargements 19 years after nephrectomy for RCC (Niikura et al., 1999).

Pulmonary infarction due to tumor emboli within pulmonary circulation is an unusual manifestation of renal cell carcinoma .The tumor emboli originates from thrombus extending along vena cava, right sided heart or proximal part of pulmonary artery (Shiono et al.,2001;Wieder et al.,2003). The disease presents with acute or sub acute cor pulmonale and cytological study of pulmonary artery sample helps diagnosis.

Despite the grave prognosis associated with pulmonary involvement in patients with RCC, there is a report by Okubo Y et al who described a patient with an obstinate cough as the sole manifestation of non- metastatic RCC .Cough disappeared after nephrectomy and recurred with tumor relapse (Okubo et al., 2007).

8. Cardiac manifestations

Heart may be involved in different manners by a non-cardiac tumor. For example, certain chemotherapeutic drugs and radiotherapy have deleterious effects on heart. Opportunistic infection of cardiac chambers has been demonstrated because of immune suppression in cancer patients. The tumor may involve the pericardium and less frequently, myoendocardium.So malignant pericardial effusion is a common finding in advanced cancer patients (Kim et al., 2010). Although uncommon, there are reports of malignant pericardial effusion secondary to RCC (Zustovich et al., 2008).

In RCC, vena cava thrombosis can extend beyond the hepatic veins into the right atrium (Kalkat et al., 2008) .However; there are reports of cardiac metastasis mimicking primary cardiac tumors without concurrent cava involvement (Aburto et al., 2009; Talukder et al., 2010). For instance, Lee HJ et al demonstrated a case of 77- year- old man with 2- month history of RCC in whom cardiac metastasis caused left ventricular outflow tract obstruction (Lee et al., 2010). Miyamoto MI et al reported a case of metastatic renal carcinoma with a left atrial mass mimicking myxoma. They demonstrated that the mass was RCC metastasis derived from pulmonary vein tumor extension. The pulmonary vein itself had been involved from adjacent mediastinal lymph nodes (Miyamoto& Picard, 2002). Cardiac metastasis in a patient with known history of primary cancer is not challenging to diagnosis. Yet it is not uncommon for a RCC to present initially with a cardiac mass (Crouch & Tak,2002).Therefore, it needs to be vigilant to the presence of an occult cancer when evaluating a cardiac mass even if it resembles a primary cardiac tumor and there is no extra cardio respratory symptom.

Not only myopericardium is involved in RCC but also the endocardium may become diseased in RCC. Non-bacterial endocarditis is a well -known disease entity in various diseases such as HIV infection, connective tissue disorders and cancers. The exact mechanism is not yet defined but thrombophilic state associated with malignancy may be responsible. The most primary cancer site is pancreas (Johnson et al., 2010). In literature review, there is few report of RCC associated with non-bacterial thrombotic endocarditis.

9. Gastrointestinal manifestations

Gastrointestinal (GI) tract is involved by RCC in different ways. Stauffer's syndrome constitutes reversible abnormalities in liver function tests including enzymes and pro thrombin time. It may present as hepatocellular or cholestatic liver disease. It is not due to liver metastasis and actually caused by humoral effects of inflammatory cytokines produced by the tumor. Therefore, the abnormalities disappear after tumor resection by nephrectomy (Kranidiotis et al., 2009). However, there are reports of renal cell carcinoma metastases to various organs of gastrointestinal tracts.

Oral cavity metastases from RCC have been demonstrated. In fact, intraoral soft tissue metastases are not common. They usually originate from lung and breast cancers. Metastatic oral cavity lesions rarely present as the initial feature of an occult cancer. For instance, Maestre-Rodríguez O reported a case of 55- year-old man who underwent resection of a gingival tumor that finally diagnosed to be metastatic RCC (Will et al., 2008; Maestre-Rodríguez et al., 2009). Esophageal metastasis producing local symptoms such as dysphagia is not surprising in a case of an advanced RCC (de los Monteros-Sanchez et al., 2004). Hematogenous spread of RCC to stomach is seen, albeit with concomitant metastases in other organs, especially lungs (Pollheimer et al., 2008).Although uncommon, gastric metastasis and upper gastrointestinal bleeding may be the initial feature of RCC. Tiwari P et al reported a 58- year-old woman with a 2-week history of melena. The source of bleeding was a 3cm×5cm vascular polypoid antral mass .She was finally diagnosed to have metastatic RCC (Tiwari et al., 2010).

Intraluminal metastases from RCC may be the source of intestinal bleeding or less commonly intussusceptions. They may behave as the leading point for an intestinal obstruction and intussusceptions. Periampullary region, duodenum and jejunum rank the most common sites .Yet, other sites as large bowel may be involved too (Eo et al., 2008; Loualidi et al., 2004; Nozawa et al., 2003; Papachristodoulou et al., 2004; Roviello et al., 2006; Sadler et al., 2007 Takeda et al., 2011). The above cases highlight the importance of considering RCC metastasis as a source of intestinal bleeding and/or obstruction, especially in patients with a known cancer history.

Liver is the organ that is frequently involved in advanced RCC (Staehler et al., 2010). Yet it is not the only solid organ within GI tract involved by RCC. Pancreatic metastasis may occur due to a close proximity to the left kidney. However, the pancreas may be involved as a nest for metastatic deposits even years after nephrectomy. Yokonishi T et al reported pancreatic metastasis in a 74 year -old man who had history of nephrectomy due to RCC 25 years before (Yokonishi et al., 2010). The physicians must be alert to pancreatic metastasis from renal cell carcinoma and differentiate it from primary tumors of the gland because the prognosis differs in each case. Ghavamian R et al reviewed 23 patients with metastatic RCC to the pancreas .They found that imaging features of metastatic RCC resembled the primary RCC and differed from pancreatic tumours such as adenocarcinoma. RCC is a hyper vascular tumour, hence the metastasis enhances in early phase of contrasted abdominal computed tomography. They also noticed that the mean interval for pancreatic metastases to develop after nephrectomy was 9.8 years (Ghavamian et al., 2000).

Budd-Chiari syndrome defined by presence of abdominal pain, hepatomegaly and ascites has also been reported as a manifestation of renal cell carcinoma. The syndrome caused by tumor thrombus extending along vena cava. As a result, hepatic venous drainage system will be blocked .It may become fulminate if not treated on time (Moragnoni et al., 2010; Shih et al., 2009).

Bowel ischemia may be seen in RCC not only as a complication of immunotherapy but also as a consequence of embolic infarcts from tumor thrombus in left heart (Low et al.,1989;Sparano etal.,1991).

Sinistral portal hypertension refers to gastric variceal hemorrhage secondary to splenic vein thrombosis. It is most common in the setting of pancreatic pathologies such as pancreatitis, pseudocysts and cancer. There is no concurrent liver dysfunction (Singhal et al., 2006). Joya Seijo MD et al reported a case of sinistral portal hypertension and gastric bleeding as the initial manifestation of left sided RCC infiltrating the pancreas (Joya Seijo et al., 2004). RCC may rarely present with variceal bleeding. A 51- year- old man presented to our hospital with an episode of upper gastrointestinal bleeding twelve years after nephrectomy for a clear cell RCC. He was diagnosed to have downhill esophageal varices. They were formed by compressing effects of enlarged mediastinal lymph nodes upon the azygous vein .Pathologic review of the lymph nodes revealed recurrence of clear cell carcinoma.

10. Endocrinologic system

Like any other organ, endocrine system is not safe from RCC. Metastatic RCC may invade pituitary gland and mimics a nonfunctional pituitary adenoma (Kramer et al., 2010). Panhypopituitarism, suprasellar extension, headache, hemianopia, galactorrhea and diabetes insipidus are reported because of RCC metastasis to pituitary gland (Gopan et al., 2007). Although uncommon, thyroid metastasis in RCC has been demonstrated that can be of diagnostic challenge to be differentiated from primary thyroid tumors (Cimino-Mathews et al,2011).Adrenal, testicular and ovarian metastases have been reported in the course of disease even years after primary nephrectomy (Guney et al.,2010;Wu et al.,2010). Toquero L et al reported a case of 54- year old woman with a pelvic mass as an initial presentation of RCC. The mass was actually ovarian metastasis from RCC (Toquero et al., 2009).Ovarian metastases usually originate from stomach, colon, breast cancers and lymphoma. However,

RCC needs to be considered in differential diagnosis. The patients with this sort of metastasis in either testis or ovary usually seek medical care because of localized symptoms rather than a symptom relevant to hypogonadism.It is may be due to age of patients who are usually in 50s-70s.

11. Paraneoplastic syndromes

There are constellation of signs, symptoms and laboratory data abnormalities not related to tumor local effect or its metastases. Some of them such as Stauffer's syndrome have been mentioned above. Most of them are cytokine mediated such as neoplastic fever (Alsirafy et al., 2011) .The remaining may be due to tumor products. Humoral hypercalcemia of malignancy is a paraneoplastic feature of various tumors. In RCC, it is multi factorial. Widespread bone metastases, parathormone-related peptide and increased production of 1, 25 hydroxyvitamin D are responsible. Therefore, hypercalcaemia in patients with RCC may respond to administration of steroids (Shivnani et al., 2009).

Glucose metabolism abnormalities have been demonstrated in association with RCC. The tumor can produce insulin like growth factor II resulting in hypoglycemia (Berman & Harland, 2001).On the other hand, hyper glycemia is reported as a paraneoplastic endocrinopathy in patients with RCC(Jobe et al.,1993).For instance, Yumura Y et al reported 2 patients whose diabetes was controlled after nephrectomy for RCC (Yumura et al.,2007).

Although hypertension is a complication of targeted therapy in RCC patients, it may develop as a paraneoplastic feature of kidney cancer not related to treatment (kirkali,2011).Some of the patients show increased blood level of renin and plasma renin activity as a possible cause of their increased blood pressure(Steffens et al.,1992).

Gynecomastia attributable to human chorionic gonadotropin overproduction has been reported as another paraneoplastic endocrinopathy in RCC (Mohammed Ilyas et al., 2008).It has also been demonstrated that expression of beta subunit of human chorionic gonadotropin is associated with adverse prognosis in RCC (Hotakainen et al., 2002, 2006).

Cancerous erythrocytosis is another rare para neoplastic disorder associated with RCC caused by over expression of erythropoietin and hypoxemia induced factor. However, only a small percentage of patients with over expression of erythropoietin develop paraneoplastic erythrocytosis (Wiesener et al., 2007).Although uncommon, paraneoplastic erythrocytosis of RCC may have grave sequels; Kruyt ND et al reported a case of 65- year - old man who presented with neurologic deficits due to multiple cerebral infarctions as the initial presentation of RCC. His erythrocytosis and cognitive dysfunction relieved after nephrectomy for newly diagnosed RCC (Kruyt & Wessels, 2006).

Although above-mentioned paraneoplastic syndromes are not common in RCC, they are of value for both diagnosis and estimating the prognosis of the primary tumor.

12. Miscellaneous abnormalities

RCC behaves unpredictably so it is common to confront its metastasis in unusual sites. The followings are some examples. It has been reported that renal cell carcinoma may initially present as an orbital mass, a mass within paranasal sinuses, gallbladder metastasis, cerebellopontine angle or superior vena cava syndrome due to supraclavicular lymph nodes involvement (Cobo-Dolset al., 2006; Fang et al., 2010; Panarese et al., 2002; sakura et al., 2007; Mudiayanselage et al., 2008).

13. Conclusion

The classic triad of flank pain, hematuria and palpable abdominal mass occurs in a small fraction of patients with renal cell carcinoma, so it is wise to be aware of various clinical presentations of the disease. The above-mentioned clinical features are summarized in Table-1.

Skin
coetaneous metastases, Skin nodules, Small vessel vasculitis, Palmar fibromatosis,Acanthosis nigricans, Hypertrichosis lanuginose,Paraneoplastic erythroderma, Bullous pemphigoid,Acquired ichthyosis
Musculoskeletal system
Bone metastases, Inflammatory myopathies, Myositis , Inclusion body myositis, Polymyalgia rheumatica- like syndrome, RS3PE (remitting symmetric sero negative synovitis with pitting edema), Metastatic monoarthritis and multi centric reticulo histiocytosis (MR)
Nervous system
Paraneoplastic neuropathy, Numb chin syndrome, Opsoclonus, Lambert-Eaton myasthenic syndrome, Encephalitis, Cerebellar ataxia, Bilateral diaphragmatic paralysis, Brain and spinal metastases
Vascular system
Renal vein and caval thromboses, Left sided varicocele, Prothrombotic state and thrombosis in unusual sites
Hematologic system
Cytopenia,Polycythemia, Micro angiopathic hemolytic anemia, Hemolytic uremic syndrome, Disseminated intravascular coagulopathy, Disturbation in fibrinolysis system
Pulmonary system
Single or multiple variable -sized pulmonary nodules, Lymphangitic carcinomatosis, Malignant pleural effusion, Mediastinal lymph adenopathy, Pulmonary infarction due to tumor emboli
Heart
Malignant pericardial effusion, Cardiac metastasis mimicking primary cardiac tumors, Non-bacterial endocarditis
Gastrointestinal tract
Stauffer's syndrome, Oral cavity metastases, Esophageal metastasis, Gastric metastasis and upper gastrointestinal bleeding, Intraluminal metastases, Hepatic and pancreatic metastases, Budd-Chiari syndrome, Bowel ischemia due to tumor emboli, Sinistral portal hypertension, Gastric variceal bleeding
Endocrinologic system
Panhypopituitarism ,Metastasis to thyroid, adrenal, ovaries and testes
Paraneoplastic syndromes
Hypercalcaemia, Hypoglycemia, Hyperglycemia, Polycythemia, Gynecomastia, Hypertension

Table 1. Clinical spectrum of patients with renal cell carcinoma

14. References

Aburto, J., Bruckner, BA. Blackmon, SH., Beyer, EA. &Reardon, MJ. (2009). Renal cell carcinoma, metastatic to the left ventricle. *Tex Heart Inst J.*, 36(1):48-9, 19436786.

Allen, JA., Yang, XJ. & Sufit, RL. (2011).Reversible demyelinating neuropathy associated with renal cell carcinoma. *Neuromuscular Disord*, 21(3):227-31, 21195618.

Alsirafy, SA., El Mesidy, SM., Abou-Elela, EN. & Elfaramawy, YI. (2011). Naproxen test for neoplastic fever may reduce suffering.*J Palliat Med.*, 14(5):665-7, 21291328.

Al-Taan, OS. Featherstone, JM., Rees, AM., Young, WT. & Stephenson TP. (2007).Renal cell carcinoma in a horseshoe kidney presenting as an acute, left sided varicocele.*Int Urol Nephrol.*, 39(2):369-71, 16835726.

Ammar, H., Brown, SH., Malani, A., Sheth, HK., Sollars, EG., Zhou, SX., Gupta ,C. &Mughal ,S. (2008 May). A case of paraneoplastic cerebellar ataxia secondary to renal cell carcinoma.*South Med J.*, 101(5):556-7, 18414160.

Amoura, Z., Duhaut ,P., Huong, DL., Wechsler, B., Costedoat-Chalumeau, N., Francès, C., Cacoub ,P., Papo ,T, Cormont ,S., Touitou, Y., Grenier, P., Valeyre, D.& Piette, JC.(2005). Tumor antigen markers for the detection of solid cancers in inflammatory myopathies.*Cancer Epidemiol Biomarkers Prev.*, 14(5):1279-82, 15894686.

Arrabal-Polo, MA. Arias-Santiago, SA. Aneiros-Fernandez, J., Burkhardt-Perez, P., Arrabal-Martin, M., &Naranjo-Sintes, R. (2009). Cutaneous metastases in renal cell carcinoma: a case report. report. Cases *J.*, 25; 2:7948-51, 19918439.

Asadi, M., Rokni-Yazdi, H., Salehinia, F. & Allameh, FS. (2009). Metastatic renal cell carcinoma initially presented with an intramedullary spinal cord lesion: a case report.*Cases J.*, 2:7805-8, 19918485.

Bell, WR. (1996). The fibrinolytic system in neoplasia.*Semin Thromb Hemost.* , 22(6):459-78, 9122711.

Berman, J. &Harland, S. (2001).Hypoglycaemia caused by secretion of insulin-like growth factor 2 in a primary renal cell carcinoma.*Clin Oncol (R Coll Radiol).* , 13(5):367-9, 11716231.

Candiano, G., Pepe, P., Grasso, G. &Aragona, F. (2010).Headache: a unique clinical presentation for renal cell carcinoma (RCC).*Arch Ital Urol Androl.* , 82(4):184-6, 21341558.

Chetcuti, K., Barnard, J., Loggos, S., Hassan, M., Srivastava, V., Mourad, F., Makhzoum, Z. & Bittar, MN. (2010). Massive hemothorax secondary to metastatic renal carcinoma.*Ann Thorac Surg.*, 89(6):2014-6, 20494072.

Choi, JW., Lee, JH., Park, HS. & Kim, YS. (2011).PAI-1 expression and its regulation by promoter 4G/5G polymorphism in clear cell renal cell carcinoma.*J Clin Pathol., July1, (Epub head of print)*, 21725041.

Cimino-Mathews, A., Sharma, R., &Netto, GJ. (2011). Diagnostic use of PAX8, CAIX, TTF-1, and TGB in metastatic renal cell carcinoma of the thyroid.*Am J Surg Pathol.* , 35(5):757-61.21451364.

Cobo-Dols, M., Alés-Díaz, I., Villar-Chamorro, E., Gil-Calle, S., Alcaide-García, J., Montesa-Pino, A., Gutiérrez-Calderón, V. & Benavides-Orgaz, M. (2006).Solitary metastasis in a nasal fossa as the first manifestation of a renal carcinoma.*Clin Transl Oncol.* , 8(4):298-300, 16648109.

Crouch, ED. & Tak, T. (2002).Renal cell carcinoma presenting as right atrial mass.*Echocardiography*, 19(2):149-51, 11926979 de los Monteros-Sanchez, AE., Medina-Franco, H., Arista-Nasr, J. & Cortes-Gonzalez ,R. (2004). Resection of an esophageal metastasis from a renal cell carcinoma.*Hepatogastroenterology,* 51(55):163-4, 15011855.

Divya, KS., Moran, NA. & Atkin, PA. (2010). Numb chin syndrome: a case series and discussion. *Br Dent J.,* 208(4):157-60, 20186196.

Donovan, DJ. &Freeman, JH. (2006). Solitary intramedullary spinal cord tumor presenting as the initial manifestation of metastatic renal cell carcinoma: case report.*Spine (Phila Pa 1976).* , 15; 31(14):E460-3., 16778676.

Dorairajan ,LN., Hemal ,AK., Aron, M., Rajeev, TP., Nair, M., Seth, A., Dogra, PN.&Gupta, NP.(1999). Cutaneous metastases in renal cell carcinoma.*Urol Int.* , 63(3):164-7, 10738187.

EO, WK., Kim, GY. & Choi, SI. (2008). A case of multiple intussusceptions in the small intestine caused by metastatic renal cell carcinoma.*Cancer Res Treat.* , 40(2):97-9, 19688056.

Fang, X., Gupta, N., Shen, SS., Tamboli, P., Charnsangavej, C., Rashid, A. & Wang, H. (2010).Intraluminal polypoid metastasis of renal cell carcinoma in gallbladder mimicking gallbladder polyp.*Arch Pathol Lab Med.,* 134(7):1003-9, 20586628.

Florcken ,A., Loew, A., Koch, M., Gebauer, B., Dorken, B. & Riess, H. (2009).Severe thrombocytopenia in a patient with metastatic renal cell carcinoma.*Onkologie.* , 32(11):670-2, 19887872.

Fottner, A., Szalantzy, M., Wirthmann, L., Stähler, M., Baur-Melnyk, A., Jansson, V. &Dürr, HR. (2010).Bone metastases from renal cell carcinoma: patient survival after surgical treatment.*BMC Musculoskelet Disord.* , 3; 11:145-50, 20598157.

Ghavamian, R., Klein, KA., Stephens, DH., Welch, TJ., LeRoy, AJ., Richardson, RL., Burch, PA. &Zincke H. (2000).Renal cell carcinoma metastatic to the pancreas: clinical and radiological features.*Mayo Clin Proc.,* 75(6) :581-5, 10852418.

Gómez de la Riva, A., Isla ,A., Pérez-López, C., Budke, M., Gutiérrez, M. & Frutos, R. (2005). [Intramedullary spinal cord metastasis as the first manifestation of a renal carcinoma].*Neurocirugia (Astur).* , 16(4):359-64, 16143809.

Gopan, T., Toms, SA., Prayson ,RA., Suh, JH., Hamrahian, AH. & Weil, RJ. (2007). Symptomatic pituitary metastases from renal cell carcinoma.*Pituitary,* 10(3):251-9, 17541748.

Guney, S., Guney, N., Ozcan, D., Sayilgan, T. & Ozakin, E. (2010).Ovarian metastasis of a primary renal cell carcinoma: case report and review of literature.*Eur J Gynaecol Oncol.* , 31(3):339-41, 21077484.

Hameed, A., Pahuja, A., Thwaini, A. &Nambirajan, T. (2011).Subclavian vein thrombosis: an unusual presentation of renal cell carcinoma. *Can Urol Assoc J.,* 5(2):E27-8, 21470547.

Hotakainen, K., Lintula, S., Ljungberg, B., Finne, P., Paju, A., Stenman, UH. &Stenman ,J. (2006).Expression of human chorionic gonadotropin beta-subunit type I genes predicts adverse outcome in renal cell carcinoma.*J Mol Diagn.* , 8(5):598-603, 17065429.

Hotakainen, K., Ljungberg, B., Paju, A., Rasmuson, T., Alfthan, H. & Stenman, UH. (2002). The free beta-subunit of human chorionic gonadotropin as a prognostic factor in renal cell carcinoma.*Br J Cancer.* , 86(2):185-9, 11870503.

Jobe BA., Bierman, MH. & Mezzacappa, FJ. (1993). Hyperglycemia as a paraneoplastic endocrinopathy in renal cell carcinoma: a case report and review of the literature.*Nebr Med J.,* 78 (11):349-51, 8309485.

Johnson, J.A., Everett, B.M., Katz, J.T. & Loscalzo, J. (2010).Clinical Problem-Solving Painful Purple Toes. *N Engl J Med.*, 362:67 – 73, 0807291.

Joya Seijo, MD., del Valle Loarte, P., Marco Martínez, J., Herrera Merino, N.& Agud Aparicio, JL.(2004). carcinoma. An *Med Interna.*, 21(6):283-4, 15283642.

Juncadella, E., Ramentol, M., Rozadilla, A., &Ferre, J . (2003). RS3PE syndrome and renal cancer. *Med Clin (Barc).*, 8;121(16):638-9, 14636547.

Kalkat, MS., Abedin, A., Rooney, S., Doherty, A., Faroqui, M., Wallace, M. & Graham, TR. (2008).Renal tumours with cavo-atrial extension: surgical management and outcome.*Interact Cardiovasc Thorac Surg.*, 7(6):981-5, 18550606.

Kim, SH., Kwak, MH., Park, S., Kim, HJ., Lee, HS., Kim, MS., Lee, JM., Zo, JI., Ro, JS. & Lee, JS. (2005). Clinical characteristics of malignant pericardial effusion associated with recurrence and survival. *Cancer Res Treat.* , 42(4):210-6, 21253323.

Kirkali, Z. (2011).Adverse events from targeted therapies in advanced renal cell carcinoma: the impact on long-term use.*BJU Int.*, 107(11):1722-32, 21251188.

Klausner, AP., Ost, MC., Waterhouse RL ,Jr. &Savage SJ. (2002). Occult renal cell carcinoma in a patient with polymyositis.*Urology.* , 59(5):773-6, 11992921.

Klein, T., Rotterdam, S., Noldus, J. &Hinkel, A. (2009). Bullous pemphigoid is a rare paraneoplastic syndrome in patients with renal cell carcinoma. *Scand J Urol Nephrol.* , 43(4):334-6, 19308806.

Koukoulis ,A., Cimas, I. &Gómara, S. (1998).Paraneoplastic opsoclonus associated with papillary renal cell carcinoma. J *Neurol Neurosurg Psychiatry.*, 64(1):137-8, 9436748.

Kramer, CK., Ferreira, N., Silveiro, SP., Gross, JL., Dora, JM. &Azevedo, MJ. (2010).Pituitary gland metastasis from renal cell carcinoma presented as a non-functioning macroadenoma.*Arq Bras Endocrinol Metabol.* , 54(5) :498-501,20694412.

Kranidiotis, GP., Voidonikola, PT., Dimopoulos, MK. & Anastasiou-Nana, MI. (2009). Stauffer's syndrome as a prominent manifestation of renal cancer: a case report. Cases *J.*, 2(1):49-52, 19144140.

Kruyt ND& Wessels PH. (2006).Cerebral infarction due to polycythaemia as the initial manifestation of renal cell carcinoma.*Ned Tijdschr Geneeskd.* , 150(17):969-72, 17225738.

Lata, J& Kumar, P. (2010). Numb chin syndrome: a case report and review of the literature. *Indian J Dent Res.* , 21(1):135-7, 20427925.

Lee, HJ., Park, JI., Lim, BH., Seo, JW., Kang, EM., Lee, BU. & Kim, YJ. (2010). Left ventricular metastasis from renal cell carcinoma causing left ventricular outflow tract obstruction. *Korean Circ J.*, 40(8):410-3, 20830256.

Lin, TK., Chen, SM. & Jung, SM. (2011).Solitary intradural extramedullary metastasis of renal cell carcinoma to the conus medullaris.*Kaohsiung J Med Sci.*, 27(1):45-8, 21329893.

Lipton, A., Colombo-Berra, A., Bukowski, RM., Rosen, L., Zheng, M. &Urbanowitz, G. (2004).Skeletal complications in patients with bone metastases from renal cell carcinoma and therapeutic benefits of zoledronic acid.*Clin Cancer Res.*, 15; 10(18 Pt 2):6397S-403S, 15448038.

Loualidi, A., Spooren, PF., Grubben, MJ., Blomjous, CE. & Goey, SH. (2004).Duodenal metastasis: an uncommon cause of occult small intestinal bleeding.*Neth J Med.*, 62(6):201-5, 15460501.

Low, DE. Frenkel, VJ., Manley, PN., Ford, SN. & Kerr, JW. (1989). Embolic mesenteric infarction: a unique initial manifestation of renal cell carcinoma. *Surgery*, 106(5):925-8, 2683176.

Lucchinetti, CF., Kimmel, DW. &Lennon, VA. (1998). Paraneoplastic and oncologic profiles of patients seropositive for type 1 antineuronal nuclear autoantibodies. *Neurology.*, 50(3):652-7, 9521251.

Marangoni, G., O'Sullivan, A., Ali, A., Faraj, W. & Heaton, N. (2010).Budd-Chiari syndrome secondary to caval recurrence of renal cell carcinoma.*Hepatobiliary Pancreat Dis Int.*, 9(3):321-4, 20525562.

Marto, G., Klitna, Z., Biléu, MC. & Barcelos, A. (2010). Remitting seronegative symmetric synovitis with pitting oedema syndrome, associated with prostate adenocarcinoma: a cse report.*Acta Reumatol Port.*, 35(3) :358-60, 20975640.

Mathai, AM., Rau, AR., Shetty, AB., Kamath, MP. & Prasad, SC. (2007). Endobronchial metastasis from renal cell carcinoma: a case report. Indian *J Pathol Microbiol.*, 50(2):379-81, 17883082.

Mattana, J., Kurtz, B., Miah, A. & Singhal, PC. (1996). Renal cell carcinoma presenting as a solitary anterior superior mediastinal mass.*J Med.*, 27(3-4):205-10, 8289968.

Maynard, JW., Christopher-Stine, L. & Gelber, AC. (2010). Testicular pain followed by microscopic hematuria, a renal mass, palpable purpura, polyarthritis, and hematochezia.*J Clin Rheumatol.*, 16 (8):388-91, 21085014.

Miyamoto, MI. & Picard, MH. (2002). Left atrial mass caused by metastatic renal cell carcinoma: an unusual site of tumor involvement mimicking myxoma.*J Am Soc Echocardiogr.*, 15(8):847-8, 12174358.

Mohammed Ilyas, MI., Turner, GD. & Cranston, D. (2008). Human chorionic gonadotropin-secreting clear cell renal cell carcinoma with paraneoplastic gynaecomastia.*Scand J Urol Nephrol.*, 42(6):555-7, 19031270.

Mueller, TJ., Wu, H., Greenberg, RE., Hudes, G., Topham, N., Lessin, SR. &Uzzo RG. (2004). Cutaneous metastases from genitourinary malignancies.*Urology*, 63 (6):1021-6, 15183939.

Niccoli, L., Salvarani, C., Baroncelli, G., Padula, A., Olivieri, I. &Cantini F. (2002).Renal cell carcinoma mimicking polymyalgia rheumatica. Clues for a correct diagnosis.*Scand J Rheumatol.*, 31(2):103-6, 12109644.

Niikura, S., Hirata, A., Kunimi, K., Yokoyama, O., Koshida, K., Uchibayashi, T., Namiki, M., Nishino, A. & Kameda, K. (1999). Renal cell carcinoma recurrence in the mediastinum lymph node 19 years after nephrectomy: a case report.*Hinyokika Kiyo.*, 45(6):419-21, 10442285.

Nozawa, H., Tsuchiya, M., Kobayashi, T., Morita, H., Kobayashi, I., Sakaguchi, M., Mizutani, T., Tajima, A., Kishida, Y., Yakumaru, K., Kagami, H. & Sekikawa, T. (2003).Small intestinal metastasis from renal cell carcinoma exhibiting rare findings.*Int J Clin Pract.*, 57(4):329-31, 12800466.

Okubo, Y., Yonese, J., Kawakami, S., Yamamoto, S., Komai, Y., Takeshita, H., Ishikawa, Y. & Fukui, I. (2007).Obstinate cough as a sole presenting symptom of non-metastatic renal cell carcinoma.*Int J Urol.*, 14(9):854-5, 17760755.

Panarese, A., Turner, J. & Fagan, PA. (2002). Renal carcinoma metastasis: an unusual cerebellopontine angle tumor.*Otolaryngol Head Neck Surg.*, 127(3):245-7, 12297820.

Papachristodoulou, A., Mantas, D., Kouskos, E., Hatzianastassiou, D. & Karatzas, G. (2004).Unusual presentation of renal cell carcinoma metastasis.*Acta Chir Belg.*, 104(2):229-30, 15154588.

Placed, IG., Alvarez-Rodriguez, R., Pombo-Otero, J., Vázquez-Bartolomé, P., Hermida-Romero, T.& Pombo-Felipe, F.(2010). Metastatic renal cell carcinoma presenting as shoulder monoarthritis: diagnosis based on synovial fluid cytology and immunocytochemistry.*Acta Cytol.* , 54(5) :730-3, 20968165.

Pollheimer, MJ., Hinterleitner, TA., Pollheimer, VS., Schlemmer, A. &Langner, C. (2008). Renal cell carcinoma metastatic to the stomach: single-centre experience and literature review. *BJU Int.* , 102 (3):315-9, 18336607.

Respicio, G., Shwaiki, W. & Abeles, M. (2007).A 58-year-old man with anti-Jo-1 syndrome and renal cell carcinoma: a case report and discussion.*Conn Med.*, 71(3):151-3, 17405398.

Rijnders, B. & Decramer, M. (2000). Reversibility of paraneoplastic bilateral diaphragmatic paralysis after nephrectomy for renal cell carcinoma. *Ann Oncol.* , 11(2):221-5, 10761760.

Roviello, F., Caruso, S., Moscovita Falzarano, S., Marrelli, D., Neri, A., Rampone, B., De Marco, G., Perrotta, ME. & Mariani, F. (2006).Small bowel metastases from renal cell carcinoma: a rare cause of intestinal intussusception.*J Nephrol.* 19(2):234-8, 16736429.

Roy, MJ., May, EF. & Jabbari B. (2002). Life-threatening polyneuropathy heralding renal cell carcinoma.*Mil Med.*, 167(12):986-9, 12502172

Russell EB. (2005). Remitting seronegative symmetrical synovitis with pitting edema syndrome: followup for neoplasia.*J Rheumatol.* , 32(9):1760-1, 16142875.

Sadler, GJ., Anderson, MR., Mos, MS. & Wilson, PG. (2007).Metastases from renal cell carcinoma presenting as gastrointestinal bleeding: two case reports and a review of the literature.*BMC Gastroenterol.* , 7:4-7, 17766757.

Sakura, M., Tsujii, T., Yamauchi, A., Tadokoro, M., Tsukamoto, T., Kawakami, S., Yonese, J. & Fukui, I. (2007). Superior vena cava syndrome caused by supraclavicular lymph node metastasis of renal cell carcinoma.*Int J Clin Oncol.* , 12(5):382-4, 17729122.

Schijns, OE., Kurt, E., Wessels, P., Luijckx, GJ. & Beuls, EA. (2000). Intramedullary spinal cord metastasis as a first manifestation of a renal cell carcinoma: report of a case and review of the literature.*Clin Neurol Neurosurg.* , 102(4):249-254, 11154816.

Shakeel, M., Kumaravel, M., Mackenzie, JM. &Knight, DJ. (2009). An uncommon cause of sciatica.*J Coll Physicians Surg Pak.*, 19(2):127-9, 19208321.

Shih, KL., Yen ,HH., Su ,WW., Soon ,MS., Hsia, CH.& Lin ,YM.(2009). Fulminant Budd-Chiari syndrome caused by renal cell carcinoma with hepatic vein invasion: report of a case.*Eur J Gastroenterol Hepatol.* , 21(2):222-4, 19212212.

Shinsaka, H., Fujimoto, N. & Matsumoto, T. (2006).A rare case of right varicocele testis caused by a renal cell carcinoma thrombus in the spermatic vein.*Int J Urol.*, 13 (6):844-5, 16834679.

Shiono, Y., Kishimoto, K., Furuta, N., Igarashi, H., Hatano, T., Miki, K., Oishi, Y.& Kiyota, H. (2001). Pulmonary infarction caused by the spontaneous migration of the vena caval tumor thrombus of right renal cell carcinoma: a case report.*Hinyokika Kiyo .Acta urologica japoniva.* , 47(11):781-4, 11771170.

Shivnani, SB., Shelton, JM., Richardson, JA. & Maalouf, NM. (2009). Hypercalcemia of malignancy with simultaneous elevation in serum parathyroid hormone--related peptide and 1, 25-dihydroxyvitamin D in a patient with metastatic renal cell carcinoma.*Endocr Pract.* , 15(3):234-9, 19364692.

Sidhom, OA., Basalaev, M. & Sigal LH. (1993). Renal cell carcinoma presenting as polymyalgia rheumatica. Resolution after nephrectomy. *Arch Intern Med.,* 13; 153(17):2043-5, 8357289.

Singhal, D., Kakodkar, R., Soin, AS., Gupta, S. & Nundy, S. (2006). Sinistral portal hypertension .a case report. *JOP.* , 10; 7(6):670-3, 17095850.

Sparano, JA., Dutcher, JP., Kaleya, R., Caliendo, G., Fiorito, J., Mitsudo, S., Shechner, R., Boley, SJ., Gucalp, R. & Ciobanu, N. (1991). Colonic ischemia complicating immunotherapy with interleukin-2 and interferon-alpha. *Cancer,* 68(7):1538-44, 1893354.

Srinivasan, N., Pakala, A., Al-Kali, A., Rathi, S. & Ahmad, W. (2010). Papillary renal cell carcinoma with cutaneous metastases. *Am J Med Sci.,* 339(5):458-61, 20234300.

Staehler, MD., Kruse, J., Haseke, N., Stadler, T., Roosen, A., Karl, A., Stief, CG., Jauch, KW. &Bruns, CJ. (2010). Liver resection for metastatic disease prolongs survival in renal cell carcinoma: 12-year results from a retrospective comparative analysis. *World J Urol.,* 28(4):543-7, 20440505.

Steffens, J., Bock, R., Braedel, HU., Isenberg, E., Bührle, CP. & Ziegler, M. (1992). Renin-producing renal cell carcinomas--clinical and experimental investigations on a special form of renal hypertension.*Urol Res.,* 20(2):111-5, 1553788.

Suyama, H., Igishi, T., Makino, H., Kaminou, T., Hashimoto, M., Sumikawa, T., Tatsukawa, T. &Shimizu, E. (2011). Bronchial artery embolization before interventional bronchoscopy to avoid uncontrollable bleeding: a case report of endobronchial metastasis of renal cell carcinoma. *Intern Med.,* 50(2):135-9, 21245638.

Takeda, T., Shibuya, T., Osada, T., Izumi, H., Mitomi, H., Nomura, O., Suzuki, S., Mori, H., Matsumoto, K., Kon, K., Abe, W., Beppu, K., Sakamoto, N., Nagahara, A., Otaka, M., Ogihara, T., Yao, T. &Watanabe S. (2011). Metastatic renal cell carcinoma diagnosed by capsule endoscopy and double balloon endoscopy. *Med Sci Monit.* , 17(2):CS15-7, 21278196.

Talukder, MQ., Deo, SV., Maleszewski ,JJ. & Park SJ. (2010). Late isolated metastasis of renal cell carcinoma in the left ventricular myocardium.*Interact Cardiovasc Thorac Surg.,* 11(6):814-6, 20847070.

Tan, BH., Barry, CI., Wick, MR., White, KP., Brown, JG., Lee, A., Litchfield, AH., Lener, EV.&Shitabata, PK.(2011). Multicentric reticulohistiocytosis and urologic carcinomas: a possible paraneoplastic association. *J Cutan Pathol.* , 38(1):43-8, 20726933.

Tebbe, B., Schlippert, U., Garbe, C. & Orfanos, CE. (1991). Erythroderma "en nappes claires" as a marker of metastatic kidney cancer. Lasting, successful treatment with rIFN-alpha-2a.*Hautarzt.* , 42(5):324-7, 1831444.

Teresa, P., Maria Grazia, Z., Doriana, M., Irene, P. & Michele, S. (2011).Malignant effusion of chromophobe renal-cell carcinoma: Cytological and immunohistochemical findings.*Diagn Cytopathol.* , Jan 6. [Epub ahead of print], 21213172.

Tiwari, P., Tiwari, A., Vijay, M., Kumar, S. & Kundu, AK. (2010). Upper gastro-intestinal bleeding - Rare presentation of renal cell carcinoma.*Urol Ann.,* 2(3):127-9, 20981203.

Toquero, L., Aboumarzouk, OM. & Abbasi, Z. (2009). Renal cell carcinoma metastasis to the ovary: a case report. *Cases J.,* 2:7472-5, 19829972.

Torvik, A. & Berntzen, AE. (1968). Necrotizing vasculitis without visceral involvement. Postmortem examination of three cases with affection of skeletal muscles and peripheral nerves.*Acta Med Scand.*, 184(1-2):69-77, 4387508.

Wallach, JB., McGarry, T. & Torres, J.(2011).Lymphangitic metastasis of recurrent renal cell carcinoma to the contralateral lung causing lymphangitic carcinomatosis and respiratory symptoms.*Curr Oncol.* , 18(1):e35-7, 21311270.

Wieder, JA., Laks, H., Freitas, D., Marmureanu, A. & Belldegrun, A. (2003). Renal cell carcinoma with tumor thrombus extension into the proximal pulmonary artery.*J Urol.* , 169(6):2296-7, 12771776.

Wiesener, MS., Münchenhagen, P., Gläser, M., Sobottka, BA., Knaup, KX., Jozefowski, K., Jürgensen, JS., Roigas, J., Warnecke, C., Gröne, HJ., Maxwell, PH., Willam, C.& Eckardt, KU. (2007). Erythropoietin gene expression in renal carcinoma is considerably more frequent than paraneoplastic polycythemia.*Int J Cancer.* , 121(11):2434-42, 17640059.

Will, TA., Agarwal, N. & Petruzzelli,GJ. (2008). Oral cavity metastasis of renal cell carcinoma: a case report.*J Med Case Reports.* , 2:313-6, 18823541.

Winter, H., Meimarakis, G., Angele, MK., Hummel, M., Staehler, M., Hoffmann, RT., Hatz, RA. &Löhe, F. (2010).Tumor infiltrated hilar and mediastinal lymph nodes are an independent prognostic factor for decreased survival after pulmonary metastasectomy in patients with renal cell carcinoma.*J Urol.*, 184(5):1888-94, 20846691.

Wu, HY., Xu, LW., Zhang, YY., Yu, YL., Li, XD. & Li, GH. (2011). Metachronous contralateral testicular and bilateral adrenal metastasis of chromophobe renal cell carcinoma: a case report and review of the literature.*J Zhejiang Univ Sci B.*, 11(5):386-9, 20443217.

Yokonishi ,T., Ito, Y., Osaka, K., Komiya, A., Kobayashi, K., Sakai, N., Noguchi, S., Kishi, H., Satomi, Y., Mogaki, M., Tsuura, Y., Mizuno, N. &Ikeda, I. (2010).Pancreatic metastasis from renal cell carcinoma 25 years after radical nephrectomy.*Hinyokika Kiyo.* , 56(11):629-33, 21187708.

Yumura, Y., Yamashita, Y., Senga, Y., Jinza, S. &Goro, A. (2007). Two cases of renal cell carcinoma with diabetes mellitus that was healed after nephrectomy.*Hinyokika Kiyo.* , 53(5):301-5, 17571714.

Zubac, DP., Wentzel-Larsen, T., Seidal, T. & Bostad, L. (2010).Type 1 plasminogen activator inhibitor (PAI-1) in clear cell renal cell carcinoma (CCRCC) and its impact on angiogenesis, progression and patient survival after radical nephrectomy.*BMC Urol.*, 10:20-4, 21129210.

Zustovich, F., Gottardo, F., De Zorzi, L., Cecchetto, A., Dal Bianco, M., Mauro, E. &Cartei, G. (2008).Cardiac metastasis from renal cell carcinoma without inferior vena involvement: a review of the literature based on a case report. Two different patterns of spread?*Int J Clin Oncol.* , 13(3):271-4, 18553240.

Maestre-Rodríguez ,O., González-García, R., Mateo-Arias, J., Moreno-García, C., Serrano-Gil, H., Villanueva-Alcojol, L., Campos-de-Orellana, AM. & Monje-Gil, F. (2009). Metastasis of renal clear-cell carcinoma to the oral mucosa, an atypical location.*Med Oral Patol Oral Cir Bucal.* , 14(11):e601-4, 19680203.

Mudiyanselage, SY., Prabhakaran, VC., Davis, GJ. & Selva, D. (2008).Metastatic renal cell carcinoma presenting as a circumscribed orbital mass.*Eur J Ophthalmol.* , 18(3):483-5, 18465741.

11

Laparoscopic Partial Nephrectomy – Current State of the Art

Paul D'Alessandro, Shawn Dason and Anil Kapoor
Divison of Urology, Department of Surgery McMaster University, Hamilton, Ontario, Canada

1. Introduction

Clayman et al described the first successful laparoscopic nephrectomy in 1991 [1]. Since that time, laparoscopic radical nephrectomy has become the standard of care for renal tumors. At the same time, the widespread use of contemporary imaging techniques has resulted in an increased detection of small incidental renal tumors. In efforts to avoid chronic kidney disease, the management of the small renal mass has trended away from radical nephrectomy toward nephron-conserving surgery. In 1993, successful laparoscopic partial nephrectomy (LPN) was first reported in a porcine model [2]. Winfield et al reported the first human LPN in 1993 [3]. From that time, centres around the world have developed laparoscopic techniques for partial nephrectomy through retroperitoneal and transperitoneal approaches. Classically, only small, peripheral, exophytic tumors were eligible for LPN, but larger, infiltrating tumors have been managed with LPN in more recent series [4].

Currently, partial nephrectomy is a standard of care treatment for the surgical management of localized renal tumors <4cm [5], and recommended in guidelines published by the American Urological Association [6] and European Association of Urology [7]. LPN combines the benefits of nephron-sparing surgery and laparoscopy to decrease the morbidity of partial nephrectomy.

The LPN technique has evolved significantly over the past decade such that its safety and efficacy rival those of open partial nephrectomy (OPN) and laparoscopic radical nephrectomy (LRN) techniques for tumors less than 4cm. LPN produces low overall morbidity, faster post-operative recovery, and comparable oncologic outcomes compared to other techniques.

Technical difficulty in LPN is encountered when securing renal hypothermia, renal parenchymal hemostasis, pelvicalyceal reconstruction, and parenchymal renorraphy by pure laparoscopic techniques. The appropriate and optimal length of warm ischemia time (WIT) remains particularly controversial. Nevertheless, ongoing advances in laparoscopic techniques and operator skills have allowed the development of a reliable technique that duplicates the established principles and technical steps underpinning open partial nephrectomy. With the advent of the da Vinci Surgical System (Intuitive Surgical, Sunnyvale, CA, USA), robot-assisted LPN (RPN) has advanced laparoscopic techniques even further. In this chapter we evaluate the role of LPN in the nephron-sparing armamentarium.

2.1 Indications and contraindications

Partial nephrectomy is performed for benign and malignant renal conditions. In the setting of malignant renal diseases, this is indicated in situations where radical nephrectomy would leave the patient anephric due to bilateral renal tumors or unilateral tumor and compromised or at risk the other side. Some investigators also defined the role of elective PN in patients with unilateral renal tumors and normal contralateral kidneys to reduce the risk of developing chronic kidney disease in the future [8].

Due to its technical limitations, LPN was initially reserved for select patients with small, peripheral, superficial, superficial, and exophytic tumors. As laparoscopic experience increased, the use of LPN was expanded to technically challenging tumors, such as tumors invading deeply into the parenchyma up to the collecting system or renal sinus, intrarenal tumors, tumors abutting the renal hilum, tumors in solitary kidneys, or tumors substantial enough to require heminephrectomies. Recent series include larger, Stage T1b tumours [9-11]; endophytic tumours near the hilum and upper pole [12]; bilateral tumors [13]; multiple ipsilateral tumors [14]; and stage T1a tumours presenting in select patients over the age of 70 [15].

General contraindications to abdominal laparoscopic surgery are applied to LPN. Specific absolute contraindications to LPN include bleeding diathesis (such as renal failure induced platelet dysfunction and blood thinners), renal vein thrombus, and aggressive locally advanced disease. Morbid obesity and a history of prior renal surgery may prohibitively increase the technical complexity of the procedure and should be considered a relative contraindication for LPN. Overall, the ultimate decision to proceed with LPN should be based on the tumor characteristics and the surgeon's skill and experience with such an approach.

2.2 Preoperative preparation

Preoperative evaluation includes routine preoperative investigations as well as a computed tomography angiogram of the abdomen to delineate renal vasculature. Renal scintigraphy is obtained if there is a question about the global renal function. Preoperative medical clearance should be obtained when there is any question of the patient's fitness for major abdominal or vascular surgery. We routinely cross-match 4 units of packed red blood cells on demand. Mechanical bowel preparation of one bottle of magnesium citrate is given the evening before the surgery, and intravenous prophylactic antibiotics are given prior to entering the operating room.

2.3 Operative technique

A substantive LPN entails renal hilar control, transection of major intrarenal vessels, controlled entry into and repair of the collecting system, control of parenchymal blood vessels, and renal parenchymal reconstruction, all usually under the pressure of minimizing warm ischemia. As such, significant experience in the minimally invasive environment, including expertise with time-sensitive intracorporeal suturing, is essential. LPN can be approached either transperitoneally (our preferred approach) or retroperitoneally based on the surgeon's experience and the tumor location. The transperitoneal approach is usually chosen for anterior, anterolateral, lateral, and upper-pole apical tumors. Retroperitoneal laparoscopy is reserved for posterior or posterolaterally located tumors. A retrospective, match-pair comparison of 105 patients who underwent either transperitoneal or retroperitoneal approaches for T1a renal masses demonstrated that both approaches provide comparable surgical and functional results [16]. Although studies report shorter operative time, decreased blood loss and shorter hospital stay with the retroperitoneal approach [16, 17], many centers prefer the transperitoneal approach for its greater working space and easy tumor accessibility[18].

After induction of general anesthesia, a Foley catheter and nasogastric tube are placed prior to patient positioning. Cystoscopy and ureteral catheter placement are performed if preoperative imaging indicates a risk of collecting system violation during resection of the lesion (a-requirement for intraparenchymal resection greater than 1.5 cm or tumor abutting the collecting system). Although many laparoscopists prefer to place their patients at a 45 to 60° angle in · the flank position, we prefer to place our patients undergoing renal surgery in the lateral flank position at 90°. This provides excellent access to the hilum and allows the bowel and spleen (on the left side) to fall off the renal hilum during procedures complicated by bowel distention.

Laparoscopic surgery is performed using a transperitoneal approach with a Veress needle, directly using the Optiview (Ethicon Endo-surgery ®) trocar system, or using the Hassan technique, to attain pneumoperitoneum. Three to four ports (including two 10-12 mm ports) are routinely placed in our technique. Exposure of the kidney and the hilar dissection are performed using a J-hook electrocautery suction probe or by using the ultrasound energy-based harmonic shears (Ethicon Endo-surgery ®) This is done by reflecting the mesocolon along the Line of Toldt, leaving Gerota's fascia intact. Mobilizing the kidney within this fascia, the ureter is retracted laterally, and cephalad dissection is carried out along the psoas muscle leading to the renal hilum. Once the tumour is localized, we dissect the Gerota's fascia and defat the kidney, leaving only the perinephric fat overlying tumor (Figure 8.1). Intraoperative ultrasonography with a Philips Entos LAP *9-5* linear array transducer (Philips ®) can be used to aid in tumor localization if it is not exophytic or if the tumor is deep into the renal parenchyma. A laparoscopic vascular clamp (Karl Storz ®) is placed around both the renal artery and the renal vein (without separation of the vessels) for hilar control in cases associated with central masses and heminephrectomy procedures, as described by Gill et al [19] (Figures 8.2-8.4).

Conversely, during a retroperitoneoscopic nephrectomy, the renal artery and vein are dissected separately to prepare for placement of bulldog clamps on the renal artery and vein individually. Mannitol may be used (0.5 g/kg intravenously) prior to hilar clamping or renal hypothermia. Resection of renal parenchyma is performed with cold scissors (Figures 8.5-8.10), and the specimen is retrieved using a 10-cm laparoscopic EndoCatch bag (US Surgical Corporation, Norwalk, Connecticut ®) and sent for frozen section analysis (sometimes with excisional biopsy from the base) to determine the resection margin status (Figures 8.17 and 8.18).

Hemostasis is accomplished using intracorporeal suturing, argon beam coagulator, and hemostatic matrix (Floseal®, Baxter, Vienna, Austria) application in a manner previously described by others (Figures 8.10-8.16) [20-23].

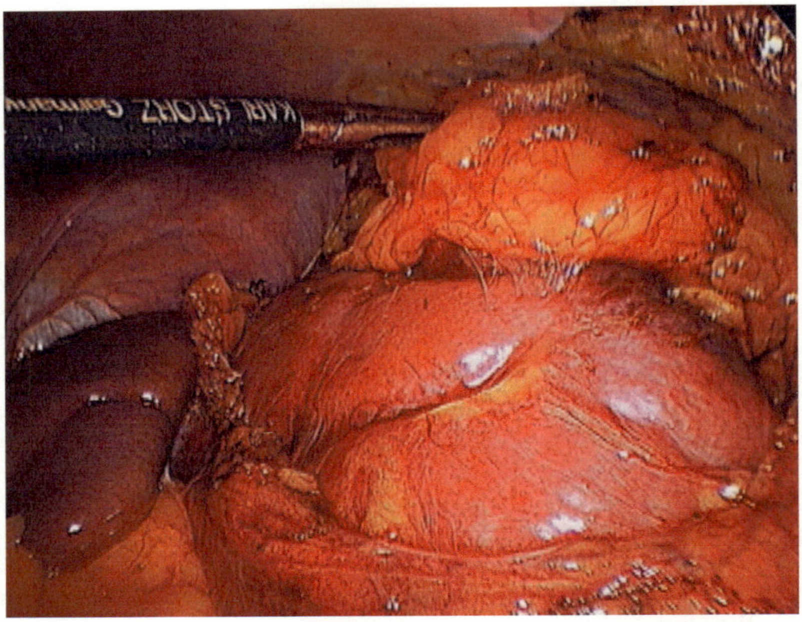

Fig. 8.1. Defatted kidney except area overlying the tumor

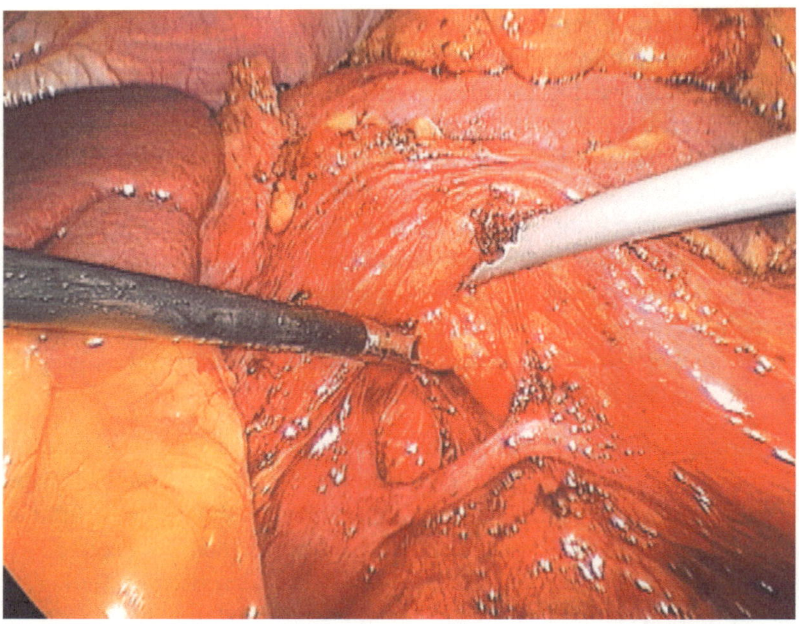

Fig. 8.2. Exposed renal hilum.

Intravenous injection of indigo carmine dye is used to delineate any collecting system violation, or retrograde injection of this dye via a ureteric catheter if it was inserted perioperatively. Any identifiable leak in the collecting system is oversewn with 4-0 absorbable sutures using the freehand intracorporeal laparoscopic technique.

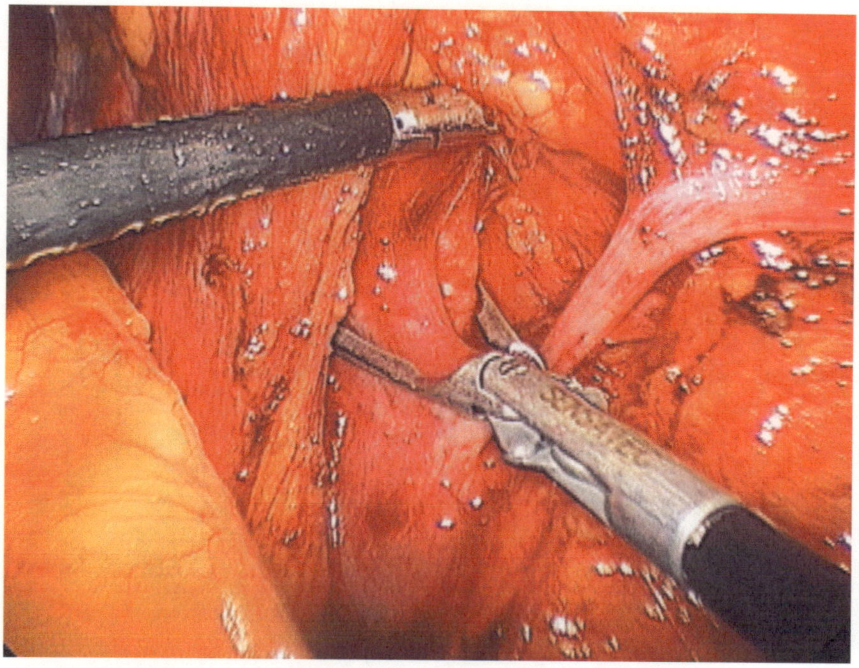

Fig. 8.3. Exposed hilum ready for clamping.

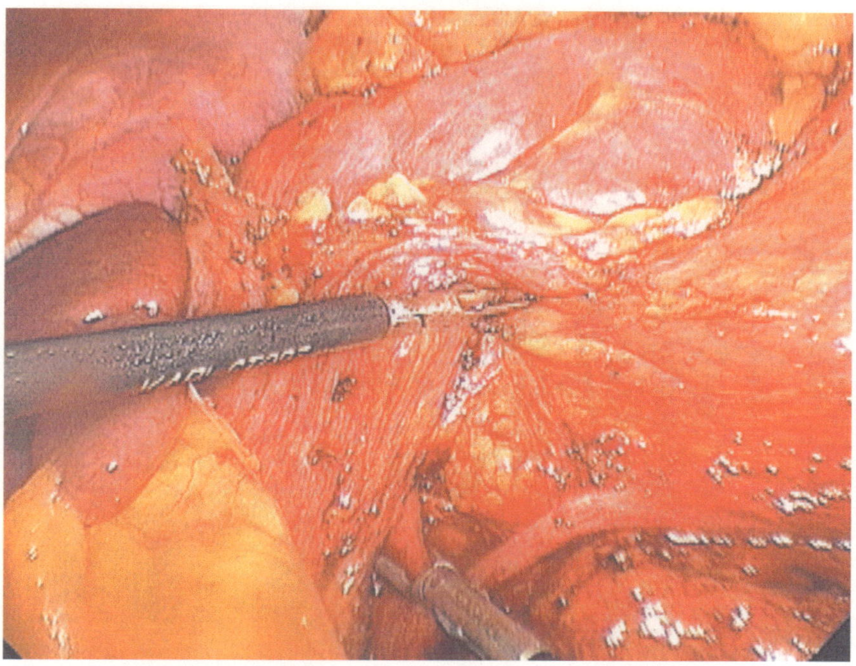

Fig. 8.4. Clamped renal hilum

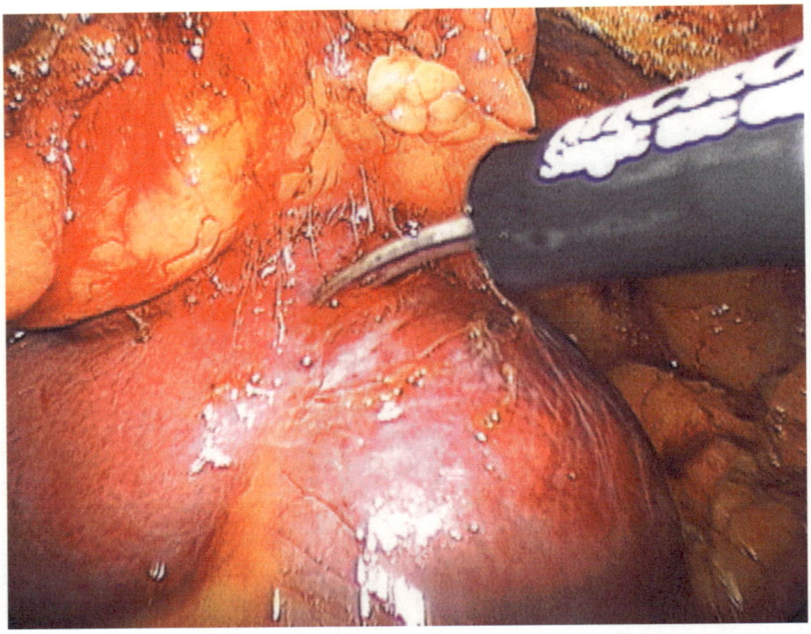

Fig. 8.5. Tumor resection using the cold scissor.

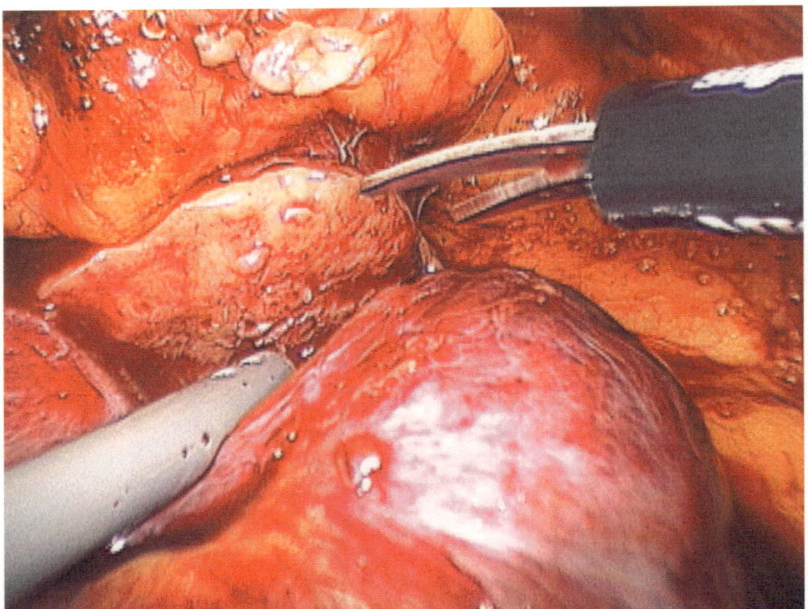

Fig. 8.6. continued tumor resection with surrounding normal parenchyma.

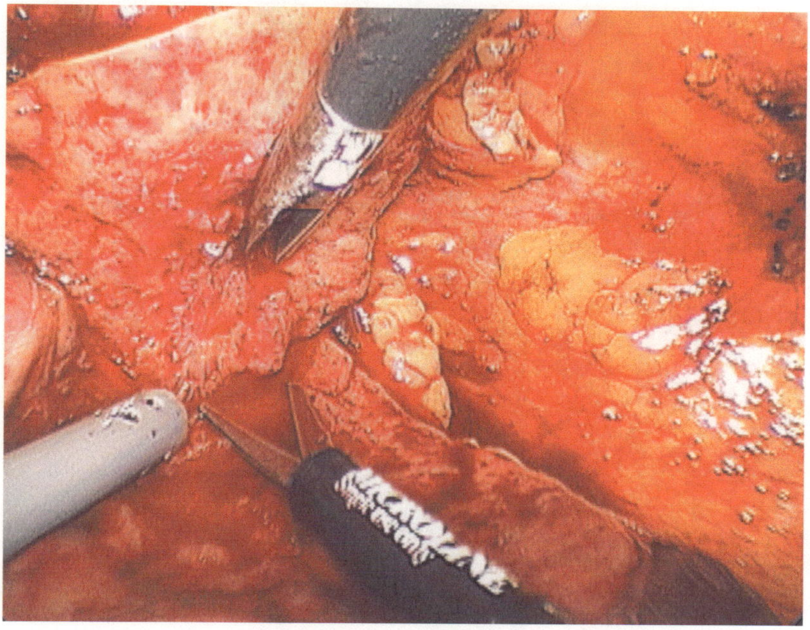

Fig. 8.7. Continued tumor resection.

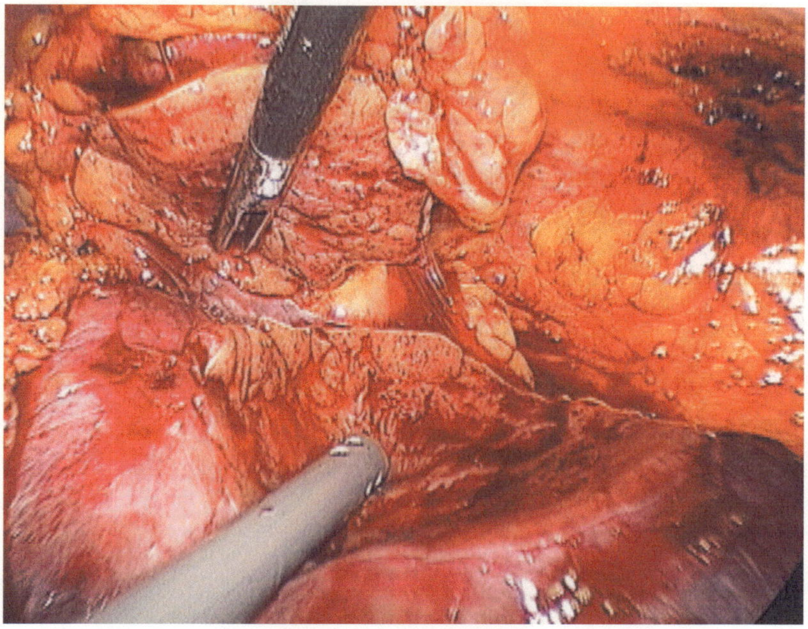

Fig. 8.8. Completely detached tumor.

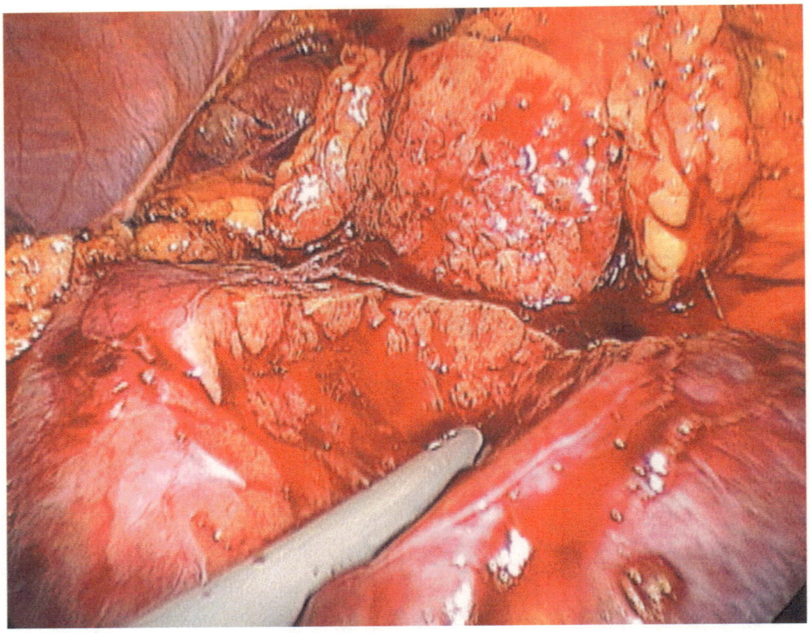

Fig. 8.9. Completely detached tumor with good surrounding parenchyma.

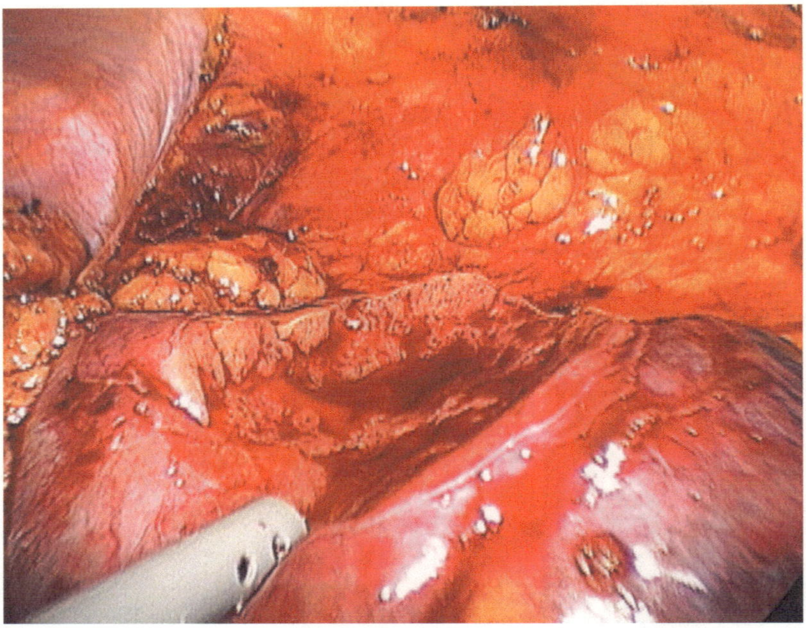

Fig. 8.10. Tumor bed.

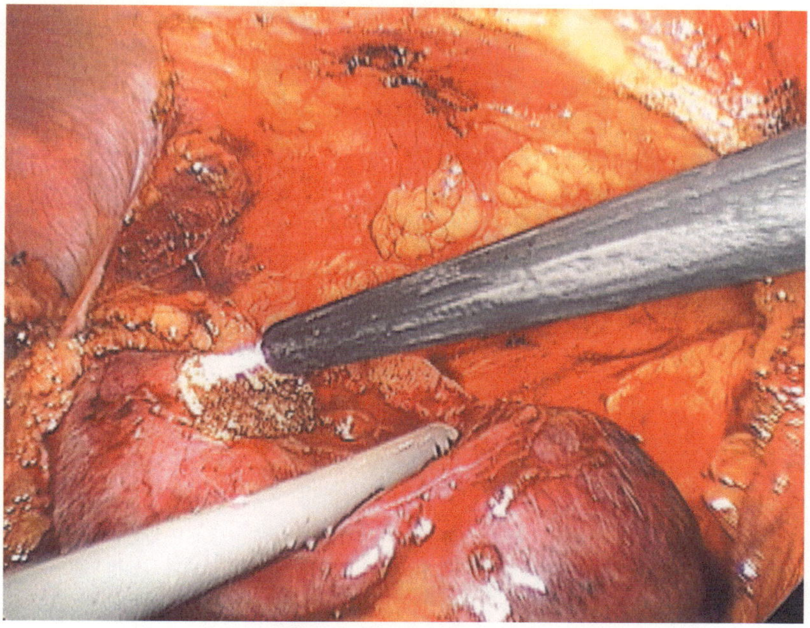

Fig. 8.11. Argon beam coagulator for bed hemostasis.

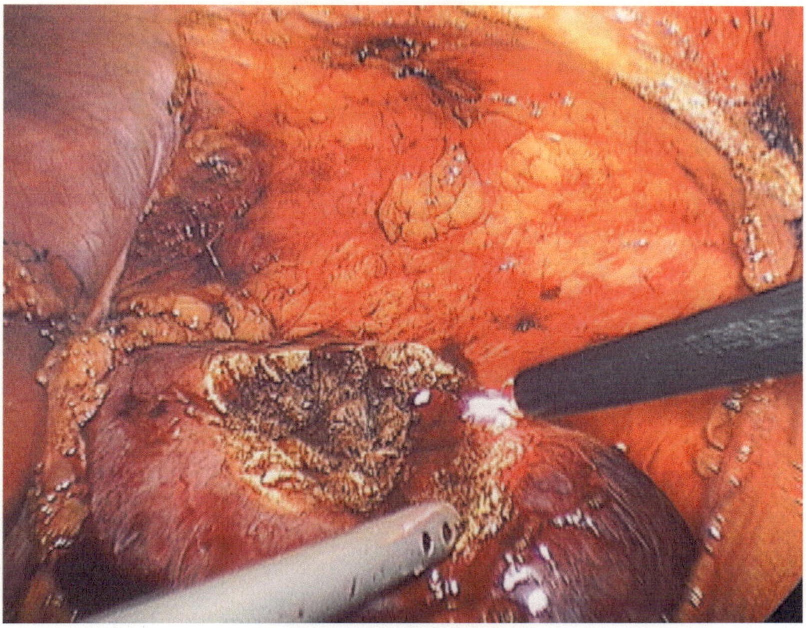

Fig. 8.12. Argon beam coagulator for bed hemostasis.

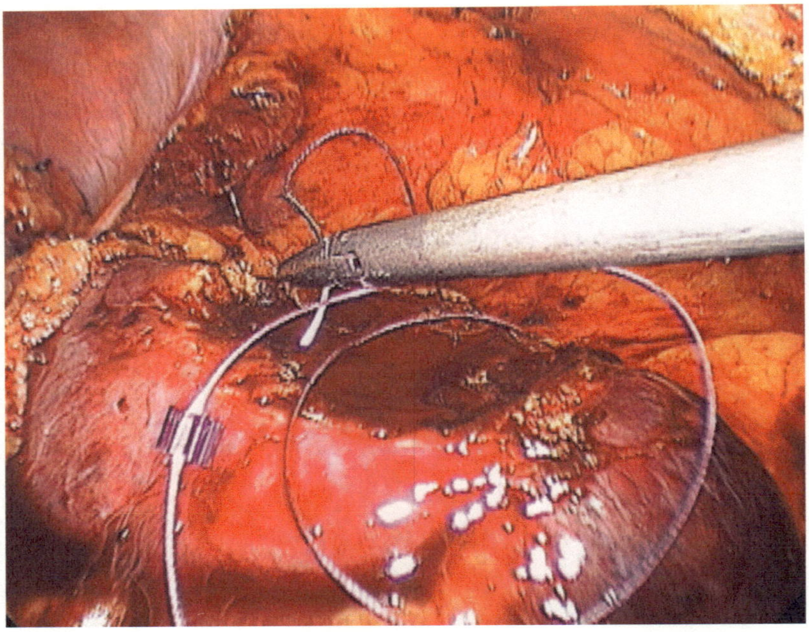

Fig. 8.13. Parenchymal intracorporeal suturing with Lapra-TY at one end.

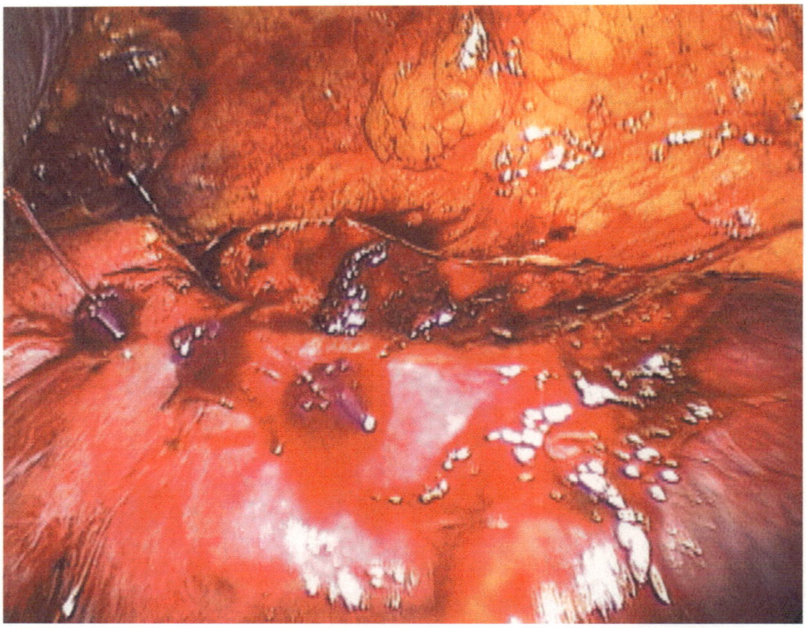

Fig. 8.14. Completed sutures with Lapra-TY on both ends.

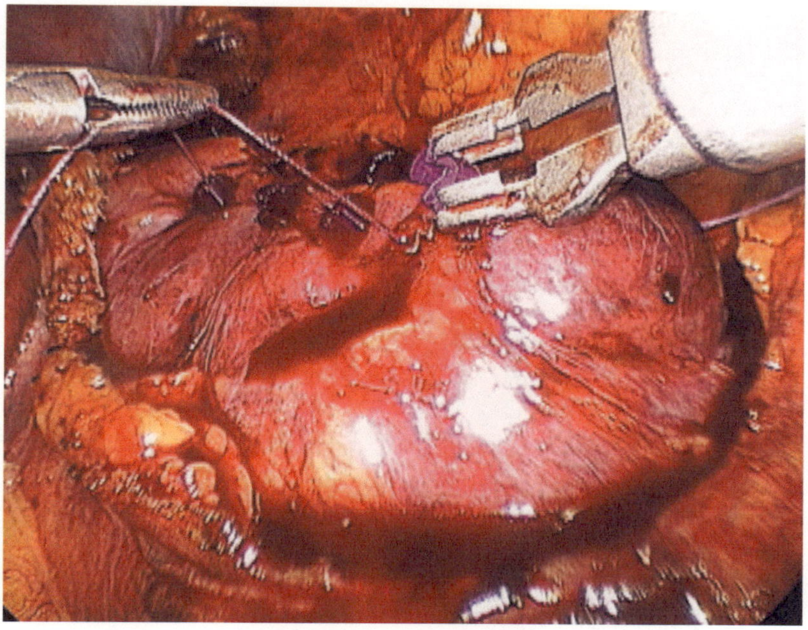

Fig. 8.15. Parenchymal suturing with Lapra-TY.

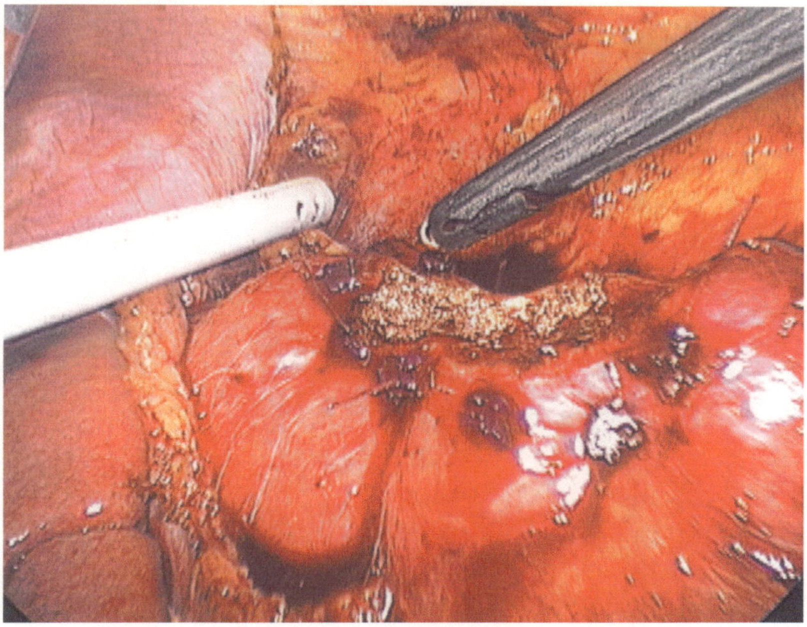

Fig. 8.16. Hemostasis with Argon beam coagulator after hilar unclamping.

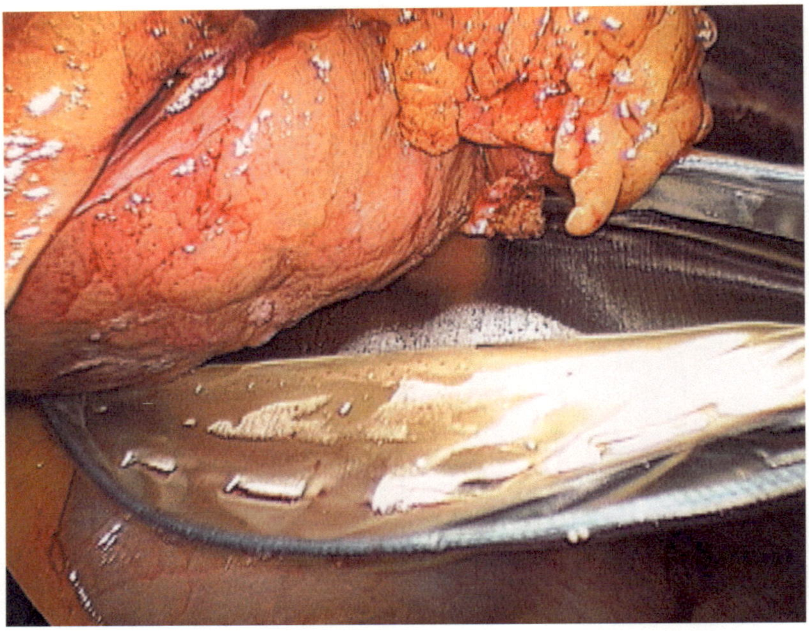

Fig. 8.17. Tumor entrapment in an Endocatch bag.

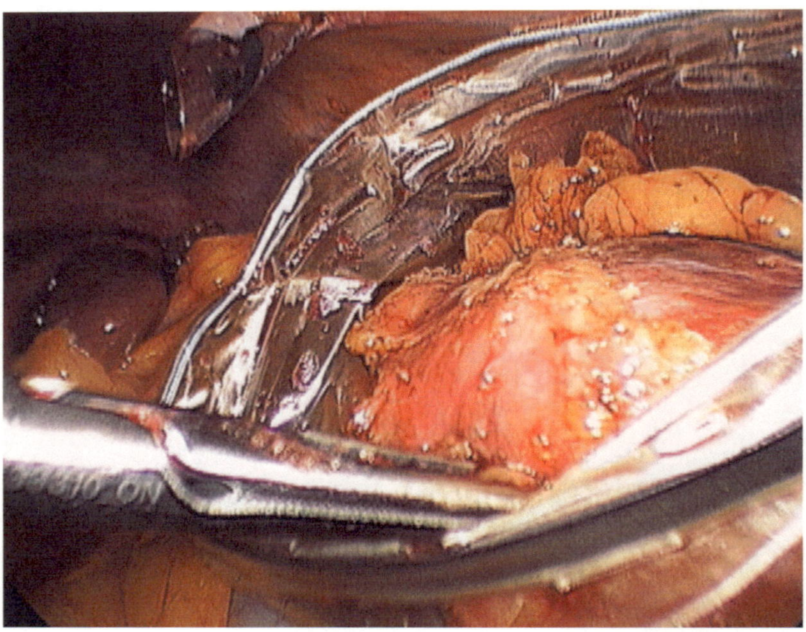

Fig. 8.18. Tumor completely entrapped.

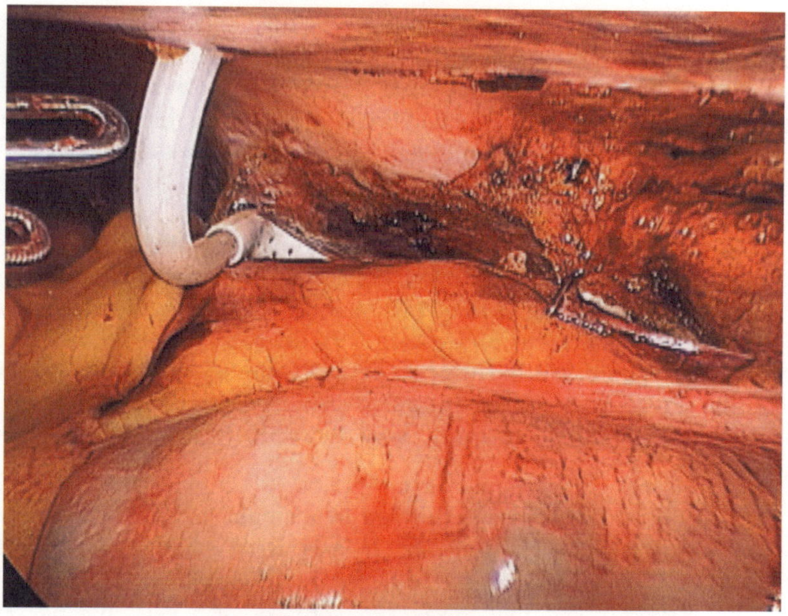

Fig. 8.19. Percutanous drain around the operated site.

If the collecting system is entered, ureteral stenting additional to a Jackson-Pratt percutanous drain placement is routinely performed (Figure 8.19). Specific figure-of-eight sutures are placed at the site of visible individual transected intrarenal vessels using a CT-1 needle and 2-0 Vicryl suture. Parenchymal closure is achieved by placing prefashioned rolled tubes or packets of oxidized cellulose sheets (Fibrillar®, Ethicon) into the parenchymal defect. Braided 2-0 absorbable sutures are used to bolster the sheets into position, and Floseal ® is applied over the operative site using a laparoscopic applicator. We perform our parenchymal repair using multiple interrupted 2-0 absorbable sutures and securing them in position using absorbable polydioxanone polymer suture clips (Lapra-TY®, Ethicon, Endosurgery). Placing one Lapra-TY clip to the end of the suture then another one to the opposite side after compressing the kidney achieves this (Figures 8.13-8.15). Surgeons can also use Hem-o-Lok ® in the place of Lapra-Ty ® for parenchymal compression, or the combination of the two for a "sliding technique".

This modification has resulted in a significant reduction of our warm ischemia time that was consumed primarily by intracorporeal suturing. Once renorrhaphy is completed, the vascular clamp is released, and the complete hemostasis and renal revascularization is confirmed. Whenever possible, the perinephric fat and Gerota's fascia is re-approximated. We extract the resected tumor along with its containing bag through a small extension of the lowermost abdominal port site incision. Laparoscopic exit under direct vision is performed once the 10-12 mm ports are closed.

3. Issues in laparoscopic partial nephrectomy

3.1 Warm ischemia and renal hypothermia

The highly differentiated cellular architecture of the kidney is dependent on the primarily aerobic renal metabolism. As such, the kidney is acutely vulnerable to the anaerobic insult conferred by warm ischemia. The severity of renal injury and its reversibility are directly proportional to the period of warm ischemia time (WIT) imposed on the unprotected kidney. The optimal warm ischemia time remains controversial. Previous studies demonstrated that recovery of renal function is complete within minutes after 10 minutes of warm ischemia, within hours after 20 minutes, within 3 to 9 days after 30 minutes, usually within weeks after 60 minutes, and incomplete or absent after 120 minutes of warm ischemia [24-26]. A 5-year, multi-centre study of WIT in LPN vs. OPN cases (n=1800) reported that the mean WIT was 30.7 minutes and 20 minutes, respectively, in each group [27]. Though the incidence of pre-operative chronic kidney disease (CKD, defined as serum creatitine >2.0 mg/dl) was measured to be 1.6% and 6.4% in each respective group, the post-operative incidence of acute renal injury was 0.9% in both groups. Unfortunately, most classic studies of WIT used crude methods of determining renal function. More recent studies, including those that implement mercaptoacetyl triglycine (MAG3) lasix renal scintigraphy to more accurately assess kidney function, have resulted in more refined guidelines.

A series of 56 consecutive LPN cases performed by a single surgeon at a single institution, using pre-operative and post-operative MAG3-lasix renal scintigraphy, demonstrated a relationship between WIT (minutes) and renal differentional function (RDF) [5]. Interestingly, the authors noted that the relationship between WIT and declining kidney function was more pronounced after 32 minutes. This suggests that within 30 minutes, focus should be on limiting resection margins, careful closure of the collecting system, and hemostasis.

Roles for cold ischemia and no ischemia have also been investigated. Also using renal scintgraphy analysis, Tatsugami and colleagues reported that, based on preoperative and postoperative analysis by renal scintigraphy of patients after OPN and LPN, cold ischemia conferred an advantage to postoperative recovery of affected renal function. The authors suggested that cold ischemia should be considered if the patient is at risk of renal function deterioration, or when warm ischemia time is expected to be >30 minutes [28]. A retrospective comparison of warm ischemia versus no ischemia during partial nephrectomy on a solitary kidney in OPN and LPN cases showed that patients with warm ischemia (median of 21 min) were more likely to develop acute renal failure (O.R. 2.1, p=0.04) and post-op GFR <15 ml/min/1.73 m^2 (OR 4.2, p=0.007) [29]. However, a surgeon selection bias was present. Patients who received warm ischemia also had significantly higher pre-op GFR and larger tumors. Even so, the authors concluded that PN without any ischemia could be considered when technically feasible.

In 2009, an expert international panel recommended that WIT be kept to <20 minutes, and that in difficult cases, cold ischemia be started immediately and should not exceed 35 minutes [30]. Currently, the debate about the appropriate and safe amount of WIT in partial nephrectomy remains unresolved. Though 30 minutes remains the acceptable limit in practice, further studies involving sophisticated means of assessing renal function may prompt changes in the future.

3.2 Hilar clamping

In LPN, clear visualization of the tumor bed is imperative. Hilar clamping achieves a bloodless operative field and decreases renal turgor. Hence, hilar clamping enhances the achievement of a precise margin of healthy parenchyma during tumor excision, suture control of transected intrarenal blood vessels, precise identification of calyceal entry followed by water-tight suture repair, and renal parenchymal reconstruction. The controlled surgical environment provided by transient hilar clamping is advantageous for a technically superior LPN. The small completely exophytic tumor with minimal parenchymal invasion may be wedge resected without hilar clamping as it would have been performed in open surgery [31, 32].

However, recent studies have demonstrated favorable results in LPN procedures conducted without hilar clamping, or by clamping only the renal artery or one of its segmental branches. Theoretically, the technique of hilar unclamping can create a less clear operative field, resulting in uncontrolled bleeding, unidentified injuries to the collecting system, and difficulty identifying the correct excisional plane. The necessity of hilar or arterial clamping becomes clear in cases where tumor resection is difficult or complex, such as tumors that are partially exophytic with a certain depth of parenchymal invasion or are large in size. A recent retrospective case series of patients who underwent LPN with or without renal artery clamping—deemed necessary when the depth of tumor invasion was greater than 50% of the renal parenchyma as seen via CT or MRI—showed that although mean operative time was longer in the clamped group ($p=0.007$), there were no significant differences in peri-operative or post-operative complications [33]. Groups were not evenly balanced, with the rate of malignant tumors confirmed via pathology being 18% in the non-clamped group, and 90% in the clamped group ($p=0.002$), suggesting. Many investigators have advocated clamping of the renal artery alone (rather than the whole pedicle. This technique facilitates precise excision, repair in a bloodless field, and continuous venous drainage to decrease venous oozing and reduce possible free-radical damage during ischemic periods. Gerber and Stockton conducted a survey to assess the trend among urologists in PN practice and found 41% of the respondents clamp the renal artery only to obtain vascular control [34]. Clamping of a segmental artery alone has also been investigated. A retrospective study at one centre has demonstrated that clamping of a single segmental artery in patients undergoing LPN for T1a or T1b tumors resulted in increased blood loss ($p<0.006$) and WI time ($p<0.001$), but equivalent post-operative complication rates, and better post-operative renal function at 3 months ($p<0.001$) compared to renal artery clamping [35]. It was noted, however, that the size (<3.5cm) and location (polar or posterior) of the tumor influenced the decision to attempt segmental artery clamping, suggesting that the novel technique was safe and feasible in select patients. Ultimately, clamping results in renal ischemia, and thus necessitates precise and expedient tumor excision and renal reconstruction. Although newer methods have been shown to be feasible, these should be reserved for select patients in the care of an experienced surgeon comfortable with these techniques.

4. Hemostasis

One of the essential elements in PN is to achieve secure renal parenchymal hemostasis. The classic technique for achieving hemostasis of the parenchymal vessels that are transected during LPN is precise suture ligation followed by a tight reapproximation of the renal parenchyma (renorrhaphy) over absorbable bolsters [36]. The renal hilum or the renal artery is cross-clamped to halt renal blood flow, similar to open PN. In efforts to decrease blood loss and warm ischemia, many hemostatic devices and materials have been reported. These are frequently used in combination and differ in their indication, efficacy, side-effects, equipment requirements and cost [34].

4.1 Hemostatic techniques

4.1.1 Parenchymal compression

Several techniques for achieving hemostasis by parenchymal compression have been described. These techniques are intended for achieving hemostasis in the resection of polar tumors. Circumferential compression of the kidney proximal to the tumor decreases blood flow to the resection site without requiring clamping.

Several recent human reports suggest that a clamping of the renal parenchyma without hilar clamping is feasible for hemostasis during LPN and open PN [37-41]. A clamp may be used on the parenchyma without dissection of the renal hilum. Clamping is limited to polar tumors and positioning the clamp can sometimes be challenging. Additionally, there are risks that the clamp may slip, causing hemorrhage, or that the pressure of the clamp may cause damage to the underlying parenchyma. Verhoest et al [42] report the use of a Satinsky clamp (Xomed Micro, France) in 5 patients undergoing LPN. The mean tumor diameter was 3.06 cm and all were polar. Mean operative time was 238 minutes and mean blood loss was 250 mL with no transfusions or other complications. Other authors have reported similar feasibility with a laparoscopic Nussbaum clamp (Aesculap AG, Tuttlingen, Germany ®) [43] and their own proprietary circumferential clamp [44].

Other methods of parenchymal compression have also been described. The double loop tourniquet technique consists of two U-loop strips of umbilical tape extending from a 17 Fr plastic sheath described by Gill et al [45] in a single LPN. McDougall et al [2] and Caddedu et al [46] have reported the use of a plastic cable tie for LPN in a pig model [2]. Compression with pledgeted sutures [47] and an Endoloop [48] have also been reported in pigs.

4.1.2 Argon beam coagulator

The argon beam coagulator (ABC) (CONMED, Utica, NY ®) is used for hemostasis along the surface of retained renal parenchyma in LPN. It is not used to coagulate larger blood vessels or for dissection. ABC works by conducting electrical current to tissue along a jet of inert, non-flammable argon gas. This gas blows away blood and other liquids on the tissue surface, enhancing visualization of the bleeding site as well as eliminating electric current dissipation in the blood. Smoke is also reduced as argon gas displaces oxygen. The surgeon should be aware of argon gas flow rates and pneumoperitoneum pressures in efforts to prevent tension pneumothorax[49] and gas embolism [50, 51]

Hernandez et al [52] have reported the successful use of the ABC for hemostasis in 25 canine partial nephrectomies without hilar clamping. The mean blood loss was 135 cc and mean depth of tissue necrosis was 2.4 mm. Meanwhile, Lucioni et al [53] have studied the use of the ABC as the sole hemostatic agent during 24 porcine laparoscopic heminephrectomies with hilar clamping. A higher power setting and completion nephrectomy were each required in one case to control bleeding.

Although no human trials reporting the efficacy of ABC have been reported, its use in conjunction with other methods is frequent [34].

4.1.3 Ultrasonic shears

Ultrasonic shears, also known as the *harmonic scalpel* (*Ultracision or Harmonic ACE*, Ethicon Endo-Surgery, Cincinnati, OH ®), allow for simultaneous tissue division and hemostasis. Hemostasis is achieved by a titanium blade vibrating at 55 000 Hz which achieves thermal denaturation of tissue into a coagulum. Animal and human studies by Jackman et al [54] and Tomita et al [55] respectively suggest that ultrasonic shears alone are insufficient for hemostasis of arcuate or larger vessels.

Harmon et al [32] evaluated its use in 15 patients undergoing LPN with small tumors (mean size 2.3 cm) without vascular clamping, and reported a mean blood loss of 368 ml and a mean operative time of 170 minutes. These investigators also employed an argon beam coagulator and oxidized cellulose gauze. Guillonneau et al [56] performed a nonrandomized retrospective comparison of two techniques for LPN, that is without and with clamping the renal vessels. In group 1 (12 patients) PN was performed with ultrasonic shears and bipolar cautery without clamping the renal vessels; while in group 2 (16 patients) the renal pedicle was clamped before tumor excision with a cold knife and hemostasis achieved by sutures and hemostatic mesh. All tumors but 1 were exophytic. Mean renal ischemia time was 27.3 minutes (range 15-47 minutes) in group 2 patients. Mean laparoscopic operating time was 179.1 minutes (range 90-390 minutes) in group 1 compared with 121.5 minutes (range 60-210 minutes) in group 2 ($p = 0.004$). Mean intraoperative blood loss was significantly higher in group 1 than in group 2 (708.3 versus 270.3 ml, $p = 0.014$). Surgical margins were negative in all specimens.

Ultrasonic shears are primarily useful in small peripheral lesions which may be excised without vascular occlusion. Disadvantages of ultrasonic shears used for this purpose include tissue charring, tissue adherence, and an inexact line of parenchymal incision with poor visualization of the tumor bed. They are also inadequate as a sole hemostatic agent and not recommended for larger or deeper tumors. The *harmonic scalpel* is not recommended when vascular clamping is employed as the harmonic scalpel is slower than other methods and may result in kidney damage secondary to increased warm ischemic time [56].

4.1.4 Water (hydro) jet dissection

Hydro-jet (Erbe Elektromedizia GmbH, Tubingen, Germany ®) involves using a high-pressure jet of saline to selectively dissect parenchymal tissue. Blood vessels and the collecting system are not penetrated if a 400-600 psi pressure is used [57]. Shekarriz et al have investigated this technology during LPN with hilar control in the porcine model[58] and reported a virtually bloodless field with the vessels and collecting system preserved. Moinzadeh et al [57] similarly evaluated hydro-jet assisted LPN in the calf model. Vessels were controlled with a BIClamp (Erbe Elektromedizia GmbH, Turbingen, Germany) bipolar instrument. Of 20 LPN, 18 were performed without hilar clamping and in 15 only the bipolar instrument was required for hemostasis. The mean Hydro-jet PN time was 63 minutes (range 13-150 minutes) and mean estimated blood loss was 174 ml (range 20 to 750 mL). Corvin et al [59] have also demonstrated the feasibility of Hydro-jet in wedge resection in the pig model.

The use of Hydro-jet dissection in LPN in humans has not been formally reported. Basting et al.[60] report the use of Hydro-jet in a series of 24 renal sparing surgeries performed for benign and neoplastic disease. Dissection took between 14 and 35 minutes and the average blood loss was 60mL with no significant complications. Shekarriz[61] describes unpublished data that hydro-dissection was successfully used in 6 open partial nephrectomies for RCC without hilar control. Dissection time was 20-30 minutes, blood loss ranged from 150-500 mL (mean 265 mL) and there were no complications.

4.1.5 Microwave coagulation

Microwave tissue coagulation (MTC) with the Microtaze device (Azwell, Osaka, Japan) utilizes a needle-type monopolar electrode which is inserted into the kidney repeatedly prior to renal incision. 2450 MHz of microwave energy is applied to tissue surrounding the electrode forming a conical-shaped wedge of coagulated tissue extending up to 10mm. Partial nephrectomy is then performed in the plane of coagulated tissue resulting in a relatively blood-free field. MTC necessitates mobilization of the entire kidney for appropriate probe insertion and has the potential for serious complications, as subsequently described.

Terai et al [62] have used MTC to perform LPN in 18 patients with peripheral tumors. They report a mean operative time of 240 minutes (range 131-390 minutes). Minimal blood loss occurred in 14 patients and 100-400mL blood loss occurred in the remaining. Postoperative complications which were managed conservatively included a hematoma in an anticoagulated patient and a 14-day urinary leak. A renal arteriovenous fistula that required embolization occurred in one patient. Finally, pelvicalyceal stenosis resulting in a nonfunctional kidney occurred in another patient. Similar complications have also been reported in OPN [63, 64]. Yoshimura et al [65], Satoh et al [66] and Itoh et al [67] have reported smaller MTC LPN series without such complications.

4.1.6 Radiofrequency ablation

Radiofrequency ablation (RFA) involves the delivery of energy via a needle causing coagulation around the inserted probe. Investigators have successfully used interstitial ablative technologies (like radiofrequency ablation and cryotherapy) as definitive in situ management of select renal lesions. Ablated tumors are left in situ, necessitating concerns about the oncologic effectiveness of ablation in the target lesion and the cost of radiographic follow-up. In RFA-assisted LPN, radiofrequency coagulation can be used prior to partial nephrectomy to achieve energy-based tissue destruction followed by resection of the ablated tissue. Resection of ablated tissue is relatively bloodless obviating the need for hilar clamping.

Wu et al [68] have recently published a series comparing 36 patients undergoing LPN with hilar clamping to 42 patients undergoing RFA-assisted robotic clampless partial nephrectomy. Tumors were larger in the RFA group (2.8 vs. 2.0cm), more often endophytic (52.6% vs. 16.1%) and collecting system reconstruction occurred more often (78.6% vs. 30.6%). Although operative time was longer in the RFA group (373 vs. 250 minutes), blood loss, transfusion rates, renal function and complication rates did not differ between groups. Zeltser et al [69] have also published a series of 32 tumors treated with RFA-assisted LPN.

Mean blood loss was 80 mL and there were no recurrences at a mean follow-up of 31 months. Other authors have also published series on this technique[70-72].

4.1.7 TissueLink

Another option that may be used for dissection and hemostasis is the TissueLink Floating Ball (TissueLink Medical, Inc., Dover, NH). This is a monopolar device that employs radiofrequency current for dissection and uses saline as a cooling medium. A total of 34 patients in several series were identified by us [73-76] which all had appropriate operative time, oncologic control, complications and blood loss when compared to other hemostatic devices.

4.2 Hemostatic materials

Hemostatic materials involve the application of a substance to the resection bed to effect hemostasis. Classes of hemostatic materials include fibrin sealants, gelatin matrix sealants, hydrogel based sealants and oxidized cellulose. The use of multiple hemostatic materials is routine in centers performing LPN [77].

These materials differ in their mechanism, cost, application conditions, uses, and tissue reaction. A rigorous comparison of these materials is beyond the scope of this chapter due to the number of products and absence of appropriate comparative studies. Concerns that arise when using these products include cost, risk allergic reaction, potential transmission of prion and other infectious diseases, and the need to mix two components and/or sequentially apply them.

Fibrin products include Tisseel (Baxter), Beriplast (CSL BehringGmbH), Hemaseel (HMN), Costasis (Cohesion Technologies), Vivostat (Vivostat A/S), and Evicel (Ethicon, Johnson & Johnson). Fibrin products must be applied to a dry surface and may offer both hemostasis and sealing of the collecting system [78]. Generally, these products include a concentrated solution of human fibrinogen which is mixed with thrombin and calcium chloride. The addition of aprotinin helps to slow the natural fibrinolysis occurring at the resection site. Natural bioabsorption eventually occurs from plasma-mediated lysis [79]. Fibrin sealants may also come in sprays [80]. Autologous fibrin sealants, such as Vivostat, have been developed in attempts to minimize this risk of infectious and allergic complications. Authors have demonstrated that fibrin sealants may be effective as the sole hemostatic technique or used in conjunction with other methods [79, 81, 82].

Gelatin matrix products provide thrombin, calcium, and bovine-derived gelatin granules. These agents include FloSeal (Baxter), which is our preferred hemostatic flowable agent to use during LPN. FloSeal may be applied to a wet surface and function only in parenchymal hemostasis. Unlike fibrin sealants, thrombin in these products converts fibrinogen from the patient's blood into a fibrin clot. The gelatin granules swell on contact with blood, creating a composite hemostatic plug with physical bulk that mechanically controls hemorrhage [83]. Gill et al [83] have reported a series of 131 patients, in which they compared their conventional technique of sutured renorraphy over a Surgicel bolster to the same technique with the addition of Floseal. FloSeal significantly reduced overall complications (37% vs. 16%) and had a trend towards lower rates of hemorrhagic complications (12% vs. 3%). Wille et al [84], Richter et al [85] and Bak et al [86] have also described positive series.

Bovine serum albumin and glutaraldehyde tissue adhesive (BioGlue, Cryolife, Kennesaw, GA) is another sealant that is applied to a dry surface and controls both the renal parenchyma and collecting system. Glutaraldehyde exposure causes the lysine molecules of the bovine serum albumin, extracellular matrix proteins, and cell surfaces to bind to each other, creating a strong covalent bond. The reaction is spontaneous without needing the patient's coagulation factors. The glue begins to polymerize within 20 to 30 seconds and reaches maximal strength in approximately 2 minutes, resulting in a strong implant. The degradation process takes approximately 2 years, and it is then replaced with fibrotic granulation tissue. Several series support the use of BioGlue [87, 88] .

Oxidized cellulose products include Surgicel (Johnson & Johnson, Somerville, NJ), Gelfoam (Pfizer, Inc., New York, NY) and Surgifoam (Johnson & Johnson). These products have hemostatic properties and can also be left as a bolster within the kidney to tamponade bleeding. Authors report the use of the bulk of these products to close fill parenchymal defects [89] although it is associated with a foreign-body reaction [90].

While numerous other hemostatic agents exist, these products represent the most frequently used materials. Newer products are currently being developed using various in vivo and in vitro models [91-93].

5. Morbidity

LPN improves upon the morbidity of open PN. Investigators from Cleveland Clinic analyzed the complications of their initial 200 cases treated with LPN for a suspected renal tumor [94] and reported that 66 (33%) patients had a complication: 36 (18%) patients had urologic complications, the majority of which was bleeding, and 30 (15%) patients had non-urologic complications. This experienced team also reported a decreased complication rate (16%) since they began using a biologic hemostatic agent as an adjunctive measure. Gill et al[19] compared 100 patients who underwent LPN with 100 patients who underwent OPN. The median surgical time was 3 hours vs 3.9 hours ($p < 0.001$), estimated blood loss was 125 ml vs 250 ml ($p < 0.001$), and mean WIT was 28 minutes vs 18 minutes ($p < 0.001$). The laparoscopic group required less postoperative analgesia, a shorter hospital stay, and a shorter convalescence. Intraoperative complications were higher in the laparoscopic group (5% vs 0%; $p = 0.02$), and postoperative complications were similar (9% vs 14%; $p = 0.27$). Functional outcomes were similar in the two groups: median preoperative serum creatinine (1.0 vs 1.0 mg/dl, $p < 0.52$) and postoperative serum creatinine (1.1 vs 1.2 mg/dl, $p < 0.65$).

Similarly, Beasley et al[95] retrospectively compared the result of laparoscopic PN to OPN using a tumor size-matched cohort of patients. Although the mean operative time was longer in the laparoscopic group (210 ± 76 minutes versus 144 ± 24 minutes; $p < 0.001$), the blood loss was comparable between the two groups (250 ± 250 ml vs 334 ± 343 ml; p = not statistically significant). No blood transfusions were performed in either group. The hospital stay was significantly reduced after LPN compared with the open group (2.9 ± 1.5 days vs 6.4 ± 1.8 days; $p < 0.0002$), and the postoperative parenteral narcotic requirements were lower in the LPN group (mean morphine equivalent 43 ± 62 mg vs 187 ± 71 mg; $p < 0.02$).

These initial results have been reproduced in recent studies. In an analysis of 1800 OPN and LPN cases for single renal T1 tumours, LPN was associated with shorter operative time, decreased operative blood loss, and shorter hospital stay ($p<0.01$) [27]. Another multicentre study of 10 years' worth of data demonstrated decreased transfusion incidence and estimated blood loss less (293 vs 418 cc) in LPN compared to OPN [96].

Interestingly, published studies have not demonstrated increased morbidity for LPN for T1b tumors. A retrospective study at a single centre compared operative and post-operative complications in patients who underwent LPN for tumors > 4cm to those who underwent LPN for tumors ≤ 4cm. The authors concluded that there were no significant differences observed with respect to operating time, transfusion requirements, post-operative complications, or hospital stay, suggesting that LPN, from a morbidity standpoint, is feasible for tumors > 4 cm in carefully selected patients [97].

Despite the absence of a prospective randomized controlled trials, these congruent series suggest improved morbidity from LPN relative to open PN.

6. Oncologic results

Longitudinal studies for LPN for tumors ≤ 4 cm and > 4 cm have demonstrated the efficacy and safety of this approach comparable to OPN and other laparoscopic techniques. The 3 year cancer-specific survival for patients with a single cT1N0M0 RCC has been reported similar for OPN and LPN (99.3% LPN and 99.2% OPN) [27]. In a 5 year, intermediate-term study, comparing laparoscopic radical nephrectomy (LRN) and LPN (n=35) for T1b-T3N0M0 RCC, overall mortality (11% in each group), cancer-specific mortality (3% in each group) and recurrence (3% vs 6%) rates (p=0.4) were equivalent [9]. Recurrence-free survival in each group was 96%. The longest follow-up study to date is a retrospective 7-year follow-up study comparing oncologic outcomes of LPN and OPN for a single cT1 cortical tumor 7cm or less. Metastases free survival with a minimum of 7 years follow-up was equivalent in both groups (97.5% LPN vs. 97.3% OPN, p=0.47.) After multivariable analysis that accounted for the propensity to undergo LPN, surgical approach was not associated with a significant difference in the odds of metastases (OR 2.18, 95% CI 0.85-5.89) [98].

Promising oncologic outcomes have also been reported for LPN with respect to more complex tumors. Porpilgia et al published a retrospective case series of 100 consecutive patients LPN for tumors ≤ 4 cm and tumors greater than 4 cm, demonstrating that in spite of statistically significant differences in tumor size and location (p=0.002), the incidence of positive surgical margins was equivalent and acceptable pathologic results were achieved in both groups [11]. Similarly, a study comparing bilateral OPN to bilateral LPN for bilateral kidney tumors demonstrated equivalent cancer-specific and recurrence-free survival rates in both groups over a mean follow-up of 5.5 years [13].

7. Emerging techniques: Robot-assisted LPN and Laproendoscopic Single-Site (LESS) surgery

Robot-assisted LPN (RPN) has recently been introduced at several centres around the world. In general, its indications are the same as for OPN and LPN[99], and the transperitoneal approach is used most often[18]. Preliminary data suggests that RPN is equivalent to LPN in terms of WIT, perioperative status, and functional outcomes, but the main drawbacks of RPN remain cost and need for trained personnel.

Studies comparing RPN to OPN, comparing RPN to LPN, and investigating the outcomes of RPN for hilar and more complex tumours suggest that RPN is safe, feasible, and provides equivalent functional outcomes to the existing standard procedures [100-103]. In some instances, it also results in a shorter hospital stay [100, 102]. A small study involving 11 patients examined the intra-operative use of indocyanine green to facilitate near infrared fluorescent imaging during RPN. The imaging was used to successfully delineate the renal vasculature in all cases. Interestingly, of the 10 patients with malignancies that were eventually confirmed via histopathology, 7 of these tumors were hyper-fluorescent compared to the surrounding renal parenchyma during the intra-operative imaging [104]. Similarly, Laparoendoscopic Single-Site (LESS) partial nephrectomy is an emerging technique that has been proven feasible for small, exophytic, easily approachable tumors [18]. Further data, prospective studies, and greater surgical experience are needed to truly realize the potential of these emerging technologies.

8. Cost effectiveness

Emerging data suggests that LPN is the most cost-effective procedure for small renal masses. A simulation analysis for cost-effectiveness– based on the case of a healthy 65-year old patient with an asymptomatic, unilateral small renal mass, and using quality adjusted life-years as a measure of benefit– concluded that immediate LPN was the most cost-effective nephron-sparing strategy [105]. In this model, LPN was favorable to OPN, laparoscopic or percutaneous ablation, active surveillance, and nonsurgical management with observation. A direct financial analysis conducted in a retrospective Canadian study demonstrated a lower total hospital cost after LPN (4839 dollars ± 1551 dollars vs. 6297 dollars ± 2972 dollars; $p < 0.05$) when compared to OPN [95]. Similarly, a retrospective meta-analysis of 2745 procedures (OPN, LPN, and RPN) confirmed that despite similar OR times, LPN was more cost effective than OPN because of a shorter length of hospital stay. Additionally, despite a longer length of stay compared to RPN, LPN was more cost effective due to lower instrumentation costs [106]. These analyses suggest that LPN currently represents the most economical option with regard to nephron-sparing procedures.

9. Summary

Partial nephrectomy is a standard of care for the surgical management small renal masses. In the past decade, laparoscopic partial nephrectomy has advanced to offer equivalent functional and oncologic outcomes, when compared to open partial nephrectomy and laparoscopic radical nephrectomy, at lower cost. Although the appropriate amount of WIT remains controversial, emerging technology (including hemostatic devices and robotic systems) will continue to facilitate improvement in the surgical management of renal masses.

10. References

[1] Clayman, R.V., et al., *Laparoscopic nephrectomy: initial case report.* J Urol, 1991. 146(2): p. 278-82.

[2] McDougall, E.M., et al., *Laparoscopic partial nephrectomy in the pig model.* J Urol, 1993. 149(6): p. 1633-6.
[3] Winfield, H.N., et al., *Laparoscopic partial nephrectomy: initial case report for benign disease.* J Endourol, 1993. 7(6): p. 521-6.
[4] Finelli, A. and I.S. Gill, *Laparoscopic partial nephrectomy: contemporary technique and results.* Urol Oncol, 2004. 22(2): p. 139-44.
[5] Pouliot, F., et al., *Multivariate analysis of the factors involved in loss of renal differential function after laparoscopic partial nephrectomy: a role for warm ischemia time.* Can Urol Assoc J, 2011. 5(2): p. 89-95.
[6] Campbell, S.C., et al., *Guideline for management of the clinical T1 renal mass.* J Urol, 2009. 182(4): p. 1271-9.
[7] Ljungberg, B., et al., *Renal cell carcinoma guideline.* Eur Urol, 2007. 51(6): p. 1502-10.
[8] Herr, H.W., *Partial nephrectomy for unilateral renal carcinoma and a normal contralateral kidney: 10-year followup.* J Urol, 1999. 161(1): p. 33-4; discussion 34-5.
[9] Simmons, M.N., C.J. Weight, and I.S. Gill, *Laparoscopic radical versus partial nephrectomy for tumors >4 cm: intermediate-term oncologic and functional outcomes.* Urology, 2009. 73(5): p. 1077-82.
[10] Kim, J.M., et al., *Comparison of Partial and Radical Nephrectomy for pT1b Renal Cell Carcinoma.* Korean J Urol, 2010. 51(9): p. 596-600.
[11] Porpiglia, F., et al., *Does tumour size really affect the safety of laparoscopic partial nephrectomy?* BJU Int, 2011. 108(2): p. 268-73.
[12] Shikanov, S., et al., *Laparoscopic partial nephrectomy for technically challenging tumours.* BJU Int, 2010. 106(1): p. 91-4.
[13] Ching, C.B., et al., *Functional and oncologic outcomes of bilateral open partial nephrectomy versus bilateral laparoscopic partial nephrectomy.* J Endourol, 2011. 25(7): p. 1193-7.
[14] Tsivian, A., et al., *Laparoscopic partial nephrectomy for multiple tumours: feasibility and analysis of peri-operative outcomes.* BJU Int, 2010.
[15] Deklaj, T., et al., *Localized T1a renal lesions in the elderly: outcomes of laparoscopic renal surgery.* J Endourol, 2010. 24(3): p. 397-401.
[16] Marszalek, M., et al., *Laparoscopic partial nephrectomy: a matched-pair comparison of the transperitoneal versus the retroperitoneal approach.* Urology, 2011. 77(1): p. 109-13.
[17] Wright, J.L. and J.R. Porter, *Laparoscopic partial nephrectomy: comparison of transperitoneal and retroperitoneal approaches.* J Urol, 2005. 174(3): p. 841-5.
[18] Lee, S.Y., J.D. Choi, and S.I. Seo, *Current status of partial nephrectomy for renal mass.* Korean J Urol, 2011. 52(5): p. 301-9.
[19] Gill, I.S., et al., *Comparative analysis of laparoscopic versus open partial nephrectomy for renal tumors in 200 patients.* J Urol, 2003. 170(1): p. 64-8.
[20] Winfield, H.N., et al., *Laparoscopic partial nephrectomy: initial experience and comparison to the open surgical approach.* J Urol, 1995. 153(5): p. 1409-14.
[21] Wolf, J.S., Jr., B.D. Seifman, and J.E. Montie, *Nephron sparing surgery for suspected malignancy: open surgery compared to laparoscopy with selective use of hand assistance.* J Urol, 2000. 163(6): p. 1659-64.
[22] Gill, I.S., et al., *Laparoscopic partial nephrectomy for renal tumor: duplicating open surgical techniques.* J Urol, 2002. 167(2 Pt 1): p. 469-7; discussion 475-6.
[23] Janetschek, G., et al., *Laparoscopic nephron sparing surgery for small renal cell carcinoma.* J Urol, 1998. 159(4): p. 1152-5.

[24] Ward, J.P., *Determination of the Optimum temperature for regional renal hypothermia during temporary renal ischaemia.* Br J Urol, 1975. 47(1): p. 17-24.

[25] Novick, A.C., *Renal hypothermia: in vivo and ex vivo.* Urol Clin North Am, 1983. 10(4): p. 637-44.

[26] McLoughlin, G.A., M.R. Heal, and I.M. Tyrell, *An evaluation of techniques used for the production of temporary renal ischaemia.* Br J Urol, 1978. 50(6): p. 371-5.

[27] Gill, I.S., et al., *Comparison of 1,800 laparoscopic and open partial nephrectomies for single renal tumors.* J Urol, 2007. 178(1): p. 41-6.

[28] Tatsugami, K., et al., *Impact of cold and warm ischemia on postoperative recovery of affected renal function after partial nephrectomy.* J Endourol, 2011. 25(5): p. 869-73; discussion 873-4.

[29] Thompson, R.H., et al., *Comparison of warm ischemia versus no ischemia during partial nephrectomy on a solitary kidney.* Eur Urol, 2010. 58(3): p. 331-6.

[30] Becker, F., et al., *Assessing the impact of ischaemia time during partial nephrectomy.* Eur Urol, 2009. 56(4): p. 625-34.

[31] McDougall, E.M., A.M. Elbahnasy, and R.V. Clayman, *Laparoscopic wedge resection and partial nephrectomy--the Washington University experience and review of the literature.* JSLS, 1998. 2(1): p. 15-23.

[32] Harmon, W.J., L.R. Kavoussi, and J.T. Bishoff, *Laparoscopic nephron-sparing surgery for solid renal masses using the ultrasonic shears.* Urology, 2000. 56(5): p. 754-9.

[33] Koo, H.J., D.H. Lee, and I.Y. Kim, *Renal hilar control during laparoscopic partial nephrectomy: to clamp or not to clamp.* J Endourol, 2010. 24(8): p. 1283-7.

[34] Gerber, G.S. and B.R. Stockton, *Laparoscopic partial nephrectomy.* J Endourol, 2005. 19(1): p. 21-4.

[35] Shao, P., et al., *Laparoscopic partial nephrectomy with segmental renal artery clamping: technique and clinical outcomes.* Eur Urol, 2011. 59(5): p. 849-55.

[36] Novick, A.C., et al., *Operative urology at the Cleveland Clinic.* 2006, Humana Press: Totowa, N.J. p. xiv, 552 p.

[37] Simon, J., et al., *Optimizing selective renal clamping in nephron-sparing surgery using the Nussbaum clamp.* Urology, 2008. 71(6): p. 1196-8.

[38] Huyghe, E., et al., *Open partial nephrectomy with selective renal parenchymal control: a new reliable clamp.* Urology, 2006. 68(3): p. 658-60.

[39] Mejean, A., et al., *Nephron sparing surgery for renal cell carcinoma using selective renal parenchymal clamping.* J Urol, 2002. 167(1): p. 234-5.

[40] Denardi, F., et al., *Nephron-sparing surgery for renal tumours using selective renal parenchymal clamping.* BJU Int, 2005. 96(7): p. 1036-9.

[41] Rodriguez-Covarrubias, F., et al., *Partial nephrectomy for renal tumors using selective parenchymal clamping.* Int Urol Nephrol, 2007. 39(1): p. 43-6.

[42] Verhoest, G., et al., *Laparoscopic partial nephrectomy with clamping of the renal parenchyma: initial experience.* Eur Urol, 2007. 52(5): p. 1340-6.

[43] Simon, J., et al., *Laparoscopic partial nephrectomy with selective control of the renal parenchyma: initial experience with a novel laparoscopic clamp.* BJU Int, 2009. 103(6): p. 805-8.

[44] Toren, P., et al., *Use of a novel parenchymal clamp for laparoscopic and open partial nephrectomy.* Can Urol Assoc J, 2010. 4(5): p. E133-6.

[45] Gill, I.S., et al., *A new renal tourniquet for open and laparoscopic partial nephrectomy.* J Urol, 1995. 154(3): p. 1113-6.

[46] Cadeddu, J.A., et al., *Hemostatic laparoscopic partial nephrectomy: cable-tie compression.* Urology, 2001. 57(3): p. 562-6.

[47] Wilhelm, D.M., et al., *Feasibility of laparoscopic partial nephrectomy using pledgeted compression sutures for hemostasis.* J Endourol, 2003. 17(4): p. 223-7.

[48] Beck, S.D., et al., *Endoloop-assisted laparoscopic partial nephrectomy.* J Endourol, 2002. 16(3): p. 175-7.

[49] Shanberg, A.M., M. Zagnoev, and T.P. Clougherty, *Tension pneumothorax caused by the argon beam coagulator during laparoscopic partial nephrectomy.* J Urol, 2002. 168(5): p. 2162.

[50] Min, S.K., J.H. Kim, and S.Y. Lee, *Carbon dioxide and argon gas embolism during laparoscopic hepatic resection.* Acta Anaesthesiol Scand, 2007. 51(7): p. 949-53.

[51] *Fatal gas embolism caused by overpressurization during laparoscopic use of argon enhanced coagulation.* Health Devices, 1994. 23(6): p. 257-9.

[52] Hernandez, A.D., et al., *A controlled study of the argon beam coagulator for partial nephrectomy.* J Urol, 1990. 143(5): p. 1062-5.

[53] Lucioni, A., et al., *Efficacy of the argon beam coagulator alone in obtaining hemostasis after laparoscopic porcine heminephrectomy: a pilot study.* Can J Urol, 2008. 15(3): p. 4091-6.

[54] Jackman, S.V., et al., *Utility of the harmonic scalpel for laparoscopic partial nephrectomy.* J Endourol, 1998. 12(5): p. 441-4.

[55] Tomita, Y., et al., *Use of the harmonic scalpel for nephron sparing surgery in renal cell carcinoma.* J Urol, 1998. 159(6): p. 2063-4.

[56] Guillonneau, B., et al., *Laparoscopic partial nephrectomy for renal tumor: single center experience comparing clamping and no clamping techniques of the renal vasculature.* J Urol, 2003. 169(2): p. 483-6.

[57] Moinzadeh, A., et al., *Water jet assisted laparoscopic partial nephrectomy without hilar clamping in the calf model.* J Urol, 2005. 174(1): p. 317-21.

[58] Shekarriz, H., et al., *Hydro-jet assisted laparoscopic partial nephrectomy: initial experience in a porcine model.* J Urol, 2000. 163(3): p. 1005-8.

[59] Corvin, S., et al., *Use of hydro-jet cutting for laparoscopic partial nephrectomy in a porcine model.* Urology, 2001. 58(6): p. 1070-3.

[60] Basting, R.F., N. Djakovic, and P. Widmann, *Use of water jet resection in organ-sparing kidney surgery.* J Endourol, 2000. 14(6): p. 501-5.

[61] Shekarriz, B., *Hydro-Jet technology in urologic surgery.* Expert Rev Med Devices, 2005. 2(3): p. 287-91.

[62] Terai, A., et al., *Laparoscopic partial nephrectomy using microwave tissue coagulator for small renal tumors: usefulness and complications.* Eur Urol, 2004. 45(6): p. 744-8.

[63] Murota, T., et al., *Retroperitoneoscopic partial nephrectomy using microwave coagulation for small renal tumors.* Eur Urol, 2002. 41(5): p. 540-5; discussion 545.

[64] Akiyama, T., et al., *Renal arteriovenous fistula developing after tumor enucleation using a microwave tissue coagulator.* Int J Urol, 2001. 8(10): p. 568-71.

[65] Yoshimura, K., et al., *Laparoscopic partial nephrectomy with a microwave tissue coagulator for small renal tumor.* J Urol, 2001. 165(6 Pt 1): p. 1893-6.

[66] Satoh, Y., et al., *Renal-tissue damage induced by laparoscopic partial nephrectomy using microwave tissue coagulator.* J Endourol, 2005. 19(7): p. 818-22.

[67] Itoh, K., et al., *Posterior retroperitoneoscopic partial nephrectomy using microwave tissue coagulator for small renal tumors.* J Endourol, 2002. 16(6): p. 367-71.

[68] Wu, S.D., et al., *Radiofrequency ablation-assisted robotic laparoscopic partial nephrectomy without renal hilar vessel clamping versus laparoscopic partial nephrectomy: a comparison of perioperative outcomes.* J Endourol, 2010. 24(3): p. 385-91.

[69] Zeltser, I.S., et al., *Intermediate-term prospective results of radiofrequency-assisted laparoscopic partial nephrectomy: a non-ischaemic coagulative technique.* BJU Int, 2008. 101(1): p. 36-8.

[70] Gettman, M.T., et al., *Hemostatic laparoscopic partial nephrectomy: initial experience with the radiofrequency coagulation-assisted technique.* Urology, 2001. 58(1): p. 8-11.

[71] Jacomides, L., et al., *Laparoscopic application of radio frequency energy enables in situ renal tumor ablation and partial nephrectomy.* J Urol, 2003. 169(1): p. 49-53; discussion 53.

[72] Oefelein, M.G., *Delayed presentation of urinoma after radiofrequency ablation-assisted laparoscopic partial nephrectomy.* J Endourol, 2006. 20(1): p. 27-30.

[73] Sundaram, C.P., et al., *Hemostatic laparoscopic partial nephrectomy assisted by a water-cooled, high-density, monopolar device without renal vascular control.* Urology, 2003. 61(5): p. 906-9.

[74] Stern, J.A., et al., *TissueLink device for laparoscopic nephron-sparing surgery.* J Endourol, 2004. 18(5): p. 455-6.

[75] Tan, Y.H., et al., *Hand-assisted laparoscopic partial nephrectomy without hilar vascular clamping using a saline-cooled, high-density monopolar radiofrequency device.* J Endourol, 2004. 18(9): p. 883-7.

[76] Coleman, J., et al., *Radiofrequency-assisted laparoscopic partial nephrectomy: clinical and histologic results.* J Endourol, 2007. 21(6): p. 600-5.

[77] Breda, A., et al., *Use of haemostatic agents and glues during laparoscopic partial nephrectomy: a multi-institutional survey from the United States and Europe of 1347 cases.* Eur Urol, 2007. 52(3): p. 798-803.

[78] Msezane, L.P., et al., *Hemostatic agents and instruments in laparoscopic renal surgery.* J Endourol, 2008. 22(3): p. 403-8.

[79] Pruthi, R.S., J. Chun, and M. Richman, *The use of a fibrin tissue sealant during laparoscopic partial nephrectomy.* BJU Int, 2004. 93(6): p. 813-7.

[80] Pick, D.L., et al., *Sprayed fibrin sealant as the sole hemostatic agent for porcine laparoscopic partial nephrectomy.* J Urol, 2011. 185(1): p. 291-7.

[81] Schips, L., et al., *Autologous fibrin glue using the Vivostat system for hemostasis in laparoscopic partial nephrectomy.* Eur Urol, 2006. 50(4): p. 801-5.

[82] Gidaro, S., et al., *Efficacy and safety of the haemostasis achieved by Vivostat system during laparoscopic partial nephrectomy.* Arch Ital Urol Androl, 2009. 81(4): p. 223-7.

[83] Gill, I.S., et al., *Improved hemostasis during laparoscopic partial nephrectomy using gelatin matrix thrombin sealant.* Urology, 2005. 65(3): p. 463-6.

[84] Wille, A.H., et al., *Laparoscopic partial nephrectomy using FloSeal for hemostasis: technique and experiences in 102 patients.* Surg Innov, 2009. 16(4): p. 306-12.

[85] Richter, F., et al., *Improvement of hemostasis in open and laparoscopically performed partial nephrectomy using a gelatin matrix-thrombin tissue sealant (FloSeal).* Urology, 2003. 61(1): p. 73-7.

[86] Bak, J.B., A. Singh, and B. Shekarriz, *Use of gelatin matrix thrombin tissue sealant as an effective hemostatic agent during laparoscopic partial nephrectomy.* J Urol, 2004. 171(2 Pt 1): p. 780-2.

[87] Hidas, G., et al., *Sutureless nephron-sparing surgery: use of albumin glutaraldehyde tissue adhesive (BioGlue).* Urology, 2006. 67(4): p. 697-700; discussion 700.

[88] Nadler, R.B., et al., *Use of BioGlue in laparoscopic partial nephrectomy.* Urology, 2006. 68(2): p. 416-8.

[89] Abou-Elela, A., et al., *Use of oxidized cellulose hemostats (surgicel) to support parenchymal closure and achieve hemostasis following partial nephrectomy.* Surg Technol Int, 2009. 18: p. 75-9.

[90] Sabino, L., et al., *Evaluation of renal defect healing, hemostasis, and urinary fistula after laparoscopic partial nephrectomy with oxidized cellulose.* J Endourol, 2007. 21(5): p. 551-6.

[91] Rane, A., et al., *Evaluation of a hemostatic sponge (TachoSil) for sealing of the renal collecting system in a porcine laparoscopic partial nephrectomy survival model.* J Endourol, 2010. 24(4): p. 599-603.

[92] Bernie, J.E., et al., *Evaluation of hydrogel tissue sealant in porcine laparoscopic partial-nephrectomy model.* J Endourol, 2005. 19(9): p. 1122-6.

[93] Murat, F.J., et al., *Evaluation of microporous polysaccharide hemospheres for parenchymal hemostasis during laparoscopic partial nephrectomy in the porcine model.* JSLS, 2006. 10(3): p. 302-6.

[94] Ramani, A.P., et al., *Complications of laparoscopic partial nephrectomy in 200 cases.* J Urol, 2005. 173(1): p. 42-7.

[95] Beasley, K.A., et al., *Laparoscopic versus open partial nephrectomy.* Urology, 2004. 64(3): p. 458-61.

[96] Park, H., et al., *Comparison of laparoscopic and open partial nephrectomies in t1a renal cell carcinoma: a korean multicenter experience.* Korean J Urol, 2010. 51(7): p. 467-71.

[97] Nouralizadeh, A., et al., *Laparoscopic partial nephrectomy for tumours >4 cm compared with smaller tumours: perioperative results.* Int Urol Nephrol, 2011. 43(2): p. 371-6.

[98] Lane, B.R. and I.S. Gill, *7-year oncological outcomes after laparoscopic and open partial nephrectomy.* J Urol, 2010. 183(2): p. 473-9.

[99] Van Haute, W., A. Gavazzi, and P. Dasgupta, *Current status of robotic partial nephrectomy.* Curr Opin Urol, 2010. 20(5): p. 371-4.

[100] Cho, C.L., et al., *Robot-assisted versus standard laparoscopic partial nephrectomy: comparison of perioperative outcomes from a single institution.* Hong Kong Med J, 2011. 17(1): p. 33-8.

[101] Dulabon, L.M., et al., *Multi-institutional analysis of robotic partial nephrectomy for hilar versus nonhilar lesions in 446 consecutive cases.* Eur Urol, 2011. 59(3): p. 325-30.

[102] Lee, S., et al., *Open versus robot-assisted partial nephrectomy: effect on clinical outcome.* J Endourol, 2011. 25(7): p. 1181-5.

[103] Rogers, C.G., et al., *Robotic partial nephrectomy for renal hilar tumors: a multi-institutional analysis.* J Urol, 2008. 180(6): p. 2353-6; discussion 2356.

[104] Tobis, S., et al., *Near infrared fluorescence imaging with robotic assisted laparoscopic partial nephrectomy: initial clinical experience for renal cortical tumors.* J Urol, 2011. 186(1): p. 47-52.

[105] Chang, S.L., et al., *Cost-effectiveness analysis of nephron sparing options for the management of small renal masses.* J Urol, 2011. 185(5): p. 1591-7.
[106] Mir, S.A., et al., *Cost comparison of robotic, laparoscopic, and open partial nephrectomy.* J Endourol, 2011. 25(3): p. 447-53.

12

Gasless Single Port Surgery for Renal Cell Carcinoma: Minimum Incision Endoscopic Surgery

Kazunori Kihara, Yasuhisa Fujii, Satoru Kawakami,
Hitoshi Masuda, Fumitaka Koga, Kazutaka Saito,
Noboru Numao, Yoh Matsuoka and Yasuyuki Sakai
Department of Urology, Graduate School,
Tokyo Medical and Dental University
Japan

1. Introduction

Advances in minimally invasive urologic surgery have accumulated rapidly in recent years with the advent of laparoscopic and robot-assisted surgeries (Clayman, 1991; Guillonneau, 1999; Dasgupta, 2009; Lee, 2009). The procedures for renal cell carcinoma (RCC), radical nephrectomy and partial nephrectomy are among those that have benefited from such innovation. Both laparoscopic surgery and robot-assisted surgery have markedly reduced the invasiveness of surgeries compared to conventional open procedures; laparoscopic surgery is characterized by the use of endoscopy, insufflation with carbon dioxide (CO_2) gas, and insertion of instruments from several trocar ports, while robot-assisted surgery also incorporates stereovision and state-of-the-art movable instruments.

At present, both branches of surgery focus mainly on further minimizing postoperative scarring by performing surgery via a single site (Figure 1) (Ponsky, 2008; Raman, 2008; Kommu, 2009; Kaouk, 2009; Han, 2011). There are currently two major obstacles to achieving the goal of minimally invasive urologic surgery, namely, the necessity of CO_2 insufflation and the high cost of the equipment. The purpose of this chapter is to present a surgery for RCC which can be performed through single-port access, under gasless conditions, and using low-cost equipment (Fig. 1). This form of surgery, which we call minimum incision endoscopic surgery (MIES) or gasless laparoendoscopic single port surgery (GasLESS), has been under development in our department since 1998; techniques have been developed for almost all urological organs (Kihara, 2002, 2004, 2007, 2009a, 2009b, 2010a, 2010b; Kageyama, 2004; Koga, 2007; Saito, 2010). MIES was certified as advanced surgery by the Japanese government in 2006, and was first covered in the Japanese universal health insurance system in 2008 (Kihara et al., 2009a). Here, we will describe the methods and results of MIES-radical nephrectomy and MIES-partial nephrectomy for RCC and discuss its advantageous features that are not associated with other forms of laparoscopic or robot-assisted surgery.

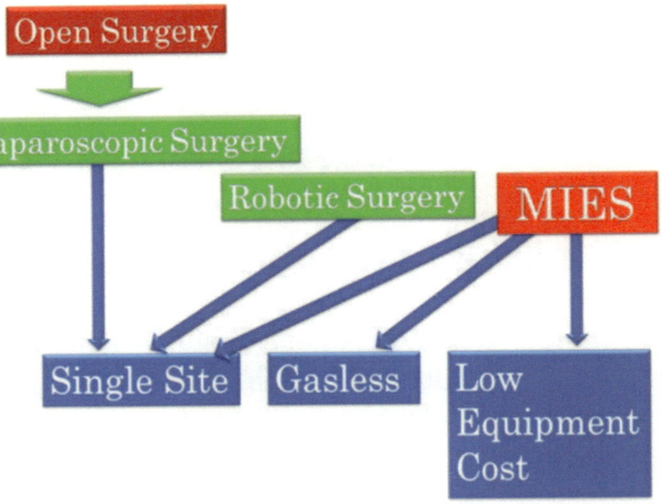

Fig. 1. Three characteristics which are currently important goals in minimally invasive urologic surgery: a single site, a gasless procedure and a low equipment cost. MIES: minimum incision endoscopic surgery.

2. Outline of procedures

2.1 Outline of minimum incision endoscopic surgery (MIES)

An outline of procedures is provided in Figure 2. 1) A minimal incision is made which will serve as a single port and permit extraction of the target specimen. 2) Through this port, a wide working space is made by separating the anatomical plane extraperitoneally; this opening is maintained with special retractors rather than gas insufflation. 3) An endoscope and all other instruments are inserted through the port. 4) Surgeons enjoy the benefits of endoscopy, especially the availability to all participants of magnified images from the beginning to the end of the operation, while the supplemental view with the naked eye remains visible through the port with stereovision and panoramic vision (Figure 3). Three dimensional high-vision endoscope is also being used at present. The size of the port can be tailored to the patient's situation before or during the operation for safety and proper practice, although this is rarely necessary. The multiple options for images and the possibility of modifying the size of the single port may mitigate technical demand and avoid patient selection. Patient position (lateral or supine) can be selected according to each patient's situation or tumour location. The operation is performed without CO_2 gas, without trocar ports, basically without antimicrobial prophylaxis, with an intact peritoneum and with minimal disposable instruments.

2.2 Representative specimen extractions

Representative extractions of various specimens are depicted. All operations were performed extraperitoneally: i) radical nephrectomy via a lumbar port in the lateral position (Figure 4), ii) radical nephrectomy through a paramedian port in the supine position (Figure 5), iii) partial nephrectomy of T1 RCC via a lumbar port (Figure 6) and iv) partial nephrectomy of T2 RCC via a lumbar port (Figure 7) .

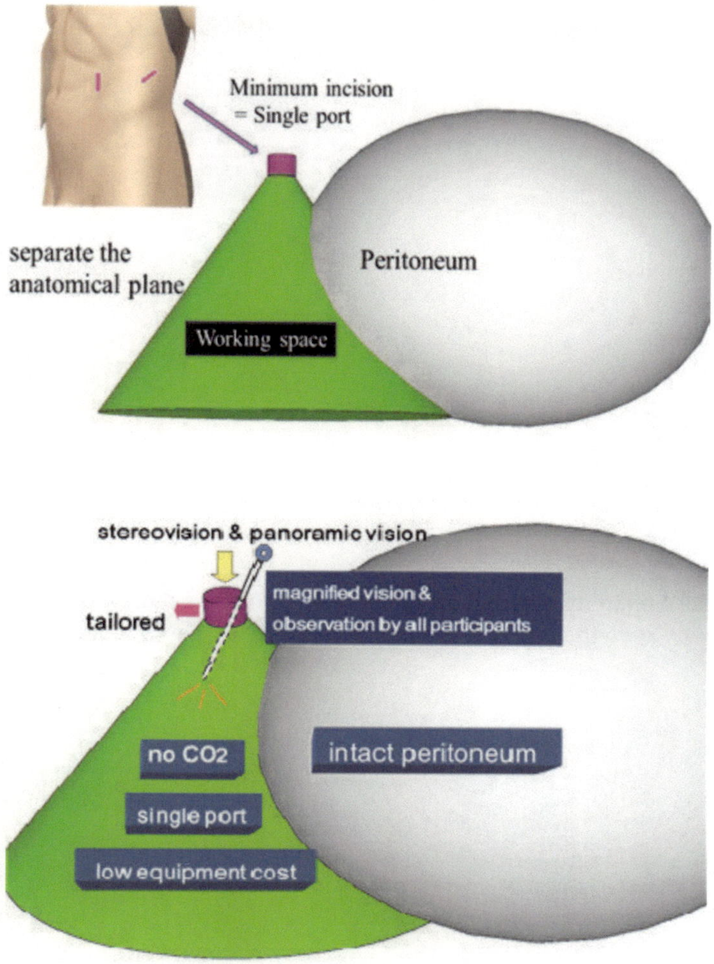

Fig. 2. Outline of the MIES procedures.

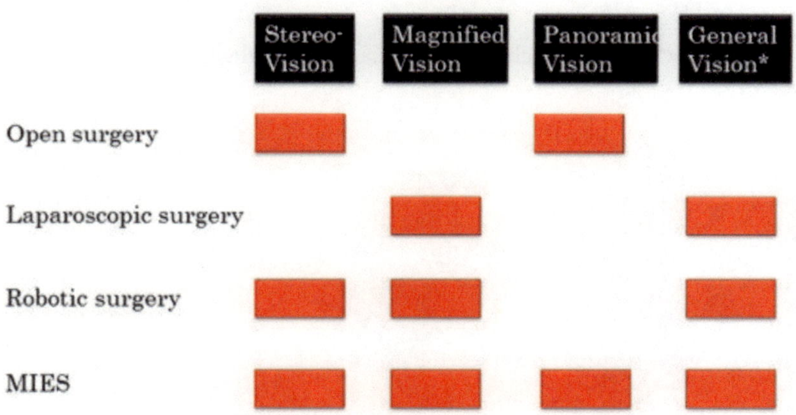

Fig. 3. Image availability in minimally invasive surgeries. *: images are available to all participants.

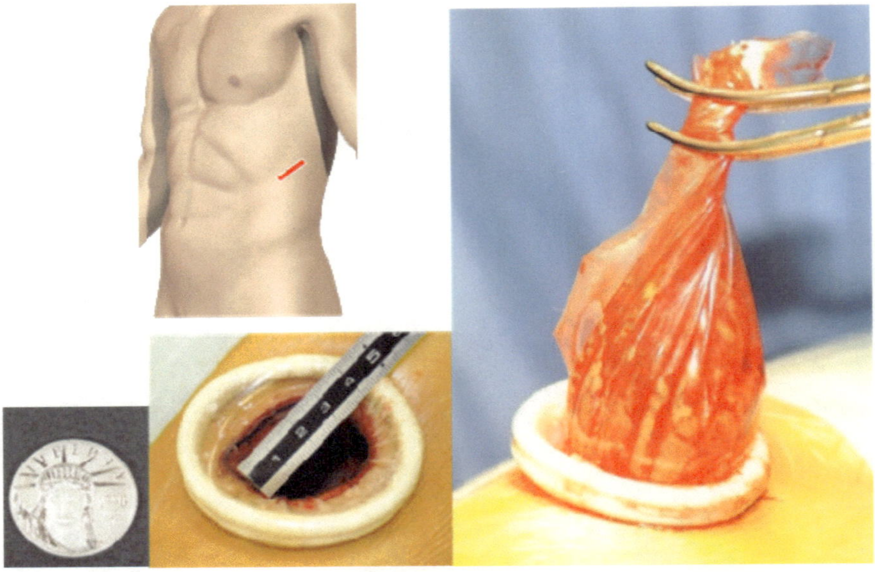

Fig. 4. Radical nephrectomy through a single lumbar port less than 4cm in diameter in the lateral position. To keep the wound open and protect it, an Alexis wound retractor® is typically used.

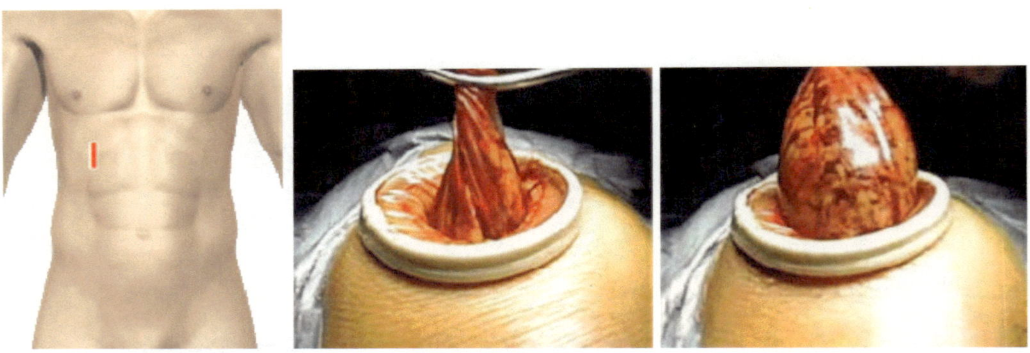

Fig. 5. Radical nephrectomy through a paramedian port in the supine position, performed extraperitoneally.

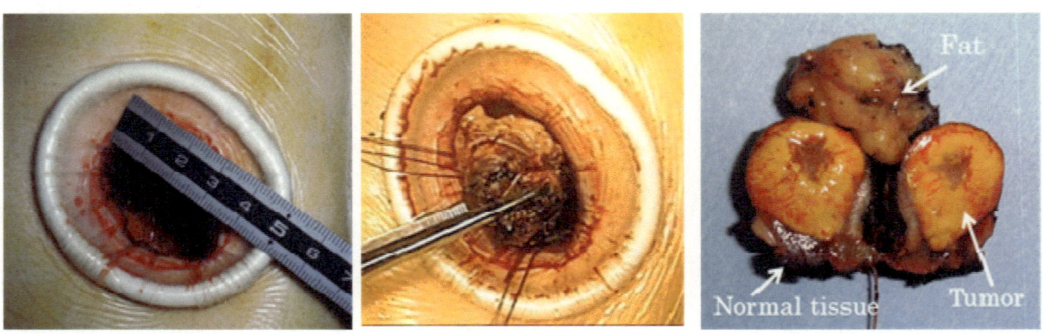

Fig. 6. Partial nephrectomy of T1 RCC via a lumbar port.

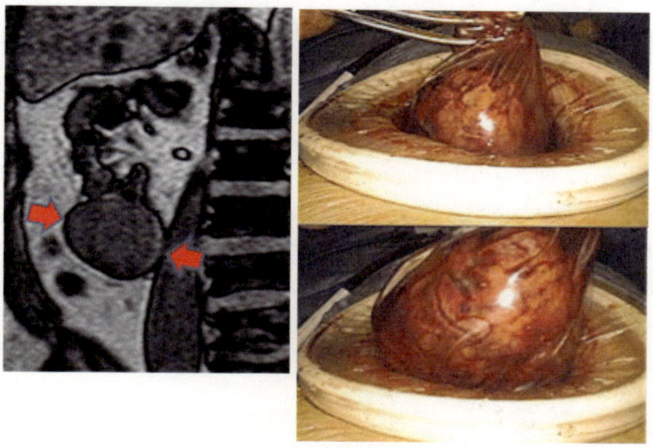

Fig. 7. Partial nephrectomy of T2 RCC through a lumbar port.

3. Methods

An outline of the technique, entitled "MIES-radical nephrectomy and MIES-partial nephrectomy", has been previously reported (kihara, 2009a, 2010a) and presented in the video library of the European Association of Urology (EAU) (Kihara, 2009b, 2010b). At our hospital, MIES-radical nephrectomy has been performed regularly over the last few years for large T1b-T3 RCC and for RCC in dialysis patients, while MIES-partial nephrectomy is performed for most (lately more than 85%) cases of T1a RCC. MIES-partial nephrectomy is typically performed without renal ischemia at our hospital to preserve renal function to as great a degree as possible.

3.1 MIES-radical nephrectomy

A lumbar or paramedian retroperitoneal approach is used. The latter approach is mainly selected when the patient has severe cardiovascular or respiratory disturbances or a large tumour adjacent to the renal pedicle. Antimicrobial prophylaxis is not used.

3.1.1 Lumbar retroperitoneal approach

After the induction of general anaesthesia, the patient is placed in the flank position over the break of the table. An incision just large enough to narrowly permit extraction of the kidney with perinephric fat, usually 3.5-6 cm, is made obliquely forward following the line of the 12th rib (Figure 4). After splitting the muscles, incising the transversalis fascia and moving the flank pad aside, the lateroconal fascia is exposed. During this procedure a small portion of the distal edge of the 12th rib may be removed if necessary. After opening the lateroconal fascia, separation is performed between the fascia of the psoas muscle posteriorly and Gerota's fascia anteriorly. During this separation procedure, the ureter can be readily identified medially. Next, an Alexis wound retractor ® is set up and the single port is prepared (Figure 4). Separation along the posterior Gerota's fascia allows immediate access to the renal artery and vein. The renal artery is circumferentially mobilized, then doubly ligated and divided (Figure 8). Next, the renal vein is freed, doubly ligated and divided. The ureter, which was identified previously, is freed as low as possible and then ligated and divided.

After the wide separation along the posterior Gerota's fascia, a similar separation is performed along the anterior Gerota's fascia, allowing immediate access to the adrenal gland. Next, the perinephric fat is transversely divided at the level of transection of the ureter and subsequently between the adrenal gland and the kidney by retracting the kidney downward with a retractor. The adrenal gland is usually preserved, but when necessary it can be removed along with the kidney. After confirming the complete isolation of the kidney with perinephric fat by passing a tube around the perinephric fat, the specimen is extracted through the single port using a Flexible catcher®. Before the wound is closed, the operative field is washed thoroughly with saline, and the subcutaneous tissue is washed again with saline before epidermal suture to avoid the need for prophylactic antimicrobial agents.

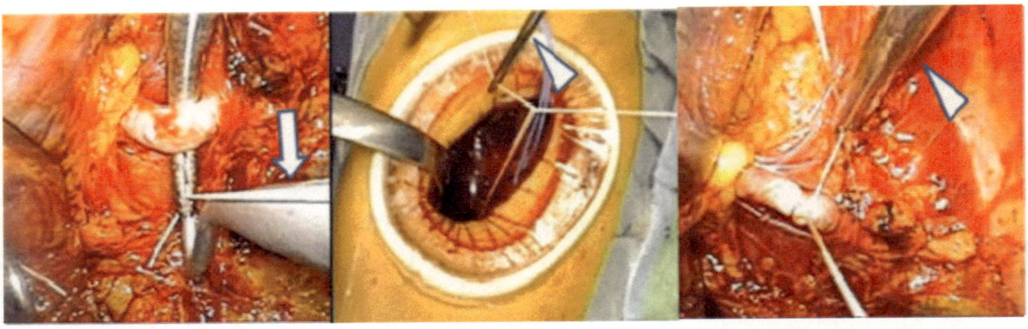

Fig. 8. Ligation of the renal artery using a Thread Pass® (arrow) and a Knot Slide® (arrowhead).

3.1.2 Paramedian retroperitoneal approach

This approach is the same as the lumbar retroperitoneal approach described above except in the following points. The patient is placed in the supine position under general anaesthesia. An incision just large enough to narrowly permit extraction of the kidney with perinephric fat is made downward on the pararectal line, 1-2 cm below the rib (Figure 5). By incising the anterior and posterior sheaths of the rectus muscle while preserving the muscle, the transversal fascia is exposed. The fascia is bluntly pushed downward off the transversal muscle to allow access to the flank pad on the lateroconal fascia. Next, the lateroconal fascia is opened and the anterior Gerota's fascia is separated medially to allow immediate access to the renal vein and artery.

After division of the renal artery and vein, wide separation along the anterior and posterior Gerota's fascia is performed. The kidney with the perinephric fat is freed from the surrounding tissue and extracted as described above, in the section on the translumbar retroperitoneal approach (Figure 5).

3.2 Partial nephrectomy

Partial nephrectomy using an MIES technique is typically performed without renal ischemia at our hospital. In some cases, such as when the tumour is adjacent to the renal pedicle, clamping of the renal vessels is performed as necessary. Either the lumbar retroperitoneal approach or the paramedian retroperitoneal approach is selected. Antimicrobial prophylaxis is not used unless the collecting system is opened.

Regardless of approach, the procedures are similar to those used in radical nephrectomy until the exposure of Gerota's fascia. After setting up the single port, separating the posterior and anterior Gerota's fascias from the surrounding tissue, and holding them back with an Alexis wound retractor®, the tumour is located within the perinephric fat by means of ultrasound (Figure 9). The surface of the kidney is exposed at some distance from the tumour, and the exposure is then extended to near the tumour.

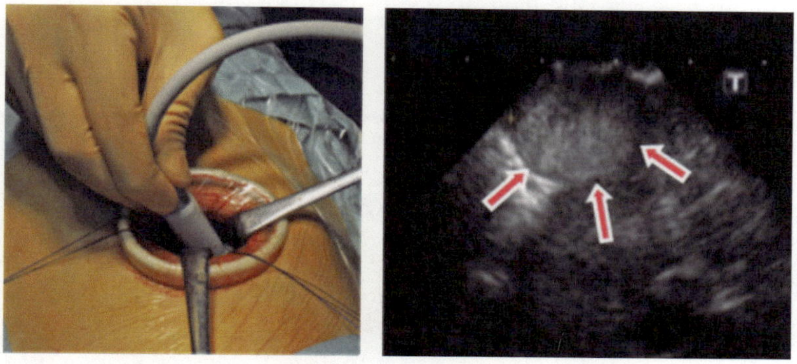

Fig. 9. Identification of the tumour using ultrasound.

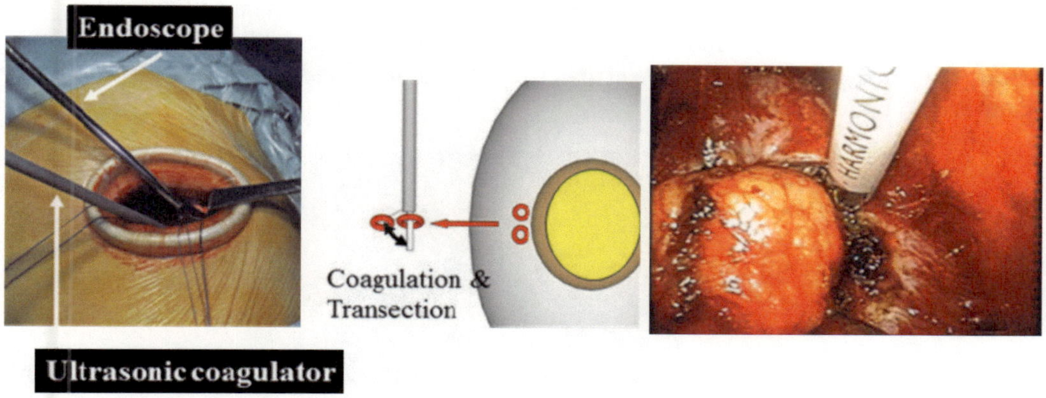

Fig. 10. Coagulation of the normal tissue around the tumour.

Using an ultrasonic coagulator, the normal tissue adjacent to the tumour is penetrated and coagulated (Figure 10). When coagulations around the tumour are completed, the tissue between coagulations is coagulated and transected. Using a suction tube, the coagulated normal tissue is shaped into the form of a pedicle connected to the tumour (Figure 11). The pedicle is tied with a rubber tape or a silk thread, with which the tumour is gently pulled up (Figure 11). After the operative field is filled with saline, the bottom of the tumour in the pedicle is identified with ultrasound. The tumour, its bottom and its transected region can be checked and the line to be transected is now identified (Figure 11).

According to the line identified, the normal tissue neighbouring the bottom of the tumour is transected using a coagulator as soon as the distance between the bottom and the collecting system is large enough. When the bottom is near the collecting system, the pedicle is transected little by little while the tissue is sutured on the calyx side. Finally, the target specimen is freed and extracted through the single port (Figure 12). Immediately after the specimen is extracted, it is split in half and the margin of the tumour is evaluated (Figure 6). When the margin seems too small, a situation which arises very rarely, adjacent normal tissue can be additionally coagulated or resected. The remaining bed is coagulated by means of an argon laser or pasted with coagulating paste, if necessary, and is carefully confirmed to be bloodless (Figure 6). Then the perinephric fat is repaired to cover the kidney defect. Before the wound is closed, the operative field is washed with 2000 ml of saline so that prophylactic antibiotics are not required. Finally, the skin is closed with an epidermal suture (Figure 12).

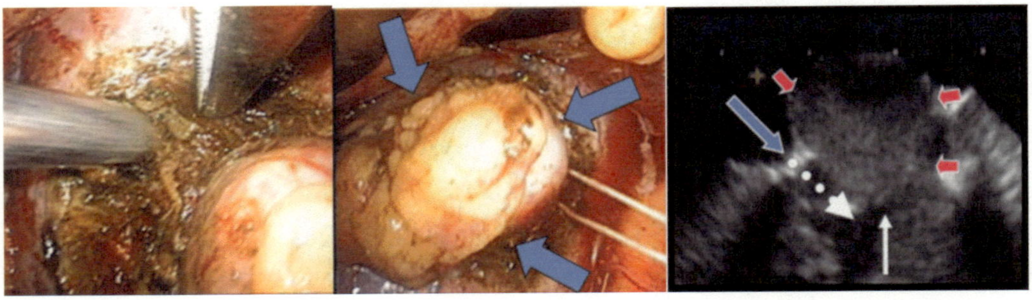

Fig. 11. Ensuring that the normal tissue beneath the tumour is clear. Transection of the normal tissue beneath the tumour is performed under ultrasound guidance. White dotted arrow, the line to be transected; blue arrow, transected normal tissue; red arrow, tumour; white arrow, bottom of the tumour.

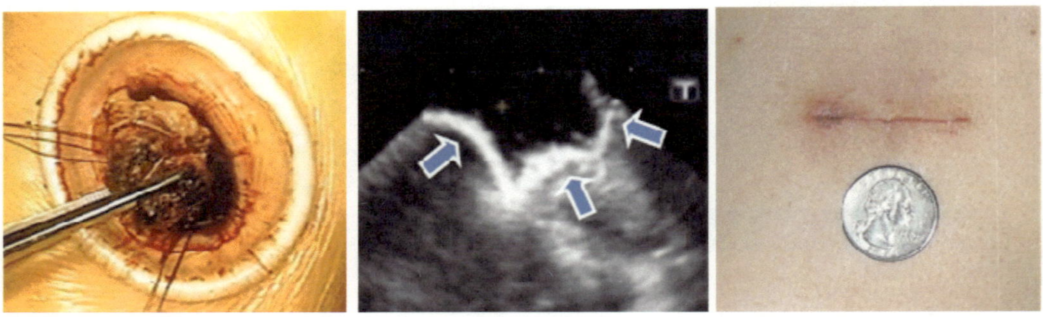

Fig. 12. Extraction of the tumour (left), remaining defect of the kidney (centre) and post-operative scar compared with a quarter (right).

3.3 Instruments

All instruments are inserted through a single port. Since this single port, usually 3-6 cm in diameter, is larger than the trocar ports typically used in laparoscopic surgery, larger instruments can be used which are not only less costly but also reusable. Representative instruments are cited. To keep the wound open as well as to protect it, an Alexis wound retractor® is usually used, but it is not always essential (Figure 4). To maintain the working space, original PLES retractors® are inserted (Figure 13). Haemostasis ligation is often achieved by means of two original devices, the Thread Pass® and the Knot Slide®, which allow easy ligation through the single port (Figure 14). A metal suction tube is useful both to clean up the operative field and to separate the anatomical plane. Transection is often performed with a reusable ultrasonic coagulation device inserted through the port. To extract the kidney, an inexpensive original Flexible catcher® is used (Figure 15). All of the original devices mentioned here are commercially available and relatively inexpensive. For radical nephrectomy, only two of the required devices are disposable, the Flexible catcher® and the Alexis wound retractor®, and both of these are inexpensive, so that the overall cost of equipment is low. For partial nephrectomy, a Sonosurg® reusable ultrasonic coagulator can be used (Figure 16).

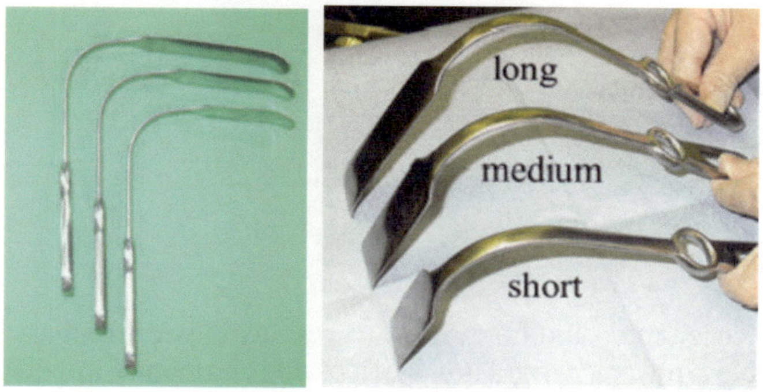

Fig. 13. Original PLES retractor®.

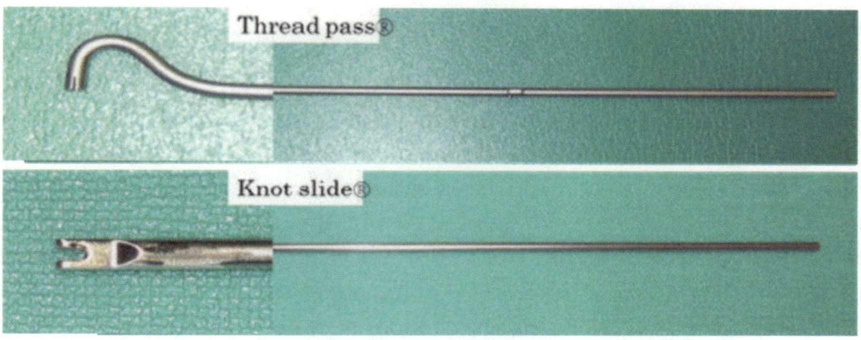

Fig. 14. Original devices for ligation: Thread Pass® and Knot Slide®. Ligation is often used for haemostasis and can be performed easily with these devices through the single port.

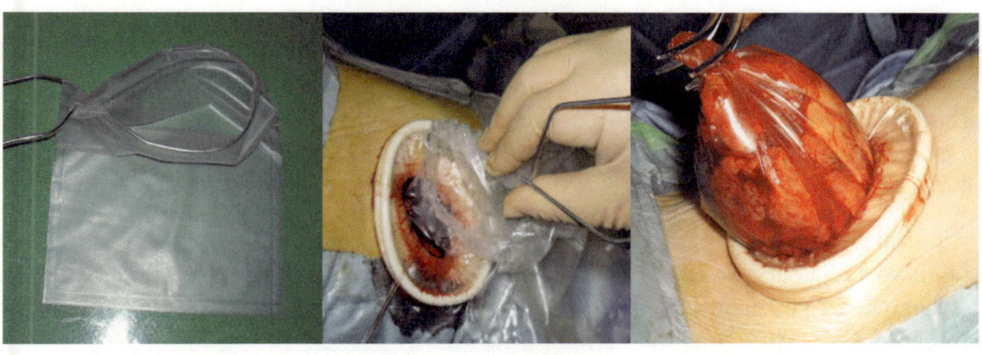

Fig. 15. The Flexible Catcher®, the original inexpensive catcher used to extract the specimen.

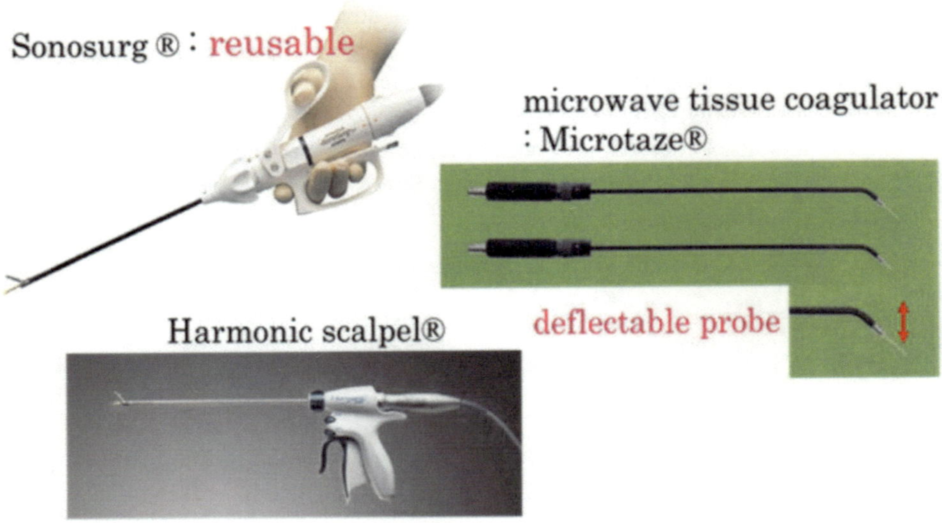

Fig. 16. For tissue coagulation and transection , especially in partial nephrectomy, a Sonosurg® reusable ultrasonic coagulator, a disposable Harmonic scalpel®, or a Microtaze® deflectable microwave tissue coagulator are used depending on the situation.

4. Results

4.1 Radical nephrectomy

The results of the initial 80 consecutive cases, performed by a small group of surgeons between August 1998 and June 2003, have been presented previously (Kihara et al., 2004). The results of 50 more recent consecutive cases, treated between 2009 and 2011, which were performed by a larger group of surgeons (including many inexperienced ones) are presented here. Patient age ranged from 35 to 85 years (mean 64). The duration of the operation was 186 min (range, 114 to 349). The median estimated blood loss was 229 ml (range, 2 to 1500). One patient subsequently received a blood transfusion. A complication arose during a single operation, namely, a small injury to the pleura which was repaired with a suture during the operation.

On the first postoperative day, oral feeding was possible in 90% of cases, and walking more than 100 m was possible in 92%. Within two postoperative days, discharge was possible for 86%. No complications ≥ grade 3a according to the Clavien-Dindo classification were observed postoperatively. The rate of surgical site infection was 4% though no antimicrobial prophylactic agents were used. All infections were successfully treated by administrating antibiotics.

Oncological outcomes of treatment for pT1-T2 RCC by means of this procedure at our hospital are as follows (Iimura et al., 2008): in 154 consecutive cases between 1998 and 2006, five-year overall survival, five-year recurrence-free survival and five-year cancer-specific survival were 95%, 91% and 96%. No local recurrence has been observed since 1998, when this procedure was introduced.

4.2 Partial nephrectomy

Between 2000 and 2011, over 150 cases of renal tumour underwent MIES-partial nephrectomy. In this chapter, we present the surgical outcomes of recent 50 consecutive cases treated between January 2009 and August 2010. Eight surgeons, including several who were inexperienced, performed these operations. The 50 cases consisted of 14 females and 36 males with a median age of 57 years (range, 36 to 79). Preoperative clinical T stage was T1a in 45 cases (90%), T1b in 3 (6%) and T2 in 1 (2%), and the median tumour size was 2.3 cm (range, 1.2 to 8.0). The location of tumour was peripheral in 37 cases (74%), central (a tumour contacting the renal sinus) in 12 (24%) and hilar (a tumour contacting the hilar vessels) in 1 (2%). The indication of partial nephrectomy was imperative in 2 cases (4%, chronic kidney disease and previous history of nephrectomy, respectively) and elective in the remaining 48 (96%).

In all cases but one, which was a central T1b tumour, partial nephrectomy was completed without clamping the hilar vessels. The median operation time was 234 min (range, 128 to 382). The median estimated blood loss was 210 ml (range, 0 to 2274). One case (2%) required allogeneic blood transfusion. No intraoperative complications were encountered.

On the first postoperative day, 47 patients (94%) resumed oral feeding. Patients were typically allowed to begin walking on the second postoperative day, when 43 patients (86%) were able to walk 100 m or farther. The median postoperative day on which the drainage tube was removed was 3 (range, 1 to 20). By postoperative day 3, 38 patients (76%) had recovered to such a degree that they no longer required inpatient care. Surgical site infection was observed in 2 cases (4%), both of which were successfully treated by administrating antibiotics. Major postoperative complications of Clavien–Dindo grade 3 or greater were observed in 2 cases (4%); both cases required retroperitoneal drainage under local anaesthesia (Clavien grade 3a) for urine leakage and retroperitoneal abscess, respectively.

Pathological examination revealed that 41 tumours (82%) were RCC while the remaining 9 (18%) were benign. Although 5 (12%) of the 41 RCC patients had a positive surgical margin as determined microscopically, tumour tissues at the margin underwent thermal denaturation applied via an ultrasonic or a microwave coagulating device. To date, none of 150 cases including these 50 patients has experienced local disease recurrence. As for renal function of the 50 cases, the median % decrease in eGFR 3 months after the operation was 5.9%.

5. Advantageous features of MIES

CO_2 gas insufflation is associated with various risks, including hypertension, hypotension, hypercapnia, pulmonary embolism, decrease of pulmonary compliance and subcutaneous emphysema (See et al., 1993; Alberto et al., 2008); these arise mainly due to the effects of insufflation on the cardiovascular, respiratory and renal systems, although clinical problems rarely arise from careful anaesthesia. Gasless surgeries, such as this operation, can reduce the above risks and might prove especially helpful in operations on aged patients who often have concurrent cardiovascular, respiratory and renal disturbances. As the global population has aged, the number of aged patients has shown rapid increase lately. A high but fortunately subclinical rate of cardiac CO_2 embolism has been reported in laparoscopic radical prostatectomy for prostate cancer which usually occurs in aged men (Hong et al.,

2010); gasless surgery could reduce this rate. From the standpoint of global warming, furthermore, a reduction in the amount of CO_2 emitted from the hospital would be welcomed. In addition, MIES is associated with a low equipment cost similar to that associated with open surgery, because neither expensive disposable instruments nor robotic assistance is necessary, and with a low admission cost similar to that associated with laparoscopic surgery, because the procedure is minimally invasive which results in earlier discharge from the hospital. For cases of T4 RCC, advanced-stage RCC invading neighbouring organs, this surgery can be modified by extending the incision as necessary. Other common modifications are described below.

5.1 Radical nephrectomy for dialysis patients

It is well known that dialysis patients have high rates of RCC. Since dialysis patients usually have various concurrent conditions, especially of their cardiovascular or respiratory systems, and often undergo bilateral radical nephrectomy due to bilateral cancers (Sakura et al., 2007), the gasless nature of MIES is preferable for these patients as it reduces the risks of complications in the above systems. The retroperitoneal approach permitted by MIES is also helpful in that it reduces the likelihood of adhesion of the peritoneum, since some of these patients undergo peritoneal dialysis. The option to use the supine position in MIES is beneficial in that it reduces the risk of shunt obstruction. Finally, the low cost of MIES may also be helpful to the patients, given the high cost of dialysis.

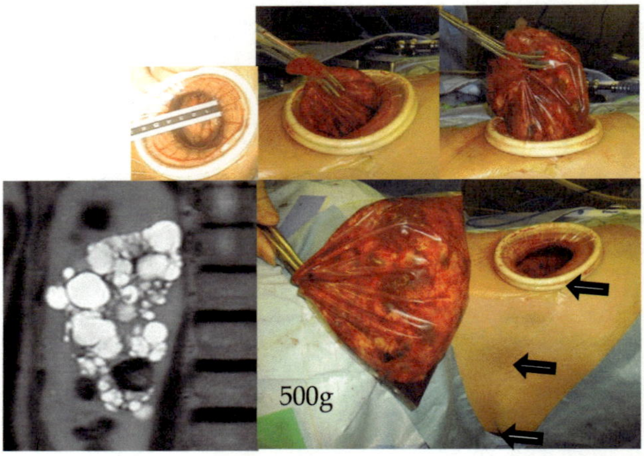

Fig. 18. Radical nephrectomy of a dialysis patient via a port 4 cm in diameter who had previously undergone partial resection of the liver. The arrows indicate the postoperative scar. The weight of the specimen extracted was 500g. CT scan shows ACDK, acquired cystic disease of the kidney, with RCC.

5.2 Modification of MIES for carcinoma of the renal pelvis

Carcinoma of the renal pelvis is considered a renal tumour and is sometimes difficult to distinguish from RCC. In other words, differential diagnosis between invasion of carcinoma of the renal pelvis into the renal parenchyma and RCC is occasionally not possible. In such cases, this procedure can be modified to allow two-port access for en-bloc extraction of the kidney and ureter (Figure 19); this is described in the EAU video library (Saito et al., 2010). The kidney is isolated and extracted through a flank port while still connected with the ureter, as in MIES-radical nephrectomy, and is immediately analyzed to determine the presence of urothelial carcinoma or RCC. When urothelial carcinoma is highly suspected, the table is rotated from a lateral position to a semioblique position, and the distal ureter with the bladder cuff is isolated through a paramedian port about 3 cm in diameter in the lower abdomen. Thereafter, the specimen is extracted en bloc through the flank port and the paramedian port is used for drainage.

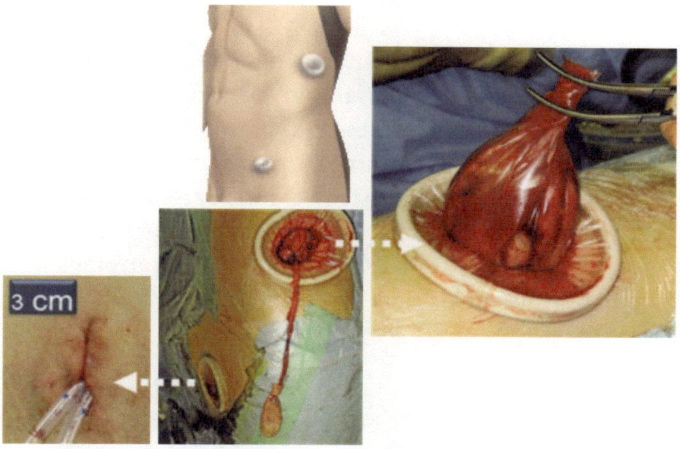

Fig. 19. MIES-total nephroureterectomy. See the text for details.

5.3 Preservation of renal function

It is essential in renal surgery to avoid the postoperative development of chronic kidney disease (Yokoyama et al., 2011a). In our analysis of 219 patients who underwent MIES-radical nephrectomy, 54 developed chronic kidney disease within 2 postoperative years. Univariate and multivariate analyses revealed that age, presence of diabetes mellitus, and preoperative estimated glomerular filtration rate were independent predictors of its development (Yokoyama et al., 2011b). Partial nephrectomy is recommended, if possible, for patients with the abovementioned risks. In order to preserve renal function insofar as it is possible during the operation, it is best to avoid clamping the renal vessels and using CO_2 insufflation which may cause compression of the renal vein. Recently, the rate of clampless MIES-partial nephrectomy at our hospital has been above 95%.

5.4 No usage of antimicrobial prophylaxis

Antimicrobial prophylaxis is associated with several negative effects, including drug-induced complications of major organs, possible introduction of drug-resistant bacteria and high cost. MIES has several features that may help reduce the incidence of infectious complications: a minimal incision, wound protection provided by the Alexis® wound retractor and completion of procedures without insertion of fingers. We prospectively evaluated the incidences of surgical site infection (SSI) after MIES for renal and adrenal tumours in the absence of antimicrobial prophylaxis (Yoshida et al., 2007; Kijima et al.,

2011). In 301 patients, the incidences of superficial SSI and deep SSI were very low, 1.3% and 0.7%, respectively. All perioperative infections were successfully treated by administrating antimicrobial agents.

Antimicrobial prophylaxis is fundamentally not necessary in MIES-radical nephrectomy or MIES-partial nephrectomy in which the urinary tract is not opened during the operation. After stopping the routine usage of antimicrobial prophylaxis, the incidence of drug-resistant bacterial infection has markedly decreased at our ward (unpublished data).

5.5 Limitations of MIES

The limitations of MIES are due to the insertion of all instruments, including the endoscope, through a small single port. It is necessary to be familiar with the handling of the instruments used in the operation. Nevertheless, inexperienced surgeons become able to deliver results similar to those of high-volume surgeons within a short period (Kihara et al., 2010a). It may be attributed to the fact that this surgery offers four visions as described above (Figure 2), and can be modified to accommodate the operator's level of experience by extending the incision as necessary. More than 2000 MIES for urological cancers have been safely performed up to now in our hospital.

6. Spread of MIES

In Japan, several regulatory requirements must be met to perform MIES, but at present more than 70 major hospitals meet these requirements, and this number is increasing year by year. This surgery has been introduced worldwide, in such places as Europe, the US, China, Korea and Brazil. MIES-radical nephrectomy, MIES-partial nephrectomy and MIES-nephroureterectomy have been cited in the video library of EAU (Kihara, 2009b, 2010b; Saito et al., 2010), and textbooks on this technique have been published in China (Kihara, 2003, 2010c).

7. MIES in the near future

The two-dimensional endoscope is being replaced by a three-dimensional endoscope in our hospital, in which case direct supplemental visualization through the port for stereovision is unnecessary. As for the size of the port, it has already been reduced to just over 2 cm in diameter for a small specimen such as the adrenal gland. The console presently used for robotic surgery may become more compact to the point of being useable as a head mount. Depending on the economic situation involved, MIES could be modified into a gasless single-port (2 cm if necessary) and conomical robotic (non-console) surgery.

8. Conclusion

MIES for RCC has several unique characteristics including its gasless nature, single-port access, the use of the retroperitoneal approach, no usage of prophylactic agents, no clamping of the renal vessels and a relatively low equipment cost. MIES shows that low invasiveness similar to that in laparoscopic surgery can be achieved in surgery for RCC without gas insufflation and without expensive disposable instruments and expensive machines.

Future work will integrate the surgical techniques described here with new devices, and perhaps robots (non-console), to fulfil additional needs in the field of surgery for urological cancers.

9. References

Alberto, R.; Bollens, R. & Cohen, B.E. (2008). Fundamentals of laparoscopic surgery. In: *Manual of laparoscopic urology*, Springer-Verlag, pp. 3-17, ISBN 978-3-540-74726-0, Berlin, Germany

Clayman, R.V.; Kavoussi, L.R.; Soper,N.J.; Dierks, S.M.; Darcy, M.D.; Long,S.R.; Roemer, F.D.; Pingleton, F.D. & Thomson, P.G. (1991). Laparoscopic nephrectomy. *N. Engl. J. Med.*, Vol.324, No.19, pp. 1370-1371

Dasgupta, P. & Kirby, R.S. (2009). Outcomes of robotic assisted radical prostatectomy. *Int. J. Urol.*, Vol.16, No.3, pp. 244-248

Guillonneau, B. & Vallancien, G. (1999). Laparoscopic radical prostatectomy: initial experience and preliminary assessment after 65 operations. *Prostate*, Vol.39, No.1, pp. 71-75

Han, W.K.; Kim, D.S.; Jeon, H.G.; Jeong, W.; Oh, C.K.; Choi, K.H.; Lorenzo, E.I. & Rha,K.H. (2011). Robot-assisted laparoendoscopic single-site surgery: partial nephrectomy for renal malignancy. *Urology*, Vol.77, No.3, pp. 612-616

Hong, J.Y.; Kim, W.O. & Kil, H.K. (2010). Detection of subclinical CO2 embolism by transesophageal echocardiography durilng laparoscopic radical prostatectomy. *Urology*, Vol.75, No.3, pp. 581-584

Iimura, Y.; Kihara, K.; Saito, K.; Masuda, H.; Kobayashi, T. & Kawakami, S. (2008). Oncological outcome of minimum incision endoscopic radical nephrectomy for pathologically organ confined renal cell carcinoma. *Int. J. Urol.*, Vol.15, No.1, pp.44-47

Kageyama, Y.; Kihara, K.; Kobayashi, T.; Kawakami, S.; Fujii, Y.; Masuda, H.; Yano, M. & Hyochi, N. (2004). Portless endoscopic adrenalectomy via a single minimum incision by retroperitoneal approach: Experience with initial 30 cases. *Int. J. Urol.* Vol.11, No.9, pp. 693-699

Kaouk, J.H. & Goel, R.K. (2009). Single-port laparoscopic and robotic partial nephrectomy. *Eur. Urol.*, Vol.55, No.5, pp. 1163-1169

Kihara, K.; Kageyama, Y.; Kobayashi, T.; Okuno, T.; kawakami, S.; Hayashi, T.; Masuda, H.; Suzuki, M.; Hyouchi N. & Arai G. (2002). *Portless endoscopic urological surgery*. Igaku-shoin, ISBN 4-260-13356-X, Tokyo, Japan (Japanese & English)

Kihara, K.; Kageyama, Y.; Kobayashi, T. ; Okuno, T.; Kawakami, S.; Hayashi, T.; Masuda, H.; Suzuki, M.; Hyouchi N. & Arai G. (2003). *Portless endoscopic urological surgery*. Liaoning Science and Technology Publishing House, pp. 10-185, ISBN 7-5381-3988-5, Liaoning, China (Chinese)

Kihara, K.; Kageyama, Y.; Yano, M.; Kobayashi, T.; Kawakami, S.; Fujii, Y.; Masuda, H. & Hyochi, N. (2004). Portless endoscopic radical nephrectomy via a single minimum incision in 80 patients. *Int. J. Urol.*, Vol.11, No.9, pp.714-720

Kihara, K. (2007). *Ilustrated minimum incision endoscopic urological surgery*. Igaku-shoin, pp. 1-130, Japanese, ISBN 978-4-260-00481-7, Tokyo, Japan (Japanese)

Kihara, K.; Kawakami, S.; Fujii, Y.; Masuda, H. & Koga, F. (2009a). Gasless single-port access endoscopic surgery in urology: minimum incision endoscopic surgery, MIES. *Int. J. Urol.*, Vol.16, No.10, pp.791-800

Kihara, K.; Kawakami, S.; Fujii, Y.; Masuda H.; Koga F. & Saito F. (2009b). Gasless single port access radical nephrectomy. *Eur. Urol. Suppl.*, Vol.8, No.4, pp. 392

Kihara, K.; Kobayashi. T.; Kawakami, S.; Fujii, Y.; Kageyama, H. & Masuda, H. (2010a). Minimum Incision Endoscopic Surgery (MIES)in Japanese Urology: Results of Adrenalectomy, radical nephrectomy and radical prostatectomy. *Aktuelle. Urol.*, Vol.41, Suppl.1, S15-S19

Kihara, K.; Tushima, S.; Kawakami, Y.; Fujii, Y.; Masuda H.; Koga F. & Saito F. (2010b). Gasless single port access ultrasound-guided clampless partial nephrectomy: MIES partial nephrectomy. *Eur. Urol. Suppl.*, Vol.9, N0.2, pp. 335-336

Kihara, K. (2010c). *Ilustrated minimum incision endoscopic urological surgery.* Guangxi Science and Technology Publishing House, pp. 1-130, ISBN 978-7-80763-578-9, Guangxi, China (Chinese)

Kijima, T.; Masuda,H.; Yoshida, S.; Tatokoro,M.; Araki, S.; Yokoyama, M.; Numao,N.; Okada,Y.; Saito, K.; Koga,F.; Fujii,Y. & Kihara,K. (2011). Antibiotic prophylaxis is not neccessary in minimally inasive surgery for renal and adrenal tumors: A prospective study of 301 consecutive patients. *J. Urol. Suppl.*, Vol.185, No.4, pp. 470-471

Koga, F.; Kihara, K.; Masuda, H.; Kageyama, Y.; Kawakami, S. & Kobayashi. T. (2007). Minimum incision endoscopic Nephrectomy for giant hydronephrosis. *Int. J. Urol.*, Vol.14, No.8, pp.774-776

Kommu, S.S.; Kaouk, J.H. & Rane, A. (2009). Laparo-endoscopic single-site surgery: preliminary advances in renal surgery. *BJU Int.*, Vol.103, No.8, pp1034-1037

Lee, R.S.; Sethi, A.S.; Passerotti, C.C.; Retik, A.B.; Borer, J.G.; Nguyen, H.T. & Peters, C.A. (2009). Robot assisted laparoscopic partial nephrectomy : a viable and safe option in children. *J. Urol.*, Vol.181, No.2, pp. 823-828

Ponsky ,L.E.; Cherullo, E.E.; Sawyer, M. & Hartke, D. (2008). Single access site laparoscopic radical nephrectomy:initial clinical experience. *J. Endourol.*, Vol.22, No.4, pp. 663-666

Raman, J.D.; Cadeddu, J.A.; Rao, P. & Rane, A. (2008). Single-incision laparoscopic surgery: initial urological experience and comparison with natural-orifice transluminal endoscopic surgery. *BJU Int.*, Vol.101, No.12, pp. 1493-14936

Saito, K.; Kihara, K.; Kawakami, Y.; Fujii, Y.; Masuda H. & Koga F. (2010). Gasless two port access total nephroureterectomy: MIES nephroureterectomy. *Eur. Urol. Suppl.*, Vol.9, No.2, pp. 335

Sakura, M.: Kawakami, S.; Masuda, H.; Kobayashi, T.; Kageyama, Y. & Kihara, K. (2007). Sequential bilateral minimum incision endoscopic radical nephrectomy in dialysis patients with bilateral renal cell carcinomas. *Int. J. Urol.*, Vol.14, No.12, pp.1109-1112

See, W.A.; Monk, T.G. & Weldon, B.C. (1993). Complications of laparoscopy. In: Clayman, R.V.; McDougall, E.M (eds). *Raparoscopic urology.* Quality Medical Publishing Inc., pp.183-206 ISBN 0-942219-41-4, St. Louis, MO, U.S.A.

Yokoyama, M.; Fujii, Y.; Iimura, Y.; Saito, K.; Koga, F.; Masuda, H.; Kawakami, S. & Kihara, K. (2011a). Longitudinal change in renal function after radical nephrectomy in Japanese patients with renal cortical tumors. *J. Urol.*, Vol.185, No.6, pp. 2066-2071

Yokoyama, M.; Fujii, Y.; Iimura, Y.; Saito, K.; Koga, F.; Masuda, H. & Kihara, K. (2011b). A nomogaram for predicting the development of chronic kidney disease within 2 years after radical nephrectomy in patients with renal cortical tumor. *J. Urol. Suppl.*, Vol.185, No.4, pp. 436

Yoshida, S.; Masuda, H.; Yokoyama, M.; Kobayashi, T.; Kawakami, S. & Kihara,K. (2007). Absence of prophylactic antibiotics in minimum incision endoscopic urological surgery(MEUS) of adrenal and renal tumors. *Int. J. Urol.*, Vol.14, No.5, pp. 384-387

13

Prognostic Impact of Perirenal Fat or Adrenal Gland Involvement in Renal Cell Carcinoma Exhibiting Venous Vascular Extension

Tetsuo Fujita, Masatsugu Iwamura, Shinji Kurosaka,
Ken-ichi Tabata, Kazumasa Matsumoto, Kazunari Yoshida and Shiro Baba
Department of Urology, Kitasato University School of Medicine
Japan

1. Introduction

Venous vascular extension is one of the aggressive tumor behaviors especially for renal cell carcinoma (RCC). It has been reported that 4% to 10% have tumor thrombus extending into the venous system among patients with newly diagnosed RCC (Marshall et al., 1970; Hoehn & Hermanek, 1983; Casanova & Zingg, 1991; Hatcher et al., 1991; Pagano et al., 1992). Compared with conservative treatment regimens, surgical resection remains the most effective treatment for these patients (Staehler & Brkovic, 2000). The mean 5-year survival rates of such patients with inferior vena cava involvement undergoing radical surgery for RCC have been reported as 32% to 64% (Neves & Zincke, 1987; Skinner et al., 1989; Montie et al., 1991; Swierzewski et al., 1994; Glazer & Novick, 1996).

Since the introduction of the tumor, node, metastasis (TNM) staging system, the pathologic stage has been considered the most important prognostic factor in RCC. According to the 2002 American Joint Committee on Cancer (AJCC) TNM staging classification (Greene et al., 2002), pT3 RCCs are subclassified into tumors invading perirenal fat and/or the ipsilateral adrenal gland (2002-pT3a), those presenting with tumor thrombus within the renal vein or the vena cava below the diaphragm (2002-pT3b) and those with vena cava thrombus above the diaphragm (2002-pT3c). This classification was very recently modified in 2009 (Edge et al., 2009), modified subclassification of pT3 RCCs are defined as tumors grossly extending into the renal vein or its segmental branches, or tumors invading perirenal and/or renal sinus fat but not beyond Gerota's fascia (2009-pT3a), those presenting with tumor thrombus within the vena cava below the diaphragm (2009-pT3b) and those with vena cava thrombus above the diaphragm or invaded the wall of the vena cava (2009-pT3c).

It has been debated that the TNM classification needs improvement in order to provide prognostic accuracy (Thompson et al., 2005; Leibovich et al., 2005; Ficarra et al., 2007). Several studies have discussed the correlation between prognosis and level of venous extension (Hatcher et al., 1991; Ljungberg et al., 1995; Tongaonkar et al., 1995; Glazer & Novick, 1996; Kuczyk et al., 1997; Staehler & Brkovic, 2000; Kim et al., 2004; Moinzadeh & Libertino, 2004). However, the prognostic impact of perirenal fat or adrenal gland involvement – based on the tumor characteristics of 2002 AJCC TNM staging classification

2002	2009
T1: Tumor 7 cm or less in greatest dimension, limited to the kidney	**T1:** Tumor 7 cm or less in greatest dimension, limited to the kidney
T1a: Tumor 4 cm or less in greatest dimension, limited to the kidney **T1b:** Tumor more than 4 cm but not more than 7 cm in greatest dimension, limited to the kidney	**T1a:** Tumor 4 cm or less in greatest dimension, limited to the kidney **T1b**: Tumor more than 4 cm but not more than 7 cm in greatest dimension, limited to the kidney
T2: Tumor more than 7 cm in greatest dimension, limited to the kidney	**T2**: Tumor more than 7 cm in greatest dimension, limited to the kidney
	T2a: Tumor more than 7 cm but less than or equal to 10 cm in greatest dimension, limited to the kidney **T2b:** Tumor more than 10 cm, limited to the kidney
T3: Tumor extends into major veins or invades adrenal gland or perinephric tissues but not beyond Gerota's fascia	**T3:** Tumor extends into major veins or perinephric tissues but not into the ipsilateral adrenal gland and not beyond Gerota's fascia
T3a: Tumor directly invades adrenal gland or perirenal and/or renal sinus fat but not beyond Gerota's fascia **T3b**: Tumor grossly extends into the renal vein or its segmental (muscle-containing) branches, or vena cava below the diaphragm **T3c:** Tumor grossly extends into the vena cava above the diaphragm or invades the wall of the vena cava	**T3a:** Tumor grossly extends into the renal vein or its segmental (muscle containing) branches, or tumor invades perirenal and/or renal sinus fat but not beyond Gerota's fascia **T3b**: Tumor grossly extends into the vena cava below the diaphragm **T3c:** Tumor grossly extends into the vena cava above the diaphragm or invades the wall of the vena cava
T4: Tumor invades beyond Gerota's fascia	**T4**: Tumor invades beyond Gerota's fascia (including contiguous extension into the ipsilateral adrenal gland)

Table 1. AJCC primary tumor staging classification of RCC

(2002-pT3a) – has not been seriously examined in patients with RCC exhibiting venous vascular extension. We hypothesized that RCC exhibiting venous vascular extension represents passive invasive features, since the low blood pressure in the renal vein allows tumors to easily extend into the venous system without aggressive characteristics, while perirenal fat or adrenal gland involvement represents active invasive features. Thus in this chapter, we describe the prognostic impact of perirenal fat or adrenal gland involvement in patients with RCC exhibiting venous vascular extension and the proposal for reclassification of the current TNM staging.

2. RCC exhibiting venous vascular extension

Forty-three patients with RCC exhibiting venous vascular extension entirely below the diaphragm were evaluated. Patients were treated by radical nephrectomy with complete resection of tumor thrombus extending into the venous system. Venous extension was defined as gross involvement. The patients included 35 males and 8 females, with median age at surgery of 62 years (range 43-82 years). The median tumor size was 8.79 cm (range 2.3-17.0 cm). The tumor site was on the right in 20 cases and on the left in 23 cases.

All patients received a preoperative evaluation that included routine blood test, chest x-rays, ultrasonography, and computerized tomography (CT), magnetic resonance imaging, or both. They then underwent radical nephrectomy with complete resection of the tumor and thrombus. Regional lymphadenectomy was performed concurrently with the radical nephrectomy. Postoperative evaluations, performed at intervals of 1 to 3 months, included blood test, chest x-rays, and CT. Bone scans were obtained when indicated. Hospital charts were retrospectively reviewed, and patient status was ascertained via office visit or telephone call to the patient.

All histological samples were reviewed by a single pathologist and were defined as tumor thrombus only or as tumor thrombus with perirenal fat or adrenal gland involvement.

Nonparametric estimates of survival were performed using Kaplan-Meier curves. Survival curves were generated based on disease-specific survival, representing patients still alive at specified intervals from the time of surgery to the date of death or the last follow-up visit. Log-rank tests were used for statistical comparisons.

Differences in identified prognostic parameters between tumor thrombus only and tumor thrombus with perirenal fat or adrenal gland involvement were analyzed using t test and chi-square test. Survival analysis regression model was assessed by Cox proportional hazards model to estimate the relative importance of the variables.

Additionally, nonparametric Kaplan-Meier survival estimates were performed to compare perirenal fat or adrenal gland involvement only (2002-pT3a), tumor thrombus only, and tumor thrombus with perirenal fat or adrenal gland involvement. The perirenal fat or adrenal gland involvement only (2002-pT3a) cohort represented 65 cases with complete resection of the tumor. Survival curves and log-rank tests were analyzed.

3. Prognostic impact of perirenal fat or adrenal gland involvement

3.1 Patient characteristics

The tumor thrombus only cohort included 21 males and 2 females (total 23 patients; 53.5%) with a median age of 61 years (range 44-78 years) and median follow-up period of 37 months (range 2-106 months). The median tumor size was 9.0 cm (range 2.3-17.0 cm); tumor site was on the right in 10 cases and on the left in 13 cases.

The tumor thrombus with perirenal fat or adrenal gland involvement cohort included 14 males and 6 females (total 20 patients; 46.5%) with a median age of 64 years (range 43-82 years) and median follow-up period of 9.5 months (range 2-45 months). The median tumor size was 8.45 cm (range 4.0-16.0 cm); tumor site was on the right in 10 cases and on the left in 10 cases.

When several parameters were analyzed for differences between tumor thrombus only cohort and tumor thrombus with perirenal fat or adrenal gland involvement cohort using *t* test or chi-square test, two parameters - Eastern Cooperative Oncology Group (ECOG) performance status (PS) 0 and histological grade 3 - proved statistically significant (P = 0.0329 and 0.0377, respectively; chi-square test).

Characteristic	Tumor thrombus only	Tumor thrombus with perirenal fat or adrenal gland involvement	*P* Value
Patients (*n*)	23	20	–
Follow-up period (month)			
Median	37	9.5	–
Range	2-106	2-45	
Age $ (year)			
Median	61	64	–
Range	44-78	43-82	
Mean ± SE	60.1 ± 1.9	64.3 ± 2.3	0.1673
Gender (*n*)			
Male	21	14	0.1180
Female	2	6	
Tumor diameter $ (cm)			
Median	9.0	8.45	–
Range	2.3-17.0	4.0-16.0	
Mean ± SE	9.0 ± 0.9	8.3 ± 0.8	0.5240
Tumor site (*n*)			
Right	10	10	–
Left	13	10	
ECOG PS 0 * (*n*)	15	6	0.0329
Initial symptom (*n*)	21	16	0.3929
Preoperative metastasis (*n*)	5	8	0.3184
Grade 3 * (*n*)	1	6	0.0377
pN (*n*)	1	5	0.0814
Clear cell (*n*)	21	14	0.1180
Spindle cell (*n*)	0	3	0.0924

KEY: ECOG PS = Eastern Cooperative Oncology Group performance status.
$ *Analysis assessed by* t *test.*
* *Statistically significant.*

Table 2. Patient characteristics and comparison among groups

3.2 Kaplan-Meier survival analysis

Nonparametric survival was analyzed by Kaplan-Meier survival curves, plotting both tumor thrombus only and tumor thrombus with perirenal fat or adrenal gland involvement.

Mean disease-specific survival time for patients with tumor thrombus with perirenal fat or adrenal gland involvement was 25.0 ± 4.4 (SE) months. On the other hand, mean survival time for those with tumor thrombus only was significantly longer at 70.9 ± 9.1 (SE) months ($P = 0.0032$, Fig. 1).

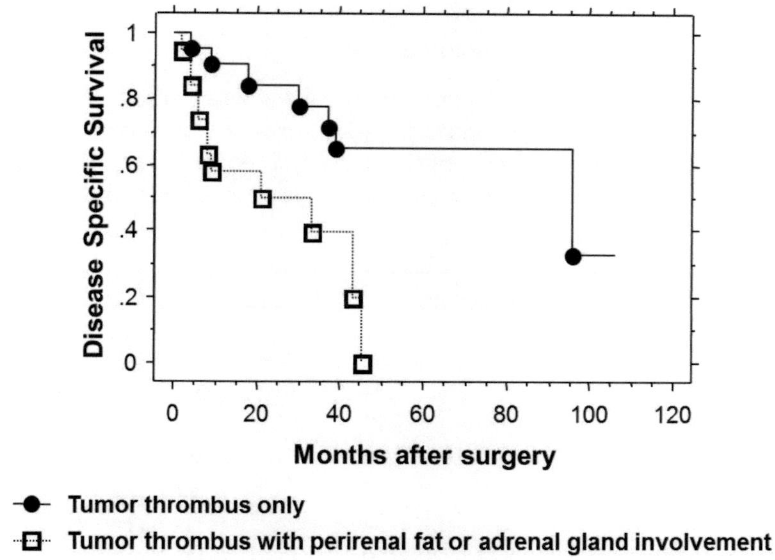

Fig. 1. Kaplan-Meier disease-specific survival after nephrectomy

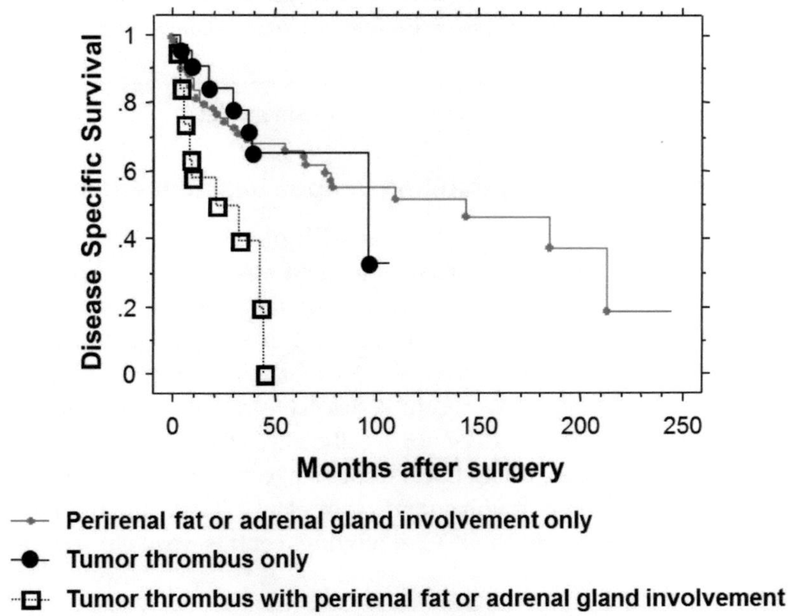

Fig. 2. Kaplan-Meier disease-specific survival after nephrectomy for those with perirenal fat or adrenal gland involvement only (2002-pT3a)

Mean disease-specific survival time for patients with perirenal fat or adrenal gland involvement only (2002-pT3a) was longer still at 116.1 ± 12.3 (SE) months. This value is significantly longer than for those with tumor thrombus with perirenal fat or adrenal gland involvement (*P* = 0.0044, Fig. 2), but not statistically significant different from that for those with tumor thrombus only.

3.3 Cox proportional hazards regression analysis

Univariate Cox proportional hazards regression analysis was performed for each variable. Significantly shorter disease-specific survival after surgery was predicted by presence of perirenal fat or adrenal gland involvement (*P* = 0.0065), preoperative metastasis (*P* = 0.0025), surgical specimens positive for lymph node metastasis (*P* = 0.0183), and spindle cell factor (*P* = 0.0233).

Variable	Hazard Ratio	95% CI	*P* Value
Perirenal fat or adrenal gland involvement *	4.11	1.49–11.4	0.0065
ECOG PS 0	1.34	0.54–3.34	0.5303
Initial symptom	2.13	0.28–16.2	0.4639
Preoperative metastasis *	4.32	1.68–11.2	0.0025
Tumor diameter	1.03	0.90–1.17	0.6984
Grade 3	0.34	0.11–1.11	0.0732
pN *	0.30	0.11–0.81	0.0183
Clear cell	1.76	0.57–5.39	0.3248
Spindle cell *	0.16	0.03–0.78	0.0233

KEY: CI = confidence interval; ECOG PS = Eastern Cooperative Oncology Group performance status.
** Statistically significant.*

Table 3. Univariate analysis by Cox proportional hazards model

4. Prognostic factors for RCC exhibiting venous vascular extension

Although the pathologic stage highly correlates with outcome in patients with RCC, the prognosis may vary even among tumors of the same stage. Thus, additional prognostic factors are needed. For RCCs exhibiting venous vascular extension, several investigators have described the prognostic significance of the level of venous extension (Hatcher et al., 1991; Ljungberg et al., 1995; Tongaonkar et al., 1995; Glazer & Novick, 1996; Kuczyk et al., 1997; Staehler & Brkovic, 2000). Most recent series have reported that the level of tumor thrombosis in the inferior vena cava does not significantly effect long-term survival (Kim et al., 2004; Moinzadeh & Libertino, 2004). Local tumor stage and grade are better predictors of prognosis than extent of venous involvement (Kim et al., 2004), but the most significant factors for survival in patients with RCC exhibiting venous vascular extension are still unknown.

The impact of perirenal fat or adrenal gland involvement in patients with RCC exhibiting venous vascular extension has not been seriously examined. Only the impact of perirenal fat involvement on prognosis of RCC patients has been documented (Gettman et al., 2003). On multivariate analyses, perirenal fat involvement led to a significantly worse prognosis, as did histological grade and metastasis (Gettman et al., 2003). However, perirenal fat involvement cannot be simply categorized, given the data we present here for the category of tumor thrombus with perirenal fat or adrenal gland involvement. This is the first investigation to specifically examine RCCs exhibiting tumor thrombus with perirenal fat or adrenal gland involvement and suggest that they represent a separate subcategory.

Tumor thrombus with perirenal fat or adrenal gland involvement has shorter disease-specific survival time than tumor thrombus only, or perirenal fat or adrenal gland involvement only (2002-pT3a). Tumors that are both tumor thrombus and perirenal fat or adrenal gland involvement are not the same as those that are only tumor thrombus. If patients with tumor thrombus also have perirenal fat or adrenal gland involvement, the prognosis is significantly poorer. The 5-year disease-specific survival estimate for tumor thrombus only was 65%, while that for tumor thrombus with perirenal fat or adrenal gland involvement was 0%. On univariate analyses, perirenal fat or adrenal gland involvement, preoperative metastasis, positive lymph node metastasis, and spindle cell factor were significant predictors of poor prognosis. Metastatic disease has been reported as an adverse predictor of disease-specific survival by several investigators (Neves & Zincke, 1987; Hatcher et al., 1991; Swierzewski et al., 1994; Tongaonkar et al., 1995; Nesbitt et al., 1997; Gettman et al., 2003). Generally, histological grade is identified as an independent prognostic factor in all RCCs (Méjean at al., 2003), but our results suggest histological grade does not affect survival in patients specifically having RCCs exhibiting tumor thrombus with perirenal fat or adrenal gland involvement.

5. Adrenal gland involvement in RCC

Patients with adrenal gland involvement have significantly worse survival than those with perirenal fat involvement (Han et al., 2003; Siemer et al., 2005). Direct ipsilateral adrenal gland involvement in RCC is rare, found in only 2.5% of radical nephrectomy specimens, and representing 13% of all 2002-pT3a lesions (Han et al., 2003). In this study, there were too few patients with RCCs exhibiting tumor thrombus with perirenal fat or adrenal gland involvement to allow a comparison of survival for patients with adrenal gland or perirenal fat involvement. However, previous investigators have emphasized that adrenal gland involvement should reclassified because of the worse prognosis (Han et al., 2003; Siemer et al., 2005; Fujita et al., 2008). According to the 2002 AJCC TNM staging classification (Greene et al., 2002), pT4 RCC is defined as tumor invades beyond Gerota's fascia. The median disease-specific survival for patients with ipsilateral adrenal gland involvement was significantly worse than that for tumor infiltrating only the perirenal fat and was similar to that for patients with 2002-pT4 RCCs (Han et al., 2003). The 5-year disease-specific survival probabilities have been reported 20.2% (Thompson et al., 2005) and 0% (Fujita et al., 2008). Primary adrenal carcinoma that invades the kidney is classified as pT4 disease (Ng & Libertino, 2003; Norton et al., 2005). A number of previous reports have suggested that, analogously, RCC with adrenal gland involvement should be reclassified as 2002-pT4 (Sandock et al., 1997; Han et al., 2003; Siemer et al., 2005; Thompson et al., 2005). Based on these investigations, adrenal gland involvement has been classified pT4 in 2009 AJCC TNM staging classification (Edge et al., 2009).

6. Proposal for reclassification of the TNM staging

According to a commentary by the Union Internationale Contre le Cancer (UICC) regarding continuous improvement of the TNM classification, the criteria for instituting changes include clinical relevance for assessment, treatment and outcome, presence of evidence for improved prognostic ability, and acceptance by the members of the UICC TNM committee (Gospodarowicz et al., 2004). The 2002 AJCC TNM system for patients with pT3 RCC incorporates the features of tumor thrombus, perirenal fat invasion and direct ipsilateral adrenal gland involvement (Greene et al., 2002). Several studies addressing 2002-pT3 staging have been reported and debated (Thompson et al., 2005; Leibovich et al., 2005; Ficarra et al., 2007; Fujita et al., 2008). And very recently, AJCC TNM staging classification was updated (Edge et al., 2009). However, tumor thrombus with perirenal fat or adrenal gland involvement was not well included in this modification. The prognosis of patients with tumor thrombus with perirenal fat or adrenal gland involvement was poor, as well as adrenal gland involvement which was subclassified as pT4 in 2009 AJCC TNM classification (Fujita et al., 2008; Edge et al., 2009). Reclassification will be still needed for tumor thrombus with perirenal fat or adrenal gland involvement RCCs. Reclassification of the current TNM staging system for RCCs according to the available clinical data and in accordance with the proposed process to update the staging system will render it a more powerful tool for predicting patient outcomes (Ficarra et al., 2006). The resultant staging system should be intended to give prognostic information that will allow accurate patient counseling, therapeutic selection, and surveillance (Howard & Wood, 2006). Our suggested revisions to the TNM classification represent a significant improvement in its prognostic accuracy.

7. Conclusion

The presence of perirenal fat or adrenal gland involvement in patients with RCC exhibiting venous vascular extension entirely below the diaphragm leads to a significantly poorer prognosis. Presence of perirenal fat or adrenal gland involvement is important for such cases and calls for active investigation. Additionally, reclassification will be needed for tumor thrombus with perirenal fat or adrenal gland involvement RCCs.

8. References

Casanova, G.A. & Zingg, E.J. (1991). Inferior Vena Caval Tumor Extension in Renal Cell Carcinoma. *Urologia Internationalis*, Vol.47, No.4, (no date), pp. 216-218, ISSN 0042-1138

Edge, S.B., Byrd, D.R., Compton, C.C., Fritz, A.G., Greene, F.L. & Trotti, A., III. (2009). *AJCC Cancer Staging Manual* (7th ed.), Springer, ISBN 978-0-387-88440-0, New York, United States of America

Ficarra, V. & Artibani, W. (2006). Staging System of Renal Cell Carcinoma: Current Issues. *European Urology*, Vol.49, No.2, (February 2006), pp. 223-225, ISSN 0302-2838

Ficarra, V., Novara, G., Iafrate, M., Cappellaro, L., Bratti, E., Zattoni, F. & Artibani, W. (2007). Proposal for Reclassification of the TNM Staging System in Patients with Locally Advanced (pT3-4) Renal Cell Carcinoma According to the Cancer-Related Outcome. *European Urology*, Vol.51, No.3, (May 2007), pp. 722-731, ISSN 0302-2838

Fujita, T., Iwamura, M., Yanagisawa, N., Muramoto, M., Okayasu, I. & Baba, S. (2008). Reclassification of the Current Tumor, Node, Metastasis Staging in pT3 Renal Cell Carcinoma. *International Journal of Urology*, Vol.15, No.7, (July 2008), pp. 582-586, ISSN 1442-2042

Gettman, M.T., Boelter, C.W., Cheville, J.C., Zincke, H., Bryant, S.C. & Blute, M.L. (2003). Charlson Co-Morbidity Index as a Predictor of Outcome after Surgery for Renal Cell Carcinoma with Renal Vein, Vena Cava or Right Atrium Extension. *Journal of Urology*, Vol.169, No.4, (April 2003), pp. 1282-1286, ISSN 0022-5347

Glazer, A.A. & Novick, A.C. (1996). Long-term Followup after Surgical Treatment for Renal Cell Carcinoma Extending into the Right Atrium. *Journal of Urology*, Vol.155, No.2, (February 1996), pp. 448-450, ISSN 0022-5347

Gospodarowicz, M.K., Miller, D., Groome, P.A., Greene, F.L., Logan, P.A. & Sobin, L.H. (2004). The Process for Continuous Improvement of the TNM Classification. *Cancer*, Vol.100, No.1, (January 2004), pp. 1-5, ISSN 1097-0142

Greene, F.L., Page, D.L., Fleming, I.D., Fritz, A.G., Balch, C.M., Haller, D.G. & Morrow M. (2002). *AJCC Cancer Staging Manual* (6th ed.), Springer-Verlag, ISBN 978-0-387-95271-0, New York, United States of America

Han, K.R., Bui, M.H., Pantuck, A.J., Freitas, D.G., Leibovich, B.C., Dorey, F.J., Zisman, A., Janzen, N.K., Mukouyama, H., Figlin, R.A. & Belldegrun, A.S. (2003). TNM T3a Renal Cell Carcinoma: Adrenal Gland Involvement is not the Same as Renal Fat Invasion. *Journal of Urology*, Vol.169, No3, (March 2003), pp. 899-904, ISSN 0022-5347

Hatcher, P.A., Anderson, E.E., Paulson, D.F., Carson, C.C. & Robertson, J.E. (1991). Surgical Management and Prognosis of Renal Cell Carcinoma Invading the Vena Cava. *Journal of Urology*, Vol.145, No.1, (January 1991), pp. 20-24, ISSN 0022-5347

Hoehn, W. & Hermanek, P. (1983). Invasion of Veins in Renal Cell Carcinoma-Frequency, Correlation and Prognosis. *European Urology*, Vol.9, No.5, (no date), pp. 276-280, ISSN 0302-2838

Howard, G.E. & Wood, C.G. (2006). Staging Refinements in Renal Cell Carcinoma. *Current Opinion in Urology*, Vol.16, No.5, (September 2006), pp. 317-320, ISSN 0963-0643

Kim, H.L., Zisman, A., Han, K.R., Figlin, R.A. & Belldegrun, A.S. (2004). Prognostic Significance of Venous Thrombus in Renal Cell Carcinoma. Are Renal Vein and Inferior Vena Cava Involvement Different? *Journal of Urology*, Vol.171, No.2 pt 1, (February 2004), pp. 588-591, ISSN 0022-5347

Kuczyk, M.A., Bokemeyer, C., Köhn, G., Stief, C.G., Machtens, S., Truss, M., Höfner, K. & Jonas, U. (1997). Prognostic Relevance of Intracaval Neoplastic Extension for Patients with Renal Cell Cancer. *British Journal of Urology*, Vol.80, No.1, (July 1997), pp. 18-24, ISSN 0007-1331

Leibovich, B.C., Cheville, J.C., Lohse, C.M., Zincke, H., Kwon, E.D., Frank, I., Thompson, R.H. & Blute, M.L. (2005). Cancer Specific Survival for Patients with pT3 Renal Cell Carcinoma–Can the 2002 Primary Tumor Classification be Improved? *Journal of Urology*, Vol.173, No.3, (March 2005), pp. 716-719, ISSN 0022-5347

Ljungberg, B., Stenling, R., Österdahl, B., Farrelly, E., Åberg T. & Roos G. (1995). Vein Invasion in Renal Cell Carcinoma: Impact on Metastatic Behavior and Survival. *Journal of Urology*, Vol.154, No.5, (November 1995), pp. 1681-1684, ISSN 0022-5347

Marshall, V.F., Middleton, R.G., Holswade, G.R. & Goldsmith, E.I. (1970). Surgery for Renal Cell Carcinoma in the Vena Cava. *Journal of Urology*, Vol.103, No.4, (April 1970), pp. 414-420, ISSN 0022-5347

Méjean, A., Oudard, S. & Thiounn, N. (2003). Prognostic Factors of Renal Cell Carcinoma. *Journal of Urology*, Vol.169, No.3, (March 2003), pp. 821-827, ISSN 0022-5347

Moinzadeh, A. & Libertino, J.A. (2004). Prognostic Significance of Tumor Thrombus Level in Patients with Renal Cell Carcinoma and Venous Tumor Thrombus Extension. Is All T3b the Same? *Journal of Urology*, Vol.171, No.2 pt 1, (February 2004), pp. 598-601, ISSN 0022-5347

Montie, J.E., el Ammar, R., Pontes, J.E., Medendorp, S.V., Novick, A.C., Streem, S.B., Kay, R. Montague, D.K. & Cosgrove D.M. (1991). Renal Cell Carcinoma with Inferior Vena Cava Tumor Thrombi. *Surgery, Gynecology and Obstetrics*, Vol.173, No.2, (August 1991), pp. 107-115, ISSN 0039-6087

Nesbitt, J.C., Soltero, E.R., Dinney, C.P., Walsh, G.L., Schrump, D.S., Swanson, D.A., Pisters, L.L., Willis, K.D. & Putnam, J.B., Jr. (1997). Surgical Management of Renal Cell Carcinoma with Inferior Vena Cava Tumor Thrombus. *Annals of Thoracic Surgery*, Vol.63, No.6, (June 1997), pp. 1592-1600, ISSN 0003-4975

Neves, R.J. & Zincke, H. (1987). Surgical Treatment of Renal Cancer with Vena Cava Extension. *British Journal of Urology*, Vol.59, No.5, (May 1987), pp. 390-395, ISSN 0007-1331

Ng, L. & Libertino, J.M. (2003). Adrenocortical Carcinoma: Diagnosis, Evaluation and Treatment. *Journal of Urology*, Vol.169, No.1, (January 2003), pp. 5-11, ISSN 0022-5347

Norton, J.A. (2005). Adrenal tumors, In: *Cancer: Principles and Practice of Oncology* (7th ed.), DeVita, V.T. Jr., Hellman, S., Rosenberg, S.A. (eds.), pp. 1528-1540, Lippincott Williams & Wilkins, ISBN 0-781-74450-4, Philadelphia, United States of America

Pagano, F., Dal Bianco, M., Artibani, W., Pappagallo, G. & Prayer Galetti, T. (1992). Renal Cell Carcinoma with Extension into the Inferior Vena Cava: Problems in Diagnosis, Staging and Treatment. *European Urology*, Vol.22, No.3, (September 1992), pp. 200-203, ISSN 0302-2838

Sandock, D.S., Seftel, A.D. & Resnick, M.I. (1997). Adrenal Metastases from Renal Cell Carcinoma: Role of Ipsilateral Adrenalectomy and Definition of Stage. *Urology*, Vol.49, No.1, (January 1997), pp. 28-31, ISSN 0090-4295

Siemer, S., Lehmann, J., Loch, A., Becker, F., Stein, U., Schneider, G., Ziegler, M. & Stöckle, M. (2005). Current TNM Classification of Renal Cell Carcinoma Evaluated: Revising Stage T3a. *Journal of Urology*, Vol.173, No.1, (January 2005), pp. 33-37, ISSN 0022-5347

Skinner, D.G., Pritchett, T.R., Lieskovsky, G., Boyd, S.D. & Stiles, Q.R. (1989). Vena Caval Involvement by Renal Cell Carcinoma. Surgical Resection Provides Meaningful Long-term Survival. *Annals of Surgery*, Vol.210, No.3, (September 1989), pp. 387-394, ISSN 0003-4932

Staehler, G. & Brkovic, D. (2000). The Role of Radical Surgery for Renal Cell Carcinoma with Extension into the Vena Cava. *Journal of Urology*, Vol.163, No.6, (June 2000), pp. 1671-1675, ISSN 0022-5347

Swierzewski, D.J., Swierzewski, M.J. & Libertino, J.A. (1994). Radical Nephrectomy in Patients with Renal Cell Carcinoma with Venous, Vena Caval, and Atrial Extension. *American Journal of Surgery*, Vol.168, No.2, (August 1994), pp. 205-209, ISSN 0002-9610

Thompson, R.H., Cheville, J.C., Lohse, C.M., Webster, W.S., Zincke, H., Kwon, E.D., Frank, I., Blute, M.L. & Leibovich, B.C. (2005). Reclassification of Patients with pT3 and pT4 Renal Cell Carcinoma Improves Prognostic Accuracy. *Cancer*, Vol.104, No.1, (July 2005), pp 53-60, ISSN 1097-0142

Thompson, R.H., Leibovich, B.C., Cheville, J.C., Lohse, C.M., Frank, I., Kwon, E.D., Zincke, H. & Blute, M.L. (2005). Should Direct Ipsilateral Adrenal Gland Invasion from Renal Cell Carcinoma be Classified as pT3a? *Journal of Urology*, Vol.173, No.3, (March 2005), pp. 918-921, ISSN 0022-5347

Tongaonkar, H.B., Dandekar, N.P., Dalal, A.V., Kulkarni, J.N. & Kamat, M.R. (1995). Renal Cell Carcinoma Extending to the Renal Vein and Inferior Vena Cava: Results of Surgical Treatment and Prognostic Factors. *Journal of Surgical Oncology*, Vol.59, No.2, (June 1995), pp. 94-100, ISSN 0022-4790

14

Health-Related Quality of Life After Radical Nephrectomy and Kidney Donation

Archil Chkhotua, Tinatin Pantsulaia and Laurent Managadze
National Center of Urology
Georgia

1. Introduction

Radical nephrectomy (RN) is a treatment of choice for the patients with renal cell carcinoma (RCC) achieving excellent results, especially in local stages of the disease. Oncological results of RN are well evaluated on a large number of patients. However, studies on a postoperative health-related quality of life (HRQol) of these patients are very limited (Novara G et al., 2010; Poulakis V et al., 2003; Clark PE et al., 2001). There are no publications available comparing the HRQoL of patients after RN with that of healthy individuals and other forms of nephrectomy.

Living kidney transplantation provides excellent results with the lowest complication and the highest graft and patient survival rates (Hariharan et al., 2000). However, it should not be forgotten that donors are healthy persons voluntarily donating an organ and their postoperative health and HRQol should be a matter of utmost importance. It has been shown that kidney donation does not cause serious medical problems like: deterioration of kidney function, arterial hypertension or proteinuria (El-Agroudy et al., 2007). Although advocated in the literature, psychosocial assessment and monitoring of living kidney donors is not yet routinely performed. There are only limited reports in the literature examining HRQol issues in the donors.

The HRQol concept is well-known in clinical medicine and is frequently applied for the assessment of surgical or other treatment modalities to determine their therapeutic success. HRQol has become a leading criteria in many outcome studies alongside with somatic and economic factors and is frequently listed as outcome parameter in many medical societies' guidelines. Despite methodological difficulties in making HRQol measurable, there are numerous surveys and questionnaires used for this purpose. The Short Form-36 (SF-36), Giessen Subjective Complaints List-24 (GBB-24) and Zerssen's Mood-Scale (Bf-S) are internationally validated and frequently used questionnaires for this purpose (Ware & Sherbourne CD, 1992; Giessing et al., 2004; Zerssen D, 1976).

The importance of this topic is underlined by the fact, that available data on psychological well-being and HRQol of the patients after RN and kidney donors are limited and somewhat controversial. It would be very interesting to know as to whether there are differences between countries, races, or social groups, with regard to HRQol of the patients and donors. While some of these studies are providing evidences that the donor HRQol is at least comparable or even better than that of the general population (Giessing et al., 2004;

Ibrahim et al, 2009; Feltrin et al, 2008; Johnson et al, 1999; Smith et al, 2003; Isotani et al, 2002; Fehrman-Ekholm et al, 2000; Tanriverdi et al, 2004; Lima et al, 2006), others are showing the negative impact of the donation on donors' HRQol (Giessing et al., 2004; Johnson et al, 1999; Smith et al, 2003; Jackobs et al., 200; Reimer et al., 2006; Schover et al., 1997; Zargooshi, 2001; Tellioglu et al., 2008). There are no studies comparing the HRQol of kidney donors with the patients who underwent neprectomy due to the urological diseases.

The aim of the current study was to assess the HRQol of the patients who underwent RN due to the RCC and compare it with age- and sex-matched healthy persons and our kidney donors.

2. Subjects and methods

The study population consisted of:

Group I: 52 patients who underwent nephrectomy due to the RCC

Group II: 120 age- and sex matched healthy individuals

Group III: The kidney donors operated at our institution from January 2005 to December 2008 (n=57).

The patients (Group I) and the kidney donors (Group III) have been followed-up prospectively. The questionnaires have been sent to them after a follow-up of at least 3 months.

The Group I consisted of the 98 consecutive patients operated at our institution for RCC. Three questionnaires (SF-36, GBB-24 and Bf-S) have been mailed to all the patients. 7 (7%) patients have been reported as dead at the time of evaluation, 10 (10%) were lost of follow-up and 29 (30%) didn't respond. We've received the completed questionnaires from 52 patients (53%). The mean follow-up was 28 months (range: 4-35 months). None of the patients had clinical signs of renal insufficiency or other substantial co-morbidities (diabetes etc). Radical or partial nephrectomy without adjuvant immunotherapy was performed in all patients. The pathological stage distribution of the tumors was the following: T1 – 21 (40%); T2 – 13 (25%); T3 – 18 (35%) patients. 14 (27%) cancers were G1, 20 (38%) - G2 and 18 (35%) - G3. Morphological evaluation revealed clear cell RCC in all 52 patients. 2 patients had lymph node and 1 patient had distant metastases at the time of surgery. 18 (34.6%) tumors were discovered incidentally, 29 (55.8%) were locally symptomatic and 5 patients (9.6%) had a systemic disease symptoms. All patients were operated on in one department.

The control group has been generated by using probability-based methods to ensure representativeness of the general population of the Country. The subjects from other psychological surveys have been provided by the national psychological association for this purpose. The control group consisted of 120 healthy volunteers with the mean age of 51±9 years (18-70 years). They were matched with the donors and patients on the basis of: age, sex, race and ethnicity. Exclusion criteria were chronic diseases, with the exception of controlled systemic hypertension and previous non-major surgical interventions.

61 living kidney transplants have been performed at our institution since January 2005 to December 2008. The mean follow-up of the donors was 32 months (range: 4-57 months). All the transplants were performed from genetically related donors. 19 donors (31%) were male and 42 (69%) were female. The mean donor age was 49±9 years. The most frequent form of donation was parent to child (86.5%). In 2.7% of cases organ was offered by sibling and in 5.4% - by cousin and uncle each.

All transplant operations were approved by the ethical committee of the Ministry of Health of Georgia. All the patients and donors were studied according to protocols accepted at our centre. Donor nephrectomy was done by open extraperitoneal approach. All transplants have been performed according to ABO compatibility and negative direct cross-match.

All the donors are alive. They have been followed either by our nephrology department or by associated institutions, with which our center cooperates closely. Three questionnaires (SF-36, GBB-24 and Bf-S) have been mailed, e-mailed, or handed out to all the donors who could be contacted, with a follow-up of at least 3 months. If no answer was returned, we called the donor, motivated him or her for participation, and sent the questionnaires again. If the donor could not be contacted, we talked to the recipient and asked for assistance. Thus, we have received answers from 57 (93%) donors who could be contacted.

The evaluation procedure was completely anonymous and all the respondents were free of any charges related to filling or sending the questionnaires.

2.1 Short form-36 questionnaire

The SF-36 questionnaire was developed in the United States (Ware & Sherbourne CD, 1992). It is a standardized instrument for measuring HRQol on eight different scales: physical function (PF), physical role (PR), social function (SF), general health perception (GH), vitality (V), bodily pain (BP), mental health (MH), and emotional role (ER). Thirty-six questions have to be answered, and a score is computed for each scale, ranging from 0 (least well-being) to 100 (greatest well-being). This form has been adapted by psychologists for use in Georgia with adequate translation and minor changes to the content of the form.

2.2 Giessen subjective complaints list-24 questionnaire

Giessen Subjective Complaints List-24 questionnaire (GBB-24) assesses physical complaints attributable to psychosomatic reasons (Giessing et al., 2004). The questionnaire has six questions, each referring to four items (cardiac complaints, gastric complaints, limb pain and fatigue tendency) for which participants are asked to rate their complaints (0-no complaints, 4-strong complaints). The sum of these four items reflects the fifth item, "overall subjective complaints" (0–96 points).

2.3 Bf-S questionnaire

Bf-S questionnaire is a self-rating scale developed by Zerssen in 1975 (Zerssen D, 1976). It is a 28 question scale designed to assess the person's mood. The questionnaire has been used for the analysis of patient's self-feeling pre- and/or post event (operation, donation etc.).

The study design was approved by the internal review board of the institution as conforming to the provisions of the Declaration of Helsinki. All participants provided written informed consent.

2.4 Statistical analysis

Statistical analysis was performed using computer software (SPSS 12.0 for Windows, Lead Technologies Inc. 2003. Chicago, IL.). Normality of data distribution was examined with

Kolmogorov-Smirnov test. The different scores in the groups were compared with ANOVA, Mann Whitney and Kruskal Wallis tests. Age-dependency of the scores was analysed by the Pearson correlation and linear regression. A p value of less than 0.05 was considered significant.

3. Results

The age, sex distribution and mean follow-up was not different between the groups. At the time of the study, 97.8% of the recipients were alive and 89% of these had a functioning graft. Overall, 12 minor complications occurred in 9 donors (15%) (table 1).

Complication	N	%
Pneumonia	1	1.7
Pneumothorax	2	3.5
UTI	3	5.2
Postoperative hernia	3	5.2
Impaired wound healing	3	5.2

Table 1. Postoperative donor complications

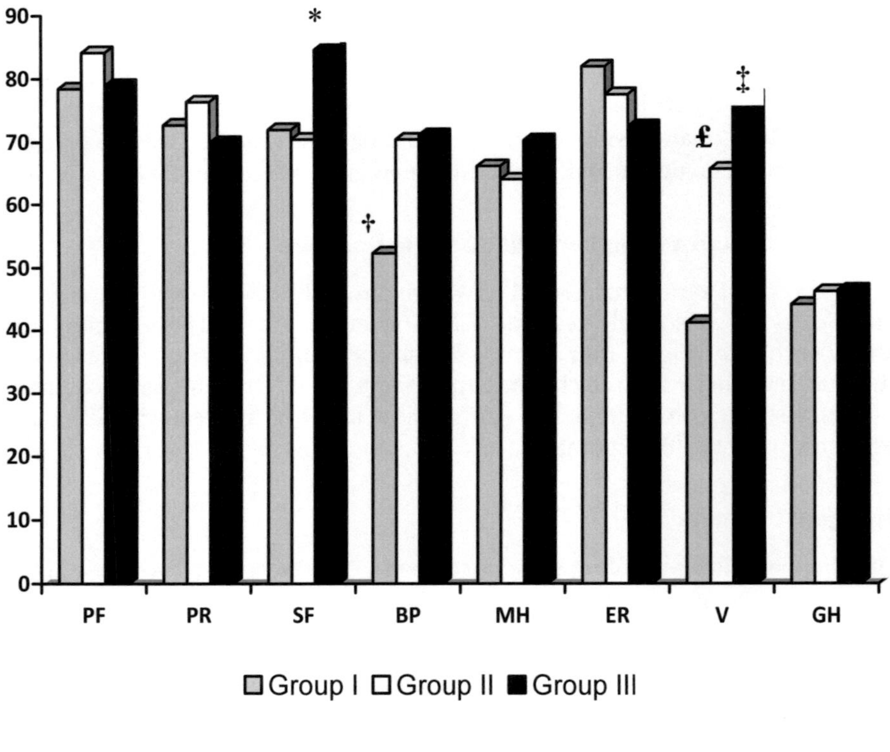

* p=0.0001vs.Group II and p=0.0209 vs. Group I
† p=0.0357 vs. Group III and p=0.0375 vs. Group II
‡ p=0.0478 vs. Group II and p=0.0006 vs. Group I
£ p=0.0128 vs. Group I

Fig. 1. Comparison of the mean (±SE) SF-36 scores between the groups

For the SF-36 items: "Social function", "Bodily pain" and "Vitality", donors scored significantly better than controls and patients. "Bodily pain" and "Vitality" indexes of the controls were significantly higher than that of the patients (Fig. 1). The SF-36 scores were not different between males and females.

We analyzed the age dependency of the SF-36 scores in all three groups. The correlation coefficients, corresponding p values and 95% CIs of the eight different SF-36 scores against age are shown in table 1. The correlation coefficients of "Social function" in Group III; "Social function", "Mental health" and "Vitality" in Group II were moderately high (-541, -0.341, -292 and -0.292, respectively); their 95% CIs were narrow (-0.768- -0.195, -0.568- -0.067, -0.530- -0.012 and -0.529- -0.011, respectively) and their p values were significant (0.0037, 0.0158, 0.0413 and 0.0416, respectively), showing a negative correlation with age. Low correlation coefficients of other SF-36 scores, especially in Group I, together with a wide range of 95% CIs including 0, indicated that these scores were not age-related (table 2).

SF-36 score	Correlation Coefficient	P value	95% Lower CI	95% Upper CI
Group I				
PF	-0.235	0.7345	-0.925	0.817
PR	-0.792	0.1282	-0.986	0.310
SF	0.334	0.6238	-0.778	0.939
BP	-0.703	0.2167	-0.978	0.472
MH	-0.326	0.6323	-0.938	0.781
ER	0.212	0.7610	-0.825	0.922
V	-0.670	0.2521	-0.976	0.520
GH	-0.312	0.6479	-0.937	0.787
Group II				
PF	-0.219	0.1307	-0.471	-0.066
PR	-0.243	0.0924	-0.491	0.041
SF	-0.341	0.0158	-0.568	-0.067
BP	-0.212	0.1439	-0.466	0.073
MH	-0.292	0.0413	-0.530	-0.012
ER	-0.017	0.4236	-0.386	0.0169
V	-0.292	0.0416	-0.529	-0.011
GH	-0.116	0.4313	-0.384	0.171
Group III				
PF	-0.045	0.8724	-0.529	0.461
PR	-0.140	0.6106	-0.595	0.382
SF	-0.541	0.0037	-0.768	-0.195
BP	-0.058	0.8340	-0.538	0.451
MH	0.008	0.9784	-0.490	0.501
ER	-0.304	0.2573	-0.695	0.226
V	0.284	0.2923	-0.246	0.684
GH	-0.068	0.8069	-0.545	0.443

Table 2. Pearson correlation analysis of the age dependency of SF-36 scores in different groups

The four scores which showed significant correlations with age ("Social function" in Group III; "Social function", "Mental health" and "Vitality" in Group II) were evaluated further with a linear regression model. Figs. 2 and 3 show the regression plots of the three scores ("Social function" in Group III; "Social function" and "Vitality" in Group II) against age. Regression analyses confirmed the results of the Pearson correlation regarding the linearity of their relationship with age. As to "Mental health" in Group II, regression analyses didn't verify linearity of the relationship.

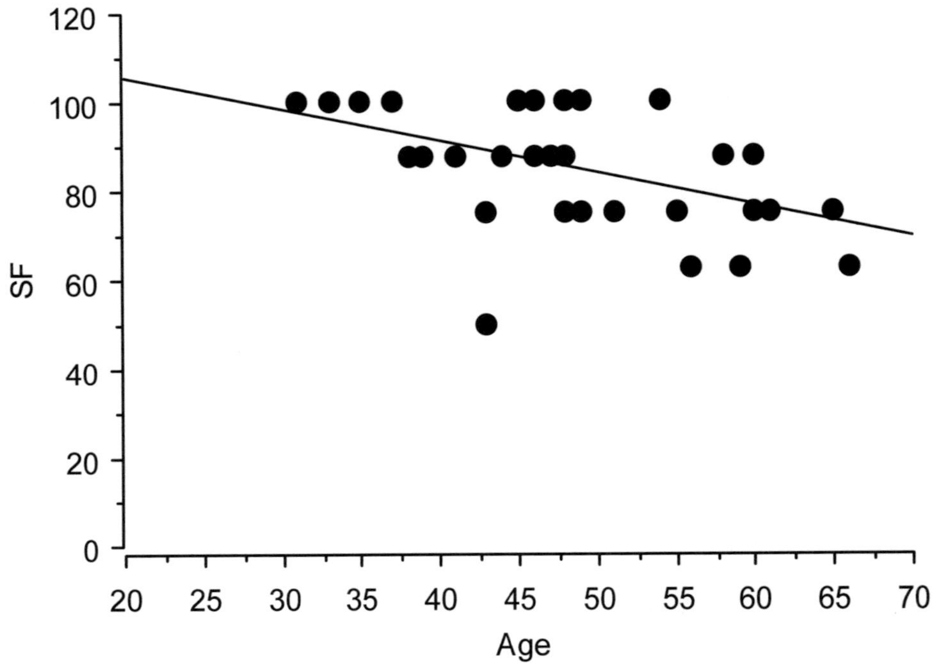

Y = 120,103 - 0,728 * X; R^2 = 0,245, p=0.0040

Fig. 2. Regression plot of SF-36 score for "social function" against age in the donors

In all five GBB-24 items the donors scored higher than the controls and patients. For the "gastric complaints" the difference was statistically significant. In this item the patients scored significantly worse than controls and donors (Fig. 4). The GBB-24 scores were not correlated with age. Comparison of the scores between males and females showed that in the Group II, in four out of five items ("Overall complaints", "Fatigue tendency", "Limb pain" and "Cardiac complaints") males scored significantly higher than females (Fig. 5). The differences in other groups were not significant (data not shown).

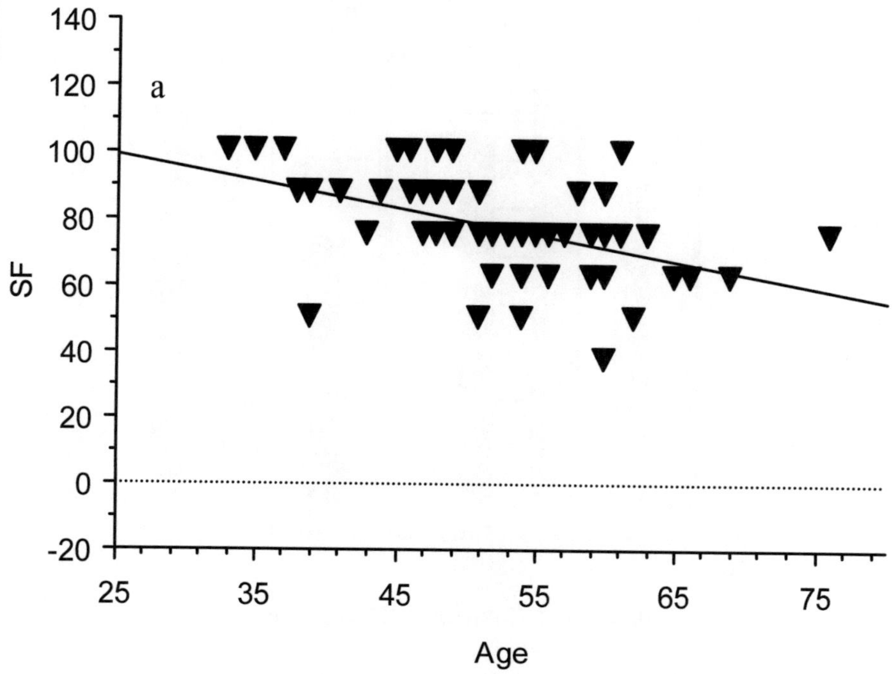

Y = 118,649 - 0,781 * X; R^2 = 0,190; p=0.0003

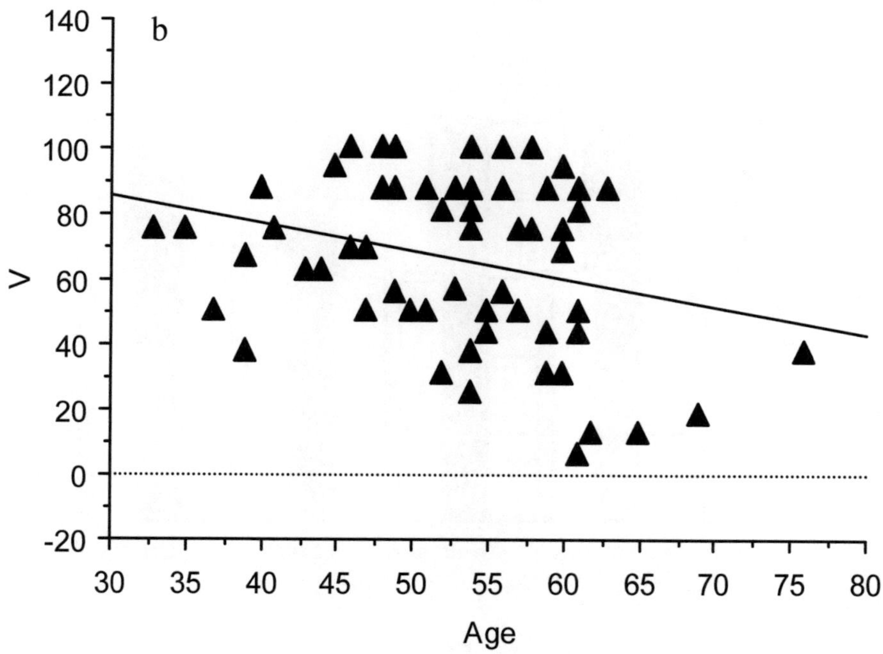

Y = 111,364 - 0,848 * X; R^2 = 0,073 ; p=0.0290

Fig. 3. Regression plots of the SF-36 scores for "social function" (a) and "vitality" (b) against age in the control group

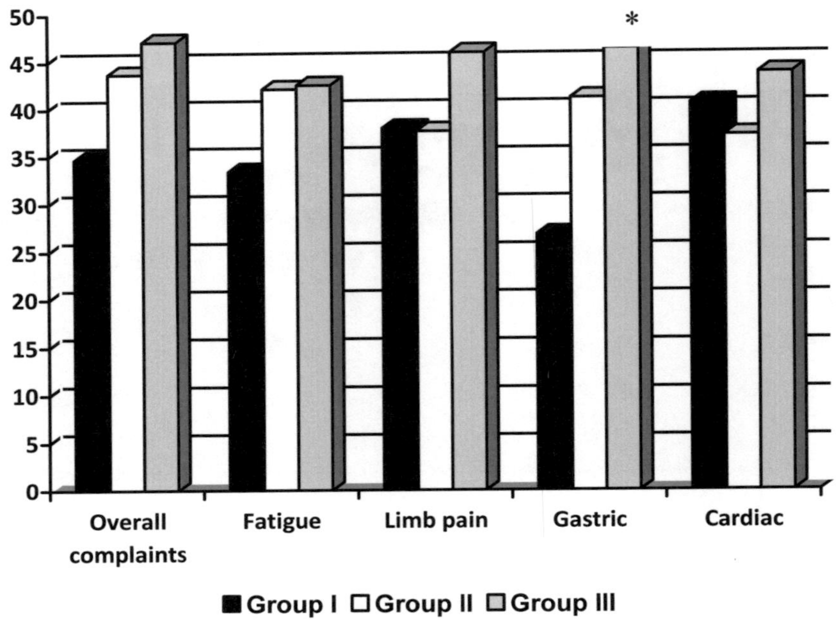

* p=0.0080 vs. Group I and p=0.0293 vs. Group II

Fig. 4. Comparison of the GBB-24 scores between the groups

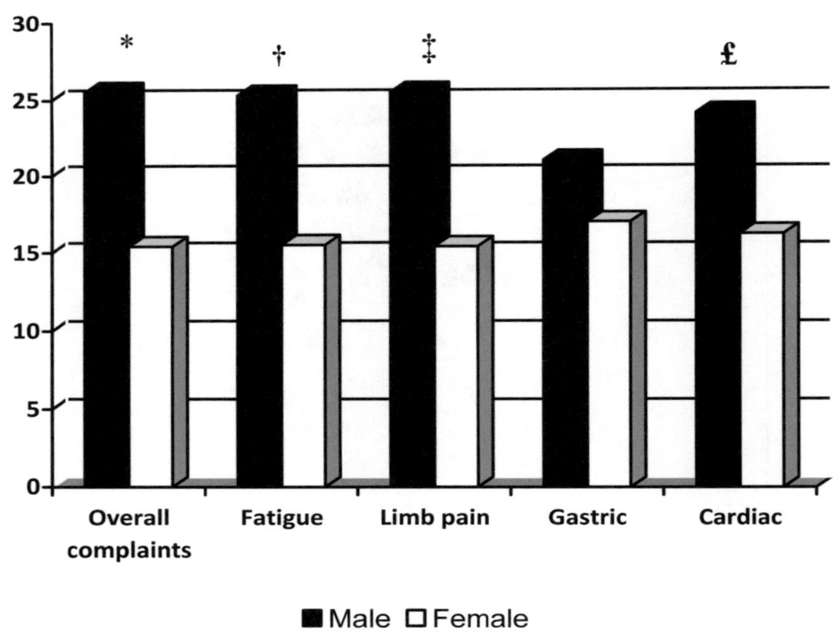

* p=0.0067, † p=0.0433, ‡ p=0.0088, £ p=0.0326.

Fig. 5. Comparison of the GBB-24 scores between males and females in the control group

The mood analyses have shown that Bf-S scores of the donors were significantly higher than that of the controls and patients. The controls scored better than the patients (Fig. 6). The Bf-S scores were not age-related and didn't differ between males and females (data not shown).

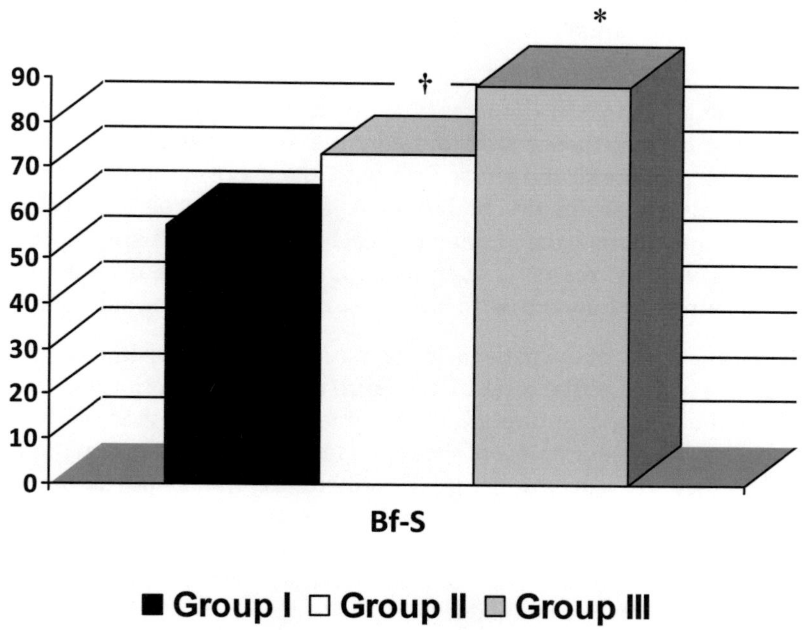

* p=0.0007 vs. Group II and p<0.0001 vs. Group I
† p=0.0183 vs. Group I

Fig. 6. Comparison of the Bf-S scores between the groups

4. Discussion

RN and nephron sparing surgery are the treatments of choice for the patients with RCC. Oncological results and complications of these forms of treatment are extensively evaluated showing excellent outcomes in the patients with local disease stages. However, information on the HRQol of these patients is scarce. There are very few publications assessing and comparing the HRQol of the patients after different forms of surgical treatment of RCC.

The studies on the donors' psychological well-being and HRQol have been conducted since the early years of kidney transplantation. Yet, this topic remains largely under-evaluated and unknown. Most of the existing studies have limitations such as: retrospective design; lack of matching the groups for age or gender; use of non-standardized and validated questionnaires; comparison of the results with references validated for another cultural background; too few participants or low response rates. Nonetheless, these studies suggest hypotheses that require evaluation in a well-designed prospective manner. It should be considered that disparities among the countries in terms of religion, culture, customs, environment, and other factors can influence the HRQol.

In this study we assessed postoperative HRQol of the patients who underwent RN in comparison with our living kidney donors and age and sex matched healthy individuals.

Three different questionnaires have been used to complexly evaluate their: postoperative HRQol (SF-36), subjective complaints (GBB-24) and mood (Bf-S). This type of design is original in existing literature and gives an opportunity to deeper analyse physical, psychosocial and spiritual well-being of the patients after RN in comparison with healthy, non-operated individuals and persons who underwent the same operation for non-medical indications.

We have shown that in three SF-36 items: "Social function", "Bodily pain" and "Vitality" donors scored significantly better than the controls and patients. In "Bodily pain" and "Vitality" items the patients scored worse than both, the donors and healthy individuals. In all five GBB-24 items the donors had higher scores than the controls and patients, but only for the "Gastric complaints" the difference reached statistical significance. Incomplete sample number may be the reason of it. In mood analyses the patients scored significantly worse than the controls and donors, with both these differences being substantial.

The reason of worse scores of the patients in comparison with the healthy subjects should be physical complains related to the main disease and/or operation performed. Also, it should be considered that after passing through the treatment process they do not feel themselves completely healthy. The better scores of the donors in somatic parameters can be explained by the fact that they are selected group of individuals, well-evaluated and with better general health than representatives of the common population. The better scores in psycho-social parameters is caused by the fact that donating an organ is associated with giving a second life to the family member and/or close relative, psycho-social mobilization of the donor and consequently, the better mood.

The new findings of this study are: negative correlation of HRQol scores with age; and gender differences in subjective complaints. We have shown that "Social function", "Mental health" and "Vitality" indexes of the healthy individuals are decreasing with age. The same was true only for the "Social function" of the donors. Significant postoperative improvement in some of the HRQol parameters could be the reason why these differences have not been detected in the donors. As to the "Social function", this domain is much more dependent on time and external factors than "Mental health" or "Vitality" and kept negative correlation with age.

Four out of five GBB-24 scores were found to be significantly higher in males as compared with females. Again, this difference was evident in the control group and disappeared in the donors and patients. This result corresponds with the outcomes of early studies showing that: a) females tend to have more health complaints than their male counterparts; b) they do receive more diagnostic workups; and c) they receive prescriptions more often during office visits than men do (Verbrugge & Steiner, 1985). Significant postoperative HRQol worsening in the patients and HRQol improvement in the donors was probably the reason why the difference was not evident in these groups. Both of these concepts need further evaluation with higher sample numbers in order to assess importance of the findings.

This study has some limitations. The most important is a lack of an ideal control group. We've used the healthy individuals from general population as controls. As far as the donors are, on the whole, healthier than representatives of the general population, it would be even more informative to compare their results with the persons who were evaluated and accepted as donors, but finally didn't donate a kidney. However, this kind of analyses would be impossible to perform with relatively small number of transplants performed in our country. An ongoing multicenter study from the US is addressing this issue and will probably come up with the results in the next few years (http://www.clinicaltrials.gov/ct2/results?term=NCT00608283). Relatively small sample number, especially in Group III, can be considered as another shortcoming of this study. Nevertheless, taking into consideration that they comprise 85% of transplants performed in Georgia, and a very high response rate, this group is representative for the Country.

Prospective design and high response rate are the most important advantages of this study. The response rate of 94% is the highest reported in the literature using these questionnaires. It was caused by the fact that the questionnaires have been handed out personally to almost all the donors by nephrologists. On the contrary, the questionnaires have been mailed to the patients (Group I) and only half of them responded. Another advantage of this study is a comparison of pairs of subjects and controls matched for gender and age. Only few studies have evaluated the matched pairs (Fehrman-Ekholm et al, 2000) whereas others have compared their findings with the scores of general population (Johnson et al, 1999; Karrfelt et al, 1998). The present study is also the first to include post-nephrectomy patients, and apply the Bf-S questionnaire to the study groups.

5. Conclusion

In conclusion, the HRQol of living kidney donors and healthy individuals is similar and better than HRQol of the patients operated due to the medical indications. The future prospective studies with higher number of participants will enhance our knowledge of factors influencing HRQol of the living kidney donors and patients after nephrectomy.

6. References

Clark, PE., et al. (2001). Quality of life and psychological adaptation after surgical treatment for localized renal cell carcinoma: impact of the amount of remaining renal tissue. *Urology,* Vol. 57, No. 2, (February 2001), pp. 252-256.

El-Agroudy, AE.; et al. (2007). Long-term follow-up of living kidney donors: a longitudinal study, *British Journal of Urology International,* Vol. 100, No. 6, (December 2007), pp. 1351-1355.

Feltrin, A.; et al. (2008). Experience of donation and quality of life in living kidney and liver donors, *Transplant International,*Vol. 21, No. 5, (may 2008), pp. 466-472.

Fehrman-Ekholm, I.; et al. (2000). Kidney donors don't regret: follow-up of 370 donors in Stockholm since 1964. *Clinical Transplantation,* Vol. 69, No. 10, (May 2000), pp. 2067-2071.

Giessing, M.; et al. (2004). Quality of Life of Living Kidney Donors in Germany: A Survey with the Validated Short Form-36 and Giessen Subjective Complaints List-24 Questionnaires. *Transplantation;* Vol. 78, No. 6, (September 2004), pp. 864-872.

Hariharan, S.; et al. (2000). Improved graft survival after renal transplantation in the United States, 1988 to 1996. *New England Journal of Medicine,* Vol. 342, No.9, (March 2000), pp. 605-612.

Ibrahim, HN.; et al. (2009). Long-Term consequences of kidney donation. *New England Journal of Medicine,* Vol. 360, No. 5, (January 2009), pp. 459-469.

Isotani, S. ; et al. (2002). Quality of life of living kidney donors: the short-form 36-item health questionnaire survey. *Urology,* Vol. 60, No. 4, (October 2002), pp. 588-592.

Jackobs, S.; et al. (2005). Quality of life following living donor nephrectomy comparing classical flank incision and anterior vertical mini-incision. *World Journal of Urology,* Vol. 23, No. 5, (November 2005), pp. 343-348.

Johnson, EM.; et al. (1999). Long-term follow-up of living kidney donors: quality of life after donation. *Transplantation,* Vol. 67, No. 5, (March 1999), pp. 717-721.

Karrfelt, HME.; et al. (1998). To be or not to be a living donor: questionnaire to parents of children who have undergone renal transplantation. *Transplantation,* Vol. 65, No. 7, (April 1998), pp. 915-918.

Lima, DX.; Petroianu A. & Hauter HL. (2006). Quality of life and surgical complications of kidney donors in the late post-operative period in Brazil. *Nephrol Dialusis and Transplantation,* Vol. 21, No. 11, (November 2006), pp. 323823-42.

Novara, G., et al. (2010). Factors predicting health-related quality of life recovery in patients undergoing surgical treatment for renal tumors: prospective evaluation using the RAND SF-36 Health Survey. *European Urology,*Vol 57, No. 1, (January 2010), pp. 112-120.

Poulakis, V., et al. (2003). Quality of life after surgery for localized renal cell carcinoma: comparison between radical nephrectomy and nephron-sparing surgery. *Urology,* Vol. 62, No. 5, (November 2003), pp. 814-820.

Reimer, J.; et al. (2006). The impact of living-related kidney transplantation on the donor's life. *Transplantation,* Vol. 81, No. 9, (May 2006), pp. 1268-1273.

Schover, LR.; et al. (1997). The psychosocial impact of donating a kidney: long-term follow-up from a urology based center. *Journal of Urology,* Vol. 157, No. 5, (May 1997), pp. 1596-1601.

Smith, GC.; et al. (2003). Prospective psychosocial monitoring of living kidney donors using the SF-36 health survey. *Transplantation,* (September 2003), Vol. 76, No. 5, pp. 807-809.

Smith, GC.; et al. (2004). Prospective psychosocial monitoring of living kidney donors using the Short Form-36 health survey: results at 12 months. *Transplantation,* Vol. 78, No. 9, (November 2004), pp. 1384-1389.

Tanriverdi, N. ; et al. (2004). Quality of life and mood in renal transplantation recipients, donors, and controls: preliminary report. *Transplant Proceedings,* Vol. 36, No. 1, (January-February 2004), pp. 117-119.

Tellioglu, G.; et al. (2008). Quality of life analysis of renal donors. *Transplant Proceedings ,* Vol. 40, No. 1, (January-February 2008), pp. 50-52.

Verbrugge, LM. & Steiner, RP. (1985). Prescribing drugs to men and women. *Health Psychology.* Vol. 4, No. 1, pp. 79-98.

Ware, JE Jr. & Sherbourne, CD. (1992). The MOS 36-item short-form health survey (SF-36). I. Conceptual framework and item selection. *Medical Care,* Vol. 30, No. 6, (June 1992), pp. 473-483.

Zargooshi, J. (2001). Quality of life of Iranian kidney donors. *Journal of Urology,* Vol. 166, No. 5, (November 2001), pp. 1790-1799.

Zerssen, D. (1976). Die Befindlichkeitsskala. - Manual. Weinheim: Beltz Test. Beltz-Test GmbH.

15

Management of Renal Cell Carcinoma Metastasis of the Spine

Alessandro Gasbarrini[1], Christiano Esteves Simões[2], Michele Cappuccio[3] and Stefano Boriani[1]
[1]Department of Oncologic and Degenerative Spine Surgery, Rizzoli Institute
[2]Department of Orthopedics and Traumatology – Spine Unit, Felício Rocho Hospital
[3]Department of Orthopedics and Traumatology – Spine Surgery, Maggiore Hospital
[1,3]Italy
[2]Brazil

1. Introduction

Renal cell carcinoma (RCC) is the most frequent malignant neoplasm of the kidneys, accounting for 85% of all renal cancers, and 2% of all adult malignancies. Forty-five percent of these tumors have been diagnosed as locally advanced or metastatic disease (Stage IV, according to the American Joint Committee on Cancer staging system), and the five-year survival rate varies between 0 to 8% according to the United States National Cancer Data Base (American Cancer Society, 2011). Bones metastases from renal cell carcinoma occur in up to 50% of patients (Swanson et al., 1981), and from this group approximately one half is located in the spine. RCC is the fourth most common metastatic tumor of the spine and the most common cancer to present as a neurologic deficit secondary to an undetected primary malignancy. According to Les et al, the prognosis is generally worse when metastases occur in the axial skeleton rather than in the extremities. In general, the average survival of all patients diagnosed with metastatic RCC is about four months and only 10% of these survive for one year (Thyavihally et al., 2005).

The RCC has a well know angiotropism associated to the anatomical and hemodynamic characteristics of the blood supply of the spine, and to the persistence of hematopoietic tissue inside the vertebral body, making this region the most susceptible localization for the metastases in the spine.

Vertebral lesions determine a severe compromise of the quality of life, with pain that can become intractable and a high risk of vertebral fracture and/or paralysis. The substitution of the healthy bone with the metastatic tissue cause a weakening of the vertebra, and sometimes an acute fracture with spinal canal invasion, that can be the most dramatic result from the clinical point of view.

Kidneys cancer cells are not usually susceptible to chemotherapy agents and traditional radiation therapy. Only a small number of patients have been shown good responses to these drugs vinblastine, floxuridine, 5-fluorouracil (5-FU), capecitabine, and gemcitabine, and therefore it should be reserved for cases in which target drugs and/or immunotherapy are not effective. Radiation therapy can be used for patients that the general health is too poor to have surgery, however it is not routinely recommended because there is no evidence that it can improve survival.

The management of bone metastasis from RCC is often a difficult task. The progressive improvement in the survival rate of the patients due to new forms of treatment, and the radiation therapy, and chemotherapy resistance associated to this tumor, imposes a great challenge to its proper treatment. The role of the spine surgeon in these cases, is to choose the best treatment considering not only the factors associated with the primary tumor, but specially the individual characteristics of every patient.

New therapies, known as "target therapies", directed to specific molecular targets implicated in angiogenesis and tumor proliferation have presented encouraging results. Even though these results coupled with a fuller understanding of molecular pathways in RCC have paved the way for new targets in the treatment of kidney cancer. These drugs are often used as the first line of treatment against advanced kidney cancers. While they may shrink or slow the growth of the cancer, it does not seem that any of these drugs can actually cure RCC (American Cancer Society, 2011). Immunotherapy associated to surgery should also be considered the first treatment of choice in selected cases or in cases of failure of previous treatment with target therapies. In the authors' experience, this treatment has been the one to show the best results so far. The surgical treatment of the spine metastasis varies from local decompression to en bloc resection of the lesion. Although the en bloc resection does not have the objective to cure the patient from the disease, it should be considered to minimize the risk of local disease progression (Les et al., 2001). However, many patients treated with en bloc resection can still develop local recurrence.

2. Metastatic pathways to the spine

The tumor dissemination to the bone can come from three pathways: direct extension, the lymphatic vessels and, the most frequent, the hematogenous pathway. The most frequent site in the vertebrae is the vertebral body, because of its abundant vascularization and the presence of bone marrow inside.

In 1928, Ewing suggested that the metastatic diffusion was influenced only by mechanical factors. The abundant tortuous vessels inside the vertebral body contribute to the metastatic embolus deposit locally and the localization of the blood vessels near the vertebral end plate can explain the normal localization of the metastases in the spine. Batson showed in 1940 the role of the paravertebral venous plexus in the metastatic dissemination of pelvic and abdominal tumors to the spine. This valveless plexus allows a retrograde blood flow from the inferior vena cava to the paravertebral venous plexus any time that the intra-abdominal or intra-thoracic pressure rises, even if temporally. This retrograde flow can deliver metastatic embolus direct to the spine, escaping from the natural filters of the organism, as the liver and lungs.

Renal cell carcinoma presents a peculiar venotropism, which is the capacity of its cells to reach the venous circulation. The diffusion can occur through an anterograde flow in the renal vein to the inferior cave vein reaching the right atrium, or through a retrograde diffusion. Moreover, the anatomical connections between the renal venous circulation and the paravertebral venous plexus through the azygos and hemiazygous systems can also favor a metastatic implantation at the spine.

The associations of the well-known angiotropism of the renal cell tumors, the anatomical and the hemodynamic characteristics of the spinal circulation, and the persistence of the hematopoietic tissue inside the vertebral spongeous bone matter are the responsible for the high frequency of metastasis of RCC.

3. Diagnosis

3.1 Clinical diagnosis

The early diagnosis of metastatic spinal disease is important because functional outcomes depend on neurologic condition at the time of presentation. The presentation of spinal metastases can vary widely from back pain to different degrees of neurologic deficit including complete paralysis at the lesion level. Pathologic fracture and a complete spinal cord lesion are the worse conditions associated to the spinal disease and, in most of the cases, can and should be avoided. Clinically, the symptoms associated to RCC spinal metastases do not differ from most of the other metastatic primary tumors. The past history of renal cell carcinoma is usually the most important clue to localize the primary site. Often, spinal metastases can occur in patients submitted in the past to nephrectomy to treat RCC, and that have been considered as "no evidence of disease" for several years.

Back pain is the most common symptom caused by spinal metastases, and often precedes the neurologic symptoms by weeks, sometimes even months. In some cases, back pain can be the first symptom related to the original cancer disease, and the primary site diagnosis is reached through a biopsy of the spinal lesion. There are mainly three different sources of back pain: mechanical, radicular and local pain. The mechanical pain is caused by the spinal instability secondary to the structural abnormality of the spine, and is also known as axial back pain (Gokaslan and York, 1998). The instability can be diagnosed because of its clinical symptoms or with obvious alterations such as pathologic fractures. This pain is movement-related and exacerbate by sitting or standing which increases the axial load on the spine. Patients presenting with pathological fractures of the spine may also present pain in recumbence and often give a history of sleeping upright in a chair for several weeks. The presumed mechanism is extension of the unstable kyphosis. At the beginning, mechanical pain maybe relieved with narcotics or an external orthosis, however it does not respond to steroids. The source of local pain can also be increased by the muscle, tendon, ligament and/or joint capsule strain that secondarily occurs from the vertebral body damage. Radicular pain may occur when spinal metastases compress or irritate an exiting nerve root, yielding pain in the dermatomal distribution of the involved nerve root. This type of pain is often described as "sharp," "shooting," or "stabbing" (Perrin et al., 1982). The periosteal stretching and/or a local inflammatory process stimulate the pain fibers within the periosteum causing local pain. It is predominantly nocturnal or early morning pain and generally improves with activity during the day, and it is usually described as a persistent "gnawing" or "aching" pain originated from the affected spinal segment. Inflammatory pain usually responds to administration of low dose steroids.

The second most common presenting complaint is motor dysfunction. Myelopathic abnormalities begins with hyperreflexia, clonus, Babisnki reflex and can progress to weakness, proprioceptive sensory loss, and loss of pain and temperature below the level of spinal cord compression. Autonomic dysfunction can occur secondarily to spinal cord compression or cauda equina compression. Bladder dysfunction is the most common autonomic finding and often correlates with the degree of motor dysfunction (Schiff 2004). The proper identification of neurologic deficit is of paramount importance, considering the motor function at the time of diagnosis correlates with the prognosis (Arguello et al., 1990). Unfortunately, the presence of back pain is extremely common in the general population, and it is likely that delay diagnoses of vertebral metastases occur in the presence of only back or neck pain. For these reasons, in every patient with a past history of RCC, the hypothesis of vertebral metastasis must be considered until proven otherwise.

Generally, the motor dysfunction is associated with sensory dysfunctions, such as anesthesia, hyperesthesia, hypoesthesia and/or paraesthesia. Complains of sensory abnormalities can occur in the dermatomal distribution of the radicular pain or weakness, while the patients with myelopathy may elicit a sensory level across the chest or abdomen.

The clinical evaluation of spinal patients should include general performance status, a pain assessment and a quantitative neurologic score. The most common method of pain assessment is the visual analog scale. The performance status reflects ambulation, medical comorbidities and extent of the disease. A patient may have normal motor strength, but be unable to walk from loss of proprioception, fracture of lower limbs or from a variety of other reasons.

The neurologic status is assessed using the modified Frankel grading system (McGuire et al., 1998) and/or the American Spinal Injury Association (ASIA) score (Table 1). Both systems assess the motor function with a score of "E" being normal and "A" being a complete paralysis.

Grade	Description
A	Complete: No motor or sensory function is preserved in the sacral segments S4-S5.
B	Incomplete: Sensory but not motor function is preserved below the neurological level and extends through the sacral segments S4-S5.
C	Incomplete: Motor function is preserved below the neurological level, and the majority of the key muscles below the neurological level have a muscle grade less than 3.
D	Incomplete: Motor function is preserved below the neurological level, and the majority of the key muscles below the neurological level have a muscle grade greater than 3.
E	Normal: Motor and sensory function is normal.

Table 1. ASIA impairment scale.

The modified Frankel score system divides the clinical-neurologic status in seven stages:

- A: Complete loss of the motor and sensitive functions.
- B: Presence of sensory but absence of voluntary motor functions.
- C: Motor deficit that allows the deambulation, but only with antibrachial support and lower limbs bracing.

- D1: High degree of motor deficit that allows deambulation using only an antibrachial support, and/or bladder or bowel paralysis.
- D2: Moderate degree of motor deficit that allows the deambulation without support or bracing, and/or bladder or bowel neurologic dysfunction.
- D3: Mild motor deficit with a normal bladder and bowel functions.
- E: Complete motor and sensitive function (osteotendinous reflexes can be abnormal)

3.2 Diagnostic imaging

Plain radiography (with or without myologram), myelography, computed tomography (CT) (with or without myelogram), magnetic resonace imaging (MRI), and positron emission tomography (PET) all play important roles in the imaging assessment of spinal cancer and metastatic lesions from RCC.

3.2.1 Plain films

Plain radiographs are readily available, easy to perform, relatively low cost, and provides a detailed assessment of osseous structures. Lytic or sclerotic areas of bone, pathologic compression fractures, deformity, and paraspinal masses can be seen, however, according to Gabriel et al., up to 50% of the bone must be eroded before there is a noticeable change on plain radiographs.

3.2.2 Computed tomography (CT)

CT provides a detailed assessment of osseous structures and the extent of tumor involvement within the bone. It is indispensible for pre-operative staging according to the Weinstein-Boriani-Biagini and surgical planning (Boriani et al., 1997). When associated to myelography, it demonstrates any suspected compression of the neural elements caused by tumor extension to the canal or osseous fragments from a pathologic fracture.

The CT is very important also to evaluate the risk of pathologic fracture based on the tumor's extension in the vertebrae.

3.2.3 Nuclear scintigraphy

Nuclear scintigraphy or bone scan demonstrates areas of active bone metabolism. A major advantage of bone scans is its cost-effective ability to scan the entire axial and appendicular skeleton at the same time and its capacity of revealing lesions at an earlier stage when compared to plain films. Its disadvantage is the low specificity, as increased metabolic activity in the presence of inflammation or infection. The image correlation with CT and MRI is necessary due to its low imaging resolution. The PET scanning with ^{18}F-fluorodeoxygucose is more sensitive and specific for whole body metastatic evaluations, but as with bone scans, it also necessitates concomitant use of CT or MRI. Koga et al, assessed the diagnostic value of bone scan in 205 patients with confirmed renal cell carcinoma, and concluded that bone scan may be omitted in patients with stages T1-3aN0M0 tumors and no bone pain because of the low proportion of missed cases with bone metastasis (Koga et al., 2001).

3.2.4 Magnetic Resonance Imaging (MRI)

MRI is currently the gold standard imaging technique for assessing the spinal metastasis. It combines excellent spatial and contrast resolution. MRI is also more sensitive than CT, and bone scans, and does not exposes patients to ionizing radiation. It provides superior resolution of soft-tissue structures such as paraspinal muscles, intervertebral disc, spinal cord and nerve roots. Standard MRI protocols include T1-weighted images (T1 WIs) without and with intravenous contrast, T2-weighted images (T2WIs) in axial, coronal and sagittal reconstructions. Fat suppression techniques are useful in evaluating osseous lesions that enhance with contrast. Disadvantages include relatively long acquisition times, insurmountable safety contra-indications in some patients, and lower sensitivity to osseous structural abnormalities.

3.2.5 Angiography

Metastasis from hypervascular tumors as RCC may have diagnostic and therapeutic benefits from angiography. Pre operative angiography can provides the knowledge about the tumors vascular supply and allows preoperative embolization, decreasing the blood loss during the intralesional excision.

3.3 Anatomopathologic diagnosis

Percutaneous biopsy to confirm the diagnosis is paramount. Although imaging modalities can provide a great definition of the anatomical aspects of the lesions the correct diagnosis is mandatory prior to the treatment planning. Patients with well-known primary cancer can present with a spinal lesion from another hidden metastatic tumor or a primary bone tumor associated. CT guided percutaneous trocar biopsies provide relatively easy access to most lesions with success rates approaching 90%. Traspedicular biopsy is the most adequate technique because of the smaller contamination of the adjacent tissues, facilitating its removal during the resection.

4. Management of spinal metastasis

When dealing with spinal metastasis factors need to be taken into consideration by the oncologist, spine surgeon, anesthesiologist and the entire multidisciplinary group involved in the caring of these patients. Considering that metastatic disease to the spine a systemic disease, at first, the curative excision of the entire secondary lesion does not seems necessary, particularly in the spine because of its anatomical characteristics and morbidity. The palliative treatment frequently applied has the primary objective to decrease the pain, stabilize the spine and, whenever is necessary, decompress the adjacent neural structures. The intralesional excision of the tumor (inadequate oncological margins) can be complete or incomplete, allowing a circumferential decompression of the spinal cord and a better local control of the disease.

RCC is well known as radiation therapy and chemotherapy resistant, and immunotherapies with cytokines based on interferon alpha and interleukin-2 (IL2) have shown poor results with significant toxicities. New therapies directed to molecular targets implicated in angiogenesis and tumor proliferation are being developed. Sunitinib is considered one of the new reference first-line treatment for RCC metastasis, however despite all the progress in recent years, complete responses are still very rare, and many important issues regarding the use of these agents in the management of metastatic renal cell cancer still need to be properly addressed.

Surgical treatment has been the only recognized therapy to improve the quality of life in the patients with RCC metastatic disease in the spine. In most of the cases the surgery does not improve the survival prognosis of these patients but it can dramatically improve the their life quality. Moreover, in a small group of patients with solitary spinal RCC metastases the en bloc resection has shown to substantially improve the overall survival time. In their retrospective work, Thyavihally et al. demonstrated the complete resection of either synchronous or metachronous solitary metastases from RCC is justified and can contribute to a long-term survival in a selective group of patients. They also concluded that patients with long interval between diagnosis and development of metastasis and early stage of the primary tumor have a better prognosis after en bloc resection of the metastases.

The treatment goals of spinal metastasis is different than the primary bone tumors, the first one aims the patient's quality of life while the main target of primary bone tumor is to preserve life. The best treatment" should include local control of the disease and restoration of the spinal function.

4.1 Treatment planning

Surgical indications for spinal metastasis in general, have been subject of controversy because the ideal moment, patient and surgical technique are still trying to be defined in the literature. Many strategies have been proposed trying to appropriately direct the best surgical treatment. In 1987 Tokuhashi et al. published a point-addition-type scoring system for the preoperative prediction of the survival period to select treatment options. This score system was later on revised and magnified its the application to the group with conservative treatment. The general condition (Karnofsky performance status), the number of extraspinal bone metastases, the number of metastases in the vertebral column, the presence of metastases to major internal organs (lungs, liver, kidneys, and brain), the primary site of cancer, and the severity of spinal cord palsy were the items evaluated. Each parameter ranged from 0 to 5 points, and the total score was 15 points. RCC was considered as moderate prognosis receiving three points in the item "primary site of cancer". Tomita et al, also have described a scoring system based on the primary tumor, the presence of metastases to the vital organs and number of bone metastases. These systems have been used among the spine surgeons with reasonable results, unfortunately the scores systems are too simple, based in numbers that allocates extremely different types of patient in the same group, and also they do not consider the clinical status and other physicians opinions involved in the patient's care before deciding the best treatment option.

In 2008, the authors published their own treatment algorithm to guide the decision planning when dealing with spine metastasis, based on a retrospective study of 43 patients (Cappuccio et al., 2008). According to Cappucio et al., multidisciplinary treatment could be beneficial, and a failure to do so, is very like to end in a suboptimum prognosis and could even lead to sever impairment. The treatment planning, including the surgical planning should involve not only the spine surgeon, but also the nonsurgical physicians (anesthetist, oncologist, radiotherapist), and it should be chosen on each individual patient. Gasbarrini et al., conducted a semi-prospective clinical study in 2010 with 202 patients to evaluate the efficacy of this algorithm which furthermore evolved to a flow chart (Figure 1).

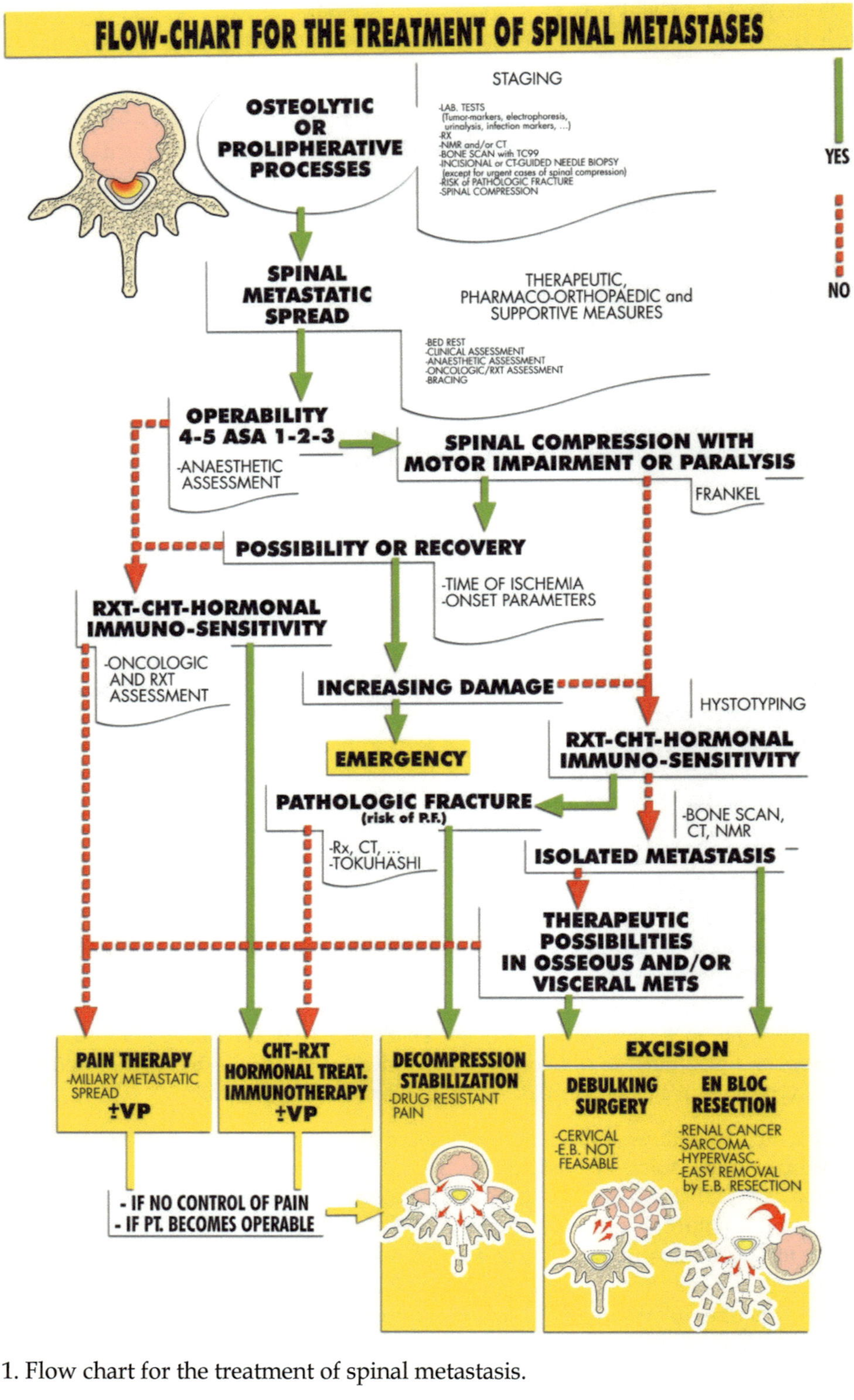

Fig. 1. Flow chart for the treatment of spinal metastasis.

According to this flow-chart, all spinal tumors must be staged, and the first question when planning the treatment is to discuss with the oncologist about the life expectancy of the patient and to reach a consensus with the anesthesiologist if the patient is operable or not (based on the ASA score). Other important items to consider is the neurological status and its capacity to deteriorate or to improve, the presence of pathologic fracture, the sensitivity of the primary tumor to non surgical therapies, and the number of spinal, bone or visceral metastasis. Following the flow chart the best therapeutic option can be achieved, ranging from only pain therapy to surgical procedures as en bloc resections.

Considering the RCC metastases, the surgical treatment is the only method that can improve the patient's quality of life, and in some well selected cases of single spinal metastases, a cure of these patients have been well documented after en bloc resections (Li et al., 2009). Patients with disseminated RCC metastasis, or clinically incapable to be submitted to surgical procedures, pain therapy is indicated.

4.2 Surgical planning

In order to apply the surgical indication determined by the oncological staging and the Gasbarrini's flow chart, it is necessary a complete work-up to evaluate the vertebral tumor that will be treated. The histological diagnosis, preferably obtained by CT-guided biopsy, is fundamental. Magnetic resonance imaging, CT-scan and in some selected cases, angiography, are the imaging techniques indicated to describe the tumor's extension on the transversal and longitudinal planes. The first attempt to determine a surgical staging system to guide the spine surgeons was made by Weistein in 1994. Boriani and Biagini modified this staging system in 1997 (Figure 2).

A. Extraosseous Soft Tissue
B. Intraosseous (Superficial)
C. Intraosseous (Deep)
D. Extraosseous (Extradural)
E. Extraosseous (Intradural)

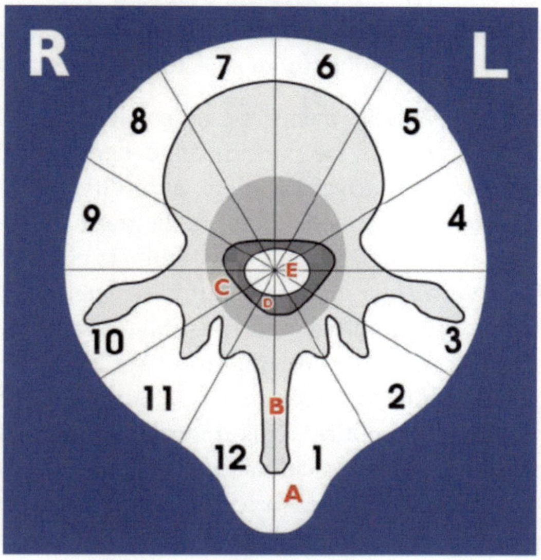

Fig. 2. WBB surgical staging system

4.2.1 Weinstein–Boriani–Biagini (WBB) surgical staging

The WBB surgical staging system is specific for spine tumors and was created to guide the planning of the surgical resection to achieve the appropriate histologic margins. It was first described to treat primary spinal tumors, but its application was later on extended to the treatment of spinal metastasis as well. Pre-operative CT-scan and MRI are required to provide detail of the lesion and the normal tissues surrounding it.

The WBB divides the axial presentation of the vertebrae involved with the tumor into 12 zones similar to a clock face. Zone 1 is located at the left half of the spinous process followed by the others in a counter clockwise sense. Zones 4 and 9 are particularly important to know because they define respectively the left and right pedicles. Vertebrectomy with adequate surgical margins depends upon one of these zones to be free of tumor. The vertebra is further divided into 5 radial zones that define the depth of tumor invasion. These zones are also known as layers, starting from layer A that corresponds to the outside surrounding tissue of the vertebra to layer E that indicates intradural involvement of the tumor. In the cervical spine there is also layer F, which corresponds to the vertebral artery involvement. It is also important to describe the longitudinal extension of the tumor.

4.2.2 Pre-operative Selective Arterial Embolization (SAE)

Vertebral metastases of renal origin are highly vascular and often cause life-threatening intraoperative bleeding. This bleeding may influence the surgeon's ability to have an adequate view of the surgical field, and thus to achieve a complete resection. Preoperative embolization facilitates resection by decreasing intraoperative blood loss, improving visualization of the tumor during surgery, and decreasing tumor size.

Embolization can also be used as a palliative treatment in patients who are poor operative candidates or have recurrent, multiple, or unresectable tumors. It can also be used to treat painful metastatic disease or for patients with neurologic compromise from metastatic lesions by reducing the tumor size, tumor growth, and spinal canal compromise.

In cases of vascular metastatic spinal lesions, as in the RCC metastasis, a preoperative angiography should be performed to demonstrate the hypervascularity of the lesion, to identify the main arterial feeders, and, ultimately, to determine whether the lesion would benefit from the embolization. Angiography of a spinal RCC metastatic lesion typically demonstrates a hyper-dynamic pathologic circulation within the vertebral tumor, enlarged feeding intercostals or lumbar arteries, angiographic blush caused by venous congestion within the tumor nidus, and, possibly, a rapid arteriovenous transit with early filling of draining venous channels (Figure 3A). The enlarged venous pool may contribute to a tumor's mass effect; therefore, embolization may decrease spinal cord compression. Before embolization procedures, it is important to identify the segmental vessels that supply the spinal cord and the radiculomedullary branch of the anterior spinal artery and to determine whether an anterior spinal artery shares the same pedicle as the feeding artery of the tumor. The presence of an anterior spinal artery, also known as artery of Adamkiewicz (Figure 3B), at the same pedicle as the feeding artery at the tumor is considered by many authors a contraindication for embolization due to the risk of spinal cord ischemia, however some authors have demonstrated in animals models that in the presence of more than one artery of Adamkiewicz artery, the embolization of the tumor feeder would not cause damage to the spinal cord. Tomita et al., published in 2009 their techniques on total en bloc spondylectomy and showed that preoperative embolization of bilateral segmental arteries at three levels (at the level of the tumor, and one segment above and another one bellow) should be tried within 48 hours before the operation.

There are many reports of surgeries on metastatic renal cell carcinoma that were aborted because of "uncontrollable bleeding" or excessive blood loss in control groups that did not have preoperative SAE, whereas no case was aborted were complete embolization was done.

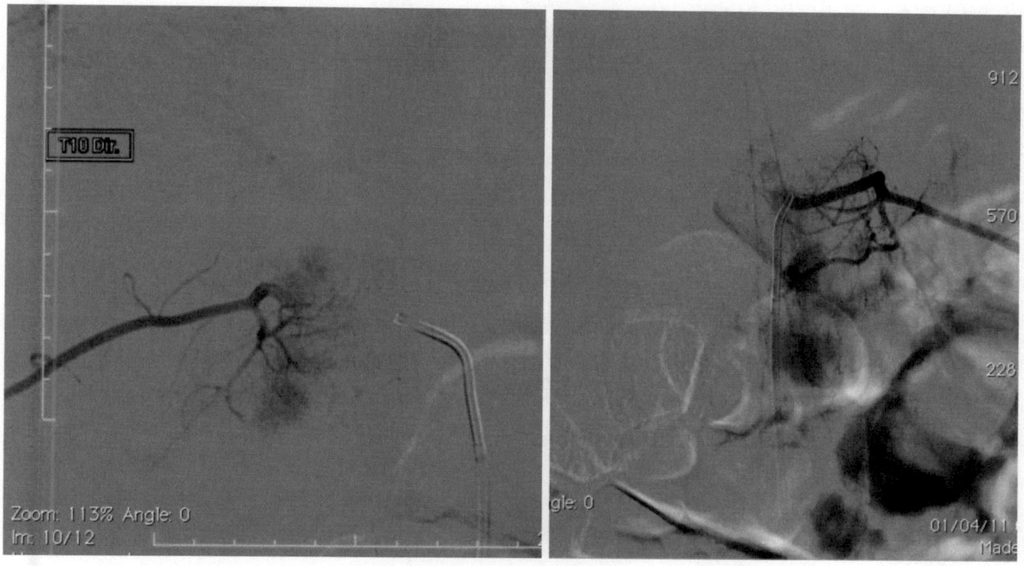

Fig. 3. A. Tumoral "blush" during angiography showing a metastatic RCC lesion in T10; 3B. Artery of Adamkiewicz.

In some cases of neurologic worsening before SAE was done the immediate surgery before the embolization can result into severe complications. Sundaresan et al., had 54% of complications in patients with RCC metastasis that were rushed into surgery without preoperative SAE. Because of this high rate of complications, some authors advocates for a delaying surgery for a few hours to perform preoperative embolization.

The choice of embolic material is based on the territory embolized, the vascular anatomy of the tumor, and the ability of selective delivery of an embolic agent via a catheter. The success of an embolization is judged by reduction in tumor vascularity and lack of tumor blush.

The timing of surgery after preoperative SAE is an important technical consideration. It is recommended that embolization be performed as close as possible to the time of surgery. Minimal blood loss occurs after embolization if surgery is performed within 24 to 48 hours after embolization. Earlier surgeries prevent the development of collateral circulation. The intraoperative blood loss can be reduced from one to two thirds in RCC metastatic lesions (Gottfried et al., 2004).

Complications rates are very low and have been reported to vary from 1% to 2%. Most complications are temporarily and are associated to a post-embolization syndrome that includes malaise, nausea, emesis, low-grade fever, elevated white blood cell count, and local pain usually lasting three to seven days. Permanent paraplegia has been reported in the literature, but fortunately it is very rare.

4.3 Surgical treatment

In the past the patients with spinal metastasis were considered as terminal patients, therefore surgical treatment was reserved for patients with uncontrollable pain with medications, or patients with high risk of pathologic fracture. The surgical approach to the spine is basically anterior or posterior. Both approaches can be also combined in the same surgery or in separated surgical procedures.

The rational behind the adequate surgical option should include:

- The best decompression possible.
- The most efficacious spinal stabilization.
- Removal of the tumor with oncological adequacy.

The correct surgical treatment does not involve simple laminectomy of the spine of any extension. The outcomes of this procedure are comparable to isolated radiation therapy and can result in a severe instability with a high risk of neurological deterioration.

The surgical techniques to be considered are:

1. Spinal decompression and stabilization.
2. Intralesional excision (debulking) and spinal column reconstruction.
3. En bloc resection and spinal column reconstruction.

4.3.1 Decompression and stabilization

This is the fastest and less aggressive surgical procedure aiming to decompress the spinal cord and to stabilize the spine. This procedure does not necessarily include a direct approach to the tumor. It is considered a palliative treatment.

The indications for decompression and stabilization are:

1. Presence, or elevated risk, of pathological fracture in the thoracic and/or lumbar spine.
2. High sensitive tumors to hormonal, chemotherapy or radiotherapy, independently of the neurological status.
3. Patients with extremely poor prognosis aiming only the improvement of the patient's quality of life.

4.3.2 Intralesional excision

Intralesional excision includes a direct approach to the tumoral mass with a partial resection of the tumor in order to reach spinal decompression and tumor mass reduction. This procedure is considered more aggressive than simple decompression and stabilization, especially when dealing with systemic diseases, and it must include a multidisciplinary approach. Selective arterial embolization should be included in the treatment to decrease the hemorrhage, very often life threatening, and also a detailed surgical planning to achieve an adequate excision and to reconstruct the spinal stability. Some times a double approach should be considered.

The indications for intralesional excision are:

1. Tumoral mass compression from radio-resistant metastasis.
2. Pathologic fractures in radio-resistant metastasis.
3. Necessity to reduce the tumoral mass ("debulking") in order to apply adjuvant therapies.

Surgical technique

The surgical technique for intralesional excision depends on the location of the metastases.

In the cervical spine the approach is always anterior, and for the thoracic and lumbar spine, a partial excision can be performed also using a posterior approach.

Cervical Spine: The anterior approach to the cervical spine (from C3 to T1) is well known among the spine surgeons. The approach to C1 and C2 can be transoral or extra-oral. An extension of this approach can be done through a very aggressive trans-mandible technique.

The vertebral arteries are a problem for the circumferential approach. The single anterior approach is indicated in the lower cervical spine for small metastasis (WBB: from sector 4 to 9). Every time that a tumor is located in the posterior elements, invading at least one articular process, a double approach not only is safer, but also indicated for the reconstruction in general.

Thoracic Spine: The metastasis in the thoracic spine can be completely excised through a thoracotomy using the classical anterolateral approach, technically challenging in the cervical-thoracic junction. Using only a posterior approach is also possible to perform a complete curettage of the lesion, legating one nerve root.

Thoracoscopy can also be used for intracapsular excision (McLain 2001).

Lumbar Spine: In the lumbar spine, the anterior approach with decompression, and reconstruction usually is the best option for an anterior lesion. A posterior approach at this level needs to scarify one or more nerve roots. The consequences of such action are persistent pain, loss of mobility and spinal cord ischemia.

4.3.3 En bloc resection

Stener in1989, and Roy-Camille in 1990, described the surgical techniques for en bloc resection in the thoracic and lumbar spine. Later in 1994, Tomita et al., described a similar technique for vertebrectomy using a posterior approach developed specially for spinal metastasis.

The preoperative planning is paramount to choose the best technique for en bloc resection. Each vertebral lesion needs to be evaluated carefully and the resection should be "customized". In order to plan the resection, all tumors should be surgically staged according to the WBB system, previously described.

The resection can be made throughout the external surface of the pseudocapsule (marginal resection), or outside of it, along with a margin of healthy tissue (wide resection).

The well accepted indications for en bloc resections are stage three benign tumors and in stage one, or stage two, primary malignant tumors. The indications for spinal metastasis are still controversial, however it should be considered in cases of a solitary metastases of primary tumors with longer life expectancy, as in the RCC.

Types of en bloc resections:

- Sagittal resection: The criteria to obtain oncologically adequate margins include: No extension to the layer D in the WBB system, or limited extension with dissection plane between the tumor's pseudocapsule and the dural sac.
- Posterior resection: According to the WBB system, the indications for posterior elements resection with oncological margins include sectors four and nine free of tumor e no extension to the layer D, or limited extension with dissection plane between the tumor's pseudocapsule and the dural sac.
- Vertebrectomy: The en bloc resection of the vertebral body is oncologically appropriate by a posterior approach only, in cases of tumors located inside the body (no invasion of layer A in the WBB system). If tumor mass is expanding anteriorly in layer A or when the tumor is located at the cervico-thoracic, thoraco-lumbar, lumbo-sacral junction, the surgical procedure should include an anterior release. In these cases, the posterior approach ends with the blunt dissection of the lateral aspect of the vertebral body not involved by the tumor, if exists. Cervical spine en bloc vertebrectomy is also feasible, however this technique is more difficult and associated to a higher morbidity and mortality because of its elevated risk of vertebral artery and spinal cord injuries.

Surgical technique

Sagittal resection: This technique aims at achieving en bloc resection of a tumor excentrically growing: it consists in the piecemeal removal of the uninvolved posterior elements in order to circumferentially release the dura and finalize the resection by a sagittal osteotomy. An anterior approach is required when the tumor is growing anteriorly and a margin of normal tissue must be left under visual control over the tumor, or vital structures must be protected. One or more neuroforamina are involved by tumor and the corresponding nerve root(s) needs to be sacrificed in order to obtain an appropriate margin. The uninvolved posterior elements are removed piecemeal. A complete release of the dural sac from the tumor should be done. Before the osteotomy, the contralateral pedicle is removed so that the dura is not retracted into its hard surface. First, the vertical cut is performed followed by the superior and inferior horizontal cut. The tumor is finally removed in one piece.

Posterior resection: The posterior resection requires both pedicles free of tumor in order to obtain an oncologically appropriate margin. The posterior arch is removed after both pedicles are transected. This technique is rarely used for RCC metastases because the great majority of spinal metastases are located anteriorly in vertebral body.

Vertebrectomy: Usually the surgical procedure is performed in two steps (first with the patient in prone decubitus position followed by a lateral oblique position at 45°), a posterior and anterior approach. For small lesions, inside the vertebral body the procedure can be done only by a posterior access with oncologically adequate margins, according to the technique described by Tomita et al. Although it is possible to perform an en bloc vertebrectomy using only the posterior approach in the lumbar spine, it should be avoided.

This technique involves a great risk of root damage and unlike the thoracic spine where one or more nerve roots can be sacrificed without causing major problems; in the lumbar spine a motor deficit can deteriorate dramatically the quality of life of these patients.

The advantages of the posterior only approach are less surgical time and blood loss, avoidance of the anterior approach and its morbidity, among others. The most important disadvantage is the high risk of spinal cord lesion and the difficult to obtain adequate cutting surfaces on the spinal column in order to reconstruct the anterior column. Nowadays several devices and techniques have been developed to overcome these problems. The use of a spinal cord protector is important in these cases, and should always be applied. In all en bloc vertebrectomies performed using only a posterior approach, the authors used a special device named PROMID®, to protect the spinal cord and guide the saw path through the vertebral body or intervertebral disc. (Figure 4) The device is positioned underneath the dural sac and secured to a rod. Once the Gigli saw passes through the spinal column, the protector restrains it. The little knots on both sides work as the saw guide, avoiding the use of chisels and scalpels that can cause a massive bone bleeding and also injure the spinal cord.

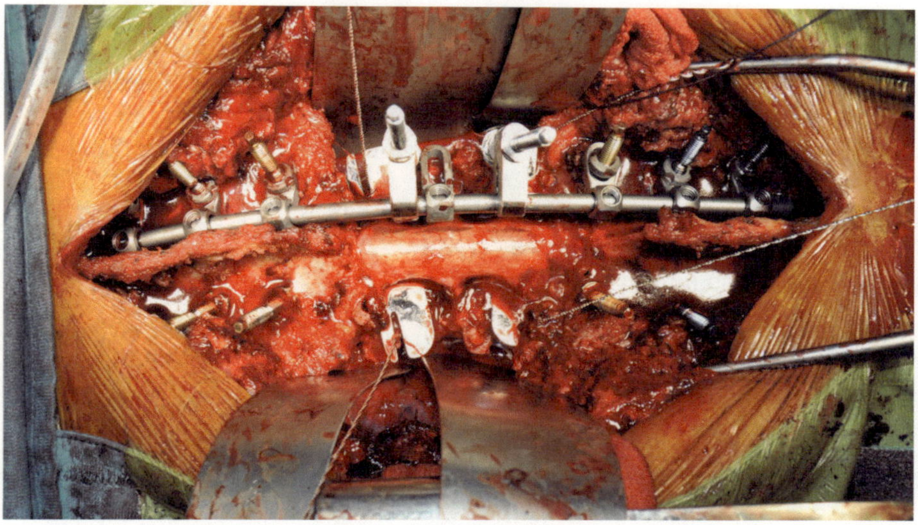

Fig. 4. The spinal cord protector and saw guide device (PROMID®) used during a posterior en bloc vertebrectomy.

The choice of the best surgical treatment is still a matter of debate, however vertebrectomy is becoming more popular among spine surgeons. This technique requires a more experienced surgical team and an adequate clinical support. It is very important to keep in mind that RCC metastases are hypervascular tumors, and intralesional excision can be associated to massive blood loss. On the other hand, en bloc resection is associated to specific techniques, sometimes a combined anterior and posterior approach, and therefore a longer surgical time. It usually requires a prolonged anesthesia, hemodynamic stability, important blood loss compensation and control of body heat loss. To overcome the necessity to complement the surgical procedure with an anterior approach and therefore to deal with its complications, the use of anterior release using thoracoscopy can be done in some selected cases with less morbidity without affecting the oncological management (Cappuccio et al., 2010).

Cappuccio et al., reported a retrospective study comparing the variation of intra-operative hemodynamic parameters (arterial blood pressure, cardiac frequency and hemoglobin levels) between a group of patients submitted to en bloc resection and a group treated by intralesional excision. Surgical timing was significantly higher in the en bloc resection group, however the cardiac frequency, hemoglobin levels and arterial blood pressure were significantly more affected in the patients submitted to intralesional excision. They concluded that constant evolution of the anesthesia techniques allows the execution of surgical treatments that have been forbidden in the past. Hemorrhagic tumors as RCC metastases can be better managed with en bloc resection, even considering that this is a more complex procedure compared to intralesional resection.

Many authors reported the comparison between the different modalities of treatments for RCC spinal metastases. En bloc spondylectomy associated to adjuvant interferon and fractionated radiation presented good results with no recurrence in cases of solitary RCC metastases with epidural extension (Sakaura et al. 2004). In an unpublished series from Boriani, 90 cases of RCC were treated with a variety of techniques, including conventional external beam radiotherapy (4 patients), palliative decompression and instrumentation (19 patients), intralesional gross total resection (42 patients), and en bloc resection (25 patients) with recurrence rates of 100%, 84%, 24%, and 4%, respectively. In the en bloc cohort, 12 patients had no evidence of disease at a median follow-up of 30 months, 5 alive with disease at a median of 28 months, and 8 dead of disease at a median of 8 months. In the en bloc group, 1 patient showed local progression of disease (Bilsky et al., 2009).

4.4 Spinal column reconstruction

The surgical treatment of bone tumors usually results in a bone defect, secondary to curettage or resection that can be reconstructed using different types of implants associated to different methods of osteosynthesis. The complexity of the spinal anatomy requires a more specific and complex technique for resection and reconstruction.

The spinal instability and the criteria for reconstruction of each patient is different case by case, and each type of resection (posterior, corpectomy or vertebrectomy) requires a specific reconstruction technique.

Denis et al., have shown that the stability of the spine is secondary to the integrity of the middle column (posterior longitudinal ligament, posterior portion of the fibrous annulus e the posterior vertebral wall) e the anterior column (anterior longitudinal ligament, anterior portion of the fibrous annulus and the anterior vertebral wall). According to Gurwitz, and Lim et al., in cases where there is a lesion of the anterior column, a posterior stabilization is not sufficiently rigid to resist all weight bearing forces and therefore, needs to be associated to an anterior stabilization. In cases of en bloc vertebrectomy, a circumferential reconstruction is indispensable, in other words, it is necessary to associate a posterior stabilization to the anterior hardware.

The posterior elements resection requires stabilization associated to a lateral arthodesis while corpectomy needs also the substitution of the vertebral body, associated to an anterior stabilization.

4.4.1 Posterior reconstruction

In the majority of the cases an oncological surgical procedure in the spine produces a wide loss of substance associated to a major instability of the spine, thus becoming necessary a rigid stabilization of it. The most indicated system is the utilization of pedicle screws and longitudinal bars above and below the defect. In association for the patients that will not be submitted to radiotherapy, autogenous bone graft should also be used to obtain a permanent postero-lateral arthrodesis.

4.4.2 Anterior reconstruction

The anterior column is responsible for 80% of body weight support in the spine and its reconstruction is mandatory after en bloc vertebrectomies. The maintenance of the biomechanical principles is paramount.

The size of the defect can be measure, and appropriately sized cage can be inserted. The reconstruction can be made using different cages (titanium, carbon fiber, etc.) or a massive allograft bone (femoral shaft). The cages or the bone shafts are filled preferably with autogenous bone. When possible, a connection between the anterior device and the posterior construct should be performed in order to enhance stability of the whole construct.

The number of options for anterior column reconstruction devices is smaller than the posterior reconstruction. They are basically bars, plates and screws or cages that are anchored to the vertebral body. In spinal oncology these implants are frequently used to achieve an anterior stabilization especially at the long term, and also to provide an early rehabilitation.

Orthopedic cement: The use of cement as a spacer, easily adaptable and with a low cost has been abandoned in the past. It has been proven not to be a reliable system at medium and long term (Boriani et al., 1996), being indicated only in selected cases of patients with short life expectancy.

Bone Graft: Bone graft represents the oldest spacer used in the oncological surgery. The bone graft can be used to obtain an interbody fusion or to replace one or more vertebral bodies. The advantage of this kind of graft is its biological integrability. The disadvantages include the necessity of a bank bone (to collect, store, and distribute), risk of infection, the necessity of a long time to consolidate and therefore it needs to be protected (body casts, bed rest, etc.). All bone grafts are somehow damaged in the biological evolution in cases of post-operative radiotherapy (Boriani et al., 1996).

Vertebral prosthesis: There are many options of vertebral body replacement prosthesis. Nowadays the most common used are made of titanium, and recently, made of carbon fibers (Figure 5). The advantages are the immediate stability, they are not damaged by radiotherapy and there is no donor site morbidity. The disadvantages include the higher cost, the necessity to have different sizes available, to be responsible for images artifacts (image distortion in the MRI or CT-s can) and to interfere as an obstacle for post-operative radiotherapy if necessary.

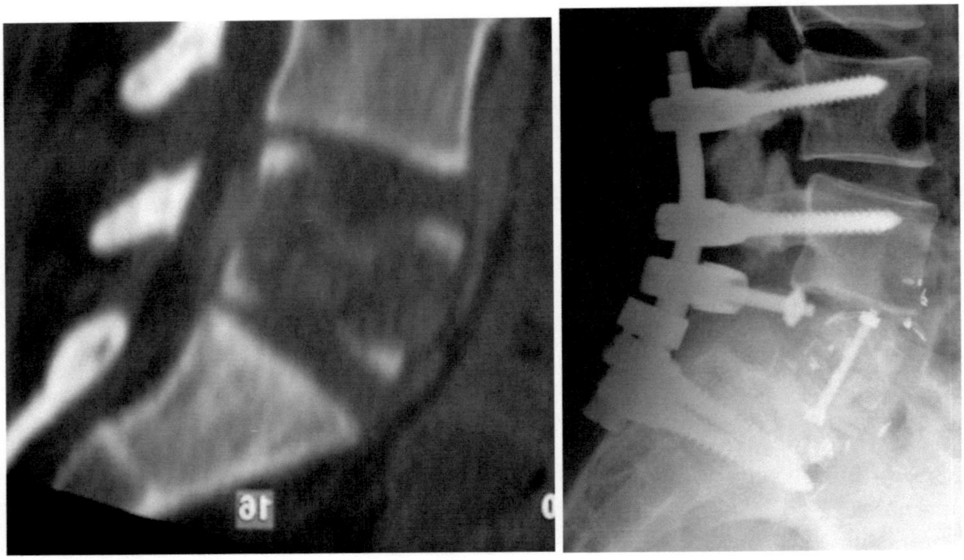

Fig. 5. A Solitary RCC metastasis of L5; 5B. 64 months of follow-up after posterior stabilization and anterior reconstruction with a carbon fiber cage filled with allograft. The bone fusion of the anterior column can be seen thorough the cage.

4.5 Stereotactic radiosurgery

Renal cell carcinoma metastases are well known to be resistant to conventional radiotherapy. In recent years, stereotactic body radiosurgery (SBRS) have allowed the safe delivery of high-dose radiation (image-guided intensity-modulated radiation therapy or spinal radio- surgery) to spinal metastases even in close proximity to the spinal cord and other paraspinal dose-sensitive organs. These treatments are often given in 1 to 5 fractions of high-dose radiation (to ensure safe doses) that are able to limit the dose to the spinal cord (Gerzsten et al., 2009). The aims of SBRS for spinal metastases are to improve on existing rates of clinical response and tumor control, and to reduce the retreatment rate by increasing the biologic equivalent dose (Sahgal et al., 2009).

According to Sahgal et al., the outcomes of spine radiosurgery can be grouped into four categories:

1. Unirradiated patients: spinal metastases in a previously unirradiated volume treated with SBRS.
2. Reirradiated patients: spinal metastases in a previously irradiated volume now containing new, recurrent, or progressive metastatic disease treated with SBRS.
3. Postoperative SBRS patients: spinal metastases treated with SBRS after open surgical intervention, with or without spinal stabilization.
4. Mixed patients: mixed populations involving patients in the previous 3 categories in which outcomes are not separately reported.

Gerzsten et al., reported a durable pain improvement in 94% of patients with RCC metastasis in the spine treated with radiosurgery. In his systematic review of the literature, radiographic control has been reported to be up to 87% in RCC (Gerzsten et al., 2009).

The use of stereotactic radiosurgery as primary option of treatment is indicated in cases of patients undergoing treatment to a symptomatic spine lesion with other significant but asymptomatic spine metastases. These asymptomatic metastases may be treated with radiosurgery to avoid further irradiation to the neural elements as well as to avoid further bone-marrow suppression and permit subsequent systemic therapy. The benefits for this approach include a single treatment that is radiobiologically larger than can be delivered with standard radiotherapy, with a minimal radiation dose to adjacent normal tissue. When used as a primary treatment modality, long- term radiographic tumor control was demonstrated in 90% of cases of isolated RCC metastases.

Stereotactic radiosurgery may be also indicated to treat patients presenting progressive neurologic deficit, where open surgery is contra-indicated, or in cases where the tumor is partially resected (intralesional resection) radiosurgery can be used to treat a residual tumor at a later date. In cases of severe compression of neural elements, the radiosurgery is not indicated and open procedure should be performed. Radiosurgery can also be used after vertebral body cement augmentation, with a local control rate as high as 92% (Gibbs et al., 2009).

Appropriate dose and fractionation schedules have not been determined and differ among institutions. There are institutions where the protocols include single-fraction radiosurgery from eight to 24 Gy or hypofractionated regimens consisting in different doses and number of fractions.

Complications associated to radiosurgery include esophagitis, mucositis, dysphagia, diarrhea, paresthesia, transient laryngitis, and transient radiculitis. Spinal cord injury has been reported, but is considered exceedingly rare.

Although the results so far reported using stereotactic radiosurgery have shown to be satisfying and promising, this technique does not treat spinal instability caused by the majority of the spinal tumors, and is contra-indicated in severe neural compression. Analysis of local tumor control rates after en bloc resection of solitary vertebral RCC metastases and after stereotactic radiosurgery appears to have comparable tumor control rates. The mean follow-up in Gerszten series of 60 patients treated with radiosurgery was 37 months and his final outcomes were comparable to the patients followed by Boriani, which showed 48% of patients with no evidence of disease after 30 months, while 52% presented systemic progression and were dead at eight to 28 months. Long-term prospective randomized studies are still to be done in order to establish to best indications and protocols for the use of stereotactic radiosurgery in RCC metastasis.

Recently, the Spine Oncology Study Group (SOSG) has conducted a systematic review trying to answer the following question "What is the optimal treatment for solitary renal cell metastases without significant epidural disease?". Their conclusion was that there is a very low quality of evidence, however stereotactic radiosurgery should be the first line therapy rather than en bloc resection (Bilsky et al., 2009).

4.6 Other treatment modalities

Radiotherapy is well known to be less effective in RCC metastases. Its use in higher doses to reach a satisfactory response increases the risk of spinal cord lesions, and also the side effects associated to it. The relationship between radiotherapy dose and duration of response has not been well studied, and the results are conflicting in the literature. The palliation of bone pain has been reported to be satisfying by Wilson et.al when compared with the palliation of symptoms at other sites of metastases, but the duration of this effect is still controversial. Higher biological effective dose does not seem to be a predictor of response or of duration of response in the palliative treatment of RCC.

The development of new management techniques of vertebral metastatic lesions has increased. Vertebroplasty, kyphoplasty, and thermablation using radiofrequency techniques have been used. Radiofrequency is fairly used throughout the world, but results evaluating the tumor necrosis have been reported by Gasbarrini et al. in 2009. The purpose of this technique is to selectively destroy the metastatic lesion with local hyperthermia as well as resulting in thrombosis of the local paravertebral veins. In their report, the authors analyzed the tumor necrosis rate under light microscope and also under electronic microscope. They found that good results can be achieved in solid tumors as liver tumors, however the necrosis rate in RCC metastases were different, showing less necrosis rates. Their possible hypothesis for the treatment failure is that in highly vascular tumors is probably difficult to maintain the necessary temperature *in situ* for adequate necrosis. Selective arterial embolization should be considered prior to radiofrequency ablation in RCC metastases.

The use of vertebroplasty, and/or kyphoplasty in spinal metastases has no effect as far as inducing tumor necrosis. Considering the heat generated by the cement and its duration as heat source, these techniques should not be used for that purpose. The use of cement inside the vertebral body is indicated in spinal oncology to increase the vertebrae's resistance and to treat spinal instability secondary to pathologic fractures.

It is very important to always keep in mind that these treatment modalities (vertebroplasty, kyphoplasty, and thermoablation are absolutely palliative and aims only to alleviate the pain.

5. Conclusion

The different therapeutic options and their indications in the treatment of patients with RCC metastatic disease can be distributed as follow:

1. Only radiotherapy:
   - Multiple osseous metastases
   - Untreatable visceral metastases
   - Untreatable primary tumor
   - Patient's poor clinical conditions
2. Decompression, and stabilization associated to radiotherapy:
   - Intractable pain and/or neurological deficit in patients with disseminated disease
   - Untreatable or treatable visceral metastases
3. Intralesional excision and radiotherapy:
   - Solitary bone metastasis (in cases where en bloc resection is contra-indicated)
   - Treatable visceral metastasis
   - En bloc resection not feasible
4. En bloc resection:
   - Solitary bone metastasis
   - Treated primary tumor
   - Absence of visceral metastasis

- Technically feasible

5. Stereotactic radiosurgery:
   - Solitary bone metastasis
   - Absence or with minimal epidural disease
   - Absence of severe spinal instability

Considering all the treatment options, the management of RCC metastases is essentially a surgical treatment. The use of stereotactic radiosurgery has proven to be effective and comparable to en bloc resection for selected cases, however we need to consider that this treatment requires a very specific technology that, so far, is not widely available for the majority of treatment centers and patients throughout the world. This technique also does not provide any kind of mechanical reinforcement to the spinal instability.

The progressive increase of the life expectancy of these patients, associated to the low sensitivity to conventional radiotherapy and the absence of a valid protocol of chemotherapy, makes surgery, associated to immunotherapy, the treatment of election, especially in cases of targeted therapies fail. Furthermore, the vertebral location of the lesion, determines a severe compromise of the quality of life often caused by intractable pain and elevated risk of paralysis and/or pathological fracture. In this last case the surgical treatment is performed in an emergency basis and therefore associated to all the anesthesiology and surgical complication that an urgent procedure can have.

The final results, comparing the en bloc resection to intralesional excision associated to radiotherapy, seems to be similar considering the local control and long term survival. The comparison between the two options as far as morbidity and cost/efficacy favors the en bloc resection.

Isolated surgery is indicated in cases of isolated metastases, and when during the preoperative planning, the procedure is planned to be outside the tumor capsule (extralesional). Selected cases of small tumors in favorable locations, where en bloc spondilectomy is feasible, associated to good prognosis of the primary disease, en bloc resection should be the treatment of choice. This is particularly true in cases of RCC metastases, because of its high risk of local recurrence, after intralesional excision even if combined with radiotherapy. In reality, the worst result after curettage occurs in cases of incomplete excisions (posterior only approach) and the effect of additional radiotherapy is incapable to eradicate the lesion. This findings confirm that the intralesional excision needs to be complete (outside the tumor capsule) in tumors partially or totally radioresitant, like the renal cell carcinoma, becoming necessary a double surgical approach.

Both palliative surgery and intralesional excision may allow, in a good amount of patients, a certain degree of neurological improvement in the short term (improving quality of life), however the survival percentage at mid term is shorter for the patients treated with simple decompression and stabilization of the spine. Although we need to consider that, in general, patients treated with palliative surgery are in worse condition compared to those treated with intralesional excision. In cases of intralesional surgery, the use of adjuvant radiation therapy is indicated even considering the low sensitivity of tumor to this treatment.

Immunotherapy should always be associated to the post-operative radiotherapy, because it has been demonstrated that the association of the adjuvant therapy increases the survival, independently of the surgical technique applied.

The use of isolated radiation therapy is indicated only in the face of multiple RCC metastases in patients with a poor prognosis. Even in those cases, when radiation therapy fails to mitigate pain and/or in the presence of a pathologic fracture with progressive neurological deterioration, a surgical intervention with decompression and stabilization should be performed.

The early diagnosis of the primary tumor, the presence and location of the metastatic disease are paramount. The possibility of detecting the metastatic lesion in an early stage allows the spine surgeon to choose the best treatment for each patient and for each lesion. Unfortunately, the identification of these patients in an advanced stage makes the surgical intervention only a palliative measure used in cases of pathological fractures or severe neurological deficit. On the other hand, the early intervention permits a better local control of the disease, increasing the success possibility as far as improving the neurological status and treating the pain.

6. References

Arguello F, Baggs RB, Duerst RE, Johnstone L, McQueen K, Frantz CN. Pathogenesis of vertebral metastasis and epidural spinal cord compression. *Cancer* 1990;65(1):98–106.

Batson OV. The function of the vertebral veins and their role in the spread of metastases. *Ann Surg* 1940; 112: 138-49.

Batson OV. The vertebral vein system as a mechanism for the spread of metastases. *Am J Roentgenol* 1942; 48: 715-8.

Batson OV. The vertebral vein system. Caldwell lecture. *Am J Roentgenol* 1957; 78:195-212.

Biagini R, Boriani S, Casadei R, Bandiera S, De Iure F, Campanacci L, Demitri S, Orsini U, Di Fiore M.; Resections techniques in the treatment of vertebral neoplasms. *Chir. Org. Mov.* 1997; 82: 341-355.

Bilsky MH, Laufer I., Burch S. Shifting paradigms in the treatment of metastatic spine disease. *Spine* 2009; 34 (22): S101-S107.

Boriani S, Biagini R, De Iure F, Andreoli I, Lari S, Di Fiore M. Lombalgia neoplastica: diagnosi e trattamento. Chir. Organi Mov. 1994; 79: 93-9.

Boriani S, Weinstein JN: Differential diagnosis and surgical treatment of primary benign and malignant Neoplasm. In Frymoyer *The adult spine; Principles and Practice.* 1996; 2nd ed. Lippincott-Raven, Philadelphia.

Boriani S, Weinstein JN, Biagini R: Spine update. Primary bone tumors of the spine. Terminology and surgical staging. 1997; Spine 22: 1036-1044.

Cappuccio M, Gasbarrini A, Van Urk P, et al. Spinal metastasis: a retrospective study validating the treatment algorithm. *Eur Rev Med Pharmaco Sci* 2008; 12:155- 60.

Cappuccio M, Gasbarrini A, Bandello L, Focarazzo E, et al. Il tratamento chirurgico delle metastasi vertebrali da carcinoma renale: problematiche anestesiologiche intraoperatorie. *Clin Ter* 2008; 159 (1): 1-6.

Cappuccio M, Gasbarrini A, Donthineni R, Beisse R, Boriani S. Thoracospcopic assisted en bloc resection of a spine tumor. *Eur Spine J* 2011; 20 (Suppl 2): S202-5.

Crockard A, Quiney R, Taylor B, Lehovsky J: 360 degree surgery for high cervical vertebral tumors. *J.Neurosurg* 1980; 53: 712-21.

Denis F: The three column spine and its significance in the classification of acute thoracolumbar spinal injuries. *Spine* 1983; 8(8): 817-831.

Duensing S, van den Berg-de Ruiter E, Störkel S, Kirchner H, Hänninen EL, Buer J, et al.: Cytogenetic studies in renal cell carcinoma patients receiving low- dose recombinant interleukin-2-based immunotherapy. *Tumour Biol.* 1996; 17: 27-33.

Gabriel K, Schiff D. Metastatic spinal cord compression by solid tumors. *Seminars in Neurology* 2004;24(4):375–83

Gasbarrini A, Cappuccio M, Mirabile L, et al. Spinal metastases: treatment evaluation algorithm. *Eur Rev Med Pharmaco Sci* 2004; 8:265–74.

Gasbarrini A, Cappucio M, Li H, Donthineni R, et al. Treatment of metastases to the vertebrae with radiofrequency ablation: determination of effectiveness by evaluation of tumor necrosis - A preliminary result. *Curr Radiopharm* 2009; 2: 191-194.

Gasbarrini A, Li H, Cappuccio M, Mirabile L, et al. Efficacy evaluation of a new treatment algorithm for spinal metastases. *Spine* 2010; 36 (2): 1466-70.

Gerszten PC, Mendel E, Yamada Y. Radiotherapy and radiosurgery for Metastatic disease: What are the options, indications, and outcomes? *Spine* 2009; 34 (22S): S78-S92.

Gibbs IC, Kamnerdsupaphon P, Ryu MR, et al. Image-guided robotic radiosurgery for spinal metastases. *Radiother Oncol* 2007; 82:185–90.

Gottfried ON, Schloesser PE, Schmidt MH, Stevens EA. Embolization of metastatic tumors. *Neurosurg Clin N Am* 2004; 15:391-99.

Gurwitz GS, Dawson JM, McNamara MJ, Federspiel CF, Spengler DM.: Biomechanical analysis of three surgical approaches for lumbar burst fractures using short-segment instrumentation. *Spine* 1993; 18 (8): 977-982.

Heldwein FL, Escudier B, Smyth G, Souto CAV, Vallancien G. Metastatic renal cell carcinoma management. *Int Braz J Urol* 2009; 35: 256-70.

Jacqmin D, van Poppel H, Kirkali Z, Mickisch G: Renal cancer. *Eur Urol.* 2001; 39: 361-9.

Jemal A, Siegel R, Ward E, Hao Y, Xu J, Murray T, et al. Cancer statistics, 2008. *CA Cancer J Clin.* 2008; 58: 71-96.

Karnofsky DA. Clinical evaluation of anticancer drugs: cancer chemotherapy. *GANN Monogr* 1967; 2: 223–31.

Kawahara N, Tomita K, Murakami H, Demura S. Total en bloc spondilectomy for spinal tumors: surgical techiniques and related basic background. *Othop Clin N Am* 2009; 40: 47-63.

Koga S, Tsuda S, Nishikido M, Ogawa Y, et al. The diagnostic value of bone scan in patients with renal cell carcinoma. *J Urol* 2001; 166(6): 2126-8.

Larkin JM, Eisen T: Kinase inhibitors in the treatment of renal cell carcinoma. *Crit Rev Oncol Hematol.* 2006; 60: 216-26.

Louis R. *Surgery of the spine.* Berlin : Springer - Verlag, 1983.

Manke C, Bretschneider T, Lenhart M, et al. Spinal metastases from renal cell carcinoma: effect of preoperative particle embolization on intraoperative blood loss. *Am J Neuroradiol* 2001; 22: 997-1003.

Marcove RC, Arlen M. *Atlas of Bone Pathology. With Clinical and Radiographic Correlations.* 1st ed. Philadelphia: J.B. Lippincot Co., 1992: 518-34.

McAfee PC, Bohlman HH, Riley LH, et al. Anterior retropharyngeal approach to the upper part of the cervical spine. *J Bone Joint Surg (Am)* 1987; 69: 1371-83.

McLain RF: Spinal cord decompression: an endoscopically assisted approach for metastatic tumors. *Spinal Cord* 2001; 39(9): 482-487.

McGuire RA: Physical examination in spinal trauma. In: Levine AM, Eismont FJ, Garfin SR, Zigler E: *Spine trauma.* W.B. Philadelphia. Saunders Company, 1998: 16-27.

Olerud C, Jonsson H, Lofberg AM, Lorelius LE, Sjostrom L. Embolization of spinal metastases reduces preoperative blood loss. 21 patients operated on for renal cell carcinoma. *Acta Orthop Scand* 1993; 64(1):9–12.

Perrin RG, Livingston KE, Aarabi B. Intradural extramedullary spinal metastasis. A report of 10 cases. *Journal of Neurosurgery* 1982;56(6):835–7.

Roy-Camille R, Mazel Ch, Saillant G, Lapresle Ph: Treatment of malignant tumors of the spine with posterior instrumentation. in: Sundaresan N., Schmidek H.H., Schiller A.L., Rosenthal D.I. (ed.) *Tumors of the Spine. Diagnosis and Clinical Management.* Philadelphia: W.B.Saunders; 1990: 473-492.

Sahgal A, Ames C, Chou D, et al. Stereotactic body radiotherapy is effective salvage therapy for patients with prior radiation of spinal metastases. *Int J Radiat Oncol Biol Phys* 2009; 74:723–31.

Sakaura H, Hosono N, Mukai Y, et al. Outcome of total en bloc spondylectomy for solitary metastasis of the thoracolumbar spine. *J Spinal Disord Tech* 2004; 17:297–300.

Schaberg J, Gainor B.J. A profile of metastatic carcinoma of the spine. *Spine* 1985; 10:19–20.

Stener B.: Complete removal of vertebrae for extirpation of tumors. *Clin Orthop Rel Res* 1989; 245: 72-82.

Sundaresan N, Choi IS, Hughes JE, Sachdev VP, Berenstein A. Treatment of spinal metastases from kidney cancer by presurgical embolization and resection. *J Neurosurg* 1990; 73(4):548–54.

Tae-Hon Lim, An HS, Hong JH, Ahn JY, You JW, Eck J, McGrady LM: Biomechanical evaluation of anterior and posterior fixations in an unstable calf spine model. *Spine* 1997; 22, 3: 261-266.

Thyavihally BY, Mahantshetty U, Chamarajanagar RS, Raibhattanavar SG, Tongaonkar HB. Management of renal cell carcinoma with solitary metastasis. *World J Surg Onc* 2005.Vol 3, No 48.

Tokuhashi Y, Kawano H, Ohsaka S, et al. A scoring system for preoperative evaluation of the prognosis of metastatic spine tumor prognosis. *J Jpn Orthop Assoc* 1989; 63:482–9.

Tokuhashi Y, Matsuzaki H, Toriyama S, et al. Scoring system for the preoperative evaluation of metastatic spine tumor prognosis. *Spine* 1990; 15:1110 –3.

Tokuhashi Y, Matsuzaki H, Sasaki M, et al. Scoring system for the preoperative evaluation of metastatic spine tumor prognosis. *Rinsho Seikei Geka* 1997;32:512–22.

Tokuhashi Y, Matsuzaki H, Okawa A, et al. Indications of operative procedures for metastatic spine tumors: a scoring system for preoperative evaluation of prognosis. *J East Jpn Orthop Traumatol* 1999; 11:31–5.

Tokuhashi Y, Matsuzaki H, Oda H, et al. A revised scoring system for preoperative evaluation of metastatic spine tumors prognosis. *Spine* 2005; 30(19): 2186-91.

Tomita K., Kawahara N., Baba H., Tsuchiya H., Nagata S., Toribatake Y.: Total en bloc spondylectomy for solitary spinal metastases. *International Orthopaedics (SICOT)* 1994; 18: 291-298.

Tomita K, Kawahara N, Baba H,etal.Total enbloc spondylectomy: a new surgical technique for primary malignant vertebral tumors. *Spine* 1997; 22:324 –33.

Tomita K, Kawahara N, Kobayashi T, et al. Surgical strategy for spinal metastases. *Spine* 2001; 26:298–306.

Weinstein JN: Primary Tumors. in: S.Weinstein: *The Pediatric Spine.* New York, Raven Press, 1994.

Wilson D, Hiller L, Gray L, Grainger M, et al. The effect of biological dose on time to symptom progression in metastatic renal cell carcinoma. *Clinical Oncology* 2003; 15: 400-4007.

Part 3

Clinical

16

Prognostic Factors in Renal Cell Carcinoma: An Evaluation of T-Stage, Histopathological Grade, p53, Ki-67, COX-2, and Her-2 Expressions

Minna Kankuri-Tammilehto
Department of Oncology and Radiotherapy, Turku University Hospital, Finland

1. Introduction

Kidney cancer[1] represents 2-3% of all diagnosed malignancies worldwide although in some Northern and Central European countries the incidence is higher, even 4-5% (Ferlay, 2010). Kidney cancer is responsible for approximately 116,000 deaths per year worldwide (Ferlay, 2010). In the European Union (EU), the annual number of new kidney cancers was 73 171 in 2008 (Ferlay, 2010). The majority of renal cell carcinomas (RCCs) arise from the cells of renal proximal tubules of nephrons, but 5% of cases from the cells of the collecting ducts (Chao *et al.* 2002, Kovacs *et al.* 1997, Störkel *et al.* 1997) (Figure 1.). Renal tumors are members of a complex family with unique histology, cytogenetic defects and variable metastatic potential (Linehan *et al.* 2003, Thoenes *et al.* 1986). Of all RCCs, 70-80% is of conventional type, also known as clear cell RCCs. Of these, approximately 75% have a mutation in the von Hippel-Lindau tumor suppressor gene (*VHL),* in the short arm of chromosome 3 (Maxwell *et al.* 1999, Gnarra *et al.* 1994).

The annual increase in RCC incidence has been 2-4% since the 1970s (Finnish Cancer Registry 2007, American Cancer Society 2004, Mathew *et al.* 2002). This has been attributed to the use of radiological imaging which is able to find presymptomatic RCC lesions (Jayson and Sanders 1998), as well as the increased prevalence of etiologic risk factors, such as obesity (Chow *et al.* 2000) and cigarette smoking (Hunt *et al.* 2005). The increase has been highest in localized disease, especially in tumors with less than 4 cm in diameter (Hollingsworth *et al.* 2006). 30-60% of RCC tumors are found incidentally in abdominal imaging performed for some other reason than suspected renal tumor, such as the evaluation of non-specific musculoskeletal or abdominal complaints (Jayson and Sanders 1998). Macroscopic hematuria, palpable tumor and pain, together called the classic triad in RCC, indicate metastatic disease (Cunningham 1938). Metastatic disease is seen in 20-30% of RCC patients at diagnosis (Janzen *et al.* 2003, Mc

[1] In epidemiological statistics, RCC and renal pelvis cancer are usually not reported separately, but combined under the heading of kidney cancer (Parkin *et al.* 2003).

Nichols *et al.* 1981). Half of the patients diagnosed with local RCC will later have a recurrence of their cancer: two thirds within the first year (Janzen *et al.* 2003), and the majority within five years (Lam *et al.* 2005, McNichols *et al.* 1981). The risk for late recurrence, at over 10 years from nephrectomy, is at least 10% (McNichols *et al.* 1981).

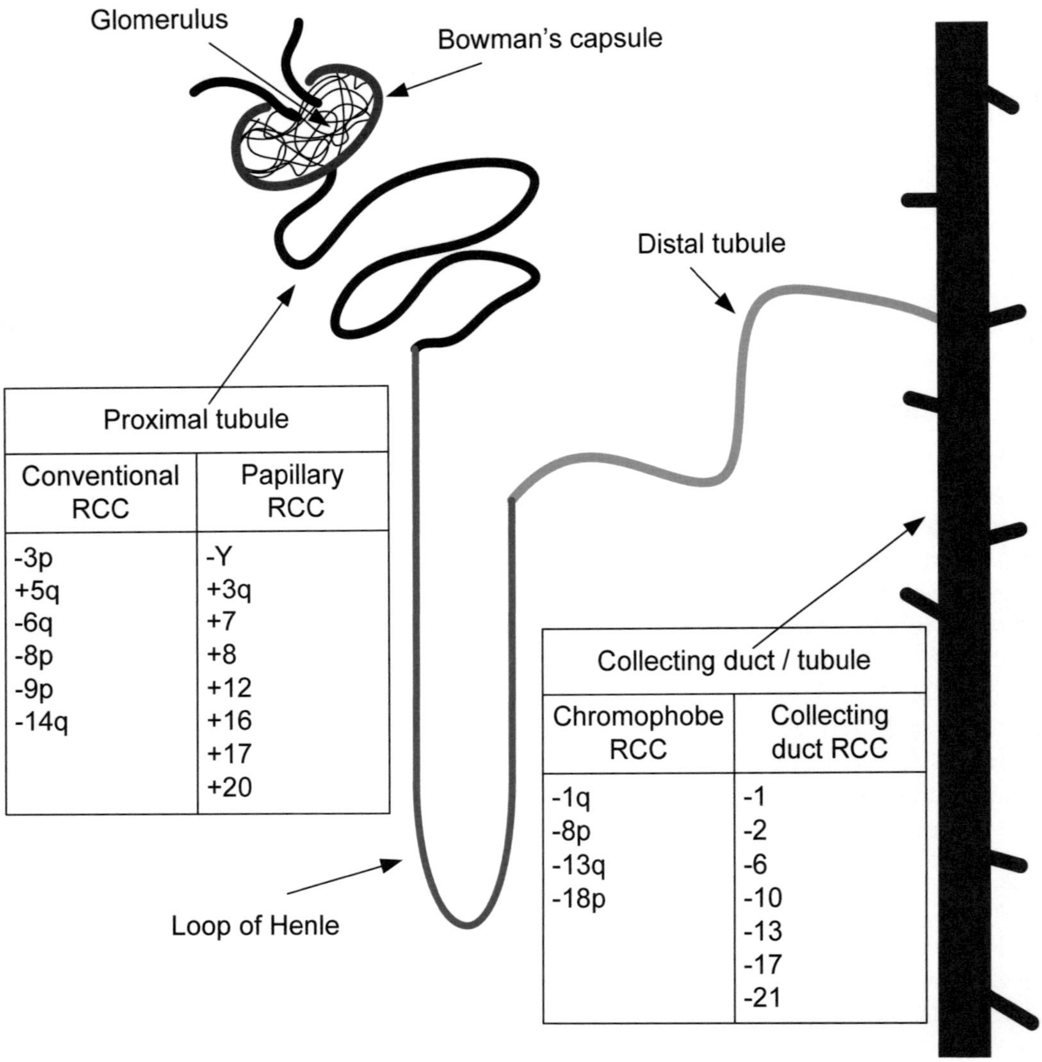

The number reflects the chromosome in which its genetic aberration is located.

- means loss of function.
+ means gain of function.
p is the short arm of the chromosome.
q is the long arm of the chromosome.

Fig. 1. The genetic changes that characterize the different RCC subtypes according to the Heidelberg classification (Modified from Bodmer *et al.* 2002).

For those RCC patients with performance status enabling current treatments the expected five-year survival rate is slightly higher than 60% (Parkin *et al.* 2003). According to a few previous studies on long-term outcome for metastatic RCC (mRCC), the five-year survival is from 3% to 16% (Atzpodien *et al.* 2002, Motzer *et al.* 2000, Minasian *et al.* 1993) if metastasectomy has not been a possible treatment. For localized RCC, nephrectomy is the only curative treatment (Robson *et al.* 2002), and currently there is no adjuvant therapy in RCC. Possible treatments for mRCC, in addition to cytoreductive nephrectomy (Flanigan *et al.* 2001, Mickisch *et al.* 2001), are immunomodulators, such as interferon-α (IFN-α) (Kankuri *et al.* 2001, Pyrhönen *et al.* 1999), interleukin-2 (IL-2) (Négrier *et al.* 2007), and more recently tyrosine kinase inhibitors, such as sunitinib (Motzer *et al.* 2007), sorafenib (Escudier *et al.* 2007), and mTOR inhibitor temsirolimus (Hudes *et al.* 2007). Everolimus, another mTOR inhibitor, has an encouraging antitumor activity against mRCC (Motzer *et al.* 2008). The efficacy of bevacizumab, an antiangiogenesis monoclonal antibody, has also been shown when used with IFN-α (Bracarda *et al.* 2011, Rini *et al.* 2010, Yang *et al.* 2003). The Food and Drug Administration (FDA) and EU have also approved pazopanib, an angiogenesis inhibitor, with advanced RCC due to the efficacy of it in RCC (Sternberg et al. 2010). Ongoing clinical trials are addressing the role of targeted agents in adjuvant therapy in RCC (Choueiri *et al.* 2011). The efficacy of many potent novel targeted agents in RCC is under investigation in phase II and III trials, among these axitinib, a multitargeted tyrosine kinase receptor inhibitor (Goldstein *et al.* 2010), tivozanib, a pan-VEGFR tyrosine kinase inhibitor (De Luca and Normanno 2010), and ipilimumab, an anti-CTLA4 antibody (Yang *et al.* 2007). Additionally, vaccine therapy in RCC is being studied (Rini *et al.* 2011). The stabilization of the disease has been shown to be beneficial for the survival of mRCC patients (Thiam *et al.* 2010, Kankuri *et al.* 2001).

2. Staging and prognostic factors in RCC

2.1 Pathological tumor staging

In the 1960's, Robson *et al*, created the staging system based on physical characteristics and tumor spread with the addition of tumor venous invasion (Robson *et al.* 2002). The poor correlation between the different Robson stages and survival led to the recommendation to use the TNM (tumor, node, metastases) staging system. Since 1978, the TNM classification system for the extent of the tumor spread has integrated characteristics such as tumor size, vascular involvement, nodal spread and distant metastases (Bassil *et al.* 1985, Harmen 1978). pTNM classification system was updated by the Union Internationale Contre le Cancer (UICC) and the American Joint Committee on Cancer (AJCC) in 1997 when the cut-off between T1 and T2 tumors was increased from 2.5 cm to 7 cm, in order to increase the difference in survival from these two tumor types. Analysis of outcome in nephrectomized patients showed that the 1997 TNM-system cut-off point between T1 and T2 tumors is too high, and a cut-off point of 4.5 – 5.0 cm has been suggested (Elmore *et al.* 2003, Zisman *et al.* 2001). In 2002, the pTNM classification system was revised: T1 was divided into T1a and T1b by a cut-off point of 4 cm, according to the suitability for partial nephrectomy, and prognostication (Sobin and Wittekind 2002, Guinan *et al.* 1997). A uniform staging classification, the TNM staging system, has improved the division of patients into radical or partial nephrectomy candidates. Additionally, it has increased the co-operation between oncologists and pathologists concerning the outcome of RCC patients (Janzen *et al.* 2003, Javidan *et al.* 1999). Howerer, modifications in the TNM system may cause difficulty in comparing outcome data in different studies (Belldegrun *et al.* 1999, Störkel *et al.* 1989).

Pathological tumor stage (T-stage) has been observed to be the most important factor for locally confined RCC in predicting the survival of patients who have undergone nephrectomy (Kankuri *et al.* 2006, Delahunt *et al.* 2002). The observed five-year survival is approximately 75-80% for stage T1, 55% for T2, 40% for T3, and 20-30% for T4 (Sunela *et al.* 2009, Tsui *et al.* 2000). For patients with stage I disease (tumor confined to the kidney) the five-year survival is approximately 90%, and for those with stage I and histologic of chromophobe type it is almost 100% (Zisman *et al.* 2001). The five-year survival rate for stage III disease is approximately 50% (Zisman *et al.* 2001). There is an 80% difference in survival rates between patients with local disease compared to those with advanced disease and distant metastases (American Cancer Society 2004). In a retrospective review of 2 473 RCC patients from 1975 - 1985, regardless of T-stage, tumor size was observed to have an inverse association with survival (Guinan *et al.* 1995). In the study of Kankuri *et al.* (2006), in the analysis of those RCC patients who later developed metastatic disease, high T-stage caused twice the risk of metastatic disease and three times the risk of death compared with low T-stage which indicates that as the tumor size increases, the more aggressive its growth becomes and the more probable is tumor cell dissemination. T-stage is a prognostic factor for both metastases-free and overall survival in RCC patients.

T-stage can be used in estimating the correct duration and frequency of surveillance of RCC patients after nephrectomy. RCC with a diameter of less than 3.0 cm grows slowly; only 2.5% have metastases during the first three years (Bosniak *et al.* 1995). Therefore, in the treatment of those in whom surgery is contraindicated, careful monitoring (watchful waiting) by computed tomography (CT scan) may be used (Roberts *et al.* 2005, Bosniak *et al.* 1995). Previously, it has been suggested that T-stage is not an important prognostic factor in the survival of patients who have neither lymph node nor distant metastases (Giuliani *et al.* 1990). The therapeutic value of lymph node dissection remains unproven (Mickish 1999). T-stage alone has been pointed to be a valuable prognostic factor for survival, even when the status of lymph nodes is unknown (Kankuri *et al.* 2006). Additionally, a high T-stage has been used as an inclusion criterion for adjuvant treatments in trials (Atzpodien *et al.* 2005, Repmann *et al.* 2003).

Moreover, T-stage is an independent prognostic factor in mRCC patients (Kankuri-Tammilehto *et al.* 2010). In the study of Kankuri-Tammilehto *et al.* (2010) high T-stage caused twice the risk of death compared with low T-stage in mRCC. The association between T-stage and overall survival was also found in those with primary metastases at the time of nephrectomy (Kankuri *et al.* 2006). T-stage is not typically used in prognostic models in mRCC, a UCLA model (Zisman *et al.* 2002) being an exception. T-stage seems to be a good tool in prognostic evaluation in mRCC patients and could be included in prognostic models.

2.2 Histopathological tumor grading

In grading systems, the major criteria are nuclear and nucleolar appearances, while in some systems, tumor architecture and cell type is also included (Mostofi *et al.* 1998, Goldstein 1997, Fuhrman *et al.* 1982, Syrjänen and Hjelt 1978, Skinner *et al.* 1971). The WHO grading system is based on the size and prominence of nucleoli (Eble *et al.* 2004, Mostofi *et al.* 1998), while the Fuhrman grading system is based on nuclear size, shape, and presence or absence of nucleoli (Fuhrman *et al.* 1982). The WHO grading system contains three grades, whereas the Fuhrman contains four.

Several studies have failed to demonstrate any statistically significant differences in the survival of patients with different grades, when all three or four grades are analyzed separately (Kankuri *et al.* 2006, Rioux-Leclercq *et al.* 2000, Usubutyn *et al.* 1998, Selli *et al.* 1983) although when analyzing only the highest and the lowest grades the statistically significant difference in survival have been found (Kankuri *et al.* 2006). This is partly because, as yet, no consensus has been reached on a universal tumor grading system (Kanamaru *et al.* 2001, Medeiros *et al.* 1997). The observed five-year disease-specific survival (DSS) rate is approximately 90% for G1, 70-85% for G2, 45-60% for G3, and 15-30% for G4 (Gudbjartsson *et al.* 2005, Ficarra *et al.* 2001). Currently, different grading systems are utilized at different institutions. Tumor-grading systems have been criticized because of their subjectivity in tumor evaluations (Lanigan *et al.* 1994), and comparison of different patient cases with respect to histopathological grade is difficult. More quantitative measures which describe the size or the shape of the nuclei have been requested by pathologists. In 1997, an international consensus conference on RCC by UICC and AJCC outlined recommendations for the grading of RCC (Goldstein 1997): the grading system should be based on standardized and reproducible criteria that reflect the heterogeneity of nuclear and nucleolar features within a tumor, and each grade should result in significant differences in patient outcome. Recently again, a joint group of urologists and pathologists has published a proposal that the criteria for nuclear grading should be different for the different histopathologic subtypes of RCC according to the Heidelberg classification (Paner *et al.* 2006). Additionally, reducing the grades in the Fuhrman system has been proposed, for better outcome stratification (Rioux-Leclercq *et al.* 2007, Lohse *et al.* 2002, Bretheau *et al.* 1995). Overall, histopathological grade seem to be imprecise for prognostic evaluation in RCC patients (Uchida *et al.* 2002, Rioux-Leclercq *et al.* 2000, Lanigan *et al.* 1994).

2.3 Heidelberg and WHO classifications for typing of renal tumors

In Heidelberg, in October 1996, the morphology was combined with genetic findings for a new classification, called the Heidelberg classification of renal tumors, in a workshop organized by the UICC and the AJCC (Kovacs *et al.* 1997, Störkel *et al.* 1997). In addition to this, in 2004, WHO published the reassessed classification which is now based on both genetic and pathological abnormalities (Eble *et al.* 2004). Progress in our knowledge of genetic alterations leads to new suggestions for RCC entities (Eble 2003). With the progress of research, the Heidelberg classification may lead to more specific treatments in different subgroups of RCC patients. The 5-year DSS for locally confined RCC is for chromophobe RCC approximately 87-100%, for papillary RCC 87%, and for conventional RCC 70-75% (Cheville *et al.* 2003, Amin *et al.* 2002). In the case of sarcomatoid change, the survival decreases with the 5-year DSS of 35% (Amin *et al.* 2002). A very rare entity of collecting duct RCC is highly aggressive with highly decreased prognosis (Antonelli *et al.* 2003). The prognostic power of the Heidelberg classification has been investigated. The current Heidelberg classification does not have independent prognostic ability, and thus it should not be considered as a major prognostic variable comparable to T-stage and histopathological tumor grade (Patard *et al.* 2005). However, Heidelberg classification associates with metastases development, indicating that unclassified tumor type metastasizes with high probability (Kankuri *et al.* 2006). In future, with the progress of research, the Heidelberg classification may lead to more specific treatments in different subgroups of RCC patients (Störkel *et al.* 1997).

2.4 Prognostic models in RCC

The heterogeneity of RCC within the same T-stage and grade (Tsui *et al.* 2000) has resulted in a need for prognostic models for prognostication and treatment modality selection. Prognostic models, anagrams and nomograms, have been developed to find those nephrectomized RCC patients who potentially have a long-term recurrence-free interval and survival, as well as those mRCC patients who have long-term survival (Table 1.). The most often represented as an independent prognostic factors in metastatic RCC (mRCC) are performance status, time to metastases, number of metastatic sites, and prior nephrectomy. Therapies for mRCC cause a wide variety of adverse effects, which reduce the quality of life. Determining the prognostic factors for survival in mRCC patients is valuable in directing therapy for those patients who would benefit from it. Several models have been developed for predicting the likelihood of response to therapy and to predict survival. However, novel biomarkers are hoped to specify the diagnosis, staging, and prognosis and to guide targeted cancer therapies. Molecular tumor markers are expected to revolutionize the staging of RCC in the future (Srigley *et al.* 1997), as nowadays stratifying the patients into risk groups is largely done on the basis of clinopathological factors, e.g. clinical stage of the disease. Still, all the molecular mechanisms that affect the development, progression and clinical behavior of RCC are not known. Advances in the understanding of the pathogenesis, behavior, and molecular biology of RCC may help to better predict tumor prognosis, and thus improve survival of RCC carcinoma patients when a more tailored therapy can be given to each individual patient. Molecular biomarkers, such as p53, Ki-67 and COX-2, are candidates for defining prognostic subgroups (Delahunt *et al.* 2002), and for guiding targeted therapies (Masters 2007), as shown in the studies, where p53, Ki-67 and COX-2 had prognostic value in predicting survival. The following chapters describe in more detail about the value of them in the prognosis in RCC.

3. Biomarkers related to molecular mechanism in RCC

3.1 pVHL, von Hippel-Lindau protein, mudulator of hypoxic response

pVHL, a tumor suppressor gene product, is expressed especially in the kidney's proximal renal tubule (Corless *et al.* 1997, Iliopoulos *et al.* 1995). Approximately 61-75% of sporadic conventional RCCs contain mutations in *VHL*, in the short arm of chromosome 3 (3p25-26) (van Houwelingen *et al.* 2005, Maxwell *et al.* 1999, Gnarra *et al.* 1994,), of which 50% show loss of heterozygosity (LOH) (Kovacs *et al.* 1997, Gnarra *et al.* 1994) and 10-20% silencing of the wild-type allele by promoter hypermethylation (Herman *et al.* 1994). VHL is associated with carcinogenesis. The function of pVHL is ubiquitylation of hypoxia-inducible factor (HIF); therefore, it modulates the hypoxic response; VHL protein can bind to hypoxia inducible factor-1 alpha (HIF-1α) and target this factor for destruction in the presence of oxygen. HIF in turn controls the expression of several proteins, including carbonic anhydrase 9 (CA9) and proteins involved in angiogenesis, i.e. vascular endothelial growth factor (VEGF) and EPO, via oxygen-dependent ubiquitination (van Houwelingen *et al.* 2005, George and Kaelin 2003). Normally, VHL down regulates vascular endothelial growth factor (VEGF) by different pathways. In VHL-defective cancer cells, increased concentrations of VEGF and EPO are observed.

Reference	Year	No. of Patients	Therapy Administered	Tumor Subtype	Prognostic Factors	Prognostic Information
Motzer *et al.* (MSKCC)	2002	463	IFN-α	All	Performance status, time from diagnosis to start of therapy, LDH, hemoglobin, corrected calcium	Survival
Zisman *et al.* (UCLA)	2002	262	IL-2 or IFN-α (197 pts), other (65 pts)	All	T-stage, nodal involvement, nuclear grade, no. of symptoms, immunotherapy	Survival
Négrier *et al.* (Group Francais d'Immunotherapie)	2002	782	IFN-α ± IL-2	All	Performance status, no. of metastatic sites, disease-free interval, signs of inflammation, hemoglobin	Survival, rapid progression
Atzpodien (Medizinische Hochschule Hannover)	2003	425	IFN-α + IL-2 ± 5-FU ± 13CRA	All	Neutrophil count , LDH, CRP, time from diagnosis to start of therapy, no. of metastatic sites, bone metastases	Survival
Motzer *et al.* (MSKCC)	2004	251	New agents	All, if cytokine refractory disease	Performance status, hemoglobin, corrected calcium	Survival for those who enter clinical trials of new agents
Choueiri *et al.* (Cleveland Clinic Foundation)	2007	358	IFN-α ± IL-2 ± chemotherapy	All	Performance status, hemoglobin, no. of metastatic sites, involved kidney of primary tumor	Long-term survival
Cho et al (Yonsei University)	2008	197	Immunotherapy	All	Performance status, N stage, no. of metastatic sites, sarcomatoid differentiation, liver metastasis	Survival
Motzer *et al.* (MSKCC)	2008	375	Sunitinib	Conventional RCC	Performance status, time from diagnosis to start of therapy, nephrectomy status, no. of metastatic sites, presence of liver or lung metastases, LDH, corrected calcium, hemoglobin, alkaline phosphatase, thrombosytosis	Probability of 12-month progression-free survival

LDH=lactate dehydrogenase
MSKCC = Memorial Sloan Kettering Cancer Center
UCLA = University of California

Table 1. Prognostic algorithms and nomograms for survival in mRCC between 2000 and 2008.

3.2 CA9, hypoxia associated enzyme

CA9, a member of the carbonic anhydrase family, is suggested to play a role in the regulation of cell proliferation in response to hypoxic conditions. Low CA9 expression associates with the absence of VHL mutation and aggressive tumor characteristics in conventional RCC (Pantuck *et al.* 2007). CA9 may indicate those patients who benefit from IL-2, as low CA9 expression associates with lower survival compared to high CA9 expression in mRCC patients who receive IL-2 (Atkins *et al.* 2005, Bui *et al.* 2003). It has also been suggested that CA9 may indicate those patients who benefit from CA9-targeted therapies. It is also being investigated whether CA9 may indicate those patients who are potential candidates for adjuvant therapy.

3.3 p53, biomarker of cell cycle point

p53, a tumor suppressor gene product, is a promoter of cell growth arrest and apoptosis (Choisy-Rossi and Yonish-Rouach 1998). Activated p53 elicits several cellular responses, including apoptosis and cell cycle arrest (Reich and Levine 1984), and responds to DNA damage at the restriction checkpoint of the G1 phase of the cell cycle (May and May 1999). In normal cells, p53 is usually undetectable (Finlay *et al.* 1988). Mutant p53 accumulates in cell nuclei and can be immunostained (Reich and Levine 1984), whereas wild-type p53, because of its short half-life, is usually undetectable by routine immunohistochemistry (Reich and Levine 1984). p53 accumulation and increased cell proliferative activity are parallel phenomena in RCC (Kankuri *et al.* 2006, Pinto *et al.* 2005). p53 may be upregulated in part by VHL, accounting for some of the tumor suppressive functions of VHL in RCC (Galban *et al.* 2003). p53 seems to associate weakly with tumor grade, as the association was seen only in univariate analysis. Nor was an association between p53 and grade observed in a previous microarray study (Zigeuner *et al.* 2004). In both studies, the nuclear grade was determined according to the WHO guidelines.

Published results on the association of p53 with survival have been controversial, some studies suggesting positive p53 associating with poor survival (Shvarts *et al.* 2005 , Zigeuner *et al.* 2004, Uchida *et al.* 2002, Haitel *et al.* 2000), while others have observed no association (Itoi *et al.* 2004, Olumi *et al.* 2001, Rioux-Leclercq *et al.* 2000, Hofmockel *et al.* 1996). In the study of Phuoc *et al.* (2007), p53 was significantly associated with survival in univariate analysis, but the association was not independent. In a tissue array study on metastasized patients, overexpression of p53 was associated with impaired DSS in renal carcinoma (Kim *et al.* 2004). In some studies, the association of p53 and survival has been investigated in a group of RCC patients with both locally confined and primary metastatic RCC; thus, patient selection varies in different studies (Olumi *et al.* 2001). The study of Kankuri *et al.* (2006) indicates that p53 is not able to predict which patients will develop metastatic disease after nephrectomy, but interestingly, they predict poor survival in mRCC patients (Figure 2.). Therefore, p53 can help in determining metastatic patients with a poor prognosis and, e.g. those who might benefit from aggressive treatment, such as high-dose interleukin-2 (Spanknebel *et al.* 2005) or temsirolimus (Hudes *et al.* 2007).

3.4 Ki-67, proliferation marker

Ki-67, a proliferation biomarker, is expressed throughout the active phases of the cell cycle, and serves as a good marker for proliferative activity in cell nuclei (Gerdes *et al.* 1984). Ki-67 accumulates during the cell cycle from G1 to mitosis, and is at its lowest level after mitosis (du Manoir *et al.* 1991). The percentage of nuclei staining by immunohistochemistry reflects Ki-67 expression (Olumi *et al.* 2001). An association between Ki-67 and high T-stage and metastases development have been observed

(Kankuri *et al.* 2006, Dudderidge *et al.* 2005, Rioux-Leclercq *et al.* 2000), indicating that Ki-67 is a marker for aggressive disease in RCC with an increased risk of early metastases development. Ki-67 has been reported to independently predict survival following nephrectomy in many studies (Dudderidge *et al.* 2005, Bui *et al.* 2004, Itoi *et al.* 2004, Rioux-Leclercq *et al.* 2000, Aaltomaa *et al.* 1997). Ki-67 has been observed to increase in sarcomatoid change (Kanamaru *et al.* 1999), indicating different protein expression profiles in different entities according to the Heidelberg classification.

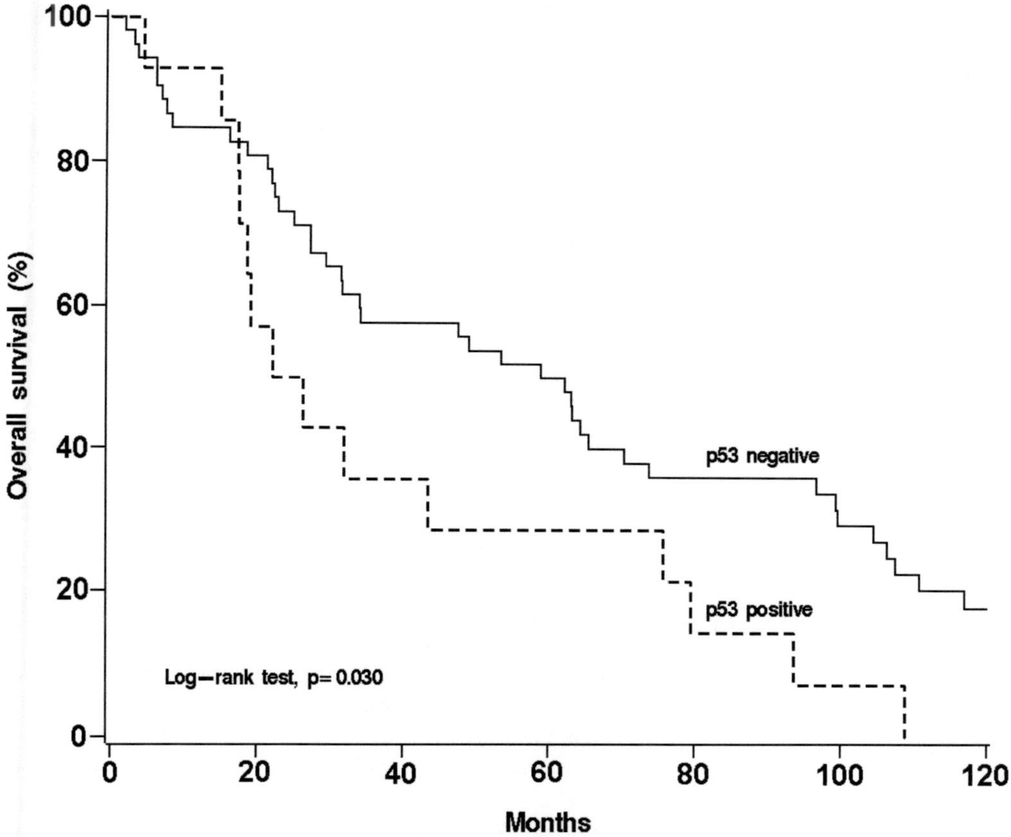

Fig. 2. Kaplan-Meier survival curve for p53 in mRCC (n=66) (Kankuri *et al.* 2006).

Dudderidge *et al.* (2005) found Ki-67 to be an independent prognostic factor for disease-free survival in nephrectomized RCC, but opposite results have also been published (Donskov *et al.* 2004, Kim *et al.* 2004, Yildiz *et al.* 2004). No association between Ki-67 alone and survival in locally confined RCC patients was found in the study of Kankuri *et al.* (2006). The differences in the classification of metastases are seen: Kim and coworkers (2004) classified both distant and local lymph node metastases as metastatic disease, whereas in the study of Kankuri *et al.* (2006), only tumors with distant metastases were classified as metastatic. However, Ki-67 predicts poor survival in mRCC patients (Figure 3.). Therefore, in addition to p53, Ki-67 can help in determining metastatic patients with a poor prognosis and, e.g. those who might benefit from aggressive treatment.

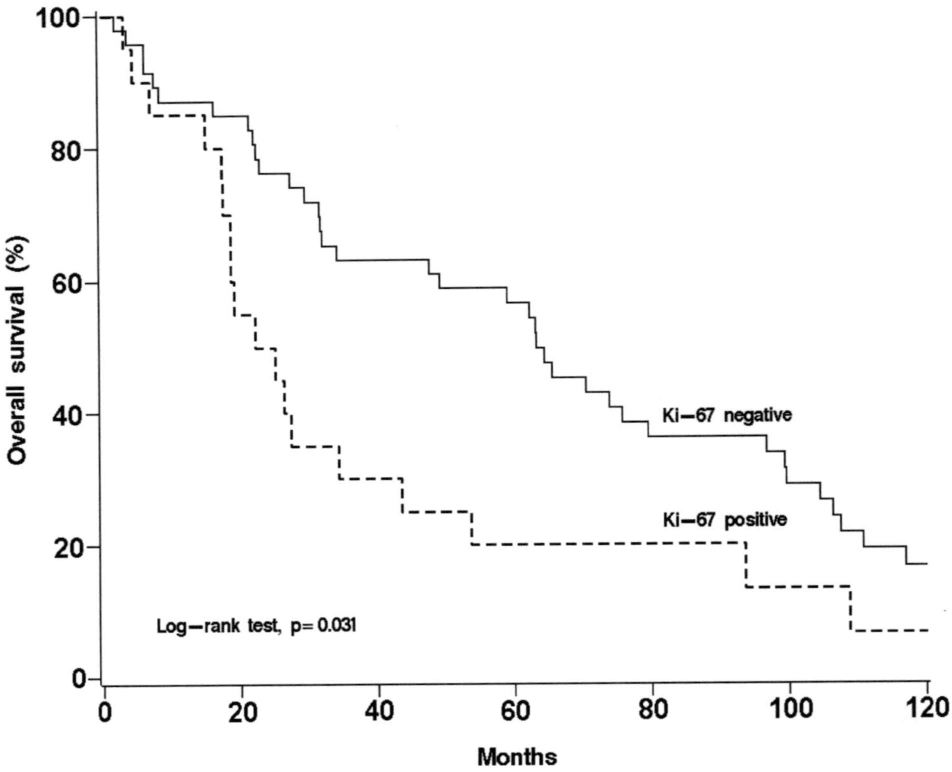

Fig. 3. Kaplan-Meier survival curve for Ki-67 in mRCC (n=66) (Kankuri *et al.* 2006).

3.5 COX-2, biomarker for inflammation and neoplasia

Cyclo-oxygenase-2 (COX-2), an isoform of the COX[3] enzyme, is an inducible form of an enzyme involved in the first steps of prostaglandins and thromboxane synthesis. COX-2 converts arachidonic acid first into prostaglandin G2, and afterwards by peroxidase activity into prostaglandin H_2, a precursor of the prostaglandins (Taketo 1998). COX-2 is suggested to play a physiological role in fetal nephrogenesis (Khan *et al.* 2001). COX-2 increases in inflammation and neoplasia (Miyata *et al.* 2003, Hara *et al.* 2002, Nose *et al.* 2002, *et al.* Taketo 1998), and is undetectable in most normal tissues (Mungan *et al.* 2006, Yoshimura *et al.* 2004). The conversion of procarcinogens to proximate carcinogens is catalyzed by the peroxidase activity of COX-2 (Elinq *et al.* 1990). COX-2 is highly induced by stimulus of oncogenes, cytokines, growth factors, and tumor promoters (Smith *et al.* 2000, Herschman 1996, Subbaramaiah *et al.* 1996). Associations between COX-2 over-expression and antiapoptotic ability, tumor invasiveness, tumor growth, angiogenesis, and immunosuppression, as well as multidrug resistance in cancer have been reported (Cao and Prescott 2002, Masferrer *et al.* 2000, Subbramaiah *et al.* 1996, Tsujii and DuBois 1995).

Cytoplasmic/membranous COX-2 staining by immunohistochemistry reflects COX-2 protein expression (Cho *et al.* 2005). The study results on associations of COX-2 with tumor stage, grade, and survival have been contradictory. Yoshimura *et al.* (2004) demonstrated that COX-2 was expressed at its highest in G1, as well as in pT1 RCC tumors, compared to other RCC tumors in grade and T-stage, while in Hashimoto *et al*'s study (2004), more COX-2 was found at the higher tumor grade, as well as stage. Kankuri-Tammilehto *et al.* (2010) found no association between COX-2 and tumor grade or T-stage. A significant association has been observed between COX-2 and Ki-67 expression in the study of Miyata *et al.* (2003), whereas Kankuri-Tammilehto *et al.* (2010) found no association between them. No association between COX-2 and p53 has been found in studies (Kankuri-Tammilehto *et al.* 2010, Cho *et al.* 2005).

Kankuri-Tammilehto *et al.* (2010) found that the proportion of COX-2 positive tumors is highest in RCC with the ability to develop later metastases, when compared to both RCC without metastatic potential and RCC with primary metastases. This finding was new. Previously, Miyata *et al.* (2003) observed that positive COX-2 expression associated with primary metastases in univariate analysis (when M0-patients were compared to M1-patients). Cho *et al.* (2005) found no association between positive COX-2 expression and metastases (when M0-patients were compared to M1-patients, or appearance of metastatic disease was compared to non-metastatic disease). In those studies, the method of analysis differs from that of the study of Kankuri-Tammilehto *et al.* (2010), where patients were divided into three categories according to the appearance of metastases. According to the study of Kankuri-Tammilehto *et al.* (2010), metastases-free survival is longer in patients with COX-2 positive tumors. The median metastases-free survival was 46 months in RCC with COX-2 positivity compared to 15 months in RCC with COX-2 negativity (Figure 4.). These

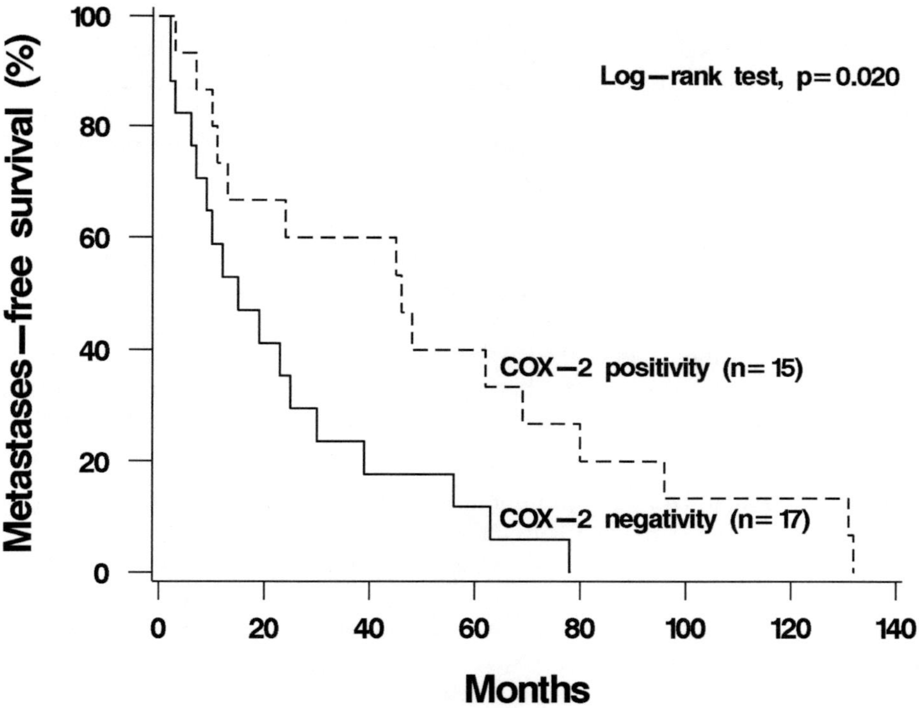

Fig. 4. The prognostic value of COX-2 for metastases-free survival from nephrectomy in RCC patients who later developed metastatic disease (n=32, Kaplan-Meier method): the median metastases-free survival time was 46 months with COX-2 positivity, and 15 months with COX-2 negativity (Kankuri-Tammilehto *et al.* 2010).

results indicate that COX-2 positivity associates with the delay of metastatic formation in RCC patients who do not have disseminated disease at presentation, and that COX-2 negativity associates with an aggressive phenotype in mRCC disease.

Few studies have reported the results of an association between COX-2 expression and survival in RCC patients. Previously, Miyata *et al.* (2003) found that the five-year survival of patients with COX-2 positive tumors from nephrectomy was 66%, and of COX-2 negative patients 91% (Miyata *et al.* 2003). In Miyata's study, the patients were 86% M0 and 14% M1 at nephrectomy. Previously, no results of COX-2 and overall survival in mRCC patients have been published. The study of Kankuri-Tammilehto *et al.* (2010) indicates that COX-2 positivity predicts improved overall survival in patients with mRCC treated with IFN-α. This is in line with the previous study of Rini *et al.* (2006), in which COX-2 positivity associated with longer time to progression in the patients treated with celecoxib plus interferon-α. Kankuri-Tammilehto *et al.* (2010) observed no association between COX-2 staining and response to IFN-α alone, while Rini *et al.* (2006) reported that all the RCC patients with objective responses to celecoxib plus interferon-α expressed COX-2 staining. Additionally, COX-2 does not associate with the Heidelberg classification (Kankuri-Tammilehto *et al.* 2010, Yoshimura *et al.* 2004).

3.6 Her-2, biomarker of proto-oncogene product

Her-2, a proto-oncogene product, is a member of the ErbB family of receptor tyrosine kinases. Her-2 functions in secretory epithelial tissues, and regulates intracellular signaling cascades (Arteaga *et al.* 2001, Olayioye *et al.* 2000). Her-2 is over-expressed in approximately 20-30% of human adenocarcinomas (Latif *et al.* 2002, Lipponen *et al.* 1994, Slamon *et al.* 1989), and the over-expression is associated with metastatic phenotype and poorer prognosis, e.g. in breast and ovarian cancer (Slamon *et al.* 1989).

Gene amplification of *Her-2* can be investigated by cytogenetic analyses, such as fluorescent *in situ* hybridization (FISH), chromogenic *in situ* hybridization (CISH), and polymerase chain reaction (PCR). In breast cancer, FISH and CISH positivity are accurate predictors of response to trastuzumab (anti-Her2 therapy) (Isola *et al.* 2004, Lebeau *et al.* 2001). Receptor-mediated targeted tumor therapy with Herceptin® (RhuMAb HER-2), a recombinant humanized monoclonal anti-Her-2 antibody, has improved the survival of breast carcinoma patients both in adjuvant therapy and in therapy for metastatic disease (Smith *et al.* 2007, Montemurro *et al.* 2003).

Membranous staining of HER-2 in immunohistochemistry reflects HER-2 protein expression (Zhang *et al.* 1997). Her-2 receptor-specific tumor toxin, in an animal model, effectively reduced pulmonary tumors of advanced RCC (Maurer-Gebhard *et al.* 1998). Parallel associations of Her-2 expression between tumor stage and grade in RCC patients have been observed in many studies (Zhang *et al.* 1997, Stumm *et al.* 1996), although in the study of Seliger *et al.* (2000) no such association was found. In the study of Hofmockel *et al.* (1997), higher tumor grades were seen when Her-2 expression was low, and higher T-stage associated with high Her-2. In the study of Phuoc *et al.* (2007), Her-2 protein expression did not correlate with Ki-67 protein expression.

In most *HER-2* gene amplification studies, *Her-2* gene amplification was observed neither by FISH analysis (Latif *et al.* 2002), messenger ribonucleic acid (mRNA) analysis (Stumm *et al.*

1996), nor PCR analysis (Selli *et al.* 1997, Zhang *et al.* 1997). Selli *et al.* (1997) found *HER-2* gene amplification in collecting duct RCC cases (45%). Therefore, *HER-2* gene amplification may be more pronounced in collecting duct RCC, than in other more common RCC types (Matei *et al.* 2005, Zhang *et al.* 1997). The association of *HER*-2 gene amplification and HER-2 protein expression with the prognosis of RCC patients has been estimated in few studies and the results have been contradictory (Phuoc *et al.* 2007, Lipponen *et al.* 1994). Further studies are needed to determine whether HER-2 protein expression or *HER-2* gene amplification may be used as prognostic factors in RCC patients.

3.7 Incidence of p53, Ki-67, and COX-2 expressions

The incidence of p53- and Ki-67-positive expression in RCC tumors was low in RCC studies (Kankuri-Tammilehto *et al.* 2010, Kirkali *et al.* 2001, Haitel *et al.* 2000, Rioux-Leclercq *et al.* 2000). It is known that in addition to melanoma, RCC belongs to tumors with a low incidence of *p53* mutations compared to, e.g. prostate and bladder cancer (Haitel *et al.* 2000, Kirkali *et al.* 2001, Rioux-Leclercq *et al.* 2000). The low *p53* mutation in different cancers (Olivier *et al.* 2002) and the low immunohistochemical staining of RCC tissue blocks for the p53 protein in studies (Haitel *et al.* 2000, Rioux-Leclercq *et al.* 2000) suggest that mutations in *p53* result in an accumulation of the p53 protein. In the study of Oda *et al.* (1995), p53 expression was found only in those components with *p53* mutations, mainly in the sarcomatoid components. The 10% cut-off value of p53 and Ki-67 was often selected to achieve statistically reliable results, and in accordance with previous studies on the subject (Kankuri *et al.* 2006, Olumi *et al.* 2001). Previously published reports indicate that the proportion of COX-2 positive cells varies in human RCCs (Cho *et al.* 2005, Miyata *et al.* 2003). In the study of Kankuri-Tammilehto *et al.* (2010), weak intensity of COX-2 staining was considered as COX-2 negative, which resulted in a lower number of positive COX-2 cells than in some other RCC studies (Tuna *et al.* 2004, Cho *et al.* 2005). For comparison, in the study of Miyata *et al.* (2003), the criterion for positive COX-2 expression was 5%, whereas in the study of Kankuri-Tammilehto *et al.* (2010), it was considered to be 10%. Also different antibodies have been used in other studies (Rini *et al.* 2006, Cho *et al.* 2005, Hashimoto *et al.* 2004). This fact and the criteria for immunohistochemical classification may contribute to the difference in the results. Validation of immunohistochemical methods is needed before the methods could be widely adopted for in clinical use.

3.8 Combining markers

In multivariate analysis, COX-2 and Ki-67 were independent variables, indicating that they are both stronger biomarkers than p53 for the development of metastases in RCC. However, combining markers may specify prognostic subgroups better than observing a single marker. As shown in a study by Haitel *et al.* (2000), p53 was not an independent predictor for survival, but p53 and mdm2, a negative regulator of p53, showed a strong association with poor survival. In the study of Kankuri *et al.* (2006), in RCC patients, double positivity for p53 and Ki-67 expression seems to indicate a higher probability of metastases than either marker alone. Additionally, combining COX-2 and Ki-67 increases their ability to predict survival in mRCC (Figure 5.). In this study, median overall survival time of RCC with COX-2 negativity/Ki-67 positivity was 19 months, which was almost five times shorter than of RCC with COX-2 positivity/Ki-67 negativity. Median overall survival time of RCC with

COX-2 negativity alone was 28 months, which was three times shorter than that of RCC with COX-2 positivity.

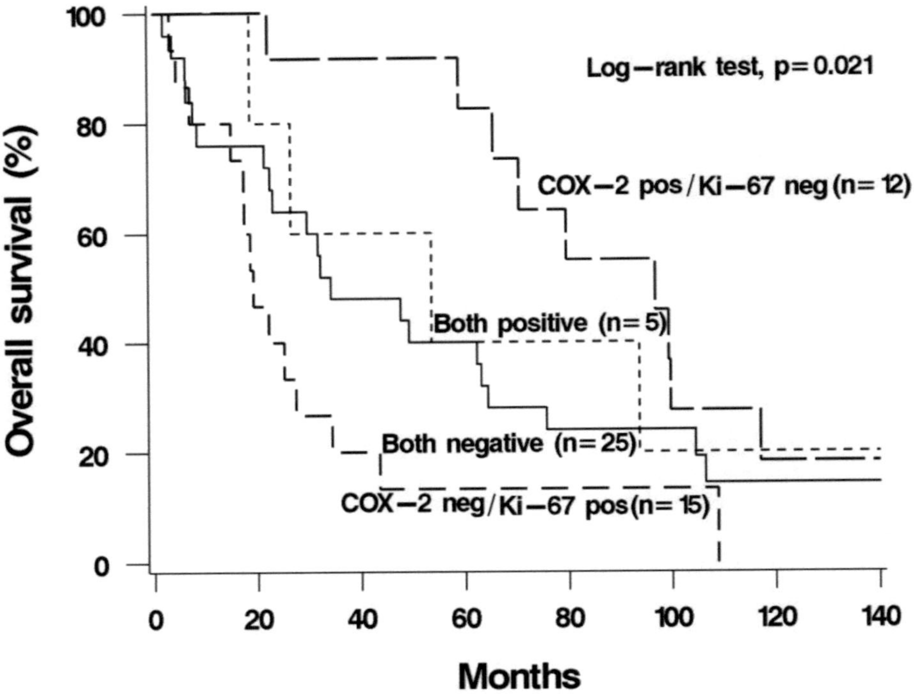

Fig. 5. The prognostic value of covariation of COX-2/Ki-67 for overall survival from nephrectomy in RCC patients with metastases (either primary presentation or later) (n=57, Kaplan-Meier method): the median overall survival time was 97 months with COX-2 positivity/Ki-67 negativity, and 19 months with COX-2 negativity/Ki-67 positivity (p=0.004) (Kankuri-Tammilehto *et al.* 2010).

Prognostic markers can be used in patient counseling, to select treatment modalities, and to determine eligibility for clinical trials. Different prognostic models have been created to specify the prognosis of RCC patients; they typically include conventional prognostic markers. However, combining biomarkers and conventional clinical markers seems to predict DSS more accurately than grade or TNM stage alone, both in locally confined and metastatic RCC (Kim *et al.* 2004).

3.9 Trends in the use of biomarkers

Prospective clinical trials on the clinical use of p53, Ki-67, and COX-2 protein expression in predicting overall survival could answer the question of whether the expression of these biomarkers can be reliably used in mRCC. These biomarkers cannot predict response to IFN-α (Kankuri-Tammilehto *et al.* 2010). Whether these biomarkers can predict response to novel targeted therapies should be investigated in trials. The new era of genetic cancer studies shows great promise in terms of patient evaluation for new targeted therapies or immunotherapy. By means of the tissue microarray technique, thousands of tumors can be investigated simultaneously to determine the protein expression profile. However, creating a consensus in the tissue microarray construction protocol is challenging, as RCC is a relatively large-size tumor of a highly heterogenous nature (Signoretti *et al.* 2008). At current, whole tissue sections are considered the gold standard, but the more cores per tumor are sampled the fewer errors are introduced by limited sampling. Using gene chips to profile kidney tumors defines the genes that determine patient survival and response to therapy, thus enabling precise prognosis determination and individual treatment planning (Tan *et al.* 2008). Additionally, tissue microarrays enable the analysis of protein expression profiles in specimens to determine their potential clinical significance and role in RCC biology.

4. Conclusion

RCC is an extremely heterogeneous disease, with patients having an overall survival from a few months to several years. For those RCC patients with performance status enabling current treatments, such as nephrectomy, immunomodulators, and more recently targeted therapies, the expected five-year survival rate has been slightly higher than 60%. Metastatic disease is seen in 20-30% of RCC patients at diagnosis. The five-year survival for metastatic RCC is from 3% to 16% if metastasectomy has not been a possible treatment. Currently, tumour (T)-stage is the best known prognostic factor for locally confined RCC. T-stage is a prognostic factor for both metastases-free and overall survival in locally confined RCC patients as well as in overall survival in metastatic RCC (mRCC). No consensus has been reached on a universal histopathologic tumor grading system. Several published reports have pointed out the differences in survival between the highest and the lowest tumor grades, even though when all three or four tumor grades were analyzed separatedly, the differences were no longer statistically significant. The heterogeneity of RCC within the same T-stage and grade has resulted in a need for more specific prognostic markers, related to molecular mechanisms of RCC, to specify diagnosis, staging and prognosis. Prognostic markers can also be used in to select treatment modalities, help in surveillance, and to determine eligibility for clinical trials. p53 associates weakly with tumor grade whereas Ki-67 associates with T-stage and metastatic development, indicating that Ki-67 is a marker for aggressive disease in RCC with an increased risk of early metastases development. The proportion of COX-2 positive tumors is highest in RCC with the ability to develop later metastases, when compared to both RCC without metastatic potential, and RCC with primary metastases. Metastases-free survival is longer in patients with COX-2 positive tumors compared to COX-2 negative tumors. These data show that COX-2 negativity associates with an aggressive phenotype in mRCC disease. COX-2 and Ki-67 alone are stronger biomarkers than p53 for the development of metastases in RCC. Her-2 seems to associate with p53 and Ki-67, but results of associations between Her-2 and survival have been contradictory. Few studies have been published on the significance of Her-2 protein expression or *Her-2* gene amplification in RCC, so more studies are warranted. p53 or Ki-67 alone are not valuable prognostic markers in locally confined RCC, but they can predict poor survival in mRCC. Therefore, p53 and Ki-67 can help in determining metastatic patients with a poor prognosis and, e.g. those who would benefit from high-dose IL-2 or temsirolimus. COX-2 positivity predicts improved overall survival in patients with mRCC treated with IFN-α. p53, Ki-67, and COX-2 cannot predict response to IFN-α. Investigating the ability of p53, Ki-67, and COX-2 protein expression to predict overall survival in a prospective clinical trial would answer the question of whether these biomarkers can be reliably used in mRCC. Combining the results of COX-2 and Ki-67 expression, may predict overall survival in mRCC. In predicting the development of metastases in nephrectomized RCC patients, COX-2 alone or a covariation of p53 and Ki-67 seem to have prognostic value. Combining p53 or COX-2 with Ki-67 may result in more specific prognosis staging in RCC than observing a single marker. In future, using the tissue microarray technique, the protein expression profile with several biomarkers can be determined quickly. Further investigations are needed on the reproducibility of staining of these novel biomarkers, and on validation of the ability of the expressions to discriminate clinical outcome in RCC. Findings on novel biomarkers have increased our understanding of the molecular biology of locally confined RCC patients and metastatic RCC patients. RCC is characterized by high resistance to radiation and chemotherapy, which may be due to the suppression of apoptotic mechanisms, such as the p53 tumour suppressor pathway. In RCC patients, Ki-67 expression is not very high, which may partly explain RCC's resistance to chemotherapy. Specification of the roles of novel tumor-related molecular prognostic factors might be translated into prognostic tools that could be used in clinical work.

5. References

Aaltomaa S et al. (1997). Prognostic value of Ki-67 expression in renal cell carcinomas. Eur Urol 31(3): 350-355

American Cancer Society (2004). Cancer facts and figures.

Amin MB et al. (2002). Prognostic impact of histologic subtyping of adult renal epithelial neoplasms: an experience of 405 cases. Am J Surg Pathol 26 (3):281-291.

Antonelli A et al. (2003). The collecting duct carcinoma of the kidney: a cytogenetical study. Eur Urol 43 (6): 680-685.

Arteaga CL et al. (2001) Inhibitors of HER2/neu (erbB-2) signal transduction. Semin Oncol 28 (6 Suppl 18): 30-35.

Atkins M et al. (2005). Carbonic anhydrase IX expression predicts outcome of interleukin 2 therapy for renal cancer. Clin Cancer Res 11: 3714-3721.

Atzpodien J et al. (2002). Thirteen-year, long-term efficacy of interferon 2alpha and interleukin 2-based home therapy in patients with advanced renal cell carcinoma. Cancer 95 (5): 1045-1050.

Atzpodien J et al.; DGCIN -- German Cooperative Renal Carcinoma Chemo-Immunotherapy Trials Group (2003).Metastatic renal carcinoma comprehensive prognostic system. Br J Cancer 88 (3): 348-353.

Atzpodien J et al.; German Cooperative Renal Carcinoma Chemo-Immunotherapy Trials Group (DGCIN) (2005). Adjuvant treatment with interleukin-2- and interferon-alpha2a-based chemoimmunotherapy in renal cell carcinoma post tumour nephrectomy: results of a prospectively randomised trial of the German Cooperative Renal Carcinoma Chemoimmunotherapy Group (DGCIN). Br J Cancer 92 (5): 843-846.

Bassil B et al. (1985).Validation of the tumor, nodes and metastasis classification of renal cell carcinoma. J Urol 134: 450-454.

Belldegrun A et al. (1999).Efficacy of nephron-sparing surgery for renal cell carcinoma: analysis based on the new 1997 tumor-node- metastasis staging system. J Clin Oncol 17: 2868-2875.

Bodmer D et al. (2002). Understanding familial and non-familial renal cell cancer. Hum Mol Genet. 11 (20): 2489-2498.

Bosniak MA et al. (1995). Small renal parenchymal neoplasms: further observations on growth. Radiology 197: 589-597.

Bracarda S et al. (2011). Overall survival in patients with metastatic renal cell carcinoma initially treated with bevacizumab plus interferon-α2a and subsequent therapy with tyrosine kinase inhibitors: a retrospective analysis of the phase III AVOREN trial. BJU Int. 107(2): 214-219.

Bretheau D et al. (1995). Prognostic value of nuclear grade of renal cell carcinoma. Cancer 76 (12): 2543-2549.

Bui MH et al. (2003). Carbonic anhydrase IX is an independent predictor of survival in advanced renal clear cell carcinoma: implications for prognosis and therapy. Clin Cancer Res 9: 802-811.

Bui MH et al. (2004). Prognostic value of carbonic anhydrase IX and KI67 as predictors of survival for renal clear cell carcinoma. J Urol 171 (6 Pt 1): 2461-2466.

Cao Y and Prescott SM (2002) . Many actions of cyclooxygenase-2 in cellular dynamics and in cancer. J Cell Physiol 190(3): 279-286.

Chao D et al. (2002). Collecting duct renal cell carcinoma: clinical study of a rare tumor. J Urol 167: 71-74.

Cheville JC et al. (2003). Comparisons of outcome and prognostic features among histologic subtypes of renal cell carcinoma. Am J Surg Pathol 27 (5): 612-624.

Cho KS et al. (2008). A comprehensive prognostic stratification for patients with metastatic renal clear cell carcinoma. Yonsei Med J 49 (3): 451-458.

Cho DS et al. (2005). Cyclooxygenase-2 and p53 expression as prognostic indicators in conventional renal cell carcinoma. Yonsei Med J 46 (1): 133-140.

Choisy-Rossi C and Yonish-Rouach E (1998). Apoptosis and the cell cycle: the p53 connection. Cell Death Differ 5: 129-131.

Choueiri M et al (2011). Adjuvant and neoadjuvant therapy in renal cell carcinoma. Curr Clin Pharmacol. 6 (3): 144-50.

Choueiri TK et al. (2007). Prognostic factors associated with long-term survival in previously untreated metastatic renal cell carcinoma. Ann Oncol 18 (2): 249-255.

Chow WH et al. (2000). Obesity, hypertension, and the risk of kidney cancer in men. N Engl J Med 343: 1305-1311.

Corless CL et al. (1997). Immunostaining of the von Hippel-Lindau gene product in normal and neoplastic human tissues. Hum Pathol. 28 (4): 459-464.

De Luca A and Normanno N (2010). Tivozanib, a pan-VEGFR tyrosine kinase inhibitor for the potential treatment of solid tumors. Idrugs 13(9): 636-645.

Cunningham J (1938). The kidney: tumors. 1938 Year book of Urology 167-192.

Delahunt B et al. (2002). Prognostic importance of tumor size for localized conventional (clear cell) renal cell carcinoma: assessment of TNM T1 and T2 tumor categories and comparison with other prognostic parameters. Cancer 94: 658-664.

Donskov F et al. (2004). In vivo assessment of the antiproliferative properties of interferon-alpha during immunotherapy: Ki-67 (MIB-1) in patients with metastatic renal cell carcinoma. Br J Cancer 90 (3): 626-631.

du Manoir S et al. (1991). Ki-67 labeling in postmitotic cells defines different Ki-67 pathways within the 2c compartment. Cytometry 12:455-463.

Dudderidge TJ et al. (2005). Mcm2, Geminin, and KI67 define proliferative state and are prognostic markers in renal cell carcinoma. Clin Cancer Res 11: 2510-2517.

Eble JN (2003). Mucinous tubular and spindle cell carcinoma and post-neuroblastoma carcinoma: newly recognised entities in the renal cell carcinoma family. Pathology 35(6):499-504.

Eble JN et al., eds. (2004). World Health Organization Classification of Tumors. Pathology and Genetics of Tumors of the Urinary System and Male Genital Organs. IARC Press, Lyon, p360.

Elinq TE et al. (1990). Prostaglandin H synthase and xenobiotic oxidation. Ann Rev Pharmacol Toxicol 30: 1-45.

Elmore JM et al. (2003). Reassessment of the 1997 TNM classification system for renal cell carcinoma. Cancer 98 (11): 2329-2334.

Escudier B et al.; TARGET Study Group (2007). Sorafenib in advanced clear-cell renal-cell carcinoma. N Engl J Med 356(2):125-134. Erratum in: N Engl J Med. 2007 357 (2): 203.

Ferlay J et al (2010). GLOBOCAN 2008 v1.2, Cancer Incidence and Mortality Worldwide: IARC CancerBase No. 10 [Internet]. Lyon, France: International Agency for Research on Cancer; 2010.

Ficarra V et al. (2001). Prognostic value of renal cell carcinoma nuclear grading: multivariate analysis of 333 cases. Urol Int 67 (2): 130-134.

Finlay C et al. (1998). Activating mutations for transformation by p53 produce a gene product that forms an hsc70-p53 complex with an altered half-life. Mol Cell Biol 8: 531-539.

Finnish Cancer Registry (2007). Institute for Statistical and Epidemiological Cancer Research: Cancer in Finland 2004 and 2005. Cancer Statistics of the National Research and Development Centre for Welfare and Health (STAKES), publication No. 72. Cancer Society of Finland, Helsinki.

Flanigan RC et al. (2001). Nephrectomy followed by interferon alfa-2b compared with interferon alfa-2b alone for metastatic renal-cell cancer. N Engl J Med 345: 1655-1659.

Fuhrman SA et al. (1982). Prognostic significance of morphologic parameters in renal cell carcinoma. Am J Surg Pathol 6: 655-663.

Galban S et al. (2003). Influence of the RNA-binding protein HuR in pVHL-regulated p53 expression in renal carcinoma cells. Mol Cell Biol 23 (20): 7083-7095.

George DJ and Kaelin WG Jr (2003). The von Hippel-Lindau protein, vascular endothelial growth factor, and kidney cancer. N Engl J Med 349 (5): 419-421.

Gerdes J et al. (1984). Cell cycle analysis of a cell proliferation-associated human nuclear antigen defined by the monoclonal antibody Ki-67. J Immunol 133: 1710-1715.

Giuliani L et al. (1990). Radical extensive surgery for renal cell carcinoma: long-term results and prognostic factors. J Urol 143: 468-473.

Gnarra JR et al. (1994). Mutations of the VHL tumor suppressor gene in renal carcinoma. Nat Genet 7: 85-90.

Goldstein NS (1997). The current state of renal cell carcinoma grading. Union Internationale Contre le Cancer (UICC) and the American Joint Committee on Cancer (AJCC) Cancer 80 (5): 977-980.

Goldstein R et al. (2010). Does axitinib (AG-01376) have a future role in metastatic renal cell carcinoma and other malignancies? Expert Rev Anticancer Ther 10(10): 1545-1557.

Gudbjartsson T et al. (2005). Histological subtyping and nuclear grading of renal cell carcinoma and their implications for survival: a retrospective nation-wide study of 629 patients. Eur Urol 48 (4): 593-600.

Guinan P et al. (1997). TNM staging of renal cell carcinoma: Workgroup No. 3. Union International Contre le Cancer (UICC) and the American Joint Committee on Cancer (AJCC). Cancer. 80: 992-993.

Guinan PD et al. (1995). Renal cell carcinoma: tumor size, stage and survival. Members of the Cancer Incidence and End Results Committee. J Urol 153: 901-903.

Hara S et al. (2002). Expression of cyclooxygenase-2 in human bladder and renal cell carcinoma. Adv Exp Med Biol 507: 123-126.

Harmen PE (1978). TNM classification of malignant tumors. Union Internationale Contre le Cancer, Geneva.

Hashimoto Y et al. (2004). Cyclooxygenase-2 expression and relationship to tumour progression in human renal cell carcinoma. Histopathology 44 (4): 353-359.

Haitel A et al. (2000). mdm2 expression as a prognostic indicator in clear cell renal cell carcinoma: comparison with p53 overexpression and clinicopathological parameters. Clin Cancer Res 6(5): 1840-4.

Herman JG et al. (1994). Silencing of the VHL tumor-suppressor gene by DNA methylation in renal carcinoma. Proc Natl Acad Sci U S A. 91 (21): 9700-9704.

Herschman HR (1996). Prostaglandin synthase 2. Biochim. Biophys Act 1299: 125-140

Hofmockel G et al. (1997). Epidermal growth factor family and renal cell carcinoma: expression and prognostic impact. Eur Urol 31 (4): 478-484.

Hofmockel G et al. (1996). Related Articles, Expression of p53 and bcl-2 in primary locally confined renal cell carcinomas: no evidence for prognostic significance. Anticancer Res 16 (6B): 3807-3811.

Hollingsworth JM et al. (2006). Rising incidence of small renal masses: a need to reassess treatment effect. J Natl Cancer Inst. 98(18):1331-1334.

Hudes G et al. ; Global ARCC Trial. (2007). Temsirolimus, interferon alfa, or both for advanced renal-cell carcinoma. N Engl J Med 356 (22): 2271-2281.

Hunt JD et al. (2005). Renal cell carcinoma in relation to cigarette smoking: meta-analysis of 24 studies. Int J Cancer. 114 (1): 101-108.

Iliopoulos O et al. (1995). Tumor suppression by the human von Hippel-Lindau gene product. Nat Med 1 (8): 822-826.

Isola J et al. (2004). Interlaboratory comparison of HER-2 oncogene amplification as detected by chromogenic and fluorescence in situ hybridization. lin Cancer Res 10 (14): 4793-4798.

Itoi T et al. (2004). Impact of frequent Bcl-2 expression on better prognosis in renal cell carcinoma patients. Br J Cancer 90 (1): 200-205.

Janzen NK et al. (2003). Surveillance after radical or partial nephrectomy for localized renal cell carcinoma and management of recurrent disease. Urol Clin North Am 30: 843-852.

Javidan J et al. (1999). Prognostic significance of the 1997 TNM classification of renal cell carcinoma. J Urol 162:1277-81.

Jayson M and Sanders H (1998). Increased incidence of serendipitously discovered renal cell carcinoma. Urology 51: 203-205.

Kanamaru H et al. (2001). Prognostic value of nuclear area index in combination with the World Health Organization grading system for patients with renal cell carcinoma. Urology 57: 257-261.

Kanamaru H et al. (1999). Immunohistochemical expression of p53 and bcl-2 proteins is not associated with sarcomatoid change in renal cell carcinoma. Urol Res 27: 169-173.

Kankuri M et al. (2001). Feasibility of Prolonged Use of Interferon-alpha in Metastatic Kidney Carcinoma. A Phase II Study. Cancer 92 (4): 761-767.

Kankuri M et al. (2006). The Association of Immunoreactive p53 and Ki-67 with T-stage, Grade, Occurrence of Metastases and Survival in Renal Cell Carcinoma. Anticancer Res 26 (5B): 3825-3833.

Kankuri-Tammilehto M et al. (2010). Prognostic Evaluation of COX-2 Expression in Renal Cell Carcinoma. Anticancer Res 30(7):3023-30.

Khan KNM et al. (2001). Expression of cyclooxygenase-2 in canine renal cell carcinoma. Vet Pathol 38: 116-119.

Kim HL et al. (2004). Using protein expressions to predict survival in clear cell renal carcinoma. Clin Cancer Res 10 (16): 5464-5471.

Kirkali Z et al. (2001). Proliferative activity, angiogenesis and nuclear morphometry n renal cell carcinoma. Int J Urol 8: 697-703.

Kovacs G et al. (1997). The Heidelberg classification of renal cell tumors. J Pathol 183: 131-133.

Lanigan D et al. (1994). A comparative analysis of grading systems in renal adenocarcinoma. Histopathology 24: 473-476.

Lam JS et al. (2005). Postoperative surveillance protocol for patients with localized and locally advanced renal cell carcinoma based on a validated prognostic nomogram and risk group stratification system. J Urol 174: 466-472.

Latif Z et al. (2002). Gene amplification and overexpression of HER2 in renal cell carcinoma. BJU Int 89 (1): 5-9.

Lebeau A et al. (2001). Her-2/neu analysis in archival tissue samples of human breast cancer: comparison of immunohistochemistry and fluorescence in situ hybridization. J Clin Oncol 19 (2): 354-363.

Linehan WM et al. (2003). The genetic basis of cancer of the kidney. J Urol 170: 2163-2172.

Lipponen P et al. (1994). Expression of proliferating cell nuclear antigen (PC10), p53 protein and c-erbB-2 in renal adenocarcinoma. Int J Cancer 57 (2): 275-280.

Lohse CM et al. (2002). Comparison of standardized and nonstandardized nuclear grade of renal cell carcinoma to predict outcome among 2,042 patients. Am J Clin Pathol 118 (6): 877-886.

Masferrer JL et al. (2000). Antiangiogenic and antitumor activities of cyclooxygenase-2 inhibitors. Cancer Res 60:1306-1311.

Masters JR (2007). Clinical applications of expression profiling and proteomics in prostate cancer. Anticancer Res 27 (3A): 1273-1276.

Matei DV et al. (2005). Synchronous collecting duct carcinoma and papillary renal cell carcinoma: a case report and review of the literature. Anticancer Res 25 (1B): 579-586.

Mathew A et al. (2002). Global increases in kidney cancer incidence, 1973-1992. Eur J Cancer Prev 11 (2): 171-178.

Maurer-Gebhard M et al. (1998). Systemic treatment with a recombinant erbB-2 receptor-specific tumor toxin efficiently reduces pulmonary metastases in mice injected with genetically modified carcinoma cells. Cancer Res 58(12): 2661-2666.

Maxwell PH et al. (1999). The tumor suppressor protein VHL targets hypoxia-inducible factors for oxygen-dependent proteolysis. Nature 399: 271-275.

May P and May E (1999). Twenty years of p53 research: structural and functional aspects of the p53 protein. Oncogene 18: 7621-7636.

McNichols DW et al. (1981). Renal cell carcinoma: long-term survival and late recurrence. J Urol 126: 17-23.

Parkin DM et al. (2003). Cancer Incidence in Five Continents Vol. VIII. The International Agency for Research on Cancer (IARC) Scientific Publication No. 155. Globocan 2002. pp.1-782.

Medeiros LJ et al. (1997). Grading of renal cell carcinoma: Workgroup No. 2. Union Internationale Contre le Cancer and the American Joint Committee on Cancer (AJCC). Cancer 80 (5): 990-991.

Mickish GH (1999). Lymphatic metastases in renal cell carcinoma. What is the value of operation and adjuvant therapy? Urologe A 38: 326-331.

Mickisch GH et al, European Organisation for Research and Treatment of Cancer (EORTC) . enitourinary Group (2001) Radical nephrectomy plus interferon-alfa-based immunotherapy compared with interferon alfa alone in metastatic renal-cell carcinoma: a randomised trial. Lancet 358 (9286): 966-970.

Minasian LM et al. (1993). Interferon alfa-2a in advanced renal cell carcinoma: treatment results and survival in 159 patients with long-term follow-up. J Clin Oncol 11: 1368-1375.

Miyata Y et al. (2003). Expression of cyclooxygenase-2 in renal cell carcinoma: correlation with tumor cell proliferation, apoptosis, angiogenesis, expression of matrix metalloproteinase-2, and survival. Clin Cancer Res 9 (5): 1741-1749.

Montemurro F et al. (2003). Safety and activity of docetaxel and trastuzumab in HER2 overexpressing metastatic breast cancer: a pilot phase II study. Am J Clin Oncol 26 (1): 95-97.

Mostofi FK and Davis CJ in Collaboration with Sobin LH and Pathologists in 6 Countries. World Health Organization (1998). Histological Typing of Kidney Tumors; in (2nd ed): International Histological Classification of Tumors. Springer 1998, Berlin Heidelberg, pp. 1-117.

Motzer RJ et al. (2002). Interferon-alfa as a comparative treatment for clinical trials of new therapies against advanced renal cell carcinoma. J Clin Oncol 20 (1): 289-296.

Motzer RJ et al. (2004). Prognostic factors for survival in previously treated patients with metastatic renal cell carcinoma. J Clin Oncol 22: 454-463.

Motzer RJ et al. (2008). Prognostic nomogram for sunitinib in patients with metastatic renal cell carcinoma. Cancer 113 (7): 1552-1558.

Motzer RJ et al.; RECORD-1 Study Group (2008). Efficacy of everolimus in advanced renal cell carcinoma: a double-blind, randomised, placebo-controlled phase III trial. Lancet 372 (9637): 449-456.

Motzer RJ et al. (2000). Effect of cytokine therapy on survival for patients with advanced renal cell carcinoma. J Clin Oncol 18 (9): 1928-1935.

Mungan MU et al. (2006). Expression of COX-2 in normal and pyelonephritic kidney, renal intraepithelial neoplasia, and renal cell carcinoma. Eur Urol 50 (1): 92-97.

Négrier S et al. (2002). Prognostic factors of survival and rapid progression in 782 patients with metastatic renal carcinomas treated by cytokines: a report from the Groupe Français d'Immunothérapie. Ann Oncol. 2002 13 (9): 1460-1468.

Négrier S et al.; For The French Immunotherapy Intergroup (2007). Medroxyprogesterone, interferon alfa-2a, interleukin 2, or combination of both cytokines in patients with metastatic renal carcinoma of intermediate prognosis: results of a randomized controlled trial. Cancer 110 (11): 2468-2477.

Nose F et al. (2002). Up-regulation of cyclooxygenase-2 expression in lymphocytic thyroiditis and thyroid tumors: significant correlation with inducible nitric oxide synthase. Am J Clin Pathol 117 (4): 546-551.

Oda H et al. (1995). Mutations of the p53 gene and p53 protein overexpression are associated with sarcomatoid transformation in renal cell carcinomas. Cancer Res 55: 658-662.

Olayioye MA et al. (2000). The ErbB signaling network: receptor heterodimerization in development and cancer. EMBO J 19 (13): 3159-3167.

Olivier M et al. (2002). The IARC TP53 database: new online mutation analysis and recommendations to users. Hum Mutat 19: 607-614.

Olumi AF et al. (2001). p53 immunoreactivity correlates with Ki-67 and bcl-2 expression in renal cell carcinoma. Urol Oncol 6: 63-67.

Paner GP et al. (2006). Immunohistochemical analysis of mucinous tubular and spindle cell carcinoma and papillary renal cell carcinoma of the kidney: significant immunophenotypic overlap warrants diagnostic caution. Am J Surg Pathol 30 (1): 13-19.

Pantuck AJ et al. (2007). Use of carbonic anhydrase IX (CAIX) expression and Von Hippel Lindau (VHL) gene mutation status to predict survival in renal cell carcinoma. Journal of Clinical Oncology, ASCO Annual Meeting Proceedings Part I. Vol 25, No. 18S: 5042.

Patard JJ et al. (2005). Prognostic value of histologic subtypes in renal cell carcinoma: a multicenter experience. J Clin Oncol 23 (12): 2763-2771.

Phuoc NB et al. (2007). Immunohistochemical analysis with multiple antibodies in search of prognostic markers for clear cell renal cell carcinoma. Urology 69 (5): 843-848.

Pinto AE et al. (2005). Prognostic biomarkers in renal cell carcinoma: relevance of DNA ploidy in predicting disease-related survival. Int J Biol Markers 20(4): 249-56.

Pyrhönen S et al. (1999). Prospective randomized trial of interferon alfa-2a plus vinblastine versus vinblastine alone in patients with advanced renal cell cancer. J Clin Oncol 17 (9): 2859-2867.

Reich NC and Levine AJ (1984). Growth regulation of a cellular tumor antigen, p53, in nontransformed cells. Nature 308: 199-201.

Repmann R et al. (2003). Adjuvant therapy of renal cell carcinoma patients with an autologous tumor cell lysate vaccine: a five-year follow-up analysis. Anticancer Res 23: 969-974.

Rini BI et al. (2011). IMA901 Multipeptide Vaccine Randomized International Phase III Trial (IMPRINT): A randomized, controlled study investigating IMA901 multipeptide cancer vaccine in patients receiving sunitinib as first-line therapy for advanced/metastatic RCC. J Clin Oncol 29: 2011.

Rini BI et al. (2010). Phase III trial of bevacizumab plus interferon alfa versus interferon alfa monotherapy in patients with metastatic renal cell carcinoma: final results of CALGB 90206. J Clin Oncol. 2010 May 1;28(13):2137-43.

Rini BI et al. (2006). Maximal COX-2 immunostaining and clinical response to celecoxib and interferon alpha therapy in metastatic renal cell carcinoma. Cancer 106 (3): 566-575.

Rioux-Leclercq N et al. (2007). Prognostic ability of simplified nuclear grading of renal cell carcinoma. Cancer 109 (5): 868-874.

Rioux-Leclercq N et al. (2000). Value of immunohistochemical Ki-67 and p53 determinations as predictive factors of outcome in renal cell carcinoma. Urol 2000: 55: 501-505.

Roberts WW et al. (2005). Pathological stage does not alter the prognosis for renal lesions determined to be stage T1 by computerized tomography. J Urol 173 (3): 713-715.

Robson CJ et al. (2002). The results of radical nephrectomy for renal carcinoma. 1969. J Urol 167 (2 Pt 2): 873-875.

Seliger B et al. (2000). HER-2/neu is expressed in human renal cell carcinoma at heterogenous levels independently of tumor grading and staging and can be recognized by HLA-A2.1 restricted cytotoxic T lymphocytes. Int J Cancer 87 (3): 345-359.

Selli C et al. (1997). Retrospective evaluation of c-erbB-2 oncogene amplification using competitive PCR in collecting duct carcinoma of the kidney. J Urol 158 (1): 245-247.

Selli C et al. (1983). Stratification of risk factors in renal cell carcinoma. Cancer 52: 899-903.

Shvarts O et al. (200).. p53 is an independent predictor of tumor recurrence and progression after nephrectomy in patients with localized renal cell carcinoma. J Urol 173: 725-728.

Signoretti S et al. (2008). Tissue-based research in kidney cancer: current challenges and future directions. Clin Cancer Res. 2008 14 (12): 3699-3705.

Skinner DG et al. (1971). Diagnosis and management of renal cell carcinoma. A clinical and pathologic study of 309 cases. Cancer 28: 1165-1177.

Slamon DJ et al. (1989). Studies of the HER2/neu protooncogene in human breast and ovarian cancer. Science 244: 707-712.

Smith WL et al. (2000). Cyclooxygenases: structural, cellular, and molecular biology. Annu Rev Biochem 69: 145-182.

Smith I et al.; HERA study team (2007). 2-year follow-up of trastuzumab after adjuvant chemotherapy in HER2-positive breast cancer: a randomised controlled trial. Lancet 369 (9555): 29-36

Sobin L and Wittekind C (2002). TNM Classification of Malignant Tumors, 6th edition. John Wiley & Sons, Inc, New York, p239.

Spanknebel K et al. (2005). Initial clinical response predicts outcome and is associated with dose schedule in metastatic melanoma and renal cell carcinoma patients treated with high-dose interleukin 2. Ann Surg Oncol 12: 381-390.

Srigley JR et al. (1997). Current prognostic factors--renal cell carcinoma: Workgroup No. 4. Union Internationale Contre le Cancer (UICC) and the American Joint Committee on Cancer (AJCC). Cancer 80: 994-996.

Sternberg CN et al. (2010). Pazopanib in locally advanced or metastatic renal cell carcinoma: results of a randomized phase III trial. J Clin Oncol 28 (6): 1061-1068. Epub 2010 Jan 25.

Stumm G et al. (1996). Concomitant overexpression of the EGFR and erbB-2 genes in renal cell carcinoma (RCC) is correlated with dedifferentiation and metastasis. Int J Cancer 20 (69): 17-22.

Störkel S et al. (1997). Classification of renal cell carcinoma: Workgroup No. 1. Union Internationale Contre le Cancer (UICC) and the American Joint Committee on Cancer (AJCC). Cancer 80: 987-989.

Störkel S et al. (1989). Prognostic parameters in renal cell carcinoma - a new approach. Eur Urol 16: 416-422.

Subbaramaiah K et al. (1996). Transcription of cyclooxygenase-2 is enhanced in transformed mammary epithelial cells.Cancer Res 56 (19): 4424-4429.

Sunela KL et al. (2009). A phase-II study of combination of pegylated interferon alfa-2a and capecitabine in locally advanced or metastatic renal cell cancer. Cancer Chemother Pharmacol.

Syrjänen K and Hjelt L (1978). Grading of human renal adenocarcinoma. Scand J Urol Nephrol 12 (1): 49-55.

Tan X et al. (2008). Global analysis of metastasis-associated gene expression in primary cultures from clinical specimens of clear-cell renal-cell carcinoma. Int J Cancer 123 (5): 1080-1088.

Thoenes W et al. (1986). Histopathology and classification of renal cell tumors (adenomas, oncocytomas and carcinomas). The basic cytological and histomorphological elements and their use for diagnostics. Pathol Res Pract 181: 125-143.

Tsui KH et al. (2000). Prognostic indicators for renal cell carcinoma. A multivariate analysis of 643 patients using the revised 1997 TNM staging criteria. J Urol 163: 1090-1095.

Tsujii M and DuBois RN (1995). Alterations in cellular adehesion and apoptosis in epithelial cells overexpressing prostaglandin endoperoxide synthase 2. Cell 83: 493-501.

Tuna B et al. (2004). Significance of COX-2 expression in human renal cell carcinoma. Urology 2004, 64(6):1116-1120.

Uchida T et al. (2002). Clinical significance of p53, mdm2, and bcl-2 proteins in renal cell carcinoma. Urology: 59: 615-620.

Usubutyn A et al. (1998). Comparison of grading systems for estimating the prognosis of renal cell carcinoma. Int. Urol. Nephrol. 30:391-397.

van Houwelingen KP et al. (2005). Prevalence of von Hippel-Lindau gene mutations in sporadic renal cell carcinoma: results from The Netherlands cohort study. BMC Cancer 5:57.

Yang JC et al. (2007). Ipilimumab (anti-CTLA4 antibody) causes regression of metastatic renal cell cancer associated with enteritis and hypophysitis. J Immunother 30 (8): 825-830.

Yang JC et al. (2003). A randomized trial of bevacizumab, an anti-vascular endothelial growth factor antibody, for metastatic renal cancer. N Engl J Med 349 (5): 427-434.

Yildiz E et al. (2004). Prognostic value of the expression of Ki-67, CD44 and vascular endothelial growth factor, and microvessel invasion, in renal cell carcinoma. BJU Int 93: 1087-1093.

Yoshimura R et al. (2004). Study of cyclooxygenase-2 in renal cell carcinoma. Int J Mol Med 13 (2): 229-233.

Zhang D et al. (1997). Vitamin E inhibits apoptosis, DNA modification, and cancer incidence induced by iron-mediated peroxidation in Wistar rat kidney. Cancer Res 57 (12): 2410-2414.

Zigeuner R et al. (2004). Value of p53 as a prognostic marker in histologic subtypes of renal cell carcinoma: a sytematic analysis of primary and metastatic tumor tissue. Urology 63: 651-655.

Zisman A et al. (2001). Re-evaluation of the 1997 TNM classification for RCC: T1 and T2 cut-off point at 4.5 cm rather than 7 cm better correlates with clinical outcome. J Urol 166: 54-58.

Zisman A et al. (2002). Mathematical model to predict individual survival for patients with renal cell carcinoma. J Clin Oncol 20: 1368-1374.

17

Contemporary Management in Metastatic Renal Cell Carcinoma

Murat Lekili
Celal Bayar University, Medical Faculty, Urology Department, Manisa Turkey

1. Introduction

In addition to advancing our understanding of RCC, improved abdominal imaging technology has caused a migration of tumor stage and alteration of surgical strategies, with tumors commonly being diagnosed at an earlier stage. Despite these advances, the prognosis for patients with metastatic RCC is poor. Of the total number of patients with renal cancer, approximately a third either presents with or later develops metastatic disease. Unfortunately, for these patients, contemporary systemic therapies are generally ineffective—median survival is less than 1 year. Despite adjuvant systemic chemotherapy, hormonal or cytokine therapies, used alone or in combination, overall response rates rarely exceed 20% and durable, complete responses are rare. Targeted therapy in the management of metastatic renal cell cancer is newly introduced to urology practise. These drugs were used in very limited number of patients and only for clear cell histology. No recommendation to use these drugs for other than clear cell histology was seen in the literature. Nevertheless, there is a encouraging responses in trials with limited number of patients in the literature. Future advances are expected.

Spontaneous remissions in 0.8–7.0% of patients are reported in surgical series of clinical trials with previous surgical intervention. The role of surgical intervention in patients with metastatic renal cancer can be twofold. First, to render a patient clinically free of all sites of metastases ('metastasectomy'). Second, to resect the primary tumor prior to initiation of systemic therapy ('cytoreductive nephrectomy').

Studies that examine combinations of surgery and systemic therapy aim to improve survival in this high-risk group. In an attempt to address this important clinical issue, two randomized, prospective clinical trials were organized in the US (Southwest Oncology Group [SWOG]) and Europe (European Organization for Research and Treatment of Cancer [EORTC]) under similar entry criteria. The trials compared treatment of metastatic renal cancer with cytoreductive nephrectomy plus IFNα-2b versus IFNα-2b alone. Median survival of patients that underwent cytoreductive nephrectomy plus IFNα-2b was significantly greater than that of those treated with IFNα-2b only.

More recent metastasectomy studies also identified favorable clinical and surgical characteristics that were associated with a positive enhancement of outcome, but metastasectomy has never been assessed in a randomized clinical trial. It is not certain that metastasectomy can be curative, but operative intervention can provide effective palliation for symptomatic metastases in sites such as bone, the brain, and the adrenal gland. Ultimately a prospective clinical trial comparing metastasectomy to best standard systemic therapy will define the exact role of this approach.The occasionally unpredictable natural history of renal cancer and varying patient selection criteria can make the interpretation of outcomes from different centers difficult. As a conclusion although there is a tendency in favor of surgery, operative intervention for metastatic renal cancer is still controversial.

The aim of this review is more recent management modalities in the management of metastatic renal cell carcinoma. In addition, the role of surgery in metastatic RCC have been emphasised.

2. The role of nephrectomy

Although it is a part of multidisciplinary approach in the management of metastatic renal cell carcinoma (RCC), the role of Cytoreducive nephrectomy is still controversial in urologic literature. Recently according to some multicentric prospective randomized trials, because of providence little survival advantage, cytoreductive nephrectomy has gained some popularity. The objectives of nephrectomy in metastatic disease are avoidance of local symptoms and negative effects of primary tumor on immunological system (asynergy) and obtaining suitable nominee for immunotherapy, increasing patient quality of life and probably increased response to systemic therapy and finally increased overall survival. On the other hand, to prevent new metastases from primary tumor, capture of circulating immune cells, especially lymphocytes, which absorbed from primary tumor and so properties of immune pressure of primary tumor on immune system. Decreasing tumor burden may help the effectiveness of systemic therapy on tumor.

Surgical mortality rates are reported as 2-11%. In NCI trial, 62% patients can take immunotherapy and response rate is 18% in 195 patients. In this trial 38% patients cannot take immunotherapy because of complications of nephrectomy or rapid deterioration in general performance after progression of the disease (6). Some oncological centers recommend primary immunotherapy in order to avoid surgical morbidity especially in patients with clinical regression in metastatic sites (7,8).

Actually, two points provide that nephrectomy is a safe procedure; one is observation of spontaneous regression phenomena in metastatic sites after nephrectomy which is very rare. Freed has reported that 51 patients presented spontaneous regression after nephrectomy in literature (9). Similarly, NCI reported 4 patients (4.4%) have demonstrated spontaneous regression in 99 patients (10). In these 4 patients have only lung metastases and they were in remission for mean 24.3 months. Although spontaneous remission rates are very low, it is still very objective data in favor of nephrectomy. The other point for nephrectomy is unresponsiveness of primary tumor to systemic therapy. Radical nephrectomy may help to increase objective responses to systemic therapy. It has been obtained 32% objective response with immunotherapy after nephrectomy in 55 patients, but 4.7% response rate has been observed with same immunotherapeutic regimen in insitu tumor (11). Recently, surgical technique for cytoreductive nephrectomy is getting importance. Minimal invasive techniques gain popularity. While laparoscopic experience increased, laparoscopic radical nephrectomy performance is increasing in literature. The surgery time is longer, but postoperative analgesic requirements and hospital stay are decreasing. Therefore patients can take systemic therapy earlier than open surgery (Mean 35 vs 67 day). Patients without immunotherapy in case of disease progression are 13-77 % in literature (16). The shared conclusion of all the reports in literature is that the patients for cytoreductive nephrectomy have to be selected and they have to be in good ECOG performance status.

The last clues for nephrectomy are quality of life. Hematuri, pain and paraneoplastic syndromes including anemia, anorexia, hypertension, hypocalcaemia etc. can be controlled with nephrectomy.

In conclusion, multidisciplinary approach including surgery stands in the forefront. But some questions are on the agenda. Timing and coordination. Which one should be the first, nephrectomy or systemic therapy?

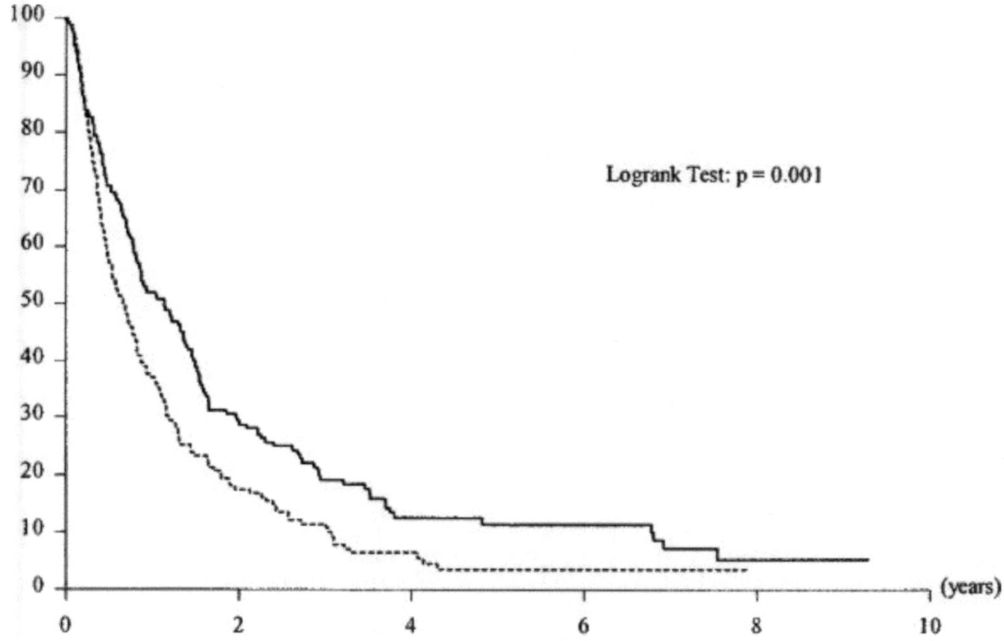

O	N	Number of patients at risk :				
141	161	46	13	9	3	—— Neph+IFN
152	163	26	7	1	0	------- IFN alone

O: Observation
N: Nephrectomy
Fig. 1. SWOG and EORTC trials

3. Metastasectomy

For a long time, if possible excision of metastases is recommended. Complete metastasectomy was performed in Kierney" report. 59% and 31% 3 and 5 years survival was obtained in 77 patients with metastatic RCC. These survivals were significantly different from patients within conservative follow (20,21). In another retrospective study with 278 patients, complete and incomplete metastasis resection can provide 44% vs 14% 5-years survival advantage (22).

In conclusion, the presence of solitary metastases and localization are important factors for clinical improvement. Resection of solitary metastases is recommended for survival and also quality of life.

4. Systemic treatments

4.1 Cytotoxic drugs

Standard cytotoxic drugs are generally ineffective. Response rates were reported below 10%. Response rate was reported 17% with Gemcitabine and 5-Florourasil combination in phase II study. Gemcitabine and capecitabine combination is effective as 20%. But grade 3-4 toxicity was reported. Same regimen reported by CALGB, Survival was 12% and stable disease rate was 59% in this study. Nevertheless toxicity was always a problem. 36% of patients could not continue the treatment protocol. The main problem is neutropenie and hand-food syndrome. Therefore, phase III studies can not be conducted.

4.2 Immunotherapy

Standard theurepathic regimen is still lack in the management of metastatic RCC. But interferon and interleukin therapy is in management list in many centers. Histological type is the most important factor for the response. The only histological type which is sensitive to immunotherapy is clear cell RCC. Granular, papillary or sarcomatoid type variants are resistant to immunotherapy. The main mechanism of cytokines is still contraversial. Cytokines are binding to specific receptors on tumor cells and initiate intracellular and intercellular signal mechanism. IL-2 is a potent stimulator of T cell proliferation. Anti-tumor T cells rapidly begin to proliferation, then tumor-specific cytotoxic T lymphocytes=CTL, natural killer lymphocytes=NK and probably intratumoral lymphocytes=TIL become active and try to kill tumor cell. However, interferons have some antiangiogenetic effects. Absence of anemia and hypocalcaemia, normal lactic dehydrogenase, prior nephrectomy and good performance status increase possibility of positive response.

The main expectations for immunotherapy in metastatic RCC

- Overhelming of T-lymphocite dysfunction, dendrtic cell dysfunction, soluble inhibitory factors secreted from tumor cells (IL-10),
- The changes of T-lymphocite antigen receptors and transmission of signals (TCRdelta, decreasing p56 levels, NFkappaB compliment changes)
- Identification of unique tumor surface antigens
- Vaccination manuplations for immun tolerence

Current immunotheraupeutic cytokines are;

- Interferons
- İnterleukins
- Colony-stimulating factors (CSF)
- Tumor necrosis factor (TNF)

4.3 Interferon

IFN-alpha is approved for the management of metastatic RCC in Europe and it is used routinely in Urological practise. Response rates are 10-25%. Recently, with recombinant forms response rates are increased to 29%. Survival advantage is 3-5 months. Toxicities are flu-like syndromes, dryness in skin and mucosal membranes, mental changes and depression. Combination with IL-2 is frequently applied in many centers. Dosage scheme is controversial.

IFN-beta and gamma are ineffective.

4.4 Interleukin-2 (IL-2)

A group of cytocine which are activated and regulated lymphocite growing and/ or differantiation

First described one is IL-2.

It is produced by activated CD4+ lymphocites.Cytotoxic T cells are stimulated by IL-2. CD8+ T cells, monocytes, lymphocyte activated killer lymphocytes (LAK) are activated and tumor necrosis factor is secreted. It is reported that IL-2 is as effective as 15% in many series. Rekombinant IL-2 (rIL-2)

- Bolus high-dose *i.v.* infusion= highly toxic
- İnhalation
- Response rate 7-27%
- Only clear cell type is respondable

Recently, there are more than 10 interleukin described other than IL-2 (IL-4; IL-7; IL-12 have been still investigating)

4.5 Cytokine combination therapy

Class I MHC Ag expression + T-lymphocite activation

- Synergy
- Mean 22% response
- Similar response rate as seen in high-dose IL-2

Phase 1 and 2 studies showed that response rates were 6-30%. Retrospective series showed that 15% and 20% response rates, but these results are not statistically significant. Nevertheless, mean survival is a little bit meaningful (9.1 vs 13 mos).

4.6 Targeted therapies

Since more new agents have been produced and limited number of prospective, randomized, placebo-controlled studies have been reported, Therefore, we have evaluated only;

1. Sorafenib (Nexavar®)
2. Sunitinib (Sutent®)
3. Bevasizumab (Avastin®) + IFN-alfa

4. Temsirolimus (Torisel®) in this review

Sorafenib and/or sunitinib, a multikinase inhibitor of tumor-cell prolferation and angiogenesis, have been shown some activity, in two double blind, placebo-controlled trial in patients with metastatic renal cell ca. All the patients' histology were clear cell ca (24,25). Renal cell carcinoma is most aggressive and mortal genitourinary cancer with more than 40% of patients dying of cancer (26). Unfortunately, no reliable treatment alternative has been still conducted for especially metastatic RCC. Recently, investigations in targeted therapy including multikinase inhibition and antiangioenesis encouraged the clinicans that they have some activity in the management of metastatic RCC. Survival benefit with the targeted therapy was demonstrated in two double blind, placebo-controlled study in the treatment of metastatic disease (24,25). Nevertheless, there are still many unresponded questions. Response rate in different histological type is not clear. We have administered sorafenib in a patient with metastatic RCC with sarcomatoid differentiation and obtained excellent result.

This case report might be an evidence that antiangiogenic agents can be used in any histologic type of renal cell carcinoma.

Additional data on the durability of the response may further clarify the complete response and survival benefit

Inactive VHL gene

↓

HIF-1-alfa↑

↓

HIF-alpha/HIF-beta complex ↑

↓

Hypoxia induced gene transcription

↓ ↓ ↓ ↓

VGEF↑ PDGF-beta↑ TGF-alpha↑ Erythropoietin ↑

Fig. 2. Loss of VHL gene and pathways

Small molecule inhibitors have mainly targeted growth factor signals, cell cycle regulatory factors and angiogenesis. Growth factors like VGEF and PDGF have been effective by transmembrane tyrzin kinase receptors which expressed in endothelial cells. They have triggered autophosphorilazition of intracellular tyrozin kinase receptors and protein activation link with the attachment of extracellular parts of receptors. Recently many small molecule inhibitors have been discovered (27,28,29). Raf kinase inhibitors like sorafenib and sunitinib, multiple kinase like VEGFR-2, VEGFR-3 and PDGFR inhibitors or mTOR inhibitors like temsirolimus, everolimus and epidermal growth factor receptor tyrosine kinase inhibitors like erlotinib and lapatinib are the most popular molecules nowadays

(30,31). Nevertheless, still prospective, placebo-controlled studies are significantly lacking in describing the most effective treatment modality in the management of metastatic RCC (32).

5. Conclusion

Cytotoxic chemotherapy and immunotherapy are less effective treatment modalities in the management of metastatic RCC. However, better understanding of promotion of RCC caused newly produced many targeted therapies. Now, it is early to say that newly introduced drugs can solve the problem, but they are encouraging. .Due to SWOG and EORTC studies which are the most reliable studies in the literature, still primary nephrectomy and combination immunotherapy modalities are the only acceptable choice in patients with good performance status for the treatment of metastatic RCC.

6. References

[1] Russo P. Renal cell carcinoma: Presentation, staging and surgical treatment. Semin Oncol 2000; 27: 160-176.

[2] Russo P. Partial nephrectomy: The contemporary gold standard operation for T1 renal masses. Am J Urol Rev 2004; 2: 214-222.

[3] Chan DY, Marshall FF. Surgery in advanced and metastatic renal cell carcinoma. Curr Opin Urol 1998; 8(5): 369-373.

[4] Motzer RJ, Russo P. Systemic therapy for renal cell carcinoma. J Urol 2000; 163: 408-417.

[5] Russo P. Surgical intervention in patients with metastatic renal cancer: current status of metastasectomy and cytoreductive nephrectomy. Nat Clin Prac Urol 2004; 1(1): 26-30.

[6] Walther MM, Yang JC, Pass HI et al. Cytoreductive surgery before high dose IL-2 based therapy in patients with metastatic renal cell carcinoma. J Urol, 1997; 158:1675-78

[7] Rackley R, Novick AC, Klein EA. The impact of adjuvant nephrectomy on multimodality treatment of metastatic renal cell carcinoma J Urol. 1994; 152:1399-403

[8] Sella A et al Surgery following response to interferon-alpha-based therapy for residual renal cell carcinoma. J Urol 1993; 149 (1): 19-21.

[9] Freed SZ, Halperin JP, Gordon M. Idioppathic regression of metastases from renal cell carcinoma. J Urol 1977; 118 (4): 538-542.

[10] Marcus SG et al. Regression of metastatic renal cell carcinoma after cytoreductive nephrectomy. J Urol 1993; 150 (2): 463-466.

[11] Mickisch GHJ. Rational selection of a control arm for randomized trials in metastatic renal cell carcinoma. Eur Urol 2003; 43: 670-9.

[12] Wagner JR et al. Interleukin-2 based immunotherapy for metastatic renal cell carcinoma with the kidney in place. J Urol 1999; 162 (1): 43-45.

[13] Bennett RT, Lerner SE, Taub HC. Cytoreductive surgery for stage IV renal cell carcinoma J Urol, 1995; 154: 32-4.

[14] Krishnamurthi V, Novick AC, Bukowski RM. Efficacy of multimodality therapy in advanced RCC. Urology 1998; 51:933-7.

[15] Finelli A, Kaouk JH, Fergany AF et al. BJU International 2004; 94(3): 291-4.

[16] Wood CG. The role of cytoreductive nephrectomy in the management of metastatic renal cell carcinoma. Urol Clin N Am 2003; 30:581-588.

[17] Mickisch G, Garin A, van Poppel H et al. Radical nephrectomy plus interferon-alfa-based immunotherapy compared with interferon-alfa alone in metastatic renal cell carcinoma: a randomized trial. Lancet 2001; 358: 966-970.
[18] Flanigan RC, Salmon SE, Blumenstein BA et al. Nephrectomy followed by interferon-alfa-2b compared with interferon alfa-2b alone for metastatic renal cell cancer. N Eng J Med, 2001; 345: 1655-9.
[19] Flanigan RC, Mickisch G, Sylvester R et al. Cytoreductive nephrectomy in patients with metastatic renal cancer: A combined analysis. J Urol, 2004; 171:1071-1076.
[20] Kierney PC, van heerden JA, Segura JW et al. Surgeon`s role in the management of solitary renal cell carcinoma metastases occuring subsequent to initial curative nephrectomy: an institutional review. Ann Surg Oncol 1994; 1:345-352.
[21] Han KR, Pantuck AJ, Bui MH et al. Number of metastatic sites rather than location dictates overall survival of patients with node-negative metastatic renal cell carcinoma. Urology 2003; 61: 314-9.
[22] Kavolius JP, Mastrorakos DP, Pavlovich C et al. Resection of metastatic renal cell carcinoma J Clin Oncol 1998; 16: 2261-6.
[23] Swanson DA. Surgery for metastases of renal cell carcinoma. Scand J Surg 2004; 93: 150-5.
[24] Pirrotta MT, Bernardeschi P, Fiorentini G. Targeted-therapy in advanced renal cell carcinoma..Curr Med Chem. 2011;18(11):1651-7.
[25] Hutson TE. Targeted therapies for the treatment of metastatic renal cell carcinoma: clinical evidence.. Oncologist. 2011;16 Suppl 2:14-22.
[26] Facchini G, Perri F, Caraglia M, Pisano C, Striano S, Marra L, Fiore F, Aprea P, Pignata S, Iaffaioli RV New treatment approaches in renal cell carcinoma.. Anticancer Drugs. 2009 Nov;20(10):893-900.
[27] Escudier B Signaling inhibitors in metastatic renal cell carcinoma.. Cancer J. 2008 Sep-Oct;14(5):325-9.
[28] Mizutani Y Recent advances in molecular targeted therapy for metastatic renal cell carcinoma.. Int J Urol. 2009 May;16(5):444-8.
[29] Motzer RJ, Bukowski RM Targeted therapy for metastatic renal cell carcinoma.. J Clin Oncol. 2006 Dec 10;24(35):5601-8.
[30] Di Lorenzo G, Scagliarini S, Di Napoli M, Scognamiglio F, Rizzo M, Carteni' G Targeted therapy in the treatment of metastatic renal cell cancer.. Oncology. 2009;77 Suppl 1:122-31.
[31] Motzer RJ, Escudier B, Oudard S, Hutson TE, Porta C, Bracarda S, Grünwald V, Thompson JA, Figlin RA, Hollaender N, Urbanowitz G, Berg WJ, Kay A, Lebwohl D, Ravaud A; RECORD-1 Study Group Efficacy of everolimus in advanced renal cell carcinoma: a double-blind, randomised, placebo-controlled phase III trial. Lancet. 2008 Aug 9;372(9637):449-56.
[32] Patard JJ, Pouessel D, Bensalah K, Culine S Targeted therapy in renal cell carcinoma. World J Urol. 2008 Apr;26(2):135-40.

18

New Systemic Approaches in the Treatment of Metastatic Renal Cell Carcinoma

Thean Hsiang Tan[1], Judith Lees[1],
Ganesalingam Pranavan[2] and Desmond Yip[2,3]
[1]*RAH Cancer Centre, Royal Adelaide Hospital,*
[2]*Medical Oncology Unit, The Canberra Hospital,*
[3]*ANU Medical School, Australian National University,*
Australia

1. Introduction

Cancer of the kidney comprises approximately 3% of all cancers in males and 2% in females according to Cancer Research UK statistics. (http://info.cancerresearchuk.org) Similar figures are seen globally. The majority (around 90%) of kidney cancers are Renal Cell Carcinomas (RCC), and clear cell carcinomas (adenocarcinomas) are the most common histological subtype. (Cohen & McGovern, 2005) The remaining 20-25% are papillary (Type I and II) (10-15%), chromophobe (4%) and collecting duct (including the rare medullary variant) (<1%) RCCs. (Cohen & McGovern, 2005) Up to a third of patients present at initial diagnosis with evidence of distant metastases, and a third of patients who undergo nephrectomy will have a recurrence within 5 years. These patients are considered candidates for systemic therapy. (Molina & Motzer, 2008)

2. Molecular pathogenesis

2.1 Clear-cell variant renal cell carcinoma

Unravelling of the biology, genetics and intracellular molecular signalling pathways of RCC has greatly improved our understanding of this disease. (Tan *et al*, 2010) The discovery of von Hippel-Lindau (VHL) tumour suppressor gene as a critical oncogene in the pathogenesis of renal cell carcinoma (clear-cell as well as some of the non-clear-cell variant) has greatly revolutionised the systemic therapy for renal-cell carcinoma where previously treatment had been disheartening. (Choueiri *et al*, 2008; Cohen & McGovern, 2005) The VHL protein (pVHL) encoded by the VHL tumour suppressor gene serves to regulate the normal cellular response to oxygen deprivation through its interaction with hypoxia-inducible factor (HIF). HIF is a heterodimeric (HIF-α/β) gene transcription factor that consists of an unstable α-subunit and a stable β-subunit. In the presence of normal oxygen tension (or normoxic state), VHL protein is the substrate recognition of an E3 ubiquitin ligase complex that targets HIF-α subunits for destruction by the proteasome as illustrated in Figure 1. (Kamura et al, 2000; Ohh et al, 2000) In the absence of functional VHL proteins, either as a result of mutation or hyper-methylation of the VHL gene as seen in majority of sporadic cases of RCC (equivalent to a physiological hypoxic state), the pVHL-HIF-α interaction is disrupted due to loss of oxygen-dependent hydroxylation of HIF-α subunits leading to their intracellular accumulation. (Maxwell et al, 1999) HIF-α subunits are able to then translocate into the nucleus where they heterodimerize with the HIF-β subunits forming transcriptional factor complexes that induce transcription of various hypoxia-response genes. (Amato, 2011) This in turn leads to the increased production of downstream pro-angiogenic factors such as vascular endothelial growth factor (VEGF), platelet-derived growth factor (PDGF) and transforming growth factor alpha and beta (TGF-α and TGF-β) as illustrated by Figure 1. (Kim & Kaelin, 2004) It is noteworthy that angiogenesis holds the key to tumour survival when the rapidly growing tumour outstrips its own existing blood supply. It utilized the effective HIF mechanism to promote its own survival, growth and progression (metastasis). (Vaupel, 2004)

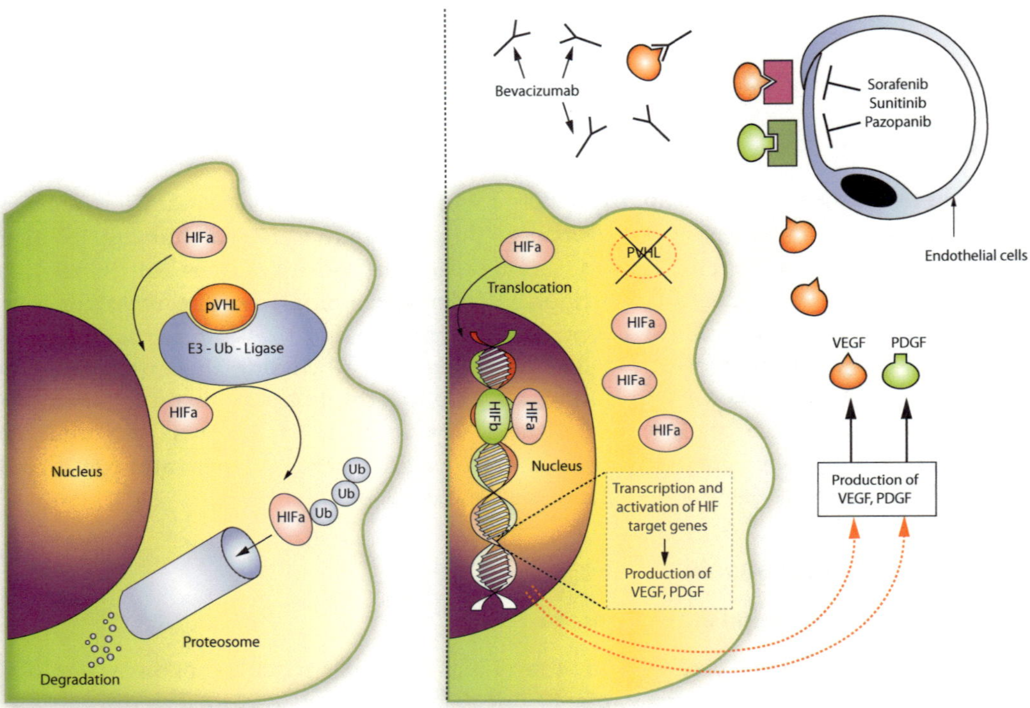

(a) (b)

Fig. 1. (a) Normoxia/normal VHL gene (b) Hypoxia/inactivated tumour suppressor VHL gene

2.2 Non clear-cell variant renal cell carcinoma

Papillary RCC is the second most common histological subtype of the non-clear cell variant of RCC. (Cohen & McGovern, 2005) It can be further categorized histologically into papillary types I and II with emerging data suggesting an underlying different genetics and molecular pathways. (Furge et al, 2010) Papillary type I RCC is associated with activating mutations of methyl-nitroso-nitroguanidine-induced (MET) oncogene. (Choi et al, 2006; Dharmawardana et al, 2004) These mutations results in ligand-independent activation of intracytoplasmic tyrosine kinase domains which subsequently activate the hepatocyte growth factor/MET pathway. (Choi et al, 2006; Sudarshan & Linehan, 2006) Papillary type II RCC, in contrast is attributed to mutation of the fumarate hydratase (FH) tumour suppressor gene. (Linehan et al, 2007) FH is a tricarboxylic acid (Kreb) cycle enzyme that has a crucial role in aerobic cellular metabolism. (Isaacs et al, 2005) Mutation of FH (inactivation) leads to the generation of a pseudo-hypoxic state with subsequent upregulation of the HIF-α subunits. The mutated FH enzyme allows the accumulation of fumarate which in turn leads to inhibition of HIF-prolyl hydroxylase (HPH), a critical enzymatic regulator of intracellular HIF-α. When HPH is inactivated, the hydroxylation of HIF is disrupted leading to failure of recognition by pVHL; thus preventing the VHL-dependent proteosomal degradation of HIFs. Accumulation of HIF-α leads to downstream transcriptional overexpression of pro-angiogenic factors as described in the previous section. (Isaacs et al, 2005)

Chromophobe RCC accounts for 4% of all RCC. (Cohen & McGovern, 2005) Whilst the exact mechanism underlying its pathogenesis is not well established, the VEGF-angiogenic pathway was again implicated in view of the elevated levels of VEGF and its receptor mRNA in this variant of RCC. The KIT oncogene and the folliculin (FLCN) gene associated with the hereditary form of chromophobe/oncocytic RCC hybrid (Birt-Hogg-Dubé Syndrome) are other molecular targets identified in this variant. (Pavlovich et al, 2002; Yamazaki et al, 2003; Zbar et al, 2002) Due to the rarity of collecting duct RCC (including the virulent medullary variant), the underlying pathogenesis has not been identify. (Oudard et al, 2007a)

3. Prognostic indicators

For patients with recurrent or metastatic disease, a question often faced by the treating physician is their prognosis as treatment is being contemplated. In metastatic RCC, numerous studies have been undertaken to investigate the prognostic markers for metastatic RCC. (Tan et al, 2010) Five prognostic markers linked to the overall survival rate of patients with metastatic RCC have been identified. These include performance status, absence or presence of prior nephrectomy, serum lactate dehydrogenase, corrected serum calcium and haemoglobin level. (Motzer *et al*, 1999) Based on these criteria, patients could be grouped into three prognostic risk categories: favourable (0 risk features), intermediate (1-2 risk features) and poor (≥3 risk features) according to the Memorial Sloan-Kettering Cancer Centre (MSKCC) risk classification. (Motzer *et al*, 1999) Previous radiotherapy, time to systemic therapy, and the presence of hepatic, pulmonary, and retroperitoneal nodal metastasis were found to be independent prognostic factors in later studies. (Mekhail *et al*, 2005) The stratification of the different prognostic factors of renal carcinoma in clinical studies is important to allow comparison of therapies and to gain insight into the cohort of patients that would most benefit from the investigational agent.

When comparing with the clear-cell variant of RCC, localized papillary RCC when resectable, has a more favourable prognosis than conventional clear cell. (Cheville *et al*, 2003; Patard *et al*, 2005) However, metastatic papillary RCC portends a worse prognosis than their clear-cell counterpart. (Margulis *et al*, 2008) The type II papillary variant is thought to be more aggressive than type I with a higher propensity to metastasize early and progress rapidly. (Motzer *et al*, 2004) Chromophobe RCC is considered a good prognostic variant and is associated with earlier stage tumour and longer overall survival compared to clear-cell RCC. In the metastatic setting, the reports from the medical literature are however conflicting. (Beck *et al*, 2004; Cindolo *et al*, 2005; Klatte *et al*, 2008; Motzer *et al*, 2002) Collecting duct RCC is associated with a grave prognosis, with up to one-third of patients presenting with metastatic disease on initial presentation. (Motzer *et al*, 2002)

4. Systemic treatment of metastatic renal cell carcinoma

Metastatic RCC is inherently refractory to chemotherapy and hormonal therapies. (Harris, 1983; Yagoda & Bander, 1989) The response rate of these treatment options are in the order of 10% thereby rendering RCC notoriously difficult to treat. (Yagoda & Bander, 1989) Solitary metastatic lesions may be surgically resected however beyond surgery, the only systemic options available prior to the era of targeted therapy were interferon alpha (IFN-α) and interleukin 2 (IL-2). (Oudard *et al*, 2007b) Allogeneic stem cell transplantation to induce a graft-versus-tumour response has also been examined but at the expense of significant life-threatening toxicities. This is therefore not recommended outside a clinical trial setting. (Barkholt *et al*, 2006; Gommersall *et al*, 2004; Rini *et al*, 2002) Patients with good prognostic features had a response rate of 10-20% to IFN-α and IL-2 and a modest improvement of median survival by ~2.5 months with IFN-α. (1999; Coppin et al, 2005) High dose IL-2 (infusion therapy requiring hospitalization) conferred a durable but small long term disease remission of ~5% in clinical responders. (Fyfe *et al*, 1995; McDermott *et al*, 2005) Both cytokine treatments especially with high dose IL-2 are toxic and difficult to administer. The classical side-effects of flu-like syndrome, depression with suicidal episodes from IFN-α; (Cohen & McGovern, 2005; Motzer *et al*, 1996) hypotension, oliguria, capillary-leak syndrome with secondary multi-organ failure, somnolence and confusion from IL-2 would render both treatments very onerous to patients. (Cohen & McGovern, 2005; Parton *et al*, 2006) Moreover the reported mortality rate of 4% from IL-2 would dilute any modest survival advantage gained. (Fyfe *et al*, 1995) Not surprisingly, the underlying enthusiasm in utilizing these agents as frontline therapy in metastatic RCC has been dampened with the advent of targeted therapies.

4.1 VEGF ligands and receptor inhibitors

Vascular endothelial growth factor (VEGF), platelet-derived growth factor (PDGF) and other angiogenic ligands once produced are able to circulate freely to to interact with cell surface receptors on the endothelial cell. Upon binding of these ligands to their cognate receptors, a cascade of intracellular signalling takes place resulting in downstream activation of Raf and mitogen-activated protein kinase (MAPK) (via phospholipase C-γ). This ultimately leads to the promotion of tumour angiogenesis, endothelial cell survival, proliferation, and migration. (Cebe-Suarez et al, 2006) The discovery of these complex VEGF signalling pathways presented an opportunity as therapeutic targets to treat metastatic RCC. VEGF signaling blockade can be achieved by either the removal of the circulating ligand with monoclonal antibody (bevacizumab) or by inhibiting its receptors with tyrosine kinase inhibitors (TKIs) as illustrated by Figure 1. (Jonasch et al, 2011) The four anti-VEGF therapies approved as of 2011: sunitinib, sorafenib, pazopanib and bevacizumab have revolutionized the treatment of metastatic RCC leading to significant improvement in progression-free survival (PFS) and in some instances overall survival (OS). (Tan et al, 2010)

4.1.1 Sunitinib

Sunitinib is an oral multi-kinase inhibitor that targets several VEGF receptors (VEGF-1, VEGF-2, VEGF-3) and other tyrosine kinase receptors (PDGFR, c-Kit, FLT-3, CSF-1R, and RET). (Abrams et al, 2003; Kim et al, 2006; Mendel et al, 2003; Murray et al, 2003; O'Farrell et al, 2003) Earlier uncontrolled trials showed sunitinib to be active in patients with advanced malignancies including RCC. (Faivre *et al*, 2006)

4.1.1.1 Sunitinib Intermittent Dosing (4 Weeks On / 2 Weeks Off)

The initial phase II study of sunitinib in patients with cytokine-refractory metastatic renal cell cancer assessed the clinical efficacy and safety of sunitinib as second-line therapy. (Motzer et al, 2006) The sixty three patients who failed cytokine-based therapy received 50mg of sunitinib for 4 weeks followed by a 2 week break (4/2), in a 6 week cycle. Forty percent (n=25) of patients had partial response (PR) and 27% (n=17) additional patients demonstrated stable disease (SD) for ≥3 months. The median time to progression and survival were 8.7 months and 16.4 months respectively. (Motzer et al, 2006)

A larger phase II multicentre trial similarly confirmed the anti-cancer efficacy of sunitinib in cytokine refractory patients with metastatic RCC. One hundred and six patients were enrolled and an overall objective response (ORR) of 44% was noted with 1% (n=1) and 43% (n=45) demonstrating a CR and PR respectively. (Motzer et al, 2007b) An additional 22% (n=23) showed SD for ≥ 3 months. The median duration of response for the 46 responding patients was 10 months whilst the median progression free survival (PFS) was 8.3 months. (Motzer et al, 2007b)

As the ORR of sunitinib seen in phase II trials far exceeded the rates previously reported for cytokine therapy as first line treatment of metastatic disease (42% vs. 10–15%), an international landmark phase III trial comparing sunitinib with INF-α for patients with metastatic clear-cell RCC was undertaken. (Costa & Drabkin, 2007; Motzer et al, 2007a) Seven hundred and fifty treatment naïve patients with clear-cell histology and good performance status (ECOG 0 or 1) were randomized in a 1:1 ratio to receive either sunitinib (dose as per earlier studies) or INF-α (9×10^6 units subcutaneously thrice weekly). (Desai *et al*, 2007; Motzer *et al*, 2007a) The median duration of treatment was 6 months (1-15 months) in the sunitinib group and 4 months (1-13 months) in the IFN-α group. The median PFS assessed by an independent third-party review was 11 months in the sunitinib group and 5 months in the IFN-α group, corresponding to a Hazard Ratio (HR) of 0.42 (95% CI 0.32–0.54; $p < 0.001$). (Motzer et al, 2007a) The investigators' assessment showed similar results, with a PFS of 11 months in the sunitinib and 4 months in the IFN-α group. An updated analysis published in 2009 has shown the ORR of 47% for sunitinib and 12% for IFN-α ($p < 0.000001$), with a median PFS of 11 months and 5 months, respectively, for sunitinib and IFN-α ($p < 0.000001$), similar to the original report. (Motzer *et al*, 2009) These results were uniformly seen, regardless of patient's age, gender and prognostic category. (Motzer *et al*, 2009) Patients on sunitinib also experienced a median OS in excess of 2 years. The OS was 26.4 months for sunitinib and 21.8 months for IFN-α ($p = 0.051$). (Motzer *et al*, 2009) A separate exploratory analysis of patients on both treatment arms who did not receive post-study cancer treatment showed the median OS with sunitinib was twice as long as IFN-α (28.1 months versus 14.1 months respectively, p=0.003). (Motzer *et al*, 2009) Based on these positive results, sunitinib has replaced INF-α in the first line treatment of metastatic RCC.

In addition to the aforesaid clinical trials, sunitinib was also evaluated in an expanded-access programme, designed to allow access to sunitinib in patients with metastatic RCC who would otherwise be excluded from the clinical trials. (Gore et al, 2009) Over 4500 patients, including older patients (≥65 years-old; n=1414), those with poorer performance status (ECOG PS ≥2; n=582), non-clear cell histology (n=288) and with brain metastases (n=320) were enrolled in this international, open-label study, thus resembling a more "real-world" setting. (Gore et al, 2009) Patients received a median of five sunitinib treatment cycles, with 56% of patients receiving more than 6 months of sunitinib therapy for a median duration of 15.6 months. In the total evaluable study population (n=4349), the median PFS was 10.9 months and median OS was 18.4 months. (Gore et al, 2009) The median PFS closely resembles the phase III study demonstrating consistent efficacy across patients within and outside clinical trials. No differences were noted in median PFS and OS between patients with or without prior cytokine therapy. Subgroup analysis of elderly patients demonstrated median PFS and OS of 11.3 and 18.2 months respectively. (Gore et al, 2009) In patients with poorer performance status, median PFS and OS were 5.1 months and 6.7 months respectively and lastly in patients with brain metastases with an overall poorer prognosis, a median PFS of 5.6 months and median OS of 9.2 months were observed. (Gore et al, 2009)

4.1.1.2 Sunitinib Continuous Dosing

Sunitinib has also been examined in an open-label multicentre phase II trial using continuous once daily dosing at a dose of 37.5 mg. (Escudier *et al*, 2009b) One hundred and seven patients were randomised equally to either morning or evening dose for a median 8.3 months. Forty three percent of patients had dose reduction to 25mg due to grade 3-4 adverse effects. (Escudier *et al*, 2009b) The ORR was 20%, with a median duration of response of 7.2 months, median PFS of 8.2 months and OS of 19.8 months. (Escudier *et al*, 2009b) The tolerability of the morning and evening dosing as well as the reporting quality of life (QoL) whilst on therapy was similar. Grade 3 diarrhoea, fatigue/asthenia and hand-foot syndrome were however noted more in the evening dosing cohort. This continuous regimen appeared promising and certainly deserves further investigation as this dosing schedule may benefit patients who are not able to tolerate the intermittent sunitinib dosing of 50mg and where one is concerned that the intermittent 37.5mg is suboptimal.

Sunitinib standard dosing schedule (50mg/day; 4 weeks on, 2 weeks off) was compared with continuous dose (37.5 mg/day) in a phase II trial (EFFECT) for patients with locally recurrent clear-cell RCC or metastatic RCC who had received no previous systemic therapy for advanced disease. The intermittent schedule when compared with the continuous schedule showed a trend to improved ORR (32.2% vs. 28.1%; p=0.444) and median PFS (8.5 months vs. 7.0 months; p=0.070). No difference were noted between the median OS (23.1 months vs. 23.5 months, p=0.615). (Motzer *et al*, 2011b) Interestingly the median OS was lower than the phase III sunitinib vs. INF-α trial which had a median OS of 26 months. The phase III trial had a higher number of patients with better baseline prognostic features (better performance status and more patients had underwent nephrectomy) which may account for better survival results. (Motzer *et al*, 2011b; Motzer *et al*, 2007a)

4.1.2 Sorafenib

Sorafenib is an oral multi-kinase inhibitor that inhibits Raf (Raf-1, B-Raf, and mutant *b-raf V600E*), VEGF (VEGF-2, VEGF-3), PDGFR (PDGFR-α, PDGFR-β), c-KIT, FLT3 and RET.

(Carlomango 2006, Wilhelm 2004) A phase II randomized discontinuation trial in 202 patients with metastatic RCC who failed previous systemic treatments were treated with sorafenib at 400 mg BD. (Ratain et al, 2006) Seventy-three patients exhibited tumour shrinkage of more than 25%. Sixty-five patients with stable disease at 12 weeks were randomly assigned to sorafenib (n=32) or placebo (n=33). Patients on sorafenib experienced prolonged median PFS (24 weeks) when compared to placebo (6 weeks) ($p = 0.087$). (Ratain et al, 2006) A second phase II trial comparing sorafenib with INF-α as first line treatment was undertaken in treatment naïve patients with metastatic RCC. Patients were randomised to receive sorafenib 400mg BD or IFN-α (9 million units thrice weekly). There was an option of dose escalation to sorafenib 600mg BD or crossover from INF-α to sorafenib upon disease progression. There was no significant improvement in PFS of sorafenib vs. placebo, 5.7 months vs. 5.8 months respectively. The ORR was 5% with sorafenib and 9% with IFN-α. (Escudier *et al*, 2009c)

A subsequent multi-centre placebo controlled phase III trial (TARGET) randomised 903 patients with metastatic clear-cell RCC on 1:1 to receive either placebo or sorafenib 400mg BD. The study cohort consisted of patients who previously received cytokine therapies with IFN-α, IL-2 or a combination of both, or radiotherapy, or had a nephrectomy. After 3 months of therapy, sorafenib resulted in a higher ORR (57% vs. 34%) and statistically significant longer PFS (5.5 months vs. 2.8 months; $p< 0.001$ with a HR of 0.44) when compared with placebo. (Escudier *et al*, 2007b) This was consistent with an earlier phase II second line trial that found PFS benefit was independent of age over or under 70 years, prognostic risk, prior cytokine therapy, lung, liver, bone or brain metastases, time from diagnosis, or whether or not the patient had clinical cardiovascular disease. (Beck *et al*, 2011; Escudier *et al*, 2007b) The latter included patients with ischemic heart disease, a previous myocardial infarction, left ventricular dysfunction, hypertension, epistaxis or central nervous system ischemia. (Beck *et al*, 2011) Patients on the placebo arm were permitted to cross over to sorafenib on diagnosis of progressive disease. In the first interim analysis, a trend towards better OS was noted in patients taking sorafenib, and this was unchanged in the final analysis (17.8 vs. 15.2 months, respectively, HR= 0.88; $p = 0.146$). (Escudier *et al*, 2007b; Escudier *et al*, 2009a) However, after placebo patients who crossed over on progression were censored, the difference in OS became significant (17.8 vs. 14.3 months; HR = 0.78; $p = 0.029$). (Escudier *et al*, 2007b)

Sorafenib has also been evaluated in two open-label expanded access studies in Europe (The European Advanced Renal Cell Carcinoma Sorafenib (EU-ARCS) and North America ARCCS (NA-ARCCS). The NA-ARCCCS offered insights into sorafenib in the real world setting. (Beck *et al*, 2008; Beck *et al*, 2011; Stadler *et al*, 2010) In Europe, about 1155 patients who failed at least one line of systemic therapy or were unsuitable for cytokine therapy received sorafenib 400mg BD until treatment intolerance or disease progression. Interim analysis revealed a median PFS of 6.9 months (95% CI: 6.2 - 7.5 months). (Beck *et al*, 2008) The North American access study enrolled 2515 patients in total with 2504 patients having received at least one cycle of sorafenib and therefore evaluable. Patients who had received no prior systemic therapy were allowed enrolment. Except for the difference in the median time from diagnosis (0.6 years vs. 2.2 years), prior nephrectomy rates (77% vs. 89%) and the incidence of >2 sites of metastatic disease prior to study entry (30% vs. 38%), the baseline characteristics were mostly balanced for patients who were treatment-naïve and patients who had at least one prior systemic treatment. The rate of disease progression was similar for fist-line sorafenib patients and patients who had received at least on e prior systemic treatment (16% vs. 17%). Similarly the rates of PFS and disease control (ORR + stable disease) were 83% vs. 84% in the first-line and prior systemic therapy cohorts, respectively. (Eisenhauer *et al*, 2009) These results demonstrate that sorafenib provides similar benefit in first- and second- or later line patient populations in a non-randomised, open access trial. (Stadler *et al*, 2010)

4.1.3 Pazopanib

Pazopanib is an oral multi-targeted receptor tyrosine kinase inhibitor that inhibits VEGF (VEGF-1, VEGF-2, VEGF-3), PDGF (PDGF-α, PDGF-β) and c-KIT. (Hutson *et al*, 2010) Pazopanib showed activity in a phase I trial with 2 partial responders and 4 patients achieving disease stability out of a total 12 patients. (Hurwitz *et al*, 2009) Subsequently, a randomised phase II study to determine the ORR, duration of response and PFS was undertaken on patients with predominantly clear-cell histology who had never been treated or had failed one line of non-multi-kinase therapy. This study was originally designed as a randomized discontinuation study but revised to an open-label study after a planned interim analysis undertaken at 12 weeks showed a response rate of 38%. (Hutson *et al*, 2010) This was confirmed to be similar on an independent review. The final analysis of this trial showed an ORR (CR + PR) of 33.8% with similar response rate between the treatment naïve cohort (34%; 95% CI 26% to 41%) and patients with one previous line of therapy (37%; 95% CI 26% to 49%). The median duration of response was 68 weeks. The estimated median PFS was 11.9 months for pazopanib vs. 6.2 months for placebo. (Rini & Al-Marrawi, 2011)

Pazopanib was subsequently tested in a phase III trial where a total of 233 treatment-naïve and 202 cytokine-pretreated patients with advanced clear-cell RCC were randomized in a 2:1 ratio to pazopanib ($n = 290$) or placebo ($n = 145$). (Sternberg *et al*, 2010) Placebo with best supportive care was thought to be an acceptable comparator arm due to the inaccessibility of other tyrosine kinase inhibitors (sunitinib or sorafenib) in some centres at the time of study initiation. Moreover, utilizing placebo control in a randomised double blind design enabled better characterization of the safety and efficacy of the profile of pazopanib. Placebo with best supportive care remained as the comparator arm as cytokines as the standard of care were challenged due to their underlying toxicities. The PFS in the pazopanib arm compared with placebo was significantly prolonged in the overall study population (9.2 months vs. 4.2 months, HR 0.46; $p < 0.0001$), in treatment naïve patients (11.1 months vs. 2.8 months, HR: 0.40, $p < 0.001$) and in cytokine-pretreated patients (7.4 months vs. 4.2 months; HR 0.54, p < 0.001). The response rate was 30% with pazopanib versus 3% in the placebo group and the median duration of response was 58.7 weeks. The final OS results were updated at the European Society of Medical Oncology meeting in 2010. A median OS of 22.9 vs. 20.5 months were noted in the pazopanib and placebo arms respectively (p=0.224). The lack of significant benefit was attributed to the early, high rate and prolonged duration of cross-over from placebo to pazopanib. In fact, more placebo than pazopanib patients received subsequent treatment (66% vs. 30% respectively) with 54% of patients on placebo crossing over to the active arm, some occurred as early as week 6 into therapy. (Rini & Al-Marrawi, 2011; Sternberg, 2010) The efficacy of pazopanib as first line therapy is comparable and is an alternative agent in patients who do not tolerate sunitinib. As yet, no head-to-head efficacy data are available to show superiority or non-inferiority between pazopanib and sunitinib and phase III trial (COMPARZ) is currently underway. (NCT00720941, 2011)

4.1.4 Bevacizumab

Bevacizumab is a humanized monoclonal antibody that uniquely targets the VEGF molecule and thus inhibiting this ligand with all of the receptors to which it binds. (Gommersall *et al*, 2004) A randomized phase II trial randomized 116 patients with metastatic clear-cell RCC to either placebo, low-dose (3 mg/kg given fortnightly) or high-dose bevacizumab (10 mg/kg given fortnightly). Accrual was halted when an interim analysis revealed a time to disease progression (TTP) benefit in the (high-dose) bevacizumab arm. A significant prolongation of TTP was observed in the high dose bevacizumab group (p<0.001; HR 2.55) compared to the placebo, and a smaller TTP benefit of borderline significance was reported for those receiving low-dose bevacizumab (p=0.053; HR 1.26). An objective partial response rate of 10.3% in the high-dose bevacizumab arm was noted. (Yang *et al*, 2003) Further data of bevacizumab as monotherapy was derived from a study comparing bevacizumab (10mg/kg; fortnightly) with placebo and bevacizumab with erlotinib (150mg bd), a small-molecule epidermal growth factor receptor (EGFR) inhibitor. Whilst the combination arm was well tolerated, it failed to demonstrate the superiority of this combination over bevacizumab alone. (Bukowski *et al*, 2007b) In both trials, the vast majority of patients treated with bevacizumab demonstrated some degree of tumour shrinkage, although in most instances the extent of tumour shrinkage did not meet the Response Evaluation Criteria in Solid Tumour (RECIST) criteria for PR. Interestingly the efficacy data from these two trials suggest the presence of clinical activity of bevacizumab monotherapy for metastatic RCC. (Elaraj *et al*, 2004) This is in clear contrast with other tumour types (non-small cell lung cancer, metastatic colorectal carcinoma, and metastatic breast carcinoma) where clinical benefit of single-agent bevacizumab without accompanying chemotherapy has been limited. (McDermott & George, 2010)

Two parallel large multicentre randomized international trials both examined the clinical efficacy of bevacizumab and IFN-α versus IFN-α alone, the previous standard of care for systemic treatment of patients with metastatic RCC. (Escudier *et al*, 2007c; Rini *et al*, 2008) Both trial (AVOREN, n=649; CALGB 90206 Intergroup Study, n=732), randomized treatment-naïve patients to IFN-α (9×10^6 units thrice weekly) and bevacizumab (10 mg/kg fortnightly) or placebo and IFN-α. The only difference was that the AVOREN study was placebo-controlled and the CALBG 90206 Intergroup study was an open labelled trial. (McDermott & George, 2010)

In the AVOREN study, the ORR was higher in the bevacizumab arm (31.4% vs. 12,8%, p=0.0001) with 70% of this group of patients demonstrating tumour shrinkage compared to 39% of patients on the IFN- α and placebo arm. The median PFS after a median follow-up of 22 months demonstrated a better median survival in the bevacizumab arm (10.2 months vs. 5.5 months; $p = 0.0001$). The improvement in PFS was evident irrespective of age, tumour subtype (clear cell or mixed), baseline VEGF level, and creatinine clearance. When stratified according to the MSKCC criteria, significant PFS benefits are seen in the low- and intermediate-risk groups but not detected in the poor risk category. As the number of patients enrolled in this poor subgroup were small (<10% of the enrolled patient), it is difficult to undertake any meaningful interpretation. (Escudier *et al*, 2007c)

A subsequent unplanned retrospective analysis revealed that PFS benefits was similar in 39% (n=131) of bevacizumab patients who received either 6 X 10^6 IU or 3 X 10^6 IU instead of 9 X 10^6 IU due to treatment related toxicity. The ORR for the reduced-dose group and full-dose group were 34% vs. 31% respectively and median duration of tumour response in turn was 13.6 months vs. 13.5 months respectively. This suggested that the dose of IFN-α could be reduced without compromising efficacy in patients who could not treatment related toxicities of IFN-α. (Melichar *et al,* 2008)

At the time of final OS analysis, only a trend towards OS was seen (23 months vs. 21.3 months, p = 0.1291). The effects of crossover to the bevacizumab arm, as well as the availability of second-line therapies where at least 35% received the TKIs (sunitinib and sorafenib) in both treatment arms, could well have compounded the results. An exploratory analysis showed that median OS was longer in patients receiving subsequent TKI therapy after bevacizumab plus IFN-α (n=113) compared with patients receiving TKIs after IFN plus placebo (n = 120) 38.6 months vs. 33.6 months respectively. (Escudier *et al,* 2007a)

In the Intergroup CALBG 90206, the ORR for active arm versus the control arm was 25.5% vs. 13.1% ($p<0.0001$) and the median PFS was in turn 8.4 months vs. 4.9 months ($p<0.0001$) respectively. (Rini *et al,* 2008) Only a trend in improved median OS was noted (18.3 months vs. 17.4 months, $p = 0.097$) and the trial did not achieve its primary end point, OS. The HR for progression was 0.71, which overlap with the AVOREN trial.

Stratification by MSKCC risk factors revealed the median PFS to be 11.1 months vs. 5.7 months in patients with absent risk factors (26%), 8.4 months vs. 5.3 months in patients with one or two risk factors (64%), and 3.3 months vs. 2.6 months in patients with three or more risk factors (10%), for the bevacizumab combination and INF-α monotherapy treatment groups, respectively. When stratified by the MKSCC risk factors, the median OS for bevacizumab / INF-α respectively was 32.5 months vs. 33.5 months for the favourable-risk group (26% of patients, p=0.524); 17.7 months vs. 16.1 months for the intermediate-risk group (64% of patients, p = 0.174) and lastly 6.6 months vs. 5.7 months for the poor risk group (p =0.25). (McDermott & George 2011, Rini *et al,* 2010)

Whilst no cross-over was allowed for the IFN-α monotherapy arm, 56% of study patients proceeded to at least one subsequent further systemic therapy in the form of a TKI. The patients who received second-line therapy were subsequently analysed and showed a median OS of 31.4 months vs. 26.8 months (p=0.079) in the bevacizumab/IFN-α and IFN-α monotherapy arms respectively. Amongst the patients who did not, the survival duration were 13.1 months vs. 9.1 months (p=0.059) respectively. (Rini *et al,* 2010)

Both trials were statistically robust and showed clear benefits in the median PFS arms with an overlapping HR and doubling of PFS when comparing the placebo/IFN-α arm with bevacizumab/IFN-α arm. (McDermott & George, 2010) The effects of crossover to the active bevacizumab arm in the AVOREN trial, as well as the permission of second-line therapies in both trials would account for the dilution of the actual overall survival benefits in both trials. (McDermott & George, 2010) Despite the lack of overall survival benefit and the notable toxicity of IFN-α with a large percentage of patients in the phase III trials undertaking dose reduction (40 – 60%), the combination of bevacizumab and IFN- α received Food and Drug Administration (FDA) approval for use as frontline of metastatic RCC.

4.2 mTOR Inhibitors

The mammalian target of rapamycin (mTOR) is a serine-threonine kinase that plays a crucial role in angiogenesis and regulation of cell cycle through a series of complex tightly regulated pathways. (Amato, 2011) mTOR activity is affected by a host of factors that influence cell functioning including nutrients (glucose, amino acid), energy depletion, as well as external signals such as cytokines, hormones, and growth factors. It also reacts to cellular stresses such as hypoxia, heat shock, oxidative stress, DNA damage and lastly a change in the microenvironment (pH or osmostic cell pressure). (Amato, 2011) The key pathway is via the phsophotidylinositol 3 kinase-protein kinase (P13K – AKT) pathway which is dysregulated in many cancers. (Amato, 2011; Beuvink *et al*, 2005) Activation of mTOR leads to phosphorylation of down-stream substrates (4E-binding protein-1 and protein S6 kinase) which in turn promotes mRNA translation, stimulation of protein synthesis and entry into the G_1 phase of cell cycle as illuastrated in figure 2. (Beuvink *et al*, 2005) Another important role of mTOR is the encoding and subsequent production of HIF-1α which drives angiogenesis, growth and survival of the cancer cells. The selective inhibition of this complex pathway by the mTOR inhibitors is achieved by binding to the intracellular protein FK506 binding protein 12 (FKBP-12) and causing inhibition of the kinase activity of the mTOR. (Amato, 2011) The two mTOR inhibitors, registered for the treatment of metastatic RCC are temsirolimus and everolimus.

4.2.1 Temsirolimus

The mTor inhibitor temsirolimus is similar to sirolimus (rapamycin) which has been used as an immunosuppressant in renal transplantation for many years. (Hudes *et al*, 2007) It affects cell division by inhibition of mTOR dependent protein translation, via binding to an intracellular protein (FK506 Binding Protein 12; FKBP12) resulting in a protein-drug complex. Temsirolimus is administered as a weekly intravenous infusion at 25mg. It is metabolised by CYP3A4 to active metabolite sirolimus and has a half-life of about 9 to 27 hours. (Hudes *et al*, 2007)

It was approved in 2007 by FDA as a first-line therapy in treatment-naïve metastatic RCC with poor prognostic features. Phase I and II trials of temsirolimus alone, or combined with IFN-α, found anti-tumour effects and stable disease in patients refractory to cytokine therapies. (Hidalgo *et al*, 2006; Raymond *et al*, 2004) In addition to that, another phase II trial on heavily pre-treated patients observed a median survival of 15 months. (Atkins *et al*, 2004) These encouraging results subsequently led to the development of an international multicentre phase III trial where 626 treatment-naïve patients with poor prognostic factors were randomized to temsirolimus (25 mg i.v. weekly), IFN-α (3×10^6 units, with an increase to 18×10^6 units s.c. thrice weekly) or the combination of temsirolimus (15 mg weekly) and IFN-α (6×10^6 thrice weekly). (Atkins *et al*, 2004) This was a pivotal trial that enrolled patients with poor prognostic factors only unlike previous studies with VEGF inhibitors which only recruited patients with good and intermediate risk features. The poor prognostic patients consisted of at least three or more of the 6 poor MSKCC prognostic factors. Another notable characteristic of recruitment is the enrolment of up to 20% of non-clear cell renal cell histological subtype. This is the only randomised study available so far for patients with the non-clear cell histology. (Atkins *et al*, 2004)

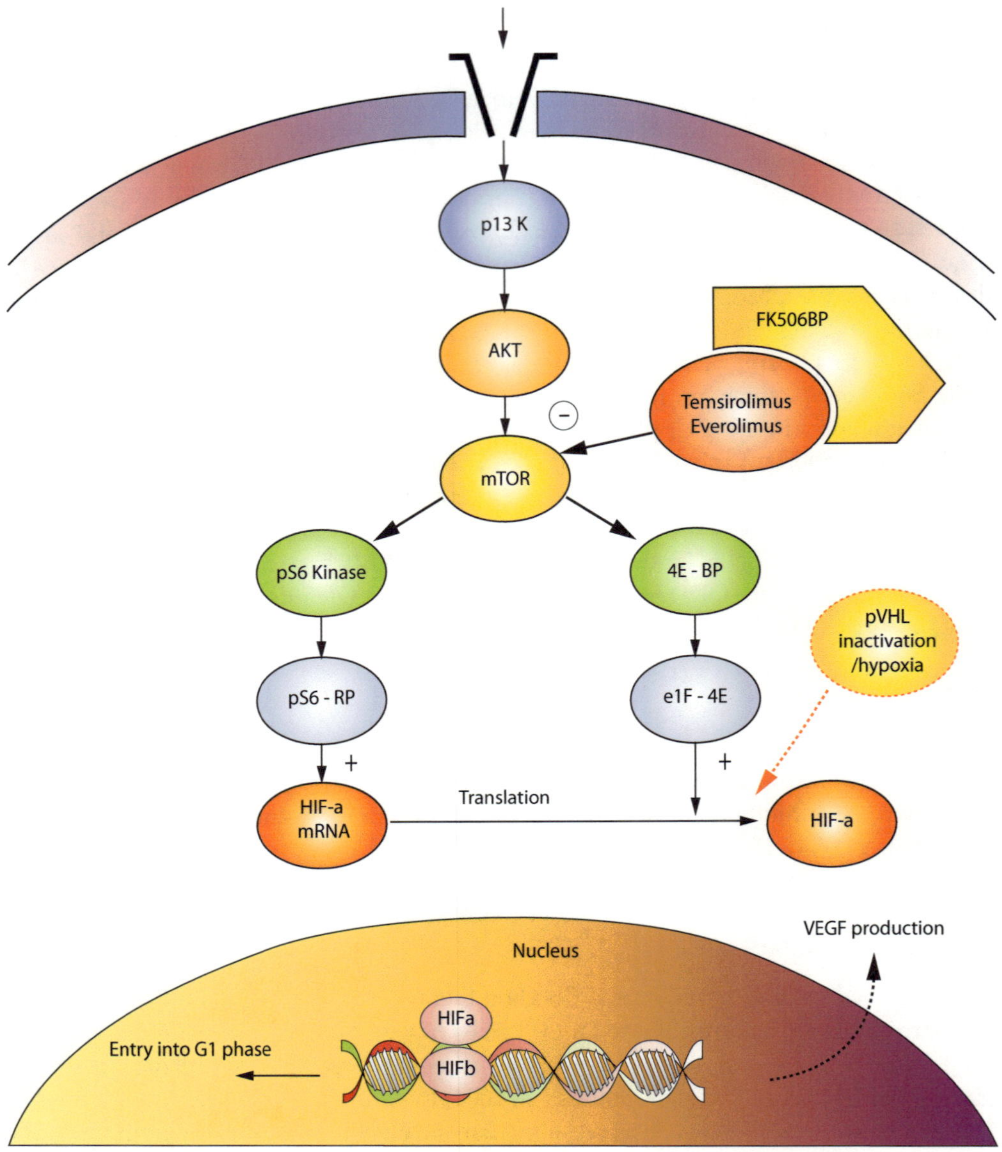

Fig. 2. External stimuli (growth factors)

Patients who received temsirolimus alone experienced a longer median OS (10.9 vs. 7.3 months; $p = 0.008$) and PFS (3.8 vs. 1.9 months; $p < 0.001$) compared with those who received INF-α alone. (Hudes *et al*, 2007) Patients in the combination therapy group had the most grade 3 or 4 adverse events leading to more dose reductions or delays. Their mean temsirolimus dose intensity was 10.9 mg per week vs. 23.1 mg per week for patients on temsirolimus alone. The median PFS in the temsirolimus, temsirolimus and IFN-α and IFN-α alone were 3.8, 3.7 and 1.9 months, respectively, and the median OS in turn was 10.9 months, 8.4 months and 7.3 months. (Hudes *et al*, 2007) Notably, older patients and patients with a higher serum LDH (> 1.5 fold the upper limit of normal) had better OS. (Hudes *et al*, 2007)

Clinicians are now faced with the challenge of treating patients who are refractory to VEGF targeted therapy as there is paucity of data in this area. The only published prospective randomised trial looking at this cohort of patients was RECORD-1 looking at everolimus vs. placebo. (Motzer *et al*, 2008) The few abstracts published on second line treatment with temsirolimus are all single institution case series confirming a modest activity in the second line setting with a median PFS of up to almost 4 months.

4.2.2 Everolimus

Everolimus is a derivative of rapamycin used in transplant medicine. Everolimus is an orally administered mTOR inhibitor with activity in patients with advanced clear-cell RCC who have failed VEGF-targeted therapies (sorafenib, sunitinib or both). (Motzer *et al*, 2008) Everolimus is converted to a main metabolite hydroxy everolimus is converted to a main metabolite hydroxy everolimus by the cytochrome 3A4 enzyme. The 30-hour half-life maintains a relative steady state achievable with the daily dosage regimen of 10mg/day. (Amato, 2011)

In RECORD-1, a double-blind placebo-controlled phase III trial, 410 patients with advanced clear-cell RCC which had progressed after sunitinib, sorafenib or both, were randomized in a 2:1 ratio to everolimus 10 mg once daily or placebo plus best supportive care. Regardless of age, gender, prognostic group, previous treatment with sorafenib, sunitinib or both, prolongation of PFS (4.9 vs. 1.9 months; $p < 0.0001$) was found with everolimus over placebo. (Motzer *et al*, 2008) However there was lack of difference for median OS (14.8 months vs. 14.4 months) as majority (80%) of patients in the placebo plus best supportive arm were allowed to cross over after the unbinding at the second interim analysis. This important landmark phase III trials proved the efficacy of mTOR inhibitors following VEGF therapy and as such received FDA registration for patients who have progressed following therapy with sunitinib and sorafenib. (Motzer *et al*, 2008)

5. New agents in clinical development

A number of second generation small molecule multi-targeted agents have been investigated in Phase II and III studies treating patients with metastatic RCC. (Fisher *et al*, 2011) These include axitinib and tivozanib which are in advanced clinical development, as well as dovitinib and others. (Fisher *et al*, 2011)

5.1 Axitinib

Axitinib is a potent oral agent that inhibits VEGFR-1, -2 and -3. It is rapidly absorbed with peak plasma concentration occurring 1 - 2 hours after administration on an empty stomach, terminal half-life of 3 – 5 hours, and bioavailability of 58%. (Pithavala *et al*, 2010) Dose-limiting toxicities seen in phase I studies were hypertension and mucositis, and in a phase II study, common adverse events also included diarrhoea and fatigue. ((Rixe *et al*, 2007b)

Axitinib has been investigated in a number of different cancers including cytokine-refractory metastatic RCC. A second line study in 52 patients using starting doses of axitinib 5 mg twice daily, resulted in two complete and 21 partial responses (ORR of 44.2%). The median response duration was 23 months and median overall survival was 29.9 months.

(Rixe *et al*, 2007b) Updated 5 year OS data from this study were presented in abstract form in 2011. (Motzer *et al*, 2011a) The 5 year survival rate was 20.6%. The ten patients surviving for more than five years had ORR 100% compared with 30% in <5 year survivors, took axitinib for longer (median 5.8 years vs. 0.67 years) and were fitter, with baseline ECOG PS of 0 in 80% of the longer term survivors compared with 53% in <5 year survivors. However they were all similar age, gender and risk factors. No unexpected new toxicities were seen with prolonged use of axitinib.

In a phase III second line study (AXIS), patients received axitinib at doses titrated up to 10mg BD or sorafenib 400mg BD. (Rini *et al*, 2011b) The 723 patients had progressive disease after one prior first line treatment (sunitinib, bevacizumab, temsirolimus or cytokines). The ORR was 19.4% for axitinib vs. 9.4% for sorafenib ($p=0.0001$) and significantly longer PFS (12.1 versus 6.5 months, $p<0.0001$) was seen in patients on the axitinib arm. Patients who had previously received cytokines were found to have significantly ($p<0.0001$) better PFS with axitinib (12.1 months) than sorafenib (6.5 months). This also occurred in those having prior sunitinib (4.8 vs. 3.4 months, $p=0.0107$). As part of the same trial, patient-reported kidney specific symptom and function assessments were secondary endpoints. (Cella *et al*, 2011) Outcomes according to validated tools were similar for both drugs during treatment, however as patients had a PFS with axitinib, this delayed worsening of the composite endpoint of cancer symptoms, progression or death compared with sorafenib.

5.2 Tivozanib

Tivozanib is an oral quinoline urea derivative small molecule TKI. It is a potent and selective inhibitor of VEGFR-1, -2 and -3 as well as inhibiting c-kit and PDGFR at higher concentrations. In 272 patients with advanced or metastatic RCC who had not received prior VEGF targeted therapy, tivozanib has shown promising efficacy and acceptable safety and tolerability in a phase II study reported in abstract form in 2011. (Nosov *et al*, 2011) All patients initially took tivozanib 1.5 mg daily for 16 weeks, and were then stratified according to response into stopping or continuing tivozanib, or if disease had stabilized, being randomised between tivozanib and placebo. Patients receiving placebo that developed progressive disease, or completed the double blind phase were allowed to restart tivozanib. Overall, 84% of patients demonstrated PR or SD by Week 16, ORR was 30%, disease control rate (DCR) was 85% and median PFS 11.7 months. Highest efficacy for tivozanib was in patients with clear-cell histology who had undergone a nephrectomy, who achieved an ORR of 36%, DCR of 88% and median PFS of 14.8 months. Commonest adverse effects included hypertension (45%) which was grade 3/4 in 12%, and dysphonia (22%). A low incidence of drug-related diarrhoea (12%), asthenia (10%), fatigue (8%), dyspnoea (6%), cough (5%), anorexia (5%), stomatitis (4%), hand-foot syndrome (4%) and proteinuria (3%) was reported. Overall median PFS, DCR and ORR were 11.7 months, 85% and 30%, respectively. Patients with clear-cell RCC who had undergone nephrectomy had PFS of 14.8 months and ORR of 36% with tivozanib. Phase III evaluation of tivozanib in nephrectomised patients with advanced clear cell RCC is on-going.

A phase Ib open-label study found tivozanib could be combined with temsirolimus at full dose/schedule in patients with advanced RCC (with clear cell component) who had failed up to one prior VEGF-targeted therapy. (Kabbinavar *et al*, 2011) Tivozanib was given orally daily for 3 weeks on, 1 week off (1 cycle) and IV temsirolimus was given once weekly. A standard 3+3 dose escalation design was used at four levels from 0.5 mg to 1.5 mg per day and 15 to 25 mg per week of tivozanib and temsirolimus, respectively. There were 28 patients (26 male) of median age 62 years and Karnofsky Performance Status from 100 to 80. Median duration of treatment was 21.1 weeks. Treatment-related adverse events seen in ≥10% of patients were: fatigue (20 all grades/4 grade 3), decreased appetite (14/0), stomatitis (13/2), thrombocytopenia (10/4), diarrhoea (16/2), nausea (13/1), constipation (10/1), and dypsnoea (10/1). There were no grade 4 events, and no dose limiting toxicities. The MTD for the combination of tivozanib and temsirolimus was 1.5 mg/day and 25 mg/week, respectively. PR was seen in 28%, SD in 64% and DCR (PR and SD>24weeks) of 48%. The combination of tivozanib with temsirolimus was well tolerated and showed encouraging clinical activity in patients with advanced RCC.

5.3 Dovitinib

Dovitinib is a potent oral inhibitor of angiogenic factors, including the fibroblast growth factor (FGFR) and VEGF receptors. The maximum tolerated dose of dovitinib is 500 mg daily on a 5 day on/ 2 day off dosing schedule in 28 day cycles. A phase II study of dovitinib in clear-cell metastatic RCC patients previously treated with a VEGFR inhibitor and/or mTOR inhibitor was reported in 2011. (Angevin *et al*, 2011) (NCT1217931, 2011) In 51 patients best overall responses were PR in 8%, and SD ≥ 4 months in 37%. Median PFS and OS were 6.1 and 16 months respectively. Fifty nine patients median age 60 years and ECOG PS 0 or 1 were evaluable for safety. The most common adverse events were nausea (73%; grade 3 : 9%), diarrhoea (64%; grade 3: 9%), vomiting (56%; grade 3: 5%), decreased appetite (48%; grade 3: 7%), asthenia (36%; grade 3: 12%), and fatigue (36%; grade 3: 10%). An on-going phase 3 trial is comparing dovitinib with sorafenib in patients who have had one previous VEFR- and mTOR-targeted therapy.

6. Combination therapy in metastatic RCC

Despite being in the era where increasing numbers of VEGF and mTOR inhibitors are at the clinician's disposal, their optimal use in patients with metastatic RCC has not been fully ascertained. Undeniably these agents have conferred significant survival benefits compared to historical series, however most patients eventually develop resistance and relapse after 6 months to 3 years of therapy. (Jonasch *et al*, 2011) This underscores the strong need to develop novel treatment strategies to achieve better clinical outcomes. This could be achieved by the use of combinations of anti-angiogenic agents or with mTOR inhibitors, chemotherapy or immunotherapy. Sequencing treatment with different anti-VEGF agents as well as with mTOR inhibitors and immunotherapeutic agents could be another solution which will be discussed subsequently. (Jonasch *et al*, 2011)

The concept of combining two (or more) targeted agents is biologically plausible as each agent may affect different targets simultaneously potentially resulting in additive or synergistic effects and achieving better clinical outcomes. (Hutson, 2011) Using a combination of drugs which target the same pathway (e.g. VEGF) at two or more different levels, has been termed "vertical blockade". In contrast, "horizontal blockade" occurs when the different pathways are blocked simultaneously by one or multiple agents in combination. (Hutson, 2011) It should be noted that combination therapy is often undertaken at the cost of increased toxicities as evidenced by some of the phase I trials where sunitinib was combined with temsirolimus, bevacizumab or everolimus. (Feldman *et al*, 2009; Rini *et al*, 2009)

6.1 VEGF-ligands or receptor inhibitors / mTOR plus immunotherapy combination

This is best illustrated by the two single arm phase II studies combining sorafenib with standard dose of IFN-α which conferred higher ORR (approximately 30%) and longer PFS (7 - 12 months) when compared with phase III data of sorafenib monotherapy. (Gollob *et al*, 2007; Ryan *et al*, 2007) However, in a randomised phase II study comparing sorafenib monotherapy with sorafenib /low-dose IFN-α combination, a very similar response rates and longer PFS were demonstrated equally in both arms. Interpretation of these phase II data required caution given the small number of patients recruited in comparison with the more robust phase III sorafenib vs. placebo trial. (Jonasch *et al*, 2010)

The AVOREN and CALBG 90206 trial demonstrated that the bevacizumab / IFN-α combination had achieved better clinical outcome when compared with IFN-α alone. (Escudier *et al*, 2007c; Rini *et al*, 2008) Unfortunately, the lack of bevacizumab as a control arm did not help address the question as to whether the addition of IFN-α to bevacizumab was able to achieve a more superior outcome compared to bevacizumab alone. A small randomised phase II study comparing erlotinib and bevacizumab with bevacizumab alone reported a non-statistical small PFS difference of 0.5 months (9.0 months vs. 8.5 months; p=0.58). Although this is small benefit may be clinically irrelevant, this trial provided insight into the clinical efficacy of bevacizumab as monotherapy. (Bukowski *et al*, 2007b)

A randomised three-arm trial was undertaken comparing temsirolimus (25mg) / bevacizumab (10mg/kg) combination with sunitinib alone and with IFN-α (9X 10^6 IU thrice weekly) / bevacizumab (10mg/kg) combination in patients with advanced RCC (TORAVA). A total of 171 treatment naïve patients were recruited in a 2:1:1 ratio and was equally distributed into the three arms. The reported median FPS was similar (8.2 months) for both temsirolimus (25mg) / bevacizumab (10mg/kg) (experimental) arm and sunitinib (comparator) arm. The duration for bevacizumab / IFN-α was however up to 16.8 months. The patients in the experimental arm experienced a high number of discontinuation from treatment for reasons other than progression (51%) when compared to the sunitinib arm (12%) and bevacizumab / IFN-α arm (38%). (Negrier *et al*, 2011) Furthermore up to 77% in the experimental arm experienced a grade 3 or higher toxicity. The trial again highlighted the lack of survival benefit due to a toxic combination that is poorly tolerated and the investigators appropriately commented that this combination would not be recommended for first-line treatment in patients with metastatic RCC. (Negrier *et al*, 2011) Similarly, when temsirolimus was prescribed in conjunction with IFN-α in a phase III trial for patients with poor prognostic advanced RCC, the overall survival benefit was worst in the tmesirolimus / IFN-α arm compared to temsirolimus monotherapy arm. Once again, toxicity prevailed in the combination arm and therefore the temsirolimus / IFN-α combination is not recommended as standard practice yet outside a clinical trial for treatment of advanced RCC. (Hudes *et al*, 2007)

6.2 VEGF-ligands or receptor inhibitors / mTOR combination

Sorafenib like sunitinib was also investigated in combination with bevacizumab in two phase I studies. In one the study of patients with metastatic RCC, the median time to progression was 11.2 months and the partial response rate was 46%. (Sosman *et al*, 2008) In the second trial which included 39 patients with solid tumours (with 3 patients with RCC), PR or disease stabilisation of ≥4 months was observed in 59% of the assessable patients, and a PR was achieved in one of the 3 patients with RCC. (Azad *et al*, 2008) The combination arm required dose reduction of both agents and resulted in a considerably lower maximum tolerated dose compared to maximal tolerated dose of the single agent. It is postulated that bevacizumab most likely enhanced the side-effects of sorafenib such as hypertension and hand-foot syndrome. (Azad *et al*, 2008; Sosman *et al*, 2008) When sunitinib was combined with bevacizumab, a high incidence of haematological and vascular toxicities (including microangiopathic haemolytic anaemia) and hypertension were observed. (Feldman *et al*, 2009) Again bevacizumab was likely responsible for the exaggeration of the side-effects of sunitinib which would have been otherwise manageable.

Finally, a phase II trial examining the feasibility, tolerability, and efficacy of multiple combinations of currently available therapies are being tested in the Eastern Cooperative Oncology BeST trial. The four arms are bevacizumab (10mg/kg), bevacizumab (5mg/kg) /temsirolimus (25 mg), bevacizumab (5mg/kg) and sorafenib (200mg twice daily)/ temsirolimus (25mg). (NCT00378703, 2006) This trial will provide insight into the efficacy of bevacizumab monotherapy and the clinical tolerability and efficacy of lowered dose of bevacizumab and sorafenib dose in conjunction with temsirolimus where previously significant toxicities was noted on the earlier phase II studies.

7. Sequencing therapy in metastatic RCC

Sequencing the systemic treatment of metastatic RCC has several potential benefits. Sequential treatment is less toxic than combination therapy and thus allowing patients to be exposed to a more optimal dose (and subsequent higher total accumulative dose) resulting in improved clinical efficacy. It also creates a treatment continuum with the goal of maintain responding patients on treatment for as long as clinically feasible. Lastly, targeting the different pathway at different point in time theoretically offers the benefit of overcoming the resistance to the individual agents. (Bellmunt, 2009)

7.1 Antiangiogenic therapy after immunotherapy

A phase II study published in 2003 examined the role of bevacizumab (10mg/kg) post progression on immunotherapy demonstrated a time-to-progression (TTP) of 4.8 months. (Yang *et al*, 2003) Two phase II trials mentioned earlier on similarly examined the efficacy of sunitinib post immunotherapy revealed promising survival benefits which subsequent led to the landmark phase III trial comparing sunitinib with IFN-α. (Motzer *et al*, 2006; Motzer *et al*, 2007b) The phase III sorafenib trial vs. placebo (TARGET) also recruited patient who had cytokine therapy and observed a doubling of PFS benefit of 2.8 to 5.6 months. (Escudier *et al*, 2007b) More recently, in a phase II trial examined the use of axitinib post cytokine therapy demonstrated a TTP of 15.7 months. (Rixe *et al*, 2007b) Whilst it is possible to compare the results of each individual phase II trials and rank them to their clinical benefit, a proper conducted phase III is essential to determine the best anti-angiogenic agent to use post-cytokine therapy.

7.2 mTOR blockade after anti-angiogenic therapy

The best illustrating example is the RECORD-1 trial which investigated the benefits of everolimus vs. placebo with best supportive care post progression on sunitinib, sorafenib or both. Of note 71% of patients had received prior sunitinib whilst 55% sorafenib. Patient that received everolimus achieved an additional of 3-month of PFS benefit regardless whether they received sunitinib or sorafenib. No overall survival benefits were noted due to large numbers of patients from placebo crossing over to everolimus arm (80%). (Motzer *et al*, 2008)

An on-going trial (RECORD-3) will randomly assign patients between either everolimus or sunitinib where at first sign of progression, patients would cross over to sunitinib if they were on everolimus and vice versa. The primary end point of this trial is to assess whether PFS after first-line treatment for patients who received everolimus will be non-inferior to patients who receive sunitinib after first-line therapy. (NCT00720941, 2011)

7.3 Serial anti-angiogenic agents

Axitinib has been investigated in both phase II and III second-line trials in advanced RCC. The results of the survival benefits have so far been encouraging especially in the phase III trial comparing with sorafenib. (Dutcher *et al*, 2008) Further trials will be undertaken clarify the outcomes. Specifically, in the Sequential Two-agent Assessment in Renal Cell Carcinoma Therapy (START) two hundred and forty treatment-naïve patients with clear-cell component mRCC will be randomly assigned to receive bevacizumab, pazopanib, or everolimus. On first progression or intolerance to therapy, patients will be randomly assigned to one of two of the remaining agents. The primary end point is the detection of the longest combination of the TTP. (NCT1217931, 2011)

A retrospective study described the efficacy of sorafenib or sunitinib in the first-line setting in 49 patients with metastatic RCC as well as the subsequent derived benefit after switching to the alternative agent on progression. (Dudek *et al*, 2009) The TTP for patients treated with sunitinib or sorafenib (after initial treatment) was 5.8 and 5.1 months respectively (p=0.299). However, sequential treatment with sorafenib followed by suntinib resulted in a trend toward improved TTP (p = 0.115). Similarly, the median OS was better for patients who received sorafenib followed by sunitinib (23.5 months) than if they received sunitinib after sorafenib (10.4 months; p=0.061). This analysis of median survival did not include patients who did not need to cross over. This retrospective study suggested the benefit of utilizing sorafenib as first line may improve duration of disease control if a subsequent agent is used and certainly warrants further investigation. (Dudek *et al*, 2009) The SWITCH trial is a prospective phase III trial which will randomize patients to upfront sunitinib and switching to sorafenib on progression versus switching from sorafenib to sunitinib on progression. The primary end point is the PFS and hopefully this trial will show further insight into which anti-VEGF treatment sequence will confer better clinical outcome in patients with metastatic RCC. (NCT00732914, 2010)

8. Systemic treatment for non-clear-cell RCC

The treatment for advanced non-clear-cell RCC is less well established than the clear-cell variants and the evidence to guide treatment is limited. Majority of the data is derived from expanded access trials, retrospective series, and subset analyses of major trials. (Tazi el *et al,* 2011) The phase III sunitinib trial virtually excluded all patients with non-clear-cell RCC. In spite of this, sunitinib was made available to all patients with clear-cell and non-clear-cell histology in a subsequent multi-centre, international, non-randomized expanded access compassionate trial. (Motzer *et al,* 2007a) A total of 588 patients with non-clear cell histology (not characterized further) received sunitinib and of that, 437 evaluable patients demonstrated an ORR of 11% (n=48) with 46 partial responders and 2 complete responders) and 57% had stable disease (n=250) for at least 3 months. (Gore *et al,* 2009) The median OS was 13.4 months. The ORR of 11% was lower than the original phase III study and was thought to due to the non-mandatory reporting of the disease response and the reliance of local practice to detect any change in the disease burden. The authors of the study therefore concluded that sunitinib is active in subjects with non-clear- cell histology amongst other subsets of patients (poor performance status, brain metastasis and patients of ≥ 65 years old) which were not enrolled in the original trial. (Motzer *et al,* 2002)

One of the largest retrospective series for papillary RCC was a multi-centre review consisting of 41 patients treated with either sunitinib or sorafenib. The response rate was disappointing with an ORR of 5% for all comers but was higher at 17% for sunitinib. The PFS was statistically longer for patients treated with sunitinib (11.9 months) when compared with sorafenib (5.1 months; $p < 0.001$). The PFS for sunitinib was comparable to the phase III clear-cell trial suggesting clinical efficacy in sunitinib for papillary carcinoma. (Choueiri *et al,* 2008) In contrast, two small phase II studies showed little-to-no clinical response and disease stability being the best clinical response for only a short duration of 1.4 to 3 months. (Plimack *et al,* 2010; Ravaud *et al,* 2009)

The efficacy of sorafenib in the treatment of advanced papillary variant is best demonstrated in the Advance Renal cell Carcinoma Sorafenib Expanded Access Program in North America. One hundred and fifty eight patients with papillary RCC were enrolled. Of the 107 patients with papillary RCC that could be evaluated, 84% (n=90) demonstrated 3 PR and 87 SD for a duration of 8 weeks or more. Sixteen percent (n=17) of patients showed early progression of disease. (Beck *et al,* 2008)

The phase III international, multicentre trial, comparing temsirolimus, IFN-α, or combination of both, is the first trial that prospectively recruited all histological subtypes of RCC. Twenty percent (n=120) were classified as non-clear cell RCC without further subclassification at the outset due to the absence central pathology review. (Hudes *et al,* 2007) An improvement in the median OS and median PFS were seen in the temsirolmus monotherapy arm compared to the combination temsirolimus/IFN-α or IFN-α monotherapy arm. Subsequent exploratory subset analyses based on tumour histology determined that 55 patients that had papillary RCC also demonstrated an OS and PFS benefit when treated with temsirolimus. (Schmidt *et al,* 2001) The OS and PFS for temsirolimus vs. IFN-α were 11.6 months vs. 4.3 months and 7.0 months vs. 1.8 months respectively. These results led to the subsequent FDA approval of temsirollimus as treatment for non-clear-cell histology in advanced RCC. Everolimus has demonstrated efficacy in the pivotal trial for patients with clear-cell RCC, post progression on sunitinib, sorafenib or both in the RECORD-1 trial. (Motzer *et al,* 2008) This has prompted the development of an open-label, single arm, multi-centre phase II examining the efficacy of everolimus as first-line systemic therapy for patients with advanced papillary RCC. (Amato,

2011) Central confirmation of histology and subclassification into type I and II will be undertaken. This trial which is still recruiting will hopefully show further insight into the treatment of papillary RCC which thus far has been disappointing.

Erlotinib was examined in a phase II study in treatment naïve patients with locally advanced or metastatic papillary RCC. (Gordon *et al*, 2009) Of the 52 registered patients, 45 were evaluable. The ORR was 11% (n=5) and the DCR was 64% with five partial responders and 24 patients with stable disease. The median OS time was 27 months with a 29% probability of freedom from treatment failure at 6 months. The presence of EGFR receptors scores and staining intensity determined by immunohistochemistry showed no correlation with TTP or OS. The estimated median survival was estimated to be 27 months. (Gordon *et al*, 2009) Combination of erlotinib with bevacizumab is currently underway designed to further evaluate the efficacy of erlotinib. (2010)

As with papillary variant of RCC, the chromophobe variant has also been excluded from many of the initial targeted therapy trials. Not surprisingly the data is even more limited. Furthermore, with the low incidence of 4% and the low likelihood of chromophobe to metastasize, any attempts to recruit patients of this type into a clinical trial is a difficult process. In the sorafenib access program described earlier, an overall DCR of 90% was noted with 5% (n=1) demonstrating partial response and 85% (n=17) of the patients experiencing disease stability for at least 2 months. (Stadler *et al*, 2010) The chromophobe variant were also included in the phase III temsirolimus versus IFN-α trial but the subgroup analysis only focused on papillary variant and the data for chromophobe was therefore not published. Nevertheless the PFS and OS were prolonged in the non-clear cell subgroup, therefore hinting some weak evidence of efficacy in this group of tumour. (Tazi el *et al*)

The strongest treatment evidence for treatment of the rare collecting duct renal cell carcinoma stemmed from a phase II multi-centre trial of 23 treatment-naïve patients who received cisplatin or carboplatin if inadequate renal function with gemcitabine. This variant is very aggressive and patient often presents with more advanced stage and succumbed earlier. This combination was selected based on some similarities in the histological features comparing with transitional cell carcinoma of the urinary bladder. In the trial, there was an observed ORR of 26%. The median PFS and OS were 7.1 months and 10.5 months. (Oudard *et al*, 2007a) To date, there is very little data to support the use of anti-VEGF therapies in this very bad prognostic cancer.

9. Side effects of targeted therapies used in renal cell carcinoma

The clinical benefit of newer targeted agents in metastatic RCC over previous conventional treatment has been shown in Sections 1 to 5 in this chapter. However as with any new treatment, sideeffects must be carefully measured and evaluated against older treatments and supportive or pharmacologic interventions developed for their prevention or control. (di Lorenzo *et al*, 2011) This is essential when considering patients' quality of life (see Section 11) and should allow patients to stay on beneficial treatment for as long as possible. (Bellmunt, 2007) Safety data from clinical trials and post-marketing surveillance have identified that many of the targeted therapies have toxicities that are different from those usually seen with conventional anticancer drugs. (di Lorenzo *et al*, 2011; Ravaud, 2011)

These angiogenesis inhibitors directly or indirectly target the VEGF pathway, and their individual mechanisms are pointers to their toxicities. (Schmidinger & Bellmunt, 2011) They share several adverse effects in common, including hypertension, fatigue, gastrointestinal, skin, and bone marrow effects. The mTOR inhibitors can cause metabolic alterations, immunosuppression and interstitial pneumonitis, whereas hypothyroidism is seen in patients taking sunitinib, potentially sorafenib and pazopanib. (di Lorenzo *et al*, 2011) Suggestions for management are shown below. The importance of patient education with respect to self-management strategies has been emphasized. (Ravaud, 2011)

9.1 Hypertension

Hypertension is a well recognised class side effect commonly observed in cancer patients treated with angiogenesis inhibitors that target the VEGF pathway, but not with mTOR inhibitors. (Izzedine *et al* 2009, diLorenzo 2011) Hypertension is reported with axitinib, bevacizumab, sorafenib, sunitinib and pazopanib. (Escudier *et al*, 2007b; Motzer *et al*, 2007a; Rini *et al*, 2011a; Rixe *et al*, 2007a; Sternberg *et al*, 2010) Hypertension has occurred whether or not the patient has a history of high blood pressure, however incidence may be higher in patients with pre-existing cardiovascular disease. Reversible posterior leukoencephalopathy syndrome is a rare association with hypertension seen with sunitinib and sorafenib where patients in addition experienced seizures and impaired vision thought to be attributed to capillary leakage and vasogenic oedema of the brain. This is reversible with cessation of the implicated agent. (Kapiteijn *et al*, 2007) Hypertension is an independent risk factor for the onset of cardio- and renovascular disease. In patients with metastatic disease, the goal of optimizing blood pressure is to allow continuous and safe administration of the anti-VEGF agents. (Izzedine *et al*, 2009; Keefe *et al*, 2011) Blood pressure monitoring (either daily or multiple times per week) is recommended and the use of antihypertensive medication may be required to avoid potential cardiovascular complications. Algorithms for hypertension management have been developed, (di Lorenzo *et al*, 2011) and treatment should be individualised to the patient. (Izzedine *et al*, 2009) The best anti-hypertensive agents is yet to be determined, however an angiotensin-converting enzyme (ACE) inhibitors is a logical choice if bevacizumab is the underlying cause as they may improve the associated proteinuria. (Keefe *et al*, 2011) Angiotensin II inhibitors, diuretics, hydropyridine calcium channel blockers (CCBs), and β-blockers are also possible anti-hypertensive agents. In patients on anti-hypertensive medications at baseline, an increase in the dose of pre-existing antihypertensive medications may be required. Temporary suspension of therapy may be required to allow for better control of the hypertension. In some cases, severe hypertension with life-threatening consequences (e.g. malignant hypertension, transient or permanent neurologic deficit, hypertensive crisis) has led to permanent discontinuation. (Keefe *et al*, 2011) The relationship between hypertension and anti-tumour effect is postulated with several of the drugs used for renal cell cancer and this will be addressed in Section 10.

9.2 Fatigue

Fatigue is the commonest of the constitutional side effects seen with the targeted agents used in metastatic RCC, but is less common than with cytokine treatment. (Adams & Leggas, 2007; di Lorenzo *et al*, 2011; Hutson, 2011; Motzer *et al*, 2007a) The incidence of fatigue in Phase III studies ranged from 14% to 51% for all grades, up to 11% for grade 3–4.

(di Lorenzo *et al*, 2011) Patients with cancer-related fatigue experience a chronic feeling of tiredness or lack of energy that is not relieved by rest. Fatigue can be caused by the targeted therapy and/or aggravated by other factors, such as anaemia, anxiety, hypothyrodism or depression, nutritional status, side effects of other medications or even organ dysfunction. (di Lorenzo *et al*, 2011; Ravaud, 2009) Patients may find it useful to record a daily fatigue diary to see when their energy levels are highest during the day in order to allow themselves time and energy for activities they enjoy. Evidence-based pharmacological interventions remain scarce, but monitoring and treating patients for any aggravating factors may help. If grade 3–4 fatigue persist, it may be necessary to dose reduce or stop treatment. (di Lorenzo *et al*, 2011; Ravaud, 2009)

9.3 Gastrointestinal side effects

Gastrointestinal toxicities are common to most of the targeted therapies for RCC but rarely lead to dose interruptions. (di Lorenzo *et al*, 2011) These include diarrhoea, nausea and to a lesser degree vomiting. Standard protocols used in prevention and treatment of these toxicities in patients having cytotoxic chemotherapy are suitable for use in this setting. Supportive medications will include loperamide (up to 16mg per day) for diarrhoea; dopamine antagonists such as metoclopramide or where necessary 5HT3 receptor antagonists for nausea and vomiting. (di Lorenzo *et al*, 2011)(di Lorenzo 2011) Oral mucositis is also reported with the mTOR inhibitors everolimus and temsirolimus, and the tyrosine kinase receptor inhibitors. Evidence-based guidelines advise good oral hygiene, local anaesthetic mouthwashes or systemic analgesics if required for mouth pain, and avoidance of alcohol based mouthwashes. (see www.mascc.org)

9.4 Dermatological side effects

Various dermatological side effects can be seen with all of the agents used in metastatic RCC. Prevention and management is important to maintain patients' health-related quality of life as well as treatment dose intensity. (Lacouture *et al*, 2011) Toxicities seen include papulopustular (acneiform) rash, hair changes (including alopecia, colour changes), dermatitis enhancement, pruritus, xerosis, skin fissures, paronychia and hand-foot skin reactions (HFSR). (di Lorenzo *et al*, 2011; Lacouture *et al*, 2011) HFSR appears as plaques or blisters with painful tingling or burning sensations in the soles of the feet or palms of the hands, and these effects are particularly common with sorafenib and sunitinib. (di Lorenzo) Avoiding tight shoes, and using moisturiser, emollient creams and topical treatment containing urea or salicyclic acid is suggested. (di Lorenzo *et al*, 2011; Ravaud, 2009) Evidence-based treatment guidelines for managing skin toxicities have recently been published by the MASCC Skin Toxicity Study Group (Lacouture *et al*, 2011) Topical hydrocortisone cream (1 %) and oral antibiotics (doxycycline or minocycline) are the mainstay of prevention of papulopustolar rash or if they are painful. (Lacouture *et al*; Ravaud, 2009)

9.5 Other reported adverse effects

Clinical hypothyroidism defined as a decrease in free thyroxine index with elevated thyroid stimulating hormone levels has been reported in patients taking sunitinib, pazopanib and sorafenib (the latter specifically in Japanese subjects). (di Lorenzo *et al*, 2011) Screening pretreatment and on days 1 and 28 each cycle, and use of thyroxine is advised. (di Lorenzo *et al*, 2011)

Heart failure is seen with a number of targeted agents including sunitinib, bevacizumab and sorafenib. (Jarkowski *et al*, 2011) Patients, especially those with pre-existing cardiovascular disease, should be closely monitored especially if they have cardiac risk factors. (Ravaud, 2011) If heart failure occurs it should be managed according to standard protocols, and the offending agent ceased. (Jarkowski *et al*, 2011) Myocardial ischaemia or infarction was significantly more frequent in patients taking sorafenib group (3%) than placebo.

Severe and fatal hepatotoxicity (boxed warning) and grade 3 or 4 proteinuria have occurred with pazopanib treatment which necessitates routine monitoring of liver function tests, and urinalyses. (Ravaud, 2011)

Venous and arterial thromboses have been reported in patients on bevacizumab. (Escudier *et al*, 2007c; Rini *et al*, 2008) Both sunitinib and sorafenib are also associated with thromboembolic events although the rates are lower to bevacizumab. (Keefe *et al*, 2011) The role of therapeutic anticoagulation for venous thrombosis and aspirin for arterial thrombosis are currently being undertaken given the increased use of the anti-VEGF agents not only in metastatic RCC but in other advance cancers such as non-small cell lung cancer and colorectal carcinoma. (Keefe *et al*, 2011) Pazopanib has also been associated with arterial thrombotic events including myocardial infarction or ischaemia, cerebrovascular accidents and transient ischaemic attacks. Incidence was 3% of patients on pazopanib compared with none in patients taking placebo. (Sternberg *et al*, 2010) The incidence of haemorrhagic events (all grades) in the pazopanib arm was 13% compared with 5% with placebo. (Sternberg *et al*, 2010)

Other agent-specific side effects include adrenal insufficiency, especially in the setting of increased physical stressors with sunitinib; (Desai *et al*, 2007) hyperglycaemia, hyperlipidaemia and acute infusion reactions with temsirolimus (Hudes *et al*, 2007); and non-infectious pneumonitis in patients receiving everolimus, or temsirolimus. (Ravaud, 2011) Patients with pneumonitis may exhibit few if any symptoms and the diagnosis is radiological. Monitoring is advisable although pneumonitis resolves spontaneously when the mTOR inhibitor is ceased and rarely requires use of corticosteroids. (Hudes *et al*, 2007)

Lastly, thrombotic microangiopathy has been reported in association with suntinib, sorafenib, and bevacizumab, either as combined or as single agents. The manifestations included thrombocytopenia, haemolytic anaemia with schistocytosis, and renal dysfunction. (Kapiteijn *et al*, 2007; Patel *et al*, 2008) The treatment of this condition would involve the cessation of the implicated agent and plasma exchange. (Frangie *et al*, 2007)

10. Hypertension as biomarker of efficacy of sunitinib

Data from the two second-line phase II trials, one first-line phase III trial, and an expanded access study of sunitinib were retrospectively analysed to determine whether there was a relationship between hypertension and anti-tumour effect. (Rini *et al*, 2011a) Hypertension in this context was defined by either maximum or mean systolic blood pressure (SBP) of ≥140 mmHg or diastolic blood pressure (DBP) of ≥ 90 mmHg, measured on days 1 and 28 of each 6-week treatment cycle at any time during the study after the first dose of sunitinib. (Rini *et al*, 2011a) The ORR was 54.8% in hypertensive patients vs. 8.7% in patients without a maximum SBP of at least 140 mmHg. Median PFS was 12.5 months vs. 2.5 months, and median OS was 30.9 months vs. 7.2 months in the same two cohorts respectively. (Rini *et al*, 2011a) Overall, a better clinical outcome was demonstrated in patients who experienced hypertension and indeed a direct correlation between SBP and DBP and clinical outcome was observed. To determine whether or not antihypertensive medications reduced the anti-tumour efficacy of sunitinib, clinical outcomes were compared in patients using medications with those that were not at baseline, after cycle 1 and cycle 2. No statistical differences were noted in the ORR or the PFS between the two cohorts regardless of the presence of anti-hypertensive treatments at baseline. The median PFS in the treated and not on antihypertensive were 11.3 months and 10.6 months respectively (p=0.20). There was however a significant difference in median OS of more than 10 months with patients on anti-hypertensive medications demonstrating a 31.8 month survival vs. 21.4 months for patients not taking anti-hypertensive agents (p <0.001). The results of median PFS and median OS measured in patients with or without hypertension at the end of cycle 1 and 2 mirrored those obtained at baseline. (Rini *et al*, 2011a) To illustrate, median PFS measured at the end of cycle 1 for patients with and without anti-hypertensive agents were 13.4 months vs. 10.8 months respectively (p=0.31) and at the end of cycle 2, the median PFS were 13.6 months vs. 10.8 months respectively (p=0.15). (Rini *et al*, 2011a)The overall survival benefit at the end of cycle 1 for patients on anti-hypertensive and not on anti-hypertensive were 30.1 months vs. 23.3 months (p=0.155) and for cycle 2 was 31.1 months vs. 23.0 months (p=0.013) respectively. When analysed according to the prognostic factors (ECOG performance status, time from diagnosis to treatment, LDH, platelet count, corrected calcium), treatment induced hypertension remained a statistically significant predictor of survival benefit (p<0.001). (Rini *et al*, 2011a) In spite of these results supporting the hypothesis that hypertension may be a viable biomarker of anti-tumour efficacy, the development of hypertension during sunitinib treatment was neither necessary nor sufficient for clinical benefit in all patients.(Rini *et al*, 2011a)

11. Drug interactions

The targeted agents are predominantly metabolized by the hepatic cytochrome P450 enzyme CYP3A4 which raises the possibility of drug- drug interactions with concomitant medications that are strong inducers or inhibitors of CYP3A4 (Table 1). (Adams & Leggas, 2007; di Lorenzo *et al*, 2011; Kollmannsberger *et al*, 2007b) For example, the CYP3A4 inhibitors that would potentially increase toxicity of targeted agents include antiretroviral agents such as ritonavir, indinavir and nelfinavir, and antibiotics/antifungals such as clarithromycin, ketoconozole, fluconazole, itraconazole and voriconazole. Potent CYP3A4 inducers that decrease therapeutic efficacy of the targeted agents would include antiepileptic medications such as phenytoin and carbamazepine; antibiotics such as rifampicin and rifabutin. (Kollmannsberger *et al*, 2007a) If the interacting concomittant agent cannot be stopped, doses of the targeted agents may need upward or downward adjustment. It is not only drug-to-drug interactions that are of concern, as many patients take supplements or complementary and alternative medicines (CAM) which they may not mention to their treating physicians. (Lees & Chan, 2011) *Hypericum perforatum*, commonly

Targeted agent	Possible clinical effect	Recommended management
sunitinib		
carbamazepine phenytoin primidone	Decreased blood levels of sunitinib, potential for reduced effect	Avoid concurrent use, choose a non-interacting anti-epileptic agent or consider increasing sunitinib dose; monitor closely for effect and tolerability
St John's Wort	Decreased blood levels of sunitinib, potential for reduced effect	Avoid concurrent use
sorafenib		
carbamazepine phenytoin primidone	Decreased blood levels of sunitinib, potential for reduced effect	Avoid concurrent use, choose a non-interacting anti-epileptic agent or consider increasing sorafenib dose; monitor closely for effect and tolerability
warfarin	Increased INR, bleeding	Monitor patient's INR closely
everolimus		
ketoconazole itraconazole fluconazole voriconazole	Increased blood levels of everolimus; potential for toxicity	Avoid concurrent use or consider reducing everolimus dose; monitor closely for effect and tolerability
phenytoin	Decreased blood levels of everolimus, potential for reduced effect	
St John's Wort	Decreased blood levels of everolimus, potential for reduced effect	Avoid concurrent use

Table 1. Selected examples of drug interactions with some targeted agents

known as St John's Wort is a herbal preparation cancer patients may well be taking for its supposed antidepressant benefits. As it is a CYP3A4 enzyme inducer if taken with sunitinib, sorafenib or everolimus, for example, their effects may be decreased. Grapefruit juice is known to be a CYP3A4 enzyme inhibitor and as such may lead to unexpected toxicity if taken with sunitinib. (Kollmannsberger *et al*, 2007a) A comprehensive full medication history incuding prescribed, self-prescribed over the counter and CAM should be taken when any patient is about to start treatment. (di Lorenzo *et al*, 2011; Lees & Chan, 2011) Drug interaction databases should be utilised, since more reports of interactions may appear as experience with these newer therapies increases.

12. Quality of life in patients with renal cell carcinoma receiving targeted therapies

Health-related quality of life (QoL) has been assessed in a number of studies of patients taking newer targeted therapies for RCC (or kidney cancer). Questionnaires used have included the Functional Assessment of Cancer Therapy-General (FACT-G), the FACT-Kidney Symptom Index-15 item (FKSI-15), the FACT-Kidney Symptom Index-Disease related Symptoms (FKSI-DRS), the European Organisation for Research and Treatment of Cancer Quality of Life Questionnaire (EORTC QLQ-C30 and the Euro QOL 5D (Index and Visual Analogue Scale) utility score (EQ-5D) Index.

Sunitinib has shown improvement over IFN-α with clinically meaningful differences both in kidney cancer related symptoms and overall QoL. (Motzer *et al*, 2007a) Sorafenib when compared with placebo, showed no difference in QoL based on the FACT-G or FKSI-15 mean scores in a sub-analysis of the TARGET trial. However certain symptoms such as fevers, ability to enjoy life, dyspnoea and cough as well as concerns for well being were reported less in the patients on sorafenib. (Bukowski *et al*, 2007a) Quality of life was assessed as a secondary end point in the pazopanib vs. placebo phase III trial (EORTC-QLQ-C30 Version 3) and EQ-5D Index. Patients on pazopanib did not have a clinically different QoL compared with placebo, despite the toxicities that may be expected with pazopanib. (Sternberg *et al*, 2010)

More recently, patient-reported kidney-specific symptom and function assessments as secondary endpoints of the AXIS trial (axitinib vs. sorafenib) were reported at ASCO 2011 (Cella *et al*, 2011). Over 700 patients randomised to axitinib or sorafenib completed FKSI-15 and its disease-related symptoms subscale FKSI-DRS with a completion rate of about 90%. (Cella *et al*, 2011) Overall estimated means in the FKSI-15 and FKSI-DRS mixed-effects models were similar between treatments. The composite time to deterioration (TTD) endpoint, using FKSI-15 or FKSI-DRS, showed a 25% risk reduction for axitinib vs. sorafenib ($p=0.0001$ for both comparisons). Axitinib treatment resulted in patient reported outcomes comparable to sorafenib in patients being treated for second-line metastatic RCC. The PFS benefit demonstrated by axitinib is accompanied by a delay in worsening of the composite endpoint of advanced RCC symptoms, progression, or death compared with sorafenib.

These data reporting on improved or unchanged QoL during treatment with anti-VEGF tyrosine kinase inhibitors (TKIs) are reassuring and may well allay any fears that patient may have and in fact encourage them to proceed on with the treatment. Indeed, the improvement of QoL with some of the TKIs may be attributed to the resolution of their cancer-related-symptoms from the treatment.

In a double-blind, placebo-controlled trial, everolimus 10 mg daily was evaluated using FKSI-DRS and EORTC QLQ-C30. (Beaumont *et al*, 2011) Longitudinal trends for FKSI-DRS scores did not differ between everolimus and placebo. For physical functioning and global QoL, a small but statistically significant decrease was seen with everolimus. All three measures were significantly related to PFS. The authors reported that even when progression of disease was delayed by the new treatment, it did not affect patients' symptoms, functioning, or their QoL, which they proposed is something patients, their family and healthcare providers might expect. (Beaumont *et al*, 2011) Furthermore,

Beaumont and colleagues suggest that for patients receiving first line treatment with a targeted agent, the prospect for clinical benefit may outweigh concerns about health-related QoL. However, in contrast, when these agents are being used in the second- and third-line settings, health-related quality of life may be of more importance to all concerned groups. Continued research is needed into the positive and negative outcomes associated with new treatments for metastatic RCC. (Beaumont *et al*, 2011)

13. Pharmacoeconomics

It is important to determine the optimal setting and sequence of new targeted agents in metastatic RCC to improve patient survival outcomes whilst considering cost-effectiveness. Comparative cost-effectiveness in the first- and second-line setting should be assessed with respect to life years gained. (Molina & Motzer, 2011) For example, Benedict and colleagues utilized a Markov model simulating disease progression, adverse events and survival to assess economic value of first-line treatments in the US and Sweden. Their analyses suggested sunitinib is cost-effective compared with sorafenib, or bevacizumab plus IFN-α for first line metastatic RCC treatment. (Benedict *et al*, 2011) In 2011 NICE, the UK National Institute for Health and Clinical Effectiveness, was unable to approve everolimus for second-line metastatic RCC as it was too expensive for the benefit provided. (http://guidance.nice.org.uk/TA219/Guidance/pdf/English accessed August 1st 2011)

14. Conclusion

The treatment landscape for metastatic RCC has dramatically changed with the development of targeted therapy. Metastatic RCC, once considered a dismal disease to treat has been transformed into a treatable cancer in the era of targeted therapy. These agents are now being investigated either in a sequential or combination fashion in an attempt to search for improved clinical efficacy. The side-effects profile is unique to each agent although there are some common class adverse effects. Careful monitoring and management of side-effects are warranted for patients on these agents to ensure good adherence and effective therapy. Further understanding and insight into the intracellular molecular signaling pathways to both clear-cell and non-clear cell RCC will hopefully lead to the discovery of agents that would confer more durable response and improved prognosis.

15. References

(1999) Interferon-alpha and survival in metastatic renal carcinoma: early results of a randomised controlled trial. Medical Research Council Renal Cancer Collaborators. *Lancet* 353: 14-7

(2010) National Institutes of Health: A phase II study of bevacizumab and erlotinib in subsets with advanced hereditary leiomyomatosis and renal cell cancer (HLRCC) or sporadic papillary renal cell cancer. Accessed Oct 2010. Available from: http://clinicaltrials.gov/ct2/show/NCT01130519?term=bevacizumab+and+erlotinib&rank=2

Abrams TJ, Murray LJ, Pesenti E, Holway VW, Colombo T, Lee LB, Cherrington JM, Pryer NK (2003) Preclinical evaluation of the tyrosine kinase inhibitor SU11248 as a single agent and in combination with "standard of care" therapeutic agents for the treatment of breast cancer. *Mol Cancer Ther* 2: 1011-21

Adams VR, Leggas M (2007) Sunitinib malate for the treatment of metastatic renal cell carcinoma and gastrointestinal stromal tumors. *Clin Ther* 29: 1338-53

Amato R (2011) Everolimus for the treatment of advanced renal cell carcinoma. *Expert Opin Pharmacother* 12: 1143-55

Angevin E, Grünwald V, Castellano DE, Lin CC, Gschwend JE, Harzstark AL, cHang J, Want Y, Shi MM, Escudier BJ (2011) A phase II study of dovitinib (TKI258), an FGFR- and VEGFR-inhibitor, in patients with advanced or metastatic renal cell cancer (mRCC). *J Clin Oncol* 29: (abstr 4551)

Atkins MB, Hidalgo M, Stadler WM, Logan TF, Dutcher JP, Hudes GR, Park Y, Liou SH, Marshall B, Boni JP, Dukart G, Sherman ML (2004) Randomized phase II study of multiple dose levels of CCI-779, a novel mammalian target of rapamycin kinase inhibitor, in patients with advanced refractory renal cell carcinoma. *J Clin Oncol* 22: 909-18

Azad NS, Posadas EM, Kwitkowski VE, Steinberg SM, Jain L, Annunziata CM, Minasian L, Sarosy G, Kotz HL, Premkumar A, Cao L, McNally D, Chow C, Chen HX, Wright JJ, Figg WD, Kohn EC (2008) Combination targeted therapy with sorafenib and bevacizumab results in enhanced toxicity and antitumor activity. *J Clin Oncol* 26: 3709-14

Barkholt L, Bregni M, Remberger M, Blaise D, Peccatori J, Massenkeil G, Pedrazzoli P, Zambelli A, Bay JO, Francois S, Martino R, Bengala C, Brune M, Lenhoff S, Porcellini A, Falda M, Siena S, Demirer T, Niederwieser D, Ringden O (2006) Allogeneic haematopoietic stem cell transplantation for metastatic renal carcinoma in Europe. *Ann Oncol* 17: 1134-40

Beaumont JL, Butt Z, Baladi J, Motzer RJ, Haas T, Hollaender N, Kay A, Cella D (2011) Patient-reported outcomes in a phase iii study of everolimus versus placebo in patients with metastatic carcinoma of the kidney that has progressed on vascular endothelial growth factor receptor tyrosine kinase inhibitor therapy. *Oncologist* 16: 632-40

Beck J, Procopio E, Verzoni S, Bajetta E, Escudier B (2008) Large open label non-comparative clinical experience trial of the multi-targeted kinase inhibitor sorafenib in European patients with advanced RCC *J Clin Oncol* 26: (Abstract 1621)

Beck J, Procopio G, Bajetta E, Keilholz U, Negrier S, Szczylik C, Bokemeyer C, Bracarda S, Richel DJ, Staehler M, Strauss UP, Mersmann S, Burock K, Escudier B (2011) Final results of the European Advanced Renal Cell Carcinoma Sorafenib (EU-ARCCS) expanded-access study: a large open-label study in diverse community settings. *Ann Oncol* 22: 1812-1813

Beck SD, Patel MI, Snyder ME, Kattan MW, Motzer RJ, Reuter VE, Russo P (2004) Effect of papillary and chromophobe cell type on disease-free survival after nephrectomy for renal cell carcinoma. *Ann Surg Oncol* 11: 71-7

Bellmunt J (2007) The Oncologist's View: Targeted Therapies in Advanced Renal Cell Carcinoma. *Eur Urol* Suppl 7: 55-62

Bellmunt J (2009) Future developments in renal cell carcinoma. *Ann Oncol* 20 Suppl 1: i13-17

Benedict A, Figlin RA, Sandstrom P, Harmenberg U, Ullen A, Charbonneau C, Sandin R, Remak E, Hariharan S, Negrier S (2011) Economic evaluation of new targeted therapies for the first-line treatment of patients with metastatic renal cell carcinoma. *BJU Int*

Beuvink I, Boulay A, Fumagalli S, Zilbermann F, Ruetz S, O'Reilly T, Natt F, Hall J, Lane HA, Thomas G (2005) The mTOR inhibitor RAD001 sensitizes tumor cells to DNA-damaged induced apoptosis through inhibition of p21 translation. *Cell* 120: 747-59

Bukowski R, Cella D, Gondek K, Escudier B (2007a) Effects of sorafenib on symptoms and quality of life: results from a large randomized placebo-controlled study in renal cancer. *Am J Clin Oncol* 30: 220-7

Bukowski RM, Kabbinavar FF, Figlin RA, Flaherty K, Srinivas S, Vaishampayan U, Drabkin HA, Dutcher J, Ryba S, Xia Q, Scappaticci FA, McDermott D (2007b) Randomized phase II study of erlotinib combined with bevacizumab compared with bevacizumab alone in metastatic renal cell cancer. *J Clin Oncol* 25: 4536-41

Cebe-Suarez S, Zehnder-Fjallman A, Ballmer-Hofer K (2006) The role of VEGF receptors in angiogenesis; complex partnerships. *Cell Mol Life Sci* 63: 601-15

Cella D, Escudier B, Rini BI, Chen HX, Bhattacharyya JC, Tarazi JC, Rosbrook B, Kim S, Motzer RJ (2011) Patient-reported outcomes (PROs) in a phase III AXIS trial of axitinib versus sorafenib as second-line therapy for metastatic renal cell carcinoma (mRCC) *J Clin Oncol* 29 (suppl) abstr 4504

Cheville JC, Lohse CM, Zincke H, Weaver AL, Blute ML (2003) Comparisons of outcome and prognostic features among histologic subtypes of renal cell carcinoma. *Am J Surg Pathol* 27: 612-24

Choi JS, Kim MK, Seo JW, Choi YL, Kim DH, Chun YK, Ko YH (2006) MET expression in sporadic renal cell carcinomas. *J Korean Med Sci* 21: 672-7

Choueiri TK, Plantade A, Elson P, Negrier S, Ravaud A, Oudard S, Zhou M, Rini BI, Bukowski RM, Escudier B (2008) Efficacy of sunitinib and sorafenib in metastatic papillary and chromophobe renal cell carcinoma. *J Clin Oncol* 26: 127-31

Cindolo L, de la Taille A, Schips L, Zigeuner RE, Ficarra V, Tostain J, Artibani W, Gallo A, Salzano L, Patard JJ (2005) Chromophobe renal cell carcinoma: comprehensive analysis of 104 cases from multicenter European database. *Urology* 65: 681-6

Cohen HT, McGovern FJ (2005) Renal-cell carcinoma. *N Engl J Med* 353: 2477-90

Coppin C, Porzsolt F, Awa A, Kumpf J, Coldman A, Wilt T (2005) Immunotherapy for advanced renal cell cancer. *Cochrane database of systematic reviews (Online)*: CD001425

Costa LJ, Drabkin HA (2007) Renal cell carcinoma: new developments in molecular biology and potential for targeted therapies. *The oncologist* 12: 1404-15

Desai J, Gurney H, Pavlakis N, McArthur GA, Davis ID (2007) Sunitinib malate in the treatment of renal cell carcinoma and gastrointestinal stromal tumor: Recommendations for patient management. *Asia-Pac J Clin Oncol* 3: 167-176

Dharmawardana PG, Giubellino A, Bottaro DP (2004) Hereditary papillary renal carcinoma type I. *Curr Mol Med* 4: 855-68

di Lorenzo G, Porta C, Bellmunt J, Sternberg C, Kirkali Z, Staehler M, Joniau S, Montorsi F, Buonerba C (2011) Toxicities of targeted therapy and their management in kidney cancer. *Eur Urol* 59: 526-40

Dudek AZ, Zolnierek J, Dham A, Lindgren BR, Szczylik C (2009) Sequential therapy with sorafenib and sunitinib in renal cell carcinoma. *Cancer* 115: 61-7

Dutcher JP, Wilding G, Hudes GR, Stadler WM, Kim S, Tarazi JC, Rosbrook B, Rini BI (2008) Sequential axitinib (AG-013736) therapy of patients (pts) with metastatic clear cell renal cell cancer (RCC) refractory to sunitinib and sorafenib, cytokines and sorafenib, or sorafenib alone. *J Clin Oncol* 26: abstr 5127

Eisenhauer EA, Therasse P, Bogaerts J, Schwartz LH, Sargent D, Ford R, Dancey J, Arbuck S, Gwyther S, Mooney M, Rubinstein L, Shankar L, Dodd L, Kaplan R, Lacombe D, Verweij J (2009) New response evaluation criteria in solid tumours: revised RECIST guideline (version 1.1). *Eur J Cancer* 45: 228-47

Elaraj DM, White DE, Steinberg SM, Haworth L, Rosenberg SA, Yang JC (2004) A pilot study of antiangiogenic therapy with bevacizumab and thalidomide in patients with metastatic renal cell carcinoma. *J Immunother* 27: 259-64

Escudier B, Bellmunt J, Negrier S, Bajetta E, Melichar B, Bracarda S, Ravaud A, Golding S, Jethwa S, Sneller V (2007a) Phase III trial of bevacizumab plus interferon alfa-2a in patients with metastatic renal cell carcinoma (AVOREN): final analysis of overall survival. *J Clin Oncol* 28: 2144-50

Escudier B, Eisen T, Stadler WM, Szczylik C, Oudard S, Siebels M, Negrier S, Chevreau C, Solska E, Desai AA, Rolland F, Demkow T, Hutson TE, Gore M, Freeman S, Schwartz B, Shan M, Simantov R, Bukowski RM (2007b) Sorafenib in advanced clear-cell renal-cell carcinoma. *N Engl J Med* 356: 125-34

Escudier B, Eisen T, Stadler WM, Szczylik C, Oudard S, Staehler M, Negrier S, Chevreau C, Desai AA, Rolland F, Demkow T, Hutson TE, Gore M, Anderson S, Hofilena G, Shan M, Pena C, Lathia C, Bukowski RM (2009a) Sorafenib for treatment of renal cell carcinoma: Final efficacy and safety results of the phase III treatment approaches in renal cancer global evaluation trial. *J Clin Oncol* 27: 3312-8

Escudier B, Pluzanska A, Koralewski P, Ravaud A, Bracarda S, Szczylik C, Chevreau C, Filipek M, Melichar B, Bajetta E, Gorbunova V, Bay JO, Bodrogi I, Jagiello-Gruszfeld A, Moore N (2007c) Bevacizumab plus interferon alfa-2a for treatment of metastatic renal cell carcinoma: a randomised, double-blind phase III trial. *Lancet* 370: 2103-11

Escudier B, Roigas J, Gillessen S, Harmenberg U, Srinivas S, Mulder SF, Fountzilas G, Peschel C, Flodgren P, Maneval EC, Chen I, Vogelzang NJ (2009b) Phase II study of sunitinib administered in a continuous once-daily dosing regimen in patients with cytokine-refractory metastatic renal cell carcinoma. *J Clin Oncol* 27: 4068-75

Escudier B, Szczylik C, Hutson TE, Demkow T, Staehler M, Rolland F, Negrier S, Laferriere N, Scheuring UJ, Cella D, Shah S, Bukowski RM (2009c) Randomized phase II trial of first-line treatment with sorafenib versus interferon Alfa-2a in patients with metastatic renal cell carcinoma. *J Clin Oncol* 27: 1280-9

Faivre S, Delbaldo C, Vera K, Robert C, Lozahic S, Lassau N, Bello C, Deprimo S, Brega N, Massimini G, Armand JP, Scigalla P, Raymond E (2006) Safety, pharmacokinetic, and antitumor activity of SU11248, a novel oral multitarget tyrosine kinase inhibitor, in patients with cancer. *J Clin Oncol* 24: 25-35

Feldman DR, Baum MS, Ginsberg MS, Hassoun H, Flombaum CD, Velasco S, Fischer P, Ronnen E, Ishill N, Patil S, Motzer RJ (2009) Phase I trial of bevacizumab plus escalated doses of sunitinib in patients with metastatic renal cell carcinoma. *J Clin Oncol* 27: 1432-9

Fisher R, Pickering L, Larkin J (2011) New targeted therapies for renal cell carcinoma. *Expert Opin Investig Drugs* 20: 933-45

Frangie C, Lefaucheur C, Medioni J, Jacquot C, Hill GS, Nochy D (2007) Renal thrombotic microangiopathy caused by anti-VEGF-antibody treatment for metastatic renal-cell carcinoma. *Lancet Oncol* 8: 177-8

Furge KA, MacKeigan JP, Teh BT (2010) Kinase targets in renal-cell carcinomas: reassessing the old and discovering the new. *Lancet Oncol* 11: 571-8

Fyfe G, Fisher RI, Rosenberg SA, Sznol M, Parkinson DR, Louie AC (1995) Results of treatment of 255 patients with metastatic renal cell carcinoma who received high-dose recombinant interleukin-2 therapy. *J Clin Oncol* 13: 688-96

Gollob JA, Rathmell WK, Richmond TM, Marino CB, Miller EK, Grigson G, Watkins C, Gu L, Peterson BL, Wright JJ (2007) Phase II trial of sorafenib plus interferon alfa-2b as first- or second-line therapy in patients with metastatic renal cell cancer. *J Clin Oncol* 25: 3288-95

Gommersall L, Hayne D, Lynch C, Joseph JV, Arya M, Patel HR (2004) Allogeneic stem-cell transplantation for renal-cell cancer. *Lancet Oncol* 5: 561-7

Gordon MS, Hussey M, Nagle RB, Lara PN, Jr., Mack PC, Dutcher J, Samlowski W, Clark JI, Quinn DI, Pan CX, Crawford D (2009) Phase II study of erlotinib in patients with locally advanced or metastatic papillary histology renal cell cancer: SWOG S0317. *J Clin Oncol* 27: 5788-93

Gore ME, Szczylik C, Porta C, Bracarda S, Bjarnason GA, Oudard S, Hariharan S, Lee SH, Haanen J, Castellano D, Vrdoljak E, Schoffski P, Mainwaring P, Nieto A, Yuan J, Bukowski R (2009) Safety and efficacy of sunitinib for metastatic renal-cell carcinoma: an expanded-access trial. *Lancet Oncol* 10: 757-63

Harris DT (1983) Hormonal therapy and chemotherapy of renal-cell carcinoma. *Semin Oncol* 10: 422-30

Hidalgo M, Buckner JC, Erlichman C, Pollack MS, Boni JP, Dukart G, Marshall B, Speicher L, Moore L, Rowinsky EK (2006) A phase I and pharmacokinetic study of temsirolimus (CCI-779) administered intravenously daily for 5 days every 2 weeks to patients with advanced cancer. *Clin Cancer Res* 12: 5755-63

Hudes G, Carducci M, Tomczak P, Dutcher J, Figlin R, Kapoor A, Staroslawska E, Sosman J, McDermott D, Bodrogi I, Kovacevic Z, Lesovoy V, Schmidt-Wolf IG, Barbarash O, Gokmen E, O'Toole T, Lustgarten S, Moore L, Motzer RJ (2007) Temsirolimus, interferon alfa, or both for advanced renal-cell carcinoma. *N Engl J Med* 356: 2271-81

Hurwitz HI, Dowlati A, Saini S, Savage S, Suttle AB, Gibson DM, Hodge JP, Merkle EM, Pandite L (2009) Phase I trial of pazopanib in patients with advanced cancer. *Clin Cancer Res* 15: 4220-7

Hutson TE (2011) Targeted therapies for the treatment of metastatic renal cell carcinoma: clinical evidence. *Oncologist* 16 Suppl 2: 14-22

Hutson TE, Davis ID, Machiels JP, De Souza PL, Rottey S, Hong BF, Epstein RJ, Baker KL, McCann L, Crofts T, Pandite L, Figlin RA (2010) Efficacy and safety of pazopanib in patients with metastatic renal cell carcinoma. *J Clin Oncol* 28: 475-80

Isaacs JS, Jung YJ, Mole DR, Lee S, Torres-Cabala C, Chung YL, Merino M, Trepel J, Zbar B, Toro J, Ratcliffe PJ, Linehan WM, Neckers L (2005) HIF overexpression correlates with biallelic loss of fumarate hydratase in renal cancer: novel role of fumarate in regulation of HIF stability. *Cancer Cell* 8: 143-53

Izzedine H, Ederhy S, Goldwasser F, Soria JC, Milano G, Cohen A, Khayat D, Spano JP (2009) Management of hypertension in angiogenesis inhibitor-treated patients. *Ann Oncol* 20: 807-15

Jarkowski A, 3rd, Glode AE, Spangenthal EJ, Wong MK (2011) Heart failure caused by molecularly targeted therapies for cancer. *Pharmacotherapy* 31: 62-75

Jonasch E, Corn P, Pagliaro LC, Warneke CL, Johnson MM, Tamboli P, Ng C, Aparicio A, Ashe RG, Wright JJ, Tannir NM (2010) Upfront, randomized, phase 2 trial of sorafenib versus sorafenib and low-dose interferon alfa in patients with advanced renal cell carcinoma: clinical and biomarker analysis. *Cancer* 116: 57-65

Jonasch E, Hutson TE, Harshman LC, Srinivas S (2011) Advanced Renal Cell Carcinoma: Overview of Drug Therapy fro the Practicing Physician. *J Clin Oncol* ASCO Education Book: 145-151

Kabbinavar FF, Srinivas S, Hauke RJ, Amato RJ, Esteves WB, Cotreau MM, Strahs AL, Bhargava P, Fishman MN (2011) Results from a phase I trial of tivozanib (AV-951) combined with temsirolimus therapy in patients (pts) with renal cell carcinoma (RCC). *J Clin Oncol* 29: abstr 4549

Kamura T, Sato S, Iwai K, Czyzyk-Krzeska M, Conaway RC, Conaway JW (2000) Activation of HIF1alpha ubiquitination by a reconstituted von Hippel-Lindau (VHL) tumor suppressor complex. *Proc Natl Acad Sci U S A* 97: 10430-5

Kapiteijn E, Brand A, Kroep J, Gelderblom H (2007) Sunitinib induced hypertension, thrombotic microangiopathy and reversible posterior leukencephalopathy syndrome. *Ann Oncol* 18: 1745-7

Keefe D, Bowen J, Gibson R, Tan T, Okera M, Stringer A (2011) Noncardiac vascular toxicities of vascular endothelial growth factor inhibitors in advanced cancer: a review. *Oncologist* 16: 432-44

Kim DW, Jo YS, Jung HS, Chung HK, Song JH, Park KC, Park SH, Hwang JH, Rha SY, Kweon GR, Lee SJ, Jo KW, Shong M (2006) An orally administered multitarget tyrosine kinase inhibitor, SU11248, is a novel potent inhibitor of thyroid oncogenic RET/papillary thyroid cancer kinases. *J Clin Endocrinol Metab* 91: 4070-6

Kim WY, Kaelin WG (2004) Role of VHL gene mutation in human cancer. *J Clin Oncol* 22: 4991-5004

Klatte T, Han KR, Said JW, Bohm M, Allhoff EP, Kabbinavar FF, Belldegrun AS, Pantuck AJ (2008) Pathobiology and prognosis of chromophobe renal cell carcinoma. *Urol Oncol* 26: 604-9

Kollmannsberger C, Soulieres D, Wong R, Scalera A, Gaspo R, Bjarnason G (2007a) Sunitinib therapy for metastatic renal cell carcinoma: recommendations for management of side-effects. *Can Urol Assoc J* 1 (Suppl 2): S41-S54

Kollmannsberger C, Soulieres D, Wong R, Scalera A, Gaspo R, Bjarnason G (2007b) Sunitinib therapy for metastatic renal cell carcinoma: recommendations for management of side effects. *Can Urol Assoc J* 1: S41-54

Lacouture ME, Anadkat MJ, Bensadoun RJ, Bryce J, Chan A, Epstein JB, Eaby-Sandy B, Murphy BA (2011) Clinical practice guidelines for the prevention and treatment of EGFR inhibitor-associated dermatologic toxicities. *Support Care Cancer* 19: 1079-95

Lees J, Chan A (2011) Polypharmacy in elderly patients with cancer: clinical implications and management. *Lancet Oncol* Epub 7 July

Linehan WM, Pinto PA, Srinivasan R, Merino M, Choyke P, Choyke L, Coleman J, Toro J, Glenn G, Vocke C, Zbar B, Schmidt LS, Bottaro D, Neckers L (2007) Identification of the genes for kidney cancer: opportunity for disease-specific targeted therapeutics. *Clin Cancer Res* 13: 671s-679s

Margulis V, Tamboli P, Matin SF, Swanson DA, Wood CG (2008) Analysis of clinicopathologic predictors of oncologic outcome provides insight into the natural history of surgically managed papillary renal cell carcinoma. *Cancer* 112: 1480-8

Maxwell PH, Wiesener MS, Chang GW, Clifford SC, Vaux EC, Cockman ME, Wykoff CC, Pugh CW, Maher ER, Ratcliffe PJ (1999) The tumour suppressor protein VHL targets hypoxia-inducible factors for oxygen-dependent proteolysis. *Nature* 399: 271-5

McDermott DF, George DJ (2010) Bevacizumab as a treatment option in advanced renal cell carcinoma: an analysis and interpretation of clinical trial data. *Cancer Treat Rev* 36: 216-23

McDermott DF, Regan MM, Clark JI, Flaherty LE, Weiss GR, Logan TF, Kirkwood JM, Gordon MS, Sosman JA, Ernstoff MS, Tretter CP, Urba WJ, Smith JW, Margolin KA, Mier JW, Gollob JA, Dutcher JP, Atkins MB (2005) Randomized phase III trial of high-dose interleukin-2 versus subcutaneous interleukin-2 and interferon in patients with metastatic renal cell carcinoma. *J Clin Oncol* 23: 133-41

Mekhail TM, Abou-Jawde RM, Boumerhi G, Malhi S, Wood L, Elson P, Bukowski R (2005) Validation and extension of the Memorial Sloan-Kettering prognostic factors model for survival in patients with previously untreated metastatic renal cell carcinoma. *J Clin Oncol* 23: 832-41

Melichar B, Koralewski P, Ravaud A, Pluzanska A, Bracarda S, Szczylik C, Chevreau C, Filipek M, Delva R, Sevin E, Negrier S, McKendrick J, Santoro A, Pisa P, Escudier B (2008) First-line bevacizumab combined with reduced dose interferon-alpha2a is active in patients with metastatic renal cell carcinoma. *Ann Oncol* 19: 1470-6

Mendel DB, Laird AD, Xin X, Louie SG, Christensen JG, Li G, Schreck RE, Abrams TJ, Ngai TJ, Lee LB, Murray LJ, Carver J, Chan E, Moss KG, Haznedar JO, Sukbuntherng J, Blake RA, Sun L, Tang C, Miller T, Shirazian S, McMahon G, Cherrington JM (2003) In vivo antitumor activity of SU11248, a novel tyrosine kinase inhibitor targeting vascular endothelial growth factor and platelet-derived growth factor receptors: determination of a pharmacokinetic/pharmacodynamic relationship. *Clin Cancer Res* 9: 327-37

Molina AM, Motzer R (2008) Current Algorithm and Prognostic Factors in the Treatment of Metastatic Renal Cell Carcinoma. *Clin Genitourinary Can* 6: S7-S13

Molina AM, Motzer RJ (2011) Clinical practice guidelines for the treatment of metastatic renal cell carcinoma: today and tomorrow. *Oncologist* 16 Suppl 2: 45-50

Motzer RJ, Bacik J, Mariani T, Russo P, Mazumdar M, Reuter V (2002) Treatment outcome and survival associated with metastatic renal cell carcinoma of non-clear-cell histology. *J Clin Oncol* 20: 2376-81

Motzer RJ, Bacik J, Mazumdar M (2004) Prognostic Factors for Survival of Patients with Stage IV Renal Cell Carcinoma. *Clin Cancer Research* 10: 6302S-6303S

Motzer RJ, Bander NH, Nanus DM (1996) Renal-cell carcinoma. *N Engl J Med* 335: 865-75

Motzer RJ, de La Motte Rouge T, Harzstark AL, michaelson MD, Liu G, Gruenwald V, Ingrosso A, Tortorici MA, Bycott PW, Kim S, Rini BI (2011a) Axitinib second-line therapy for metastatic renal cell carcinoma (mRCC): Five-year (yr) overall survival (OS) data from a phase II trial. *J Clin Oncol* 29: (suppl; abstr 4527)

Motzer RJ, Escudier B, Oudard S, Hutson TE, Porta C, Bracarda S, Grunwald V, Thompson JA, Figlin RA, Hollaender N, Urbanowitz G, Berg WJ, Kay A, Lebwohl D, Ravaud A (2008) Efficacy of everolimus in advanced renal cell carcinoma: a double-blind, randomised, placebo-controlled phase III trial. *Lancet* 372: 449-56

Motzer RJ, Hutson TE, Olsen MR, Hudes GR, Burke JM, Edenfield WJ, Wilding G, Martell B, Hariharan S, Figlin RA (2011b) Randomized phase II multicenter study of the efficacy and safety of sunitinib on the 4/2 versus continuous dosing schedule as first-line therapy of metastatic renal cell carcinoma: Renal EFFECT Trial. *J Clin Oncol* 29: (suppl 7; abstrc LBA308)

Motzer RJ, Hutson TE, Tomczak P, Michaelson MD, Bukowski RM, Oudard S, Negrier S, Szczylik C, Pili R, Bjarnason GA, Garcia-del-Muro X, Sosman JA, Solska E, Wilding G, Thompson JA, Kim ST, Chen I, Huang X, Figlin RA (2009) Overall survival and updated results for sunitinib compared with interferon alfa in patients with metastatic renal cell carcinoma. *J Clin Oncol* 27: 3584-90

Motzer RJ, Hutson TE, Tomczak P, Michaelson MD, Bukowski RM, Rixe O, Oudard S, Negrier S, Szczylik C, Kim ST, Chen I, Bycott PW, Baum CM, Figlin RA (2007a) Sunitinib versus interferon alfa in metastatic renal-cell carcinoma. *N Engl J Med* 356: 115-24

Motzer RJ, Mazumdar M, Bacik J, Berg W, Amsterdam A, Ferrara J (1999) Survival and prognostic stratification of 670 patients with advanced renal cell carcinoma. *J Clin Oncol* 17: 2530-40

Motzer RJ, Michaelson MD, Redman BG, Hudes GR, Wilding G, Figlin RA, Ginsberg MS, Kim ST, Baum CM, DePrimo SE, Li JZ, Bello CL, Theuer CP, George DJ, Rini BI (2006) Activity of SU11248, a multitargeted inhibitor of vascular endothelial growth factor receptor and platelet-derived growth factor receptor, in patients with metastatic renal cell carcinoma. *J Clin Oncol* 24: 16-24

Motzer RJ, Michaelson MD, Rosenberg J, Bukowski RM, Curti BD, George DJ, Hudes GR, Redman BG, Margolin KA, Wilding G (2007b) Sunitinib efficacy against advanced renal cell carcinoma. *J Urol* 178: 1883-7

Murray LJ, Abrams TJ, Long KR, Ngai TJ, Olson LM, Hong W, Keast PK, Brassard JA, O'Farrell AM, Cherrington JM, Pryer NK (2003) SU11248 inhibits tumor growth and CSF-1R-dependent osteolysis in an experimental breast cancer bone metastasis model. *Clin Exp Metastasis* 20: 757-66

NCT00378703 Cgi (2006) Bevacizumab, Sorafenib, and Temsirolimus in Treating Patients With Metastatic Kidney Cancer (BeST) *[cited 16 Dec 2010]*. Available from http://clinicaltrials.gov/ct2/show/NCT00378703

NCT00720941 Cgi (2011) Pazopanib Versus Sunitinib in the Treatment of Locally Advanced and/or Metastatic Renal Cell Carcinoma (COMPARZ) *[cited 21 July 2011]*. Available from: http://clinicaltrials.gov/ct2/show/NCT00720941

NCT00732914 Cgi (2010) Sequential Study to Treat Renal Cell Carcinoma *[cited 18 Oct 2010]*. Available from:
http://clinicaltrials.gov/ct2/show/NCT00732914?term=NCT00732914&rank=1

NCT1217931 Cgi (2011) Sequential Two-agent Assessment in Renal Cell Carcinoma Therapy *[cited 17 May 2011]*. Available from:

http://clinicaltrials.gov/ct2/show/NCT01217931?term=NCT01217931&rank=1

Negrier S, Gravis G, Perol D, Chevreau C, Delva R, Bay JO, Blanc E, Ferlay C, Geoffrois L, Rolland F, Legouffe E, Sevin E, Laguerre B, Escudier B (2011) Temsirolimus and bevacizumab, or sunitinib, or interferon alfa and bevacizumab for patients with advanced renal cell carcinoma (TORAVA): a randomised phase 2 trial. *Lancet Oncol* 12: 673-80

Nosov D, Bhargava P, Esteves WB, Strahs AL, Lipatov ON, Lyulkp OO, Anischenko AO, Chacki RT, Doval D, Slichenmyer WJ (2011) Final analysis of the phase II randomized discontinuation trial (RDT) of tivozanib (AV-951) versus placebo in patients with renal cell carcinoma (RCC). *J Clin Oncol* 29: (suppl; abstr 4503)

O'Farrell AM, Abrams TJ, Yuen HA, Ngai TJ, Louie SG, Yee KW, Wong LM, Hong W, Lee LB, Town A, Smolich BD, Manning WC, Murray LJ, Heinrich MC, Cherrington JM (2003) SU11248 is a novel FLT3 tyrosine kinase inhibitor with potent activity in vitro and in vivo. *Blood* 101: 3597-605

Ohh M, Park CW, Ivan M, Hoffman MA, Kim TY, Huang LE, Pavletich N, Chau V, Kaelin WG (2000) Ubiquitination of hypoxia-inducible factor requires direct binding to the beta-domain of the von Hippel-Lindau protein. *Nat Cell Biol* 2: 423-7

Oudard S, Banu E, Vieillefond A, Fournier L, Priou F, Medioni J, Banu A, Duclos B, Rolland F, Escudier B, Arakelyan N, Culine S (2007a) Prospective multicenter phase II study of gemcitabine plus platinum salt for metastatic collecting duct carcinoma: results of a GETUG (Groupe d'Etudes des Tumeurs Uro-Genitales) study. *J Urol* 177: 1698-702

Oudard S, George D, Medioni J, Motzer R (2007b) Treatment options in renal cell carcinoma: past, present and future. *Ann Oncol* 18 Suppl 10: x25-31

Parton M, Gore M, Eisen T (2006) Role of cytokine therapy in 2006 and beyond for metastatic renal cell cancer. *J Clin Oncol* 24: 5584-92

Patard JJ, Leray E, Rioux-Leclercq N, Cindolo L, Ficarra V, Zisman A, De La Taille A, Tostain J, Artibani W, Abbou CC, Lobel B, Guille F, Chopin DK, Mulders PF, Wood CG, Swanson DA, Figlin RA, Belldegrun AS, Pantuck AJ (2005) Prognostic value of histologic subtypes in renal cell carcinoma: a multicenter experience. *J Clin Oncol* 23: 2763-71

Patel TV, Morgan JA, Demetri GD, George S, Maki RG, Quigley M, Humphreys BD (2008) A preeclampsia-like syndrome characterized by reversible hypertension and proteinuria induced by the multitargeted kinase inhibitors sunitinib and sorafenib. *J Natl Cancer Inst* 100: 282-4

Pavlovich CP, Walther MM, Eyler RA, Hewitt SM, Zbar B, Linehan WM, Merino MJ (2002) Renal tumors in the Birt-Hogg-Dube syndrome. *Am J Surg Pathol* 26: 1542-52

Pithavala YK, Tortorici M, Toh M, Garrett M, Hee B, Kuruganti U, Ni G, Klamerus KJ (2010) Effect of rifampin on the pharmacokinetics of Axitinib (AG-013736) in Japanese and Caucasian healthy volunteers. *Cancer Chemother Pharmacol* 65: 563-70

Plimack ER, Jonasch E, Bekele bN, Qiao W, Ng CS, Tannir NM (2010) Sunitinib in papillary renal cell carcinoma (pRCC): Results from a single-arm phase II study. *J Clin Oncol* 28: (suppl; abstr 4604)

Ratain MJ, Eisen T, Stadler WM, Flaherty KT, Kaye SB, Rosner GL, Gore M, Desai AA, Patnaik A, Xiong HQ, Rowinsky E, Abbruzzese JL, Xia C, Simantov R, Schwartz B,

O'Dwyer PJ (2006) Phase II placebo-controlled randomized discontinuation trial of sorafenib in patients with metastatic renal cell carcinoma. *J Clin Oncol* 24: 2505-12

Ravaud A (2009) How to optimise treatment compliance in metastatic renal cell carcinoma with targeted agents. *Ann Oncol* 20 (Suppl 1): i7-12

Ravaud A (2011) Treatment-Associated Adverse Event Management in the Advanced Renal Cell Carcinoma Patient Treated with Targeted Therapies. *Oncologist* 16(suppl 2): 32-44

Ravaud A, Oudard S, Gravis-Mescam G, Sevin E, Zanetta S, Théodore C, de Fromont M, Mahier-Aït Oukhatar C, Chêne G, Escudier B (2009) First-line sunitinib in type I and II papillary renal cell carcinoma (PRCC): SUPAP, a phase II study of the French Genito-Urinary Group (GETUG) and the Group of Early Phase trials (GEP). *J Clin Oncol* 27: (suppl; abstr 5146)

Raymond E, Alexandre J, Faivre S, Vera K, Materman E, Boni J, Leister C, Korth-Bradley J, Hanauske A, Armand JP (2004) Safety and pharmacokinetics of escalated doses of weekly intravenous infusion of CCI-779, a novel mTOR inhibitor, in patients with cancer. *J Clin Oncol* 22: 2336-47

Rini B, Al-Marrawi MY (2011) Pazopanib for the treatment of renal cancer. *Expert Opin Pharmacother* 12: 1171-89

Rini BI, Cohen DP, Lu DR, Chen I, Hariharan S, Gore ME, Figlin RA, Baum MS, Motzer RJ (2011a) Hypertension as a biomarker of efficacy in patients with metastatic renal cell carcinoma treated with sunitinib. *J Natl Cancer Inst* 103: 763-73

Rini BI, Escudier B, Tomczak P, Kaprin A, Hutson TE, Szczylik C, Tarazi JC, Rosbrook B, Kim S, Motzer RJ (2011b) Axitinib versus sorafenib as second-line therapy for metastatic renal cell carcinoma (mRCC): Results of phase III AXIS trial. *J Clin Oncol* 29: (suppl; abstr 4503)

Rini BI, Garcia JA, Cooney MM, Elson P, Tyler A, Beatty K, Bokar J, Mekhail T, Bukowski RM, Budd GT, Triozzi P, Borden E, Ivy P, Chen HX, Dolwati A, Dreicer R (2009) A phase I study of sunitinib plus bevacizumab in advanced solid tumors. *Clin Cancer Res* 15: 6277-83

Rini BI, Halabi S, Rosenberg JE, Stadler WM, Vaena DA, Archer L, Atkins JN, Picus J, Czaykowski P, Dutcher J, Small EJ (2010) Phase III trial of bevacizumab plus interferon alfa versus interferon alfa monotherapy in patients with metastatic renal cell carcinoma: final results of CALGB 90206. *J Clin Oncol* 28: 2137-43

Rini BI, Halabi S, Rosenberg JE, Stadler WM, Vaena DA, Ou SS, Archer L, Atkins JN, Picus J, Czaykowski P, Dutcher J, Small EJ (2008) Bevacizumab plus interferon alfa compared with interferon alfa monotherapy in patients with metastatic renal cell carcinoma: CALGB 90206. *J Clin Oncol* 26: 5422-8

Rini BI, Zimmerman T, Stadler WM, Gajewski TF, Vogelzang NJ (2002) Allogeneic stem-cell transplantation of renal cell cancer after nonmyeloablative chemotherapy: feasibility, engraftment, and clinical results. *J Clin Oncol* 20: 2017-24

Rixe O, Billemont B, Izzedine H (2007a) Hypertension as a predictive factor of Sunitinib activity. *Ann Oncol* 18: 1117

Rixe O, Bukowski RM, Michaelson MD, Wilding G, Hudes GR, Bolte O, Motzer RJ, Bycott P, Liau KF, Freddo J, Trask PC, Kim S, Rini BI (2007b) Axitinib treatment in patients with cytokine-refractory metastatic renal-cell cancer: a phase II study. *Lancet Oncol* 8: 975-84

Ryan CW, Goldman BH, Lara PN, Jr., Mack PC, Beer TM, Tangen CM, Lemmon D, Pan CX, Drabkin HA, Crawford ED (2007) Sorafenib with interferon alfa-2b as first-line treatment of advanced renal carcinoma: a phase II study of the Southwest Oncology Group. *J Clin Oncol* 25: 3296-301

Schmidinger M, Bellmunt J (2011) Plethora of agents, plethora of targets, plethora of side effects in metastatic renal cell carcinoma. *Cancer Treat Rev* 36: 416-24

Schmidt LS, Warren MB, Nickerson ML, Weirich G, Matrosova V, Toro JR, Turner ML, Duray P, Merino M, Hewitt S, Pavlovich CP, Glenn G, Greenberg CR, Linehan WM, Zbar B (2001) Birt-Hogg-Dube syndrome, a genodermatosis associated with spontaneous pneumothorax and kidney neoplasia, maps to chromosome 17p11.2. *Am J Hum Genet* 69: 876-82

Sosman JA, Flaherty KT, Atkins MB, McDermott DF, Rothenberg WL, Vermeulen WL, Harlacker K, Hsu A, Wright JJ, Puzanov I (2008) Updated results of phase I trial of sorafenib (S) and bevacizumab (B) in patients with metastatic renal cell cancer (mRCC). *J Clin Oncol* 26 (May 20 Suppl): Abstr 5011

Stadler WM, Figlin RA, McDermott DF, Dutcher JP, Knox JJ, Miller WH, Jr., Hainsworth JD, Henderson CA, George JR, Hajdenberg J, Kindwall-Keller TL, Ernstoff MS, Drabkin HA, Curti BD, Chu L, Ryan CW, Hotte SJ, Xia C, Cupit L, Bukowski RM (2010) Safety and efficacy results of the advanced renal cell carcinoma sorafenib expanded access program in North America. *Cancer* 116: 1272-80

Sternberg CN (2010) Randomised, double-blind phase III study of pazopanib in patients with advaced/metastatic renal cell carcinoma (MRCC), ESMO: Pazopanib in advanced MRCC - late breaker published 11/10/2011 by cancer reported Jo Armstrong.

Sternberg CN, Davis ID, Mardiak J, Szczylik C, Lee E, Wagstaff J, Barrios CH, Salman P, Gladkov OA, Kavina A, Zarba JJ, Chen M, McCann L, Pandite L, Roychowdhury DF, Hawkins RE (2010) Pazopanib in locally advanced or metastatic renal cell carcinoma: results of a randomized phase III trial. *J Clin Oncol* 28: 1061-8

Sudarshan S, Linehan WM (2006) Genetic basis of cancer of the kidney. *Semin Oncol* 33: 544-51

Tan TH, Pranavan G, Haxhimolla HZ, Yip D (2010) New systemic treatment options for metastatic renal-cell carcinoma in the era of targeted therapies. *Asia Pac J Clin Oncol* 6: 5-18

Tazi el M, Essadi I, Tazi MF, Ahellal Y, M'Rabti H, Errihani H (2011) Advanced treatments in non-clear renal cell carcinoma. *Urol J* 8: 1-11

Vaupel P (2004) The role of hypoxia-induced factors in tumor progression. *Oncologist* 9 Suppl 5: 10-7

Yagoda A, Bander NH (1989) Failure of cytotoxic chemotherapy, 1983-1988, and the emerging role of monoclonal antibodies for renal cancer. *Urol Int* 44: 338-45

Yamazaki K, Sakamoto M, Ohta T, Kanai Y, Ohki M, Hirohashi S (2003) Overexpression of KIT in chromophobe renal cell carcinoma. *Oncogene* 22: 847-52

Yang JC, Haworth L, Sherry RM, Hwu P, Schwartzentruber DJ, Topalian SL, Steinberg SM, Chen HX, Rosenberg SA (2003) A randomized trial of bevacizumab, an anti-vascular endothelial growth factor antibody, for metastatic renal cancer. *N Engl J Med* 349: 427-34

Zbar B, Alvord WG, Glenn G, Turner M, Pavlovich CP, Schmidt L, Walther M, Choyke P, Weirich G, Hewitt SM, Duray P, Gabril F, Greenberg C, Merino MJ, Toro J, Linehan WM (2002) Risk of renal and colonic neoplasms and spontaneous pneumothorax in the Birt-Hogg-Dube syndrome. *Cancer Epidemiol Biomarkers Prev* 11: 393-400

19

Sequential Use of Targeted Therapies (TT) in Metastatic Renal Cell Cancer (mRCC): Overall Results of a Large Experience

G. Procopio, E. Verzoni, R. Iacovelli,
F. Gelsomino, M. Catanzaro and L. Mariani
'IRCCS 'Istituto Nazionale dei Tumori', Medical Oncology, Milan
Italy

1. Introduction

Renal cell carcinoma accounts for 80% of all kidney cancers -worldwide; the tumor staging at diagnosis ranges from small, low-stage tumors to more advanced neoplasms [1-5]. The survival rate has increased in recent years: nowadays, patients with localized disease have a 5-year survival >80% but in those with distant metastatic RCC, 5-year survival is <10% [6-8]. The increase in overall survival was due, at least in part, to improved surgical techniques [9,10]. Until recently cytokines (interleukin-2 or interferon-alpha), were the mainstay of systemic treatment despite low response rates and significant toxicity [11,12].

Since 2005, six targeted therapies for advanced/metastatic RCC were approved by both the FDA and EMA: three are multitargeted tyrosine kinase inhibitors (TKIs), sorafenib (SO), sunitinib (SU) and pazopanib (PZ), two are oral mTOR inhibitors, temsirolimus (TS) and everolimus (EV) and one is the anti-VEGF monoclonal antibody bevacizumab (BV), administered in combination with IFN-alpha [13]. These new agents improved the progression free survival (PFS) and the overall survival (OS) in several subgroups of patients; however, expert opinion on the optimal therapeutic strategy is divided.

Two main therapeutic approaches—use of these new agents in combination or sequentially—have been studied to increase efficacy and tolerability. Sequential therapy is the current standard of care in the treatment of advanced RCC as existing combination regimens have a high incidence of adverse events without a substantial increase in efficacy. The use of sequential therapy provides a number of important advantages: patients who are refractory to one or more targeted agent(s) may benefit from treatment with a different agent; there is no/limited cross-resistance between agents and patients experiencing disease progression with one anti-angiogenic agent can subsequently benefit from treatment with another [14,15].

The results of recent phase III randomized controlled trials (RCTs) prompted the National Comprehensive Cancer Network (NCCN) and the European Association of Urology (EAU) to update their clinical practice guidelines for the treatment of metastatic RCC [16,17]. The EAU recommended SU as a first-line therapy in low- and intermediate-risk patients and concluded that SO is effective as second-line treatment after failure of cytokine therapy or in patients unfit for cytokines [18]. Clinical evidence supports the efficacy of sequential treatment with SU/SO [19]; however, the optimal sequence for SO and SU is still under debate, and additional evidence on the optimal use of sequential targeted therapies is advocated.

In this retrospective study - the preliminary results of which have been previously presented [20] - the safety and efficacy of different sequential schemes of targeted therapies, in patients with advanced/metastatic RCC were studied.

2. Methods

2.1 Patients

This retrospective study was conducted at the 'Istituto Nazionale Tumori of Milan' (National Institute of Tumors, Milan, Italy) - one of the most important Italian institutions for cancer diagnosis and treatment - between January 2004 and July 2010. Patients were patients aged ≥18 years with advanced/metastatic RCC and a life expectancy of >3 months who had been treated with antiangiogenic therapy (one or more) were eligible for enrollment in this retrospective study. Patients with Eastern Cooperative Oncology Group (ECOG) performance status (PS) of 0, 1 or 2 were included. A number of patients enrolled in this study had previously taken part in a range of prospective trials including TARGET , the EU-ARCCS , RECORD-1 , AXIS , AVOREN and ROSORC at our centre.

3. Treatment

Patients received a range of different systemic agents – SO, SU, BV, EV, TS and axitinib (AX) alone or in combination, and could have received a previous treatment with cytokines. SO was administered orally at a dose of 400 mg twice daily and SU at a daily dose of 50 mg orally with a 4 weeks on 2 weeks off schedule. BV was administered iv at 10 mg/Kg every 2 weeks in combination with Interferon-a subcutaneously, EV was administered orally at 10 mg daily continuously, TS iv weekly at 25 mg/dose and AX at 10 mg/daily orally continuously. Patients received systemic therapy until disease progression or the presence of serious adverse events.

4. Study assessments

Study assessments were conducted at baseline and once a month thereafter. Baseline characteristics were taken ≤28 days after the start of treatment. Drug safety and tolerability were assessed using the National Cancer Institute Common Terminology Criteria for Adverse Events (NCTCA version 3). Efficacy was assessed by progression-free survival (PFS) and overall survival (OS) according to the Motzer classification [21]. PFS was defined as the time from start of systemic treatment to death or disease progression whichever occurred first. Disease progression was evaluated using the Response Evaluation criteria in Solid Tumours (RECIST, version 1.0) by the treating physician. Assessments were performed monthly (every 3 weeks for patients on sunitinib, due to the schedule of administration for this drug). Patients with Bellini duct RCC were excluded from the efficacy analysis, due to the different histology of the tumor.

5. Statistical analyses

All clinical and instrumental variables and toxicity data were analyzed by descriptive statistics: mean, standard deviation, minimum, and maximum values for continuous variables, and absolute and relative frequencies for categorical variables. Curves relevant to OS (overall, Motzer and according to therapy option) were estimated by the Kaplan–Meier method and compared by means of the log-rank test. Reports of AEs were categorized according to type, severity, and outcome. A p value <0.05 was considered statistically significant.

6. Results

A total of 310 patients with metastatic RCC were observed, and followed-up for a median of 37 months (range 21–49 months). Patient characteristics at baseline are shown in **Table 1**.

Patients included in database	310	
Median age (years)	62	
Range	55–69	
Male	229	(74%)
Female	81	
ECOG PS		
0	168	(54%)
1	123	(40%)
2	19	(6%)
Histology		
Clear-cell	268	(86.4%)
Papillary	27	(8.7%)
Bellini	7	(2.2%)
Chromophobe	6	(1.9%)
Oncocytoma	1	(0.3%)
UNK	1	(0.3%)
Previous nephrectomy, %	273	(88.1%)
Fuhrman grade, %		
1	15	(5.58%)
2	93	(34.57%)
3	118	(43.87%)
4	43	(15.99%)
Missing	41	
Motzer criteria		
High	64	(20.6%)
Low	100	(32.3%)
Intermediate	146	(47.10%)
Targeted therapies %		
1	163	(52.6%)
2	113	(36.5%)
3	30	(9.7%)
4	4	(1.29%)

Number of disease sites		
1	121	(39.0%)
2	107	(34.5%)
3	67	(21.2%)
4	12	(3.9%)
5	3	(0.9%)
Sites of disease (n=599)		
Bone	88	(28.39%)
Brain	16	(5.16%)
Liver	59	(19.03%)
Lung	204	(65.81%)
Lymph nodes	119	(38.39%)
Pancreas	15	(4.84%)
Thyroid	4	(1.29%)
Other	94	(30.32%)

Table 1. Patient characteristics at baseline

Overall the majority of patients (163; 53.9%) received one treatment line with systemic agents while 113 (36.5%) received two, 30 (9.7%) received three line and four patients (1.3%) received four. One-sided analysis of variance showed that the Motzer classification/score was predictive regarding the number of therapy lines (Fisher 8.49, $p<0.01$) with the mean number of treatments significantly lower in the high-risk group ($p<0.05$) than in the low/intermediate risk groups (t-tests). Overall the majority of patients 196/310 received SO as first line followed by SU in 96 cases or SU, in 63 cases followed by SO in 13 cases). The remaining 51/310 received other systemic agents in sequence (BV, TS, AX alone or in sequence/combination with SO and SU).

Median OS was 22 months and the 5-year OS was 23.4% (95% CI 16.7, 30.0%) (**Figure 1**).

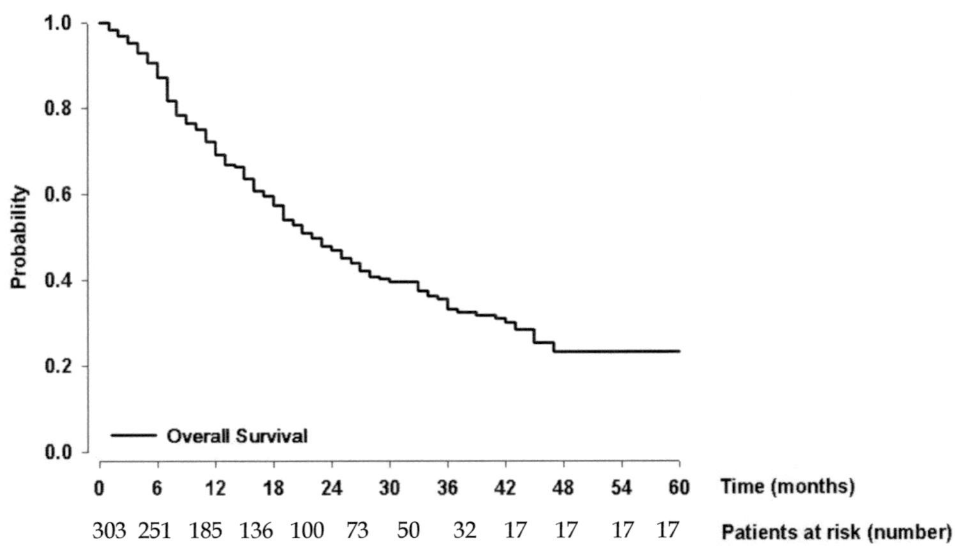

Fig. 1. Overall survival

The Motzer criteria were validated as prognostic factors in both the uni- and multi-variate analysis ($p<0.001$). The median and 5-year OS was 43 months and 42.8% in low-risk patients, 21 months and 15.9% in intermediate risk patients and 8 months in patients with poor risk (**Figure 2**).

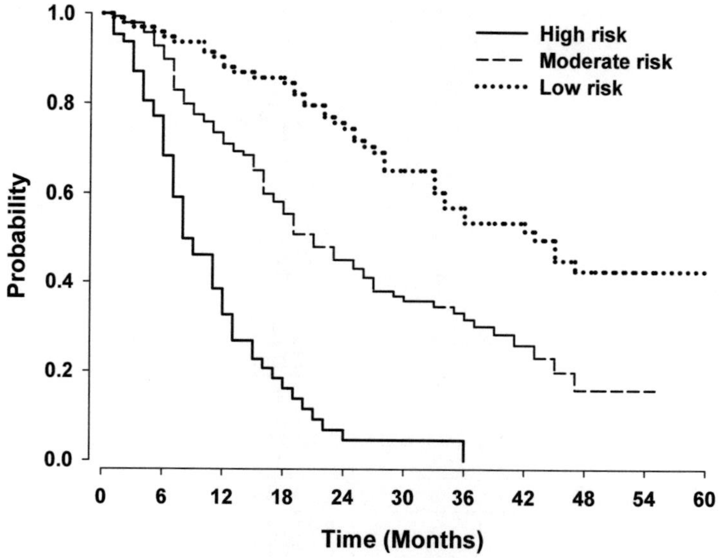

Fig. 2. Overall survival according to Motzer classification

Interestingly in both the multi- and uni-variate analysis there were no significant differences in the hazard ratios when SO+SU are compared with SU+SO and with other therapies (**Table 2, 3 and Figure 3**).

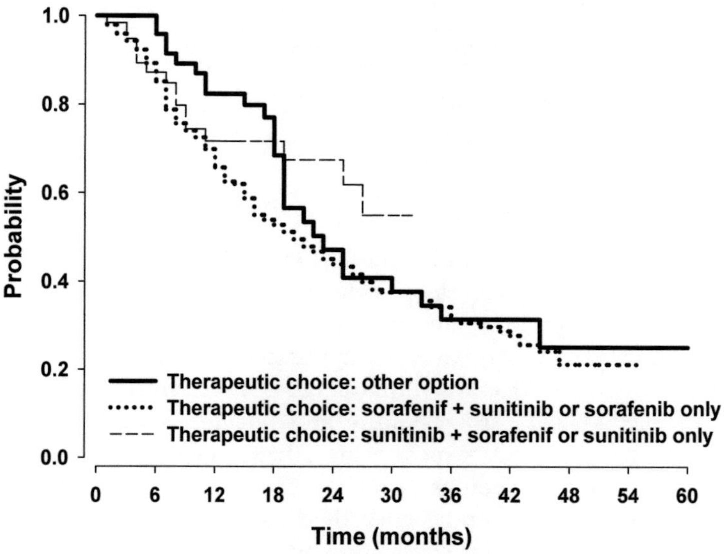

Fig. 3. Overall survival with sorafenib and sunitinib compared with other therapies

In detail, the PFS was 17 months with the specific sequence of SO+SU (9 months + 8 months) and 16 months with SU+SO (12 months + 4 months). The median PFS of first line treatment with either SO or SU was 10.5 months.

Furthermore in the multivariate overall survival analysis un-adjusted for the Motzer classification (**Table 3**) the risk was nearly 1.5 times higher in those patients who had previously been treated with cytokines compared with those who had not received cytokines (p<0.033).

	Hazard ratio (95% CI)	p
Age		
10 years increasing	0.98 (0.86; 1.11)	0.735
Sex		
Male vs. female	1.09 (0.77; 1.55)	0.635
ECOG PS		
1 vs. 0	1.69 (1.25; 2.29)	**<0.001**
2 vs. 0	2.62 (1.39; 4.95)	
Cytokine		
Yes vs. no	1.28 (0.95 ; 1.72)	0.101
Histology		
Papillary vs. clear cell	1.39 (0.85; 2.27)	0.247
Non clear cell vs. Clear cell	1.47 (0.75; 2.89)	
Nephrectomy		
Yes vs. no	0.41 (0.26; 0.65)	**<0.001**
Motzer criteria		
Intermediate vs. low risk	2.30 (1.57; 3.35)	**<0.001**
High vs. low risk	7.90 (5.07;12.31)	
Therapeutic choice		
Other option vs. Sorafenib+sunitinib	0.77 (0.51;1.17)	0.212
Sunitinib+sorafenib vs. sorafenib+sunitinib	0.69 (0.41;1.16)	

ECOG PS = Eastern Cooperative Group Performance Score

Table 2. Univariable overall survival analysis

7. Adverse events

The most commonly reported treatment-related all grade adverse events (AEs) were typical of those reported with TKIs including asthenia, hand-foot syndrome, hypertension, diarrhea, mucositis, hypothyroidism and most of these were mild or moderate in intensity (Grade 1 or 2). Overall, 61 (19.68%) patients experienced AEs Grade ≥3 (**Table 4**) and there were a total of 65 Grade ≥3 AEs, and three patients experienced a Grade 4 event (two patients receiving SU+SO had cardiac failure and one receiving SO+SU had a cardiac stroke). The percentage of patients experiencing adverse events Grade ≥3 was similar in patients treated when SO was given as in those treated first with SU then SO (18.88 and 17.46%). In those treated with other systemic therapies there was a tendency to a higher incidence of AEs (25.5%). Furthermore the nature and severity of AEs groups did not differ if SO or SU was given first.

	Adjusted for Motzer criteria		Not adjusted for Motzer criteria	
	Hazard ratio (95% CI)	p	Hazard ratio (95% CI)	p
Age				
10 years increasing	0.98 (0.85; 1.12)	0.767	0.91 (0.80; 1.04)	0.180
Sex				
Males vs. females	0.91 (0.62; 1.32)	0.611	1.09 (0.76; 1.59)	0.631
ECOG PS				
1 vs. 0	1.09 (0.78; 1.54)	0.838	1.53 (1.11; 2.12)	**0.003**
2 vs. 0	0.95 (0.48; 1.89)		2.42 (1.27; 4.59)	
Cytokine				
Yes vs. no	1.26 (0.91; 1.75)	0.169	1.41 (1.03; 1.94)	**0.033**
Histology				
Papillary vs. clear cell	1.35 (0.81; 2.24)	0.478	1.42 (0.86; 2.35)	0.285
Non clear cell vs. clear cell	1.19 (0.60; 2.39)		1.38 (0.69; 2.74)	
Nephrectomy				
Yes vs. no	0.59 (0.35; 0.98)	**0.041**	0.40 (0.24; 0.67)	**0.001**
Motzer criteria				
Intermediate vs. low risk	2.15 (1.44; 3.21)	**<0.001**	-	-
High vs. low risk	7.23 (4.42; 11.83)		-	
Therapeutic choice				
Other options vs. sorafenib+sunitinib	0.84 (0.55; 1.29)	0.388	0.85 (0.56; 1.30)	0.675
Sunitinib+sorafenib vs. Sorafenib+sunitinib	0.70 (0.40; 1.23)		0.85 (0.49; 1.47)	

ECOG PS = Eastern Cooperative Group Performance Score

Table 3. Multivariable overall survival analysis

Adverse event	N	% (N/310)
Asthenia	36	11.61
Hand-foot syndrome	13	4.19
Anemia	4	1.29
Cardiac failure	2	0.65
Hypertension	2	0.65
Mucositis	2	0.65
Abdominal pain	1	0.32
Cardiac stroke	1	0.32
Fever	1	0.32
Macroematuria	1	0.32
Nausea	1	0.32
Rash	1	0.32

Table 4. Adverse events Grade ≥3 (patients may have experienced one or more events)

8. Discussion

Despite improvements in therapy, RCC eventually progresses during therapy and other agent(s) need to be administered in an attempt to control the disease.

This large-scale retrospective analysis was carried out to investigate the effects of systemic therapy in general and in particular to compare the efficacy and safety of different sequential approaches with targeted therapies in controlling the disease progression of patients with RCC. Importantly, our results show that treatment with TKIs improves survival. In fact the median OS for patients with advanced RCC has increased from around 13 months before the introduction of TKIs to around 22 months in the last decade and the median OS of 22 months observed in the present study provides further evidence to support the importance of use of TKI in patients with advanced RCC. In addition, to our knowledge most studies have considered PFS, and not OS, as the major determinant of clinical efficacy of any sequential therapy for the treatment of RCC: our study provides new evidence on OS even in a large unselected population from a single institution. Of note, a relevant proportion of patients received sorafenib as a first-line agent, despite current recommendations suggest this molecule as a second-line treatment, and sunitinib at progression of disease. This therapeutic strategy did not result in any worsening of clinical outcomes and in a similar tolerability with respect to the other therapeutic strategies assessed. Even if this study was not designed to evaluate the feasibility of sorafenib as a first-line agent, and therefore we are unable to draw any conclusion, we believe that this finding could be of some interest in the current therapeutic scenario of RCC patients.

In addition, the Motzer criteria resulted significant prognostic factors in both the uni- and multi-variate analysis. On this basis, we suggest that these criteria should – at present - be regarded to as the most useful tool for the definition of prognosis and, as a consequence, for the optimization of therapy for every single patient.

Of note, the findings reported in the present report were obtained in a real-life scenario, on a large population of unselected patients: it has been suggested that observational trials can expand upon outcomes of randomized controlled trials, which are necessarily conducted in highly-selected patients [22].

In most patients with advanced RCC the objective of treatment is to stabilize disease and prolong survival and there is good evidence that this can be achieved with sequencing systemic agents. The use of this therapeutic approach, in fact, may determine a relevant benefit in terms of OS and quality of life, independently from the specific sequence of targeted therapies used.

Our study confirms the suitability of a TKI sequential therapy. This finding is in line with recent evidence, albeit collected in retrospective studies, which seems to support that the use of SO before SU, rather than vice versa may be more effective in extending PFS (**Table 5**). In addition, some studies suggest that SO may be associated with a more favorable safety profile than more potent SU, in terms of incidence of changes in blood counts and anemia [23,24].

The major limitations of the current study was that the sample size was not randomized and the data were collected retrospectively. In addition the study populations were very hoeterogenous with much patients received the sequence TKI followed TKI and only few cases treated with bevacizumab, everolimus, temsirolimus and axitinib.

Source	*n*	1st PFS (months)	2nd PFS (months)
Sorafenib→Sunitinib			
Eichelberg et al.	30	8.7	10.3
Dudek et al.	29	5.1	18.0
Porta et al.	83	9.8	8.4
Procopio et al.	50	9.5	8.3
Sablin et al.	68	6.0	6.5
Zimmerman et al.	22	11.5	5.0
Sunitinib→Sorafenib			
Dudek et al.	20	5.8	8.5
Porta et al.	87	8.3	3.7
Sablin et al.	22	5.1	3.9
VEGFi→Sorafenib			
Garcia et al	48	8.7	3.7

PFS = progression-free survival; TTP = time to progression.

Table 5. Summary of sorafenib and sunitinib sequence data (reproduced from ref 24)

In conclusion, despite the major breakthrough introduced by targeted therapies, further research is necessary to shed new lights on the most effective use of these drugs in clinical practice: in particular, the optimal sequence of TKIs has yet to be established.

Our study supports - however - the importance of TKI treatment in RCC patients to improve OS. In addition, it suggests that factors other than the specific sequence of treatment, like the Motzer classification, influence the OS in a large unselected population from clinical practice collected in a single institution. On the basis of these results and of current evidence reported in literature is now clear that there is not one therapy that will benefit all patients and treatment should be tailored to meet individual circumstances and needs. Physicians should therefore base their treatment decisions not only on data from RCTs but also on clinical experience and judgment

9. References

[1] Lindblad P. Epidemiology of renal cell carcinoma. *Scand. J. Surg.* 93(2), 88–96 (2004).
[2] Chow WH, Devesa SS, Warren JL, Fraumeni Jr JF. Rising incidence of renal cell cancer in the United States. *JAMA*. 281(17), 1628–1631 (1999).
[3] Bos SD, Mellema CT, Mensink HJ. Increase in incidental renal cell carcinoma in the northern part of the Netherlands. *Eur. Urol.* 37 (3), 267–270 (2000).
[4] Mevorach RA, Segal AJ, Tersegno ME, Frank IN. Renal cell carcinoma: incidental diagnosis and natural history: review of 235 cases. *Urology*, 39 (6), 519–522 (1992).
[5] Hock LM, Lynch J, Balaji KC. Increasing incidence of all stages of kidney cancer in the last 2 decades in the United States: an analysis of surveillance, epidemiology and end results program data. *J. Urol.* 167 (1), 57–60 (2002).
[6] Pantuck AJ, Zisman A, Belldegrun AS. The changing natural history of renal cell carcinoma. *J. Urol.*166 (5), 1611–1623 (2001).
[7] Atzpodien J, Royston P, Wandert T, Reitz M. Metastatic renal carcinoma comprehensive prognostic system. *Br. J. Cancer* 88 (3), 348–353 (2003).

[8] Cheville JC, Lohse CM, Zincke H, Weaver AL, Blute ML. Comparisons of outcome and prognostic features among histologic subtypes of renal cell carcinoma. Am. J. Surg. Pathol. 27 (5), 612–624 (2003).

[9] Jemal A, Tiwari RC, Murray T, et al. Cancer statistics, 2004. *CA Cancer. J. Clin.* 54(1), 8–29 (2004).

[10] Motzer RJ, Russo P. Systemic therapy for renal cell carcinoma. *J. Urol.* 163 (2), 408–417 (2003).

[11] Oudard S, George D, Medioni J et al. Treatment options in renal cell carcinoma: past, present and future. *Ann. Oncol.* 18 (suppl 10), 25–31 (2007).

[12] Atkins MB, Regan M, McDermott D. Update on the role of interleukin 2 and other cytokines in the treatment of patients with stage IV renal carcinoma. *Clin. Cancer. Res.* 10 (suppl), 6342–6346 (2004).

[13] Hutson TE. Targeted Therapies for the Treatment of Metastatic Renal Cell Carcinoma: Clinical Evidence. *The Oncologist.* 16 (suppl 2), 14–22 (2011).

[14] Dudek AZ, Zolnierek J, Dham A, Lindgren BR, Szczylik C. Sequential therapy with sorafenib and sunitinib in renal cell carcinoma. *Cancer.* 115 (1), 61–67 (2009).

[15] Motzer RJ, Escudier B, Oudard S, Hutson TE, Porta C, Bracarda S et al. Efficacy of everolimus in advanced renal cell carcinoma: a double-blind, randomised, placebo-controlled phase III trial. *Lancet.* 372 (9637), 449–456 (2008).

[16] National Comprehensive Cancer Network. NCCN Clinical Practice Guidelines in Oncology. Kidney Cancer. V. 2.2010. Available at http://www.nccn.org/professionals/physician_gls/PDF/kidney.pdf. Accessed March 22, 2011.

[17] Ljungberg B, Cowan N, Hanbury DC et al. European Association of Urology Guidelines on Renal Cell Carcinoma. 2010. Available at http://www.uroweb.org/gls/pdf/Renal%20Cell%20Carcinoma%202010.pdf. Accessed March 22 2011.

[18] Hutson TE, Bukowski RM, Cowey CL, Figlin R, Escudier B, Sternberg CN. Sequential use of targeted agents in the treatment of renal cell carcinoma. *Crit. Rev. Oncol. Hematol.* 77 (1), 48–62 (2011).

[19] Beck J,Procopio G,Bajetta E et al. Final results of the European Advanced Renal Cell Carcinoma Sorafenib (EU-ARCCS) expanded-access study: a large open-label study in diverse community settings. *Ann. Oncol.* 2011; Epub ahead of print.

[20] Procopio G,Verzoni E, Guadalupi V, Pietrantonio F, Salvioni R, Nicolai N, et al. Sequential use of sorafenib (So) followed by sunitinib (Su) in metastatic renal cell cancer (mRCC): a single-institution experience [abstract]. Genitourinary Cancers Symposium. Orlando, FL, February 26–28; 2009 [Abstract 319].

[21] Motzer RJ, Mazumdar M, Bacik J, Berg W, Amsterdam A, Ferrara J. Survival and prognostic stratification of 670 patients with advanced renal cell carcinoma. *J. Clin. Oncol.* 17 (8): 2530-40 (1999).

[22] Silverman SL. From randomized controlled trials to observational studies. *Am. J. Med.* 122 (2), 114-20 (2009).

[23] Grünwald V, Heinzer H, Fiedler W. Managing side effects of angiogenesis inhibitors in RCC. *Onkologie* 30, 519–524 (2007).

[24] Ivanyi P, Winkler T, Ganser A, Reuter C, Grünwald V. *Dtsch. Arztebl. Int.* 105 (13): 232–237 (2008).

20

Treatment of Renal Cell Carcinoma in Elderly and Frail Patients

Mirjana Rajer
Institute of Oncology Ljubljana
Slovenia

1. Introduction

Renal cell carcinoma (RCC) is the most common cancer of the kidney (Motzer et.al., 1999). In the United States each year 57.000 new patients are being diagnosed with RCC resulting in 12.900 deaths (Linehan et.al., 2011). The median age at diagnosis today is 64 years and even though it represents only 3% of all cancers, the incidence is increasing steadily. With rising prevalence of some known risk factors like hypertension and population ageing, the incidence of RCC is expected to be rising even more in subsequent years. With increasing incidence of renal cell carcinoma (RCC) combined with population ageing, questions about the treatment of elderly and frail patients with RCC are becoming more and more relevant. Many of the patients with newly diagnosed RCC are in advanced age and/or have some major co-morbidities which often results in their poor performance status. Elderly or frail patients are frequently excluded from clinical trials, because the results of their treatment are often difficult to interpret. This is also true for patients with heart, lung, liver or other major co-morbidities. Excluding these patients from clinical trials leads to lack of evidence-based guidelines for their treatment and often poses to oncologists a difficult dilemma when they need to decide what treatment options to offer to patients (Scuch et.al., 2008). In the present chapter we would like to present current recommendations for diagnostics and treatment of elderly and frail patients with RCC. In the second part of the chapter results of the analysis of metastatic RCC patients treated in a single institution with emphasis on differences in the treatment between good and poor performance status patients are presented.

2. Age, performance status, co-morbidities and prognostic models

2.1 Age

Ageing is a complex process that affects every aspect of life. The US department of Health and Human Services Administration of Ageing estimates that 1 in every 8 Americans is older than 65 years. In 2006 this group represented 12,4% of the population, but by 2030 this number is expected to increase to 20%. With population ageing, incidence of all cancers is supposed to be rising in the next years and RCC is no exception (Neustadt et.al., 2008).

It is well known that the actual age is determined by physiology rather than chronology. Factors of biological aging include changes in the physical structure of the body as well as changes in the performance of motor skills and sensory awareness. These changes can lead to multiple adverse events during the hospitalisation of an elderly patient especially in the postoperative period. Delirium episodes (acute decline of attention and cognition) can occur in 15-35% of patients during hospitalisation in the postoperative period and as high as 70-78% of patients in intensive care units. Prolonged hospitalisation is also associated with falls at rate 4-10/1000 patient-days. Other common adverse events are functional decline in 32% and adverse events of drugs in 10-15% of patients (Pushkar & Govorov, 2008).

Organs have a certain capacity to resist to stress and return to normal functioning after the stress on them has passed. This concept is termed "organ reserve". This reserve diminishes with age and may explain some functional deterioration in the elderly. Organ reserve in the young is supposed to be 7-11 times greater than in the advanced age person. Declining of organ reserve with age can not be predicted properly because it is subject to individual variation. Still, it has to be taken into account in treatment decision making (Neustadt et.al., 2008).

The patient's age is incorporated in the development of treatment decision and often is an inclusion /exclusion criterion of clinical trials. For a long time it was believed that older patients may tolerate treatment less well and may develop more adverse events compared to younger patients. Consequently, many treatments were not offered to older patients only on the basis of their chronological age without any strong evidence gained from clinical trials. It is becoming more and more clear that older patients may tolerate available treatments as well as younger ones and that treatments are being equally effective in both groups. Still, not all available treatments can be given without causing harm to all patients and some prudence is needed. Evaluation of functional organ reserve, evaluation of co-morbidities and performance status is of utmost importance (Calvo et.al., 2010).

2.2 Performance status

Beside accurate diagnostics and staging of tumours, before the decision on treatment modalities, performance status needs to be assessed in all cancer patients. Importance of pre-treatment performance status evaluation has been determined on the basis of several clinical trials that confirmed its prognostic value. Performance status can be assessed based on several different scales. In oncology the most commonly used are Karnofsky scale and the ECOG score (published by Oken et al. in 1982), also named WHO or Zubrod score. Scores and their comparisons are shown in Tables1 and 2.

Percentage	*Description*
100%	Normal, no complaints, no signs of disease
90%	Capable of normal activity, few symptoms or signs of disease
80%	Normal activity with some difficulty, some symptoms or signs
70%	Caring for self, not capable of normal activity or work
60%	Requiring some help, can take care of most personal requirements
50%	Requiring help often, requires frequent medical care
40%	Disabled, requires special care and help
30%	Severely disabled, hospital admission indicated but no risk of death
20%	Very ill, urgently requiring admission, requires supportive measures or treatment
10%	Moribund, rapidly progressive fatal disease processes

Table 1. Karnofsky performance status scale

WHO/ECOG	Description
0	Fully active, able to carry on all predisease activities without restriction
1	Restricted in physically strenuous activity but ambulatory and able to carry out work of a light or sedentary nature. For example, light housework, office work
2	Ambulatory and capable of all self care but unable to carry out any work activities. Up and about more than 50% of waking hours
3	Capable of only limited self-care, confined to bed or chair 50% or more of waking hours
4	Completely disabled. Cannot carry on any self-care. Totally confined to bed or chair

Table 2. WHO performance status scale

Karnofsky score of 90-100% corresponds to 0 on WHO scale, 70-80% to 1, 50-60% to 2, 30-40% to 3 and 10-20% to WHO grade 4. Patient death corresponds to 0% or 5 on Karnofsky and WHO scale respectively (Pushkar & Govorov, 2008).

Poor performance status in patients with RCC can be the result of one or multiple causes leading to a heterogeneous group of patients. Causes of poor PS (> 1 WHO) may be directly connected to RCC and metastases or may be the result of co-morbidities not directly connected to cancer (e.g. cardiovascular or hepatic diseases). Causes of poor PS related to tumour may be: pain from primary tumour or metastases, pleural effusion or ascites, brain metastases, anaemia, cachexia, gastrointestinal symptoms or fatigue (Pushkar&Govorov, 2008).

In measuring PS of the patient on WHO or Karnofsky scale some caution is needed because there are some situations where assessment of patient's functional status may require more than PS values written in numbers. For example, bone metastases: involvement of pelvis, femur or spine can force the patient to become bedridden, and the evaluation of PS in those patients can be difficult. Other criticism to the PS scales is that they do not include patient's nutritional status and they don't assess cachexia. Although performance status assessed with WHO or Karnofsky scales may not always reflect the actual functional status of the patient it is a most useful tool and should be utilized before and during the treatment of all cancer patients (Shuch et.al., 2007).

2.3 Co-morbidities

Outcome of therapy is depended not only on type and tumour aggressiveness but also on functional status of the patient and co-morbidities. In predicting possible outcome in elderly patients, evaluating performance status may not be enough and a thorough evaluation of their co-morbidities and organ functional reserve is mandatory. It is estimated that five years after the diagnosis of RCC, 30% of patients die because of conditions other than RCC. There are several ways to evaluate co-morbidities like American society of anaesthesiology (ASA) score used before surgery. Even though none of them is universally accepted, they may help us to determine the functional status of the patient (Pushkar & Govorov, 2008).

Evaluation of co-morbidities is and important part in the treatment decision process; but not only that, some of them may even predict the higher risk of developing RCC. The number of patients with end stage renal disease has increased markedly and haemodialysis is the most widely used form of renal replacement therapy in the elderly. It has been demonstrated that patients on haemodialysis have a higher probability of developing RCC (Ishikawa et.al., 1990). The overall relative risk of RCC is 5-10-times higher in patients with end-stage renal failure (Levine et.al., 1992). To detect RCC early in the course of the disease, these patients should have regular urologic follow-ups. The incidence of RCC is also high in patients after kidney transplantation. Murphy reported that post-transplant patients have a 1,85 times higher risk of development of RCC that their matched controls in the general population. This higher risk was not affected by age, gender, ethnical group and time since transplantation (Pushkar & Govorov, 2008).

Neuzillet et.al. evaluated clinicopathologic characteristics and treatment outcome in 1250 RCC patients with end stage renal disease in comparison with RCC patients without end stage renal disease (ESRD). They found that ESRD patients with RCC were younger (55 vs. 62 years, p<0,01), were more frequently discovered incidentally (87% vs 44%, p<0,01), had less local and systemic symptoms and were males (76,5% vs 61,9%, p<0,01) at rate compared to RCC patients without ESRD. Tumours were detected at lower stage in patients with ESRD, had lower grade and were papillary higher in higher percentage (37% vs 7%, p<0,01) in ESRD. Interestingly, more patients with ESRD were in good performance status (ECOG 0) (76% vs 63%). Authors conclude that better tumour and patient's characteristics are the results of more abdominal imaging performed in these patients. Consequently, more incidental tumours are being diagnosed (Neuzillet et.al., 2011).

2.4 Prognostic models

In the treatment decision making process it is very important to predict the patient's survival. Patients with short predicted survival time should be evaluated carefully and best quality of life should be the primary goal of their treatment (Bukowski & Negrier, 2004).

Motzer et.al. conducted a retrospective trial to identify prognostic factors and to find predictive model of survival of patients with metastatic RCC. Pretreatment factors were evaluated. They identified five prognostic factors on the basis of which patients can be divided into three risk groups (low, intermediate or high) for which the median survival time was separated by six months. Patients with zero risk factors (low risk group) had median survival of 20 months, those with one or two risk factors (intermediate risk group), had median survival time of 10 and those with three or more risk factors (high risk group) had survival time of 4 months. The identified prognostic factors (called also Memorial Sloan Kettering prognostic factors) were (Motzer et.al., 1996):

- Lactate dehydrogenase levels > 1,5 times upper limit of normal
- Haemogloben level < lower limit of normal
- Corrected serum calcium level > 10 mg/dl (2,5mmol/l)
- Interval of less than a year from original diagnosis to the start of systemic treatment
- Karnofsky performance status < 80
- Absence of prior nephrectomy

In another trial conducted in the year 2004, Motzer evaluated survival in previously treated patients with metastatic RCC. 251 patients were included in the trial. Identified prognostic factors were:

- low (<80) Karnofsky performance status
- low haemoglobin levels
- high corrected serum calcium.

Based on these three factors he divided patients into three groups regarding their prognosis. The median survival in patients without any of the factors present was 22 months, with one factor 11,9 months and those with two or three 5,4 months. Even though his intent was to categorize patients into risk groups to better interpret the results of clinical trials, we can use this categorisation in assessing predicted survival in our every day clinical practice (Motzer et.al., 2004).

To evaluate Memorial Sloan Kettering prognostic factors, researchers at the Cleveland Clinic Taussig Center retrospectively evaluated 353 patients with metastatic RCC that were included in clinical trials between 1987 and 2002. Four of the five prognostic factors identified by Motzer were independent predictors of survival. In addition, prior radiotherapy and presence of hepatic, lung, and retroperitoneal nodal metastases were found to be independent prognostic factors. Using these expanded criteria, favorable risk is defined as zero or one poor prognostic factor, intermediate risk is two poor prognostic factors, and poor risk is more than two poor prognostic factors. Median overall survival times of these groups were 26.0, 14,4, and 7,3 months, respectively (P < ,0001) (Bukowski & Negrier, 2004, Mekhail et.al, 2005).

Different models predicting survival other than those developed by Motzer and Cleveland group have been proposed. Bamias studied prognostic factors in patients treated with sunitinib. He identified three prognostic factors: time from diagnosis to the start of sunitinib therapy, number of metastatic sites and performance status (Bamias et.al., 2010). Hudes et.al. in a trial with temsirolimus used slightly modified Motser's factors in selecting poor prognosis patients. Instead of absence of prior nephrectomy, metastases in multiple organs were included and Karnofsky performance status <70 was used (Hudes et.al., 2007).

2.5 Definitions of elderly and frail patients

Elderly population is not an uniform entity, since chronological and biological age can differ considerably (Neustadt et.al., 2008). On a basis of the observation that active oncological treatment can be outweighed by increased treatment toxicity in this patient population, age of 75 years was determined as a milestone for defining elderly patients population (Lane et.al., 2010). Frail patients are considered those in poor performance status (WHO>1) (Pushkar & Govorov, 2008). According to MSK model, patients with Karnofsky PS<80%had worse survival compared to patients with higher score (Motzer, et.al. 1996)

3. Tumour evaluation

3.1 Diagnostic procedures

In tumour evaluation, the diagnostic tests do not differ much between older and younger patient populations. In both groups CT is necessary for accurate detection of tumour and nodal extension. In patients with renal insufficiency, CT without contrast media or magnetic resonance imaging instead of CT is being performed in order to prevent further damage to kidneys by using a nephrotoxic contrast media. Abdominal ultrasound is another very useful diagnostic tool that can easily be performed in all patients regardless of their age or performance status. The role of percutaneous tumour biopsy is limited in all patients. It may be of value in frail patients or in patients with overt metastatic disease to make a diagnosis of RCC and to avoid radical nephrectomy (Pushkar & Govorov, 2008).

3.2 Differences in tumour characteristics between young and elderly patients

Renal carcinoma is the most common renal parenchymal malignancy. Most of the patients are elderly with only 3-7% of RCC occurring in patients younger than 40 years. Trials performed in patients with breast, colon and prostate carcinomas showed that younger patients have a biologically more aggressive disease that leads to worse prognosis compared to elderly patients (Denzinger et.al., 2009).

To explore this issue in RCC, Denzinger retrospectively evaluated 1042 patients that were treated between 1992 and 2005. He compared patients younger than 45 years to patients aged over 75. In a multivariate analysis lower age was associated with higher 5-years cancer specific survival (95,2% vs 72,3% p=0,009) and lower 5-y progression rate (11,3% vs 42,5% p=0,002) (Denzinger et.al., 2009). Komai et.al. also found younger age to be a favourable prognostic factor. The 5-year cancer-specific survival rate was significantly better for the younger patients than for the older patients (p = ,049). Multivariate analysis showed that age was significantly associated with cancer specific survival (Komai et. al. 2011). Similar results were obtained in a trial of Jung and co-workers on low stage RCC patients (Jung et.al., 2009). These and other trials show uniformly, that younger RCC patients have better prognosis compared to the elderly (Denzinger et.al., 2009).

Trials also uniformly showed that younger patients are more likely to have a lower disease stage, lower nuclear grade, and smaller tumor size than older patients (Denzinger et.al., 2009, Komai et.al., 2011, Jung et.al., 2009).

4. Surgical treatment of elderly and frail patients

4.1 Radical and nephron sparing surgery in localized disease

Surgical resection is effective therapy for clinically localized RCC; with options including radical nephrectomy and nephron-sparing surgery. Radical nephrectomy (RN) was for many years considered the "gold standard" in the treatment of locally advanced RCC and nephron sparing surgery (NSS) was suggested when radical nephrectomy would render the patient functionally anephric. These cases included RCC in a solitary kidney, RCC in one kidney and the other non functioning and bilateral RCC (NCCN, 2011).

In recent years nephron-sparing surgery has become more and more popular (NCCN, 2011). Several trials showed that in patients with small tumours (<7 cm) the same oncological results can be achieved with NSS compared to RN (NCCN, 2011, Leibovich et.al, 2006, Becker et.al., 2006). In the trial of Leibowich the results of 91 patients treated with NSS and 841 patients treated with RN for 4 to 7 cm RCC between 1970 and 2000 have been compared. Cancer specific survival rates at 5 years for patients treated with NSS and RN for 4 to 7 cm RCC were 98% and 86%, respectively, the difference was not statistically significant (risk ratio 1,60, 95% CI 0,50-5,12, p = 0,430). Differences were not statistically significant even when authors compared the occurrence of local relapse or distant metastases (Leibovich et.al, 2006).

Nephrectomy (radical or nephron-sparing) should be considered as part of treatment decision process in all patients with stage I-III disease fit for surgical procedure (NCCN, 2011). In elderly or poor performance status patients still amenable for surgery nephron-sparing nephrectomy rather than radical nephrectomy should be performed whenever possible (Lane et.al., 2009). In patients with decreased life expectancy and/or extensive co-morbidities, surgery represents excessive risk and other options like tumour termoablation or active surveillance should be considered (NCCN, 2011)

4.2 Cytoreductive nephrectomy in patients with metastatic disease

Multimodality treatment in patients with metastatic RCC consists of surgery combined with systemic therapy. Surgical approach consists of cytoreductive nephrectomy often combined with metastasectomy of distant metastases. This approach in cancer therapy is distinctly different from treatment of other types of cancer. The rationale for nephrectomy is multiple: enhancing the effects of systemic therapy, removing the source of distant metastases and providing additional tissue for evluation in targeted therapy (Kutikov et.al., 2010).

To assess the benefit of cytoreductive surgery in patients with poor performance status (PS WHO 2 or 3), Shuch et.al. performed a retrospective analysis of all patients who underwent CN surgery at the University of California in between 1989 and 2006. They compared the results of patients in good (WHO 0,1) with those in poor performance status (WHO 2,3). Patients with poor PS had shorter disease-specific survival compared to patients with better PS (6 months vs. 27 months). Systemic treatment in CN was administered to only 57,5% of patients in poor performance status and no objective response was seen in these patients. CN in these patients may be used only to palliate haematuria or pain, but survival benefit of CN in poor PS patients is limited. (Scuch et.al., 2008, Kutikov et.al., 2010, Pushkar & Govorov, 2008, Chouieri, 2010).

Cytoreductive surgery should be offered to patients in good performance status only. Beside these, patients with lung metastases only and those with good prognostic features benefit most from it. The role of CN in the era of targeted therapy has not been defined jet. Randomized trials are ongoing and should answer this dilemma (NCCN, 2011).

4.3 Observation and palliative surgical aproaches

Observation (so called watchful waiting or active surveillance) is a less aggressive treatment modality and should be considered as an option in elderly patients with or without major co-morbidities, especially those with small incidentally found tumours and in those with larger tumours, but very short life expectancy. For the latter, surgery represents a greater risk compared to observation alone. Kassouf et.al. demonstrated that observation is a safe option, most of the tumours observed did not show signs of growth and none of the 24 patients in the trial developed metastases during the 31.6 months of median follow-up (Pushkar & Govorov, 2008).

One question still open is whether to perform tumour biopsy to prove malignity before active therapy is delivered. In the past this approach was not frequently adopted, mainly because a lot of false negative results found and because of the fear of side effects connected to biopsy of renal mass. In recent years renal biopsy became relevant. This is due to the fact that 20% of small renal tumours are benign or have low malignant potential. Biopsy should be considered whenever some doubt exists in decision to perform surgery, minimally invasive procedures or to observe the patient (Lazzeri et.al., 2010).

Paliative nephrectomy should be considered in patients with gross haematuria or other symptoms related to primary tumour that can not be controlled by non invasive measures, like uncontrollable pain (NCCN, 2011). Moreover, it may palliate pain and treat paraneoplastic syndromes associated with metastatic RCC (Kutikov et.al., 2010).

Tumour transarterial embolisation (TAE) in RCC patients has an established role in palliative treatment. It can be used to diminish patient's suffering from pain, haematuria or paraneoplastic symptoms. It can be offered as a sole treatment option or preoperatively to diminish the blood loss during nephrectomy. Although it is considered a palliative measure, 80% of patients to whom TAE has been performed, remain disease free after the procedure (Lane et.al., 2010). TAE should be offered to patients with short life expectancy, since neovascularisation is expected to occur some time after the procedure (de Reijke et.al., 2010). Munro et.al evaluated 25 patients treated with TAE. In this survey TAE was performed in two groups of patients. The first group consisted of patients with stage IV disease (median age 73 years) and the second of mainly elderly (median age 80 years) patients stage I-III disease who were unable or unwilling to receive nephrectomy. Authors analysed the usefulness of TEA regarding symptom control, hospital stay and survival. The conclusion was that embolisation is a good treatment option for palliating symptoms derived from primary tumour in patients with advanced disease and those with localized disease and poor general condition (Pushkar & Govorov, 2008). Other palliative measures available today are cryoablation, radiofrequency ablation, high-intensity focused US; microwave thermotherapy and radiosurgery. Results with all these techniques, even if studied in trials with small included number of patients, are promising not only in terms of palliation, but also in terms of disease free and cancer related survival (Lazzeri et.al., 2010).

5. Systemic therapy of metastatic disease

Despite advances in RCC detection, still 20-30% of patients present with metastatic disease. Treatment of metastatic disease in elderly and frail patients represents a big challenge for medical oncologists. Until recently there was a widely accepted belief that the treatment may not be effective in older patients and that they may be at higher risk of developing adverse events than younger patients. Consequently, they were often excluded or inadequately represented in clinical trials. However, recent evidence indicates that available treatments may be tolerated and effective in all patients regardless of age. Metastatic RCC is a chemotherapy resistant disease and until recently treatment options of these patients were limited. With the development of targeted therapies, new treatment options became available. Yet the question of efficiency and tolerability of this agents in elderly and frail patients arose (NCCN, 2011, Scuch et.al., 2008).

5.1 Treatment with immunotherapy

Immunotherapy with interferon alfa and interlekin-2 was for a long period the cornerstone of systemic treatment of metastatic RCC. Nowadays immunotherapy is being successfully replaced by less toxic and more effective targeted therapies. Trials performed with immunotherapy have shown that patients with worse performance not only had shorter survival, but also had a decreased response rate to immunotherapy and greater frequency 3 and 4 toxicity. Decreased response to immunotherapy is supposed to be due to the fact that patients with PS>1 have a compromised immune system; immunotherapy success is clearly related to a good immune system. Nevertheless, it is difficult to determine whether the treatment is less effective because the performance status is low or whether the performance status is low because tumour is more aggressive (Pushkar & Govorov, 2008). This, together with tumour characteristics, is the reason why immunotherapy was not approved in the treatment of patients with poor performance status (Scuch et.al., 2008).

5.2 Treatment with targeted therapies

In recent years a whole new spectrum of treatments with targeted drugs became available in the treatment of metastatic RCC. These new drugs were tested to treat elderly and frail patients with promising results (Bellmunt et.al., 2011).

Sunitinib targets a number of receptor tyrosine kinases including platlet-derived growth factor receptors, vascular endothelial growth factor receptors, stem cell factor receptor, FMS-like tyrosine kinase, colony stimulating receptor and neurotropic factor receptor (NCCN, 2011). Sunitinib has established role in the treatment of metastatic RCC (Gore et.al., 2009). The efficacy and safety of sunitinib in elderly and poor prognosis patients was assessed in an expanded-access trial. Of 4371 included patients 582 (13%) had PS 2 or higher and 1418 (32%) were aged 65 or more. Results showed a 17% objective response rate in the elderly and a 9% rate in PS≥2 patients. Median progression free survival was 11,3 months (95% in elderly and 5,1 months in poor performance group). Side effects were few and tolerable. Authors concluded that sunitinib is effective and safe even in groups of patients that are supposed to tolerate treatment less well and are usually excluded from clinical trials (Gore et.al., 2009, NCCN, 2011, Calvo et.al., 2010).

Sorafenib is a small molecule that inhibits multiple tyrosine kinase receptors (NCCN, 2011). Treatment with sorafenib is considered to be equally effective in elderly and younger patients. Retrospective subgroup analysis of data from TARGET (Treatment Approach in Renal Cancer Global Evaluation) trial showed similar clinical benefit in patients aged 70 years or more compared to younger ones (83,5% in older and 84,3% in younger patients) (Calvo et.al., 2010). Incidence of adverse events were not significantly higher in elderly patients receiving sorafenib. Thus sorafenib represents an important treatment option for elderly patients with RCC (Dutcher et.al., 2010).

Temsirolimus was tested in a phase 3 trial comparing it to interferone therapy in patients with poor prognosis. Patients included in the trial had at least three of the 6 criteria for poor prognosis according to the modified MSCC. Patients were randomized to one of the three arms (temsirolimus alone, interferone alone or both treatments given together). Patients that received temsirolimus alone had longer overall survival compared to other two groups. (OS 10,9 months temsirolimus alone, 7,3 interferone, 8,4 combination). The main conclusion of this trial is that treatment with temsirolimus alone leads to moderate prolongation of survival compared to treatment with interferon in patients with poor prognosis. Based on this trial, temsirolimus is indicated in the first line of therapy in poor prognosis patients (Hudes et.al., 2009, Rejike et.al., 2010).

Bevacisumab is an recombinant humanized monoclonal antibody that binds and neutralizes circulating VEGF-A. Bevacisumab was approved by FDA for first line treatment in combination with IFN-α (NCCN, 2011). Concerns about administering bevacisumab in elderly, have been diminished by retrospective trials that showed similar efficacy and toxicity profiles compared with younger patients. Billemont et.al. presented data regarding treatment of elderly patients with all antiangiogenic therapies (sunitinib, sorafenib, bevacisumab). There were no toxic deaths, most common grade 3 or 4 were skin toxicity and mucositis. Authors conclude that antiangiogenic therapy including bevacisumab, can be administered safely to patients older than 75 years (Billemont et.al., 2010). Other retrospective trials similarly conclude that side effects, while more pronounced in the elderly, are well tolerated and not dose-limiting (Calvo, 2010).

Pazopanib is an oral VEGFR-1 and 2, PDGFR-α and β. It was approved for treatment of metastatic RCC in 2009 (NCCN, 2011). The most common side effects of pazopanib are diarrhoea, fatigue and hair depigmentation. The most worrying side effect is hepatotoxicity grade 3 present in 12% aldough fatal events are rare (0,05% of cases). Even if only 6% of patients included in the trials with pazopanib were aged > 75 years, no differences in safety and effectiveness was observed in comparison with younger ones (Calvo et.al., 2010, FDA, 2009, Bukowski, 2011).

Everolimus is an inhibitor of mTOR. It was approved for the treatment of metastatic RCC after failure of sunitinib or sorafenib in 2009 based on a phase III trial named RECORD 1 wich compared treatment with everolimus to placebo (NCCN, 2011). To assess the efficacy and safety of everolimus in elderly patients (>70 years), Hutson et.al. performed an exploratory analysis of RECORD-1 trial data. Everolimus prolonged PFS in this group of patients, compared to placebo. Some adverse events (eg, cough, diarrhea, asthenia, fatigue) were more frequent in the elderly subset vs. the overall RECORD-1 population (median age, 61 y); but this is likely related to the intrinsic characteristics of this subpopulation, given that these adverse events also were more frequent in the elderly subgroup receiving placebo (Hutson et.al., 2010).

According to the data obtained from trials published until now, most of the targeted therapies are equally effective and safe in elderly and/or frail or in young and good performance status patients. In most cases dose reduction is not necessary and some of the targeted therapies (i.e. everolimus) may even prevent worsening of renal function in transplant patients and those with multiple co-morbidities. The conclusion of multiple trials is that newer targeted drugs should be offered to elderly and/or patients with multiple co-morbidities. It can not be stressed enough that including these patients in clinical trials is mandatory (Calvo et.al., 2010).

6. Treatment with radiotherapy

In the rare case of inoperable RCC, radiotherapy can be administered with promising results. In a trial of Wersall, 58 patients with inoperable or metastatic RCC received high dose stereotactic radiotherapy (32Gy in 4 fractions, 40Gy in 4 fractions or 45Gy in 3 fractions). Partial response or stable disease was observed in 90% of patients and local control rate of 90-98% was achieved. Radiotherapy can be safely administered to elderly and frail patients and should be considered whenever radical therapy is not applicable (Wersall et.al., 2005, de Rejike et.al., 2010).

For patients with brain metastases, radiotherapy has an important role in their treatment. Using stereotactic radiotherapy similar results can be achieved as with surgical removal of brain metastases. The stereotactic radiotherapy is non-invasive, outpatient and can be applied in patients in lower PS, without worsening their condition (de Rejike et.al., 2010).

Bone metastases represent a special problem. Patients with bone metastases are often symptomatic; pathological fractures, spinal cord compression and the need for surgery are common, and nearly 80% of untreated patients experience skeletal-related events. Until recently treatment options for these patients were scarce because of the chemo and ratio-resistance of RCC. With the development of new agents like biphosphonates and targeted agents, better results in treatment of bone metastases regarding pain control and pathologic fractures can be achieved. Yuasa showed that combining radiotherapy with biphosphonates administration leads to higher objective response and less skeletal related events compared to radiation therapy alone. In administering biphosphonates caution is needed because of the renal impairment (Yuasa et.al., 2010).

7. Treatment of elderly and frail metastatic RCC patients at the Institute of Oncology Ljubljana

To explore the treatment approach in every-day practice we retrospectively evaluated T_{any} N_{any} M1 RCC patients that were treated at the Institute of Oncology Ljubljana, Slovenia, between 2006 and 2009 and for whom appropriate data were available. A patient was considered to have a metastatic disease if it was confirmed by biopsy or clear signs of metastatic disease were present on radiographic evaluation. Staging was performed by using CT imaging of thorax and abdomen. If needed other diagnostic tests were performed. Surgical procedures were done in hospitals other than Institute of Oncology. Performance status was assessed according to WHO scale. The aim was to assess possible differences in the treatment strategy decisions in good (WHO 0 or 1) versus poor (WHO>1) performance status patients.

Medical records of 368 patients were reviewed. Patients with incomplete records were excluded. Patient and tumour characteristics are presented in Table 3.

Variable	*Metastatic RCC patients No=368*
Male	268 (72,8%)
Female	100 (27,2%)
Median age	63.3 (34-86) years
Histology	
Clear cell	228 (62%)
Papillary	37 (10,0%)
RCC not other specified	64 (17.4%)
Sarcomatoid	26 (7,1%)
Other rare (chromophobe, collecting duct, mixed…)	13 (3,5%)

Performance status	
0	89 (24,2%)
1	108 (29,3%)
2	57 (15,5%)
3	70 (19,0%)
4	38 (10,3%)
Unknown	6 (1,6%)
Co-morbidities	
Present	93 (25,3%)
Absent	262 (71,2%)
Unknown	13 (3,5%)

Table 3. Patient and tumour caracteristics

All patients were reviewed by the multidisciplinary board that consists of an urologist, a medical oncologist and a radiation oncologist. All patients had proven metastatic disease before presentation to the board. Administered treatment is shown in Table 4.

Treatment mode	*Number of patients treated (percentage)*
Surgery	
Nephrectomy with radical intent (performed before metastatic disease was present)	162 (44,1%)
Cytoreductive nephrectomy	106 (28,8%)
Tumour embolisation	43 (11,6%)
Systemic therapy	
Immunotherapy	50 (13,6%)
Targeted therapy	156 (42,4%)
Watchful waiting	12 (3,3%)
Best supportive care	150 (40,0%)

Table 4. Treatment options

To establish possible differences in the decision of treatment strategy in different groups of patients, a comparison was made. All treatment decisions were made by a multidisciplinary team of oncologists on the basis of medical documentation and clinical examination of the patient by a member of the team. Comparison between groups was done with X^2 test. Differences between patients in good vs. poor performance status, patients with or without major co-morbidities and younger vs. elderly patients is shown in Table 5.

	Systemic therapy *(immunotherapy or targeted therapy)*	*Best supportive care or observation*	
Performance status			
PS 0,1	179 (90,8%)	18 (9,2%)	
PS>1	26 (15,7%)	139 (84,3%)	p<0,01
Co-morbidities			
Not present	160 (61%)	102 (39%)	
Present	50 (53,7%)	43 (46,3%)	p=0,76
Age			
< *75 years*	151 (72,7%)	57 (27,3%)	
≥ *75 years*	12 (7,5%)	148 (92,5)%	p<0,01

Table 5. Differences in treatment decisions

As expected, the patient's performance status has an important impact on treatment decision. Patients in good PS receive systemic therapy in much greater percentage of cases than patients in poor PS. Patients in poor PS are more likely to tolerate less well systemic therapy and treatment decisions in every-day practice reflects the knowledge of this fact. Defining PS, even if it is a subjective measure, is very important and should be made by an experienced clinician. Still, some patients in good PS do not get the systemic therapy and some in poor PS get it. This reflects the influence of other factors, like age of the patients and co-morbidities on treatment decisions.

The difference between treatment decisions based on co-morbidities is not clear. In our review, systemic treatment was administered to many patients with co-morbidities. An explanation for this is, that according to known data, most of the available targeted therapies are effective and safe for the majority of patients with co-morbidities. Nevertheless, half of the patients with co-morbidities present do not get the specific therapy.

With evolving results from clinical trials, new data on safety and efficacy will become available which will help clinicians in treatment decisions.

Age has a huge impact on treatment decisions. Less than 10% of metastatic RCC patients older than 75 years get systemic therapy prescribed. Prescribing targeted therapies to elderly patients still represents a challenge to clinicians. This is in accordance with the widely established tendency to believe that older patients tolerate the treatment less well and develop adverse events in higher percentage and at greater degree. Recent evidence shows that available treatments (targeted therapy) are safe and efficient in elderly as well as young patients (Calvo et.al., 2010).

8. Conclusions

Longer life expectancy together with the growing incidence of RCC has raised the number of elderly and frail patients with this malignancy. Tailoring treatment to the individual patient according to the tumour stage and patient general condition is the primary goal of treatment. Treatment options for the elderly and frail are multiple and vary in their aggressiveness. Finding the right treatment for the right patient can be a difficult task for oncologists. Improvement in all fields from surgery to targeted therapies led to broader treatment choice. The problem that remains is that often no evidence exists which treatment combination to use, since much too often these patients are excluded form clinical trials. How to encourage investigators to design clinical trials so as that these patients can be included in greater numbers, remains a difficult open question especially in large trials testing new drugs. Conducting trials addressing these populations after the drug has been approved for use in good prognosis-good performance patients deprives others of a new drug which is often well tolerable and effective.

9. References

Bellmunt, J.; Eisen, T.; Szczylk, C.; et.al. A new patient-focused approach to the treatment of metastatic renal cell carcinoma: establishing customized treatment options. *British Journal of Urology International,* Vol.107, No.8, (April 2011), pp. 1190-99, ISSN 2042-2997

Bamias, A.; Karadimou, A.; Lampaki, S.; et.al. Prognostic stratification of patients with advanced renal cell carcinoma treated with sunitinib: comparison with the Memorial Sloan-Kettering prognostic factors model. *BMC Cancer,* Vol.10, No.45, (published online February 2010), pp. 1-12, ISSN 1471-2407

Becker, F.; Siemer, S.; Humke, U.; et.al. Elective nephron sparing surgery should become standard treatment for small unilateral renal cell carcinoma: survival data of 216 patients. *European Urology,* Vol.49, No.2, (February 2006), pp. 308-13, ISSN 1871-2592

Billemont, B.; Massard, S.; Negrier, M.; et.al. Antiangiogenic treatment in elderly patients (>75 years) with metastatic RCC: Experience from the French Renal Group. Poster presented at the American Society of Clinical Oncology conference 2010.

Bukowski, RM.; Negrier, S. Prognostic factors in patients with advanced renal cell carcinoma. Development of an International Kidney Cancer Working Grup. *Clinical Cancer Research,* Vol.15, No.10, (September 2004), pp. 6310-14, ISSN 1078-0432

Bukowski, RM. Critical appraisal of pazopanib as treatment for patients with advanced metastatic renal cell carcinoma. *Cancer Management and Research,* Vol.3, (August 2011), pp. 273-85, ISSN 1179-1322

Calvo, E.; Maroto, P.; Garcia del Moro, X.; et.al. Update from the Spanish Oncology Genitourinary Group on the treatment of advanced renal cell carcinoma: focus on special populations. *Cancer metastasis review,* Vol.29 (Suppl 1) (July 2010), pp. 11-20, ISSN 0167-7659

Choueiri, TK.; Wanling, X.; Kollmansberger, C.; et.al. The Impact of cytoreductive Nephrectomy on Survival of Patients With Metastatic Renal Cell Carcinoma Receiving Vascular Endothelial Growth Factor Targeted Therapy. *The Journal of Urology,* Vol.185, No.1 (November 2010), pp. 60-6, ISSN 0022-5347

Denzinger, S.; Otto, W.; Burger, M.; et.al. Sporadic renal cell carcinoma in young and elderly patients: are the different clinicopathological features and disease specific survival rates?. *World Journal of Surgical Oncology,* Vol.5, No.16, (February 2009), pp. 5-16, ISSN 1477-7819

Dutcher, JP.; Tannir, N.; Bellmunt, J.; et.al. Experience with sorafenib and the elderly patients. *Medical oncology,* Vol.27, No.4, (December 2010), pp. 1359-70, ISSN 1357-0560

de Rejike, TM.; Bellmunt, J.; van Poppel, H.; et.al. EORTC-EU group expert opinion on metastatic renal cell cancer. *European journal of cancer,* Vol.45, No.2 (January 2009), pp. 766-73, ISSN 0959-8049

FDA prescribing information: http://www.accessdata.fda.gov/drugsatfda_docs/label/2009/022465lbl

Gore, ME.; Szczylik, C.; Porta, C.; et.al. Safety and efficacy of sunitinib for metastatic renal-cell carcinoma: an expanded-access trial. *The Lancet Oncology,* Vol.10, No.8 (August 2009), pp. 757-63, ISSN 1470-2045

Hudes, M.; Carducci, M.; Zomczak, M.; et.al. Temsirolimus, Interferon Alfa or Both for Advanced Renal-Cell Carcinoma. *The New England Journal of Medicine,* Vol.356, No.22, (May 2007), pp. 2271-81, ISSN 0028-4793

Hutson, TE.; Calvo, BJ.; Escudier, S.; et.al. Everolimus in elderly patients with metastatic renal cell carcinoma: An exploratory analysis of the RECORD-1 study. Poster presented at the American Society of Clinical Oncology conference, 2010

Ishikawa, I.; Saito, Y.; Shikura, N.; et.al. A ten year prospective study on the development of renal cell carcinoma in dialysis patients. *American Journal on Kidney Diseases,* Vol.16, No.5, (November 1990), pp.452-8, ISSN 0272-6386

Jung, EJ.; Lee, HY.; Kwak, C.; et.al. Young age is independent prognostic factor for cancer specific survival of low-stage clear cell renal cell carcinoma. *Urology,* Vol.73, No.1, (January 2009), pp. 1341-8, ISSN 0090-4295

Kutikov, A.; Uzzo, RG.; Caraway, A.; et.al. Use of systemic therapy and factors affecting survival for patients undergoing cytoreductive nephrectomy. *British Journal of Urology International,* Vol.106, No.2, (July 2010), pp. 218-23, ISSN 2042-2997

Komai, Y.; Fujii, Y.; Tatokoro, M.; et.al. Young age as favorable prognostic factor for cancer-specific survival in localized renal cell carcinoma. *Urology,* Vol. 77, No.4, (April 2011), pp. 847-8, ISSN 0090-4295

Lane, BR.; Abouassaly, R.; Tianning, G.; et.al. Active Treatment of Localized Renal Tumours May Not Impact Overall Survival in Patients Aged 75 Years or Older. *Cancer,* Vol.116, No.13, (July 2010), pp. 3119-26, ISSN 1097-0142

Lazzeri, M. & Guazzoni P. Early 21st Century Renal Cell Carcinoma. *Cancer,* Vol.116, No.13, (July 2010), pp. 3135-42, ISSN 1097-0142

Leibovich, BC.; Blute, ML.; Cheville, JC.; et.al. Nephron sparing surgery for appriopriately selected renal cell carcinoma between 4 and 7 cm results in outcome similar to radical nephrectomy. *The Journal of Urology,* Vol.172, No.3 (September 2004), pp. 1066-70, ISSN 0022-5347

Levine, E. renal cell carcinoma in uremic acquired renal cystic disease: incidence, detection and management. *Urologic Radiology,* Vol.13, No.2, (December 1992), pp. 203-10, ISSN 0171-1091

Linehan, WM.; Rini, AV.; Yang JC. (2011). Cancer of the kidney, In: *Cancer. Principles and Practice of Oncology,* DeVita, VT.; Lawrence, TS; Rosenberg, SA. (Ed.), 1161-91, Lipincott Williams & Wilkins, ISBN 978-1-4511-1813-1, Philadelphia, USA

Macfarlane, R.; Heng, DYC.; Xie, W.; et.al. The Impact of Kidney Function on the Outcome of Metastatic Renal Cell Carcinoma Patients Treated With Vascular Endothelial Growth Factor-Targeted Therapy. *Cancer,* (published online August 2011), pp. 1-6, ISSN 1097-0142

Mekhail, TM.; Abu-Jawde, BM.; Boumerhi, G.; et.al. Validation and extension of the Memorial Sloan-Kettering prognostic factors model for survival in patients with previously untreated metastatic renal cell carcinoma. *Journal of Clinical Oncology,* Vol.23, No.4 (February 2005), pp. 832-41, ISSN 0732-183X

Motzer, RJ.; Baick, Y.; Lawrence, W.; et.al. Prognostic Factors for Survival in Previously Treated Patients With Metastatic Renal Cell Carcinoma. *Journal of Clinical Oncology,* Vol.22, No.3 (February 2004), pp. 454-63, ISSN 0732-183X

Motzer, RJ.; Mazumdar, M.; Baick, J.; et.al. Survival and Prognostic Stratification of 670 Patients With Advanced Renal Cell Carcinoma. *Journal of Clinical Oncology,* Vol.17, No.8 (August 1999), pp. 2530-40, ISSN 0732-183X

NCCN clinical practice guidelines in oncology: Kidney cancer, Version 2 (2011): http://www.nccn.org

Neustadt, Y. and Pieczenik, S. Organ Reserve and Healthy Ageing. *Integrative Medicine,* Vol.7, No.3, (Jun/Jul 2008), pp. 50-2, ISSN 1543953X

Neuzillet, J.; Tillou, X.; Mathieu, R. Renal Cell Carcinoma (RCC) in Patients With End-Stage Renal Disease Exhibits Many Favourable Clinical, Pathologic, and Outcome Features Compared With RCC in the General Population. *European Urology,* Vol.60, No.2, (August 2011), pp. 366-73, ISSN 1871-2592

Pushkar, D. & Govorov, AV. (2008). Old and Fragile Patients, In: *Renal Cell Cancer,* J. De la Rosette, CN. Sternberg, H. van Poppel (Ed.), 353-64, Springer, ISBN 978-84628-763-3, London, England

Shuch, B.; La Rochelle, JC.; Wu, J.; et.al. Performance Status and Cytoreductive Nephrectomy. *Cancer,* Vol.113, No.6, (September 2008), pp. 1324-31, ISSN 1097-0142

Wersäll, PJ.; Blomgren, H.; Lax, I.; et.al. Extracranial stereotactic radiotherapy for primary and metastatic renal cell carcinoma. *Radiotherapy and Oncology,* Vol.77, No.1, (June 2005), pp. 88-95, ISSN 0167-8140

Yuasa, T.; Urakami, S.; Yamamoto S.; et.al. Treatment outcome and prognostic factors in renal cell cancer patients with bone metastases. *Clinical and experimental metastasis,* Vol.42, No.8, (August 2010), pp. 299-303, ISSN 0262-0898

Part 4

Case Reports

21

Simultaneous Nephron-Sparing Surgery and Caesarian Section for the Treatment of Renal Cell Carcinoma in Pregnancy: Case Report and Review of the Literature

Ambrosi Pertia, Laurent Managadze and Archil Chkhotua
National Center of Urology
Georgia

1. Introduction

Renal cell carcinoma (RCC) accounts for about 3% of all adult malignancies and is the most lethal urological cancer. Although extremely rare in pregnant women, it is the commonest urological neoplasm in pregnancy occurring in 1 in 1000 cases (Walker, JL., & Knight, EL., 1986). It is potentially curable with prompt diagnosis and correct management. However, treatment of the disease is a substantial challenge for both, urologist and obstetrician.

Over 70 cases of RCC in pregnancy have been reported in literature. 95% of them are clear cell type, with a poorer prognosis than the rest 5% that are chromophobe type. Women with these tumors may present at any stage of the pregnancy. Only 26% of them describe the classical triad of: loin pain, palpable mass and haematuria. The most common mode of presentation of the disease is a palpable mass (88%) and pain (50%). Haematuria implies collecting system invasion and occurs in 50% of the cases. However, haematuria in pregnant women is faint due to other possible causes, including: urinary tract infection, calculi and hydronephrosis (Pearson, GAH., & Eckford, SD., 2009). Other rare forms of presentations are: hypertension, haemolytic anaemia and hypercalcaemia (Monga, et al., 1995; Usta, IM., et al., 1998). With the advent of ultrasound there has been a change in presentation of the disease with diagnosis more frequently made incidentally during ultrasound examination performed for other reasons (Fynn, J., & Venyo, AKG., 2004).

Diagnostic evaluation of a pregnant woman with renal mass requires special consideration combining non-invasive techniques with as little radiation exposure as possible to the mother and fetus. As a first step, urine has to be sent for cytology. Abdominal CT and intravenous pyelography (IVP) are frequently used in the evaluation of non-pregnant patients and should be avoided due to the unsafe radiation exposure to fetus. Renal radionuclide scans being used to determine function of a contralateral kidney has to be replaced by Doppler scan. Ultrasonography (US) is the safest method for diagnosis of the renal mass in pregnant woman with the similar to IVP and CT sensitivity of 85% (Warshauer, DM., et al., 1988). Magnetic resonance imaging (MRI) is also suitable, due to the least radiation exposure and no harm to pregnant woman. However, it should be stressed that chest CT remains the most sensitive method for diagnosis of pulmonary metastases. The US and MRI are the investigations of choice adequately identifying, differentiating and staging the solid renal masses in pregnancy.

The management of RCC in pregnant woman should depend on tumor biology and age of gestation. Decision to operate and prevent further tumor spread should be taken in consideration of the degree of fetal maturity. The impact of surgical and adjuvant therapy on the potential for future pregnancies should be also considered.

The most frequent form of treatment of RCC in pregnancy is open or laparoscopic radical nephrectomy (RN) followed-up by spontaneous delivery (Pearson, GA., & Eckford, SD., 2009; Gnessin, E., et al., 2002; Qureshi, F., et al., 2002; Monga, M., et al., 1995; O'Connor, JP., et al., 2004; Lee, D., & Abraham, N., 2008). RN with or without termination of pregnancy (Loughlin, KR., 1995; Usta, IM., et al., 1998; Simon, I., et al., 2008), Caesarean section (CS) followed-up by RN (Stojnić, J., et al., 2009) and simultaneous RN and CS (Kobayashi, T., et al., 2000) have also been reported in the literature. There are no reports on the simultaneous nephron sparing surgery (NSS) and CS in the pregnant women.

Here we report the first case of NSS performed together with CS for the treatment of RCC in the second trimester of pregnancy. The review of the literature discussing the tretment options, timing of the surgery and multidisciplinarity of approach is also given.

2. Case history

A 33 years old female was referred to our center at 24 weeks' gestation without previous history of urological diseases and any subjective complaints. The right renal mass has been found on routine sonography. A 6X6X4.5 cm. solid tumor has been detected on MRI arising from the upper pole of the right kidney (figure 1). Regional lymph nodes were negative. Hepatic and pulmonary metastases have been excluded by abdominal and chest MRI. Renal biopsy has not been performed due to the following reasons: a) the positive predictive value of the imaging findings is so high that a negative biopsy result would not alter the management strategy; b) 10-20% of biopsies are reported to be non-conclusive; c) high risk of complications associated with biopsy (Silverman, SG., et al., 2006).

The tumor was graded according to the Padua anatomical classification and assigned the score 6. According to this score the risk of surgical complications related to the NSS was considered as low. There were no radiological signs of local extension and/or distant metastases. Clinically the tumor was staged as: T1b, N0, M0.

After extensive counseling and consultation with the obstetrician decision has been taken to postpone the operative treatment until the third trimester of gestation as recommended in the literature. The patient was followed-up by: regular urological and obstetrical checkup; sonography once per month; and weekly urinalysis, until maximal chance of fetal viability. The patient was stable without any signs of disease progression until 33rd week of gestation. After re-consulting with obstetric staff, simultaneous NSS and caesarian section was planned at this time point.

Caesarian section has been performed first under epidural anesthesia. A healthy girl weighing 2.4 kg was delivered without any surgical difficulties. The patient was intubated and operation was continued with open NSS through flank incision. Enucleoresection was performed with arterial clamping and local hypothermia. Cold ischemia time was 15 min. Duration of the NSS was 115 min. Blood loss was less than 100 cc. The renal capsular defect has been covered with free peritoneal graft.

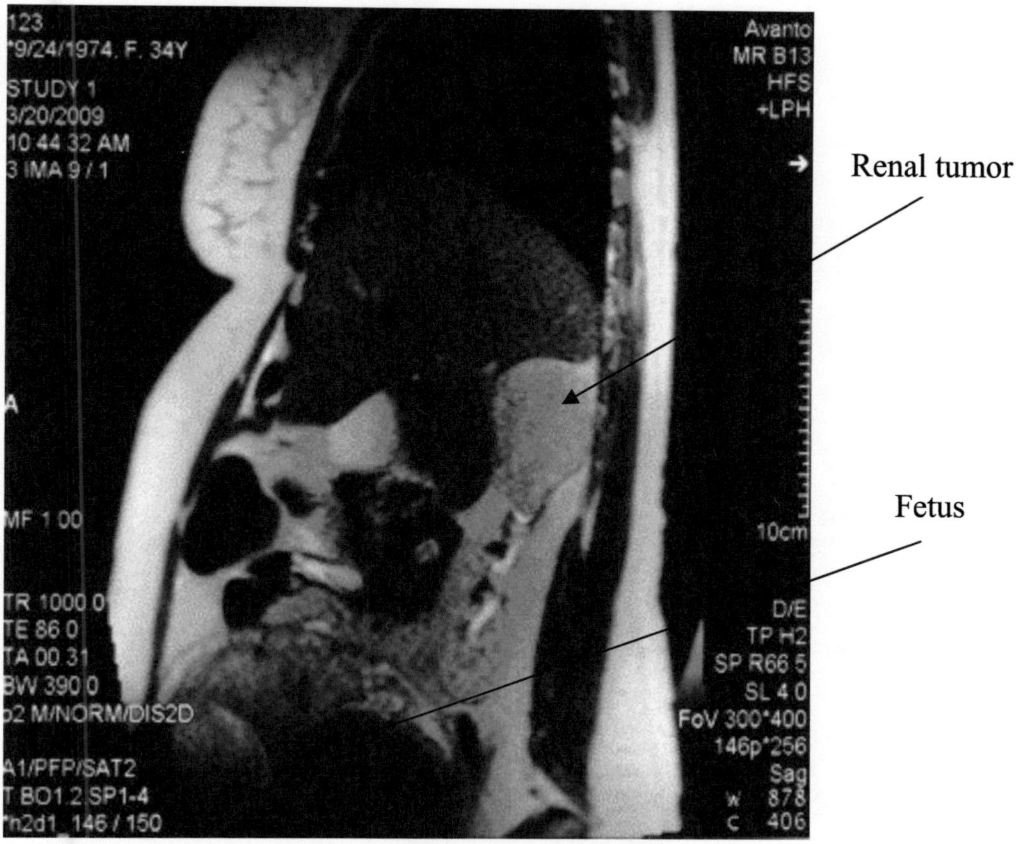

Fig. 1 MRI scan demonstrating right renal mass and the fetus

Postoperative course was uneventful for both, the mother and child. The patient made a good recovery with normal obstetric examinations. Morphology revealed clear cell RCC pT1bN0M0, grade 1. After the follow-up of 30 months the patient is doing well without any signs of the disease recurrence. The child is healthy with normal physical and mental development.

3. Discussion

RN and NSS are the treatments of choice for the patients with RCC. Oncological results and complications of the treatments are extensively evaluated showing excellent outcomes in the patients with local stages of the disease. However, management of RCC in pregnant women is extremely challenging due to the rarity and difficulty of the situation. There are several reports in the literature about the treatment of RCC at different time points of pregnancy. Table 1 describes the cases of the treatment of RCC in pregnancy reported in the literature.

Author	Year of publication	N of cases	Age of gestation at diagnosis	Stage	Treatment	Age of gestation at treatment	Pregnancy outcome
Gladman, MA., et al.	2002	2	14th and 24th weeks	T2N0Mx	RN	17th and 25th weeks	1. Spontaneous delivery at 40th weeks; 2. CS at 40th weeks
Fynn, J., Venyo, AK.	2004	1	12th week	T2N0M0	RN	24th week	CS at 24th weeks
Fazeli-Matin, S., et al.	1998	1	13th week	T2N0M0	NSS	13th week	Spontaneous delivery
Gnessin, E., et al.	2002	2	18th and 16th weeks	T1N0M0 and T2N0M0	RN	18th and 16th weeks	Spontaneous deliveries
Qureshi, F., et al.	2002	1	I trimester	T2N0MX	RN	I trimester	Spontaneous delivery
Lee, D., & Abraham, N.	2008	1	I trimester	-	Lap. nephrectomy	19th week	Spontaneous delivery
O'Connor, J., et al.	2004	1	11th week	T1N0M0	Lap. nephrectomy	19th week	Spontaneous delivery at 38 week
Simon, I., et al.	2008	1	I trimester	-	RN	I trimester	Pregnancy interruption
Pearson, GAH., Eckford, SD.	2009	1	28th week	T2	RN	CS at 34th week	CS at 32nd week
Stojnić, J., et al	2009	1	I trimester	-	RN	II trimester	CS in II trimester
Kobayashi, T., et al.	2000	1	22nd week	T2N0M0	RN	28th week	CS at 28th week

Table 1. Cases of the treatment of RCC in pregnancy reported in the literature

It was believed for a long time that there is no association between RCC and pregnancy. However, more recent studies discovered new facts. Lambe, M., et al. in a Swedish population-based study, found a strong association between the number of births and the risk of RCC. They have shown that the parous women were at a 40% increased risk of RCC compared to nulliparous women (Lambe, M., et al., 2002). It is known that both, normal and malignant renal cells contain oestrogen and progesterone receptors (Ronchi, E., et al., 1984). Chow, WH., et al. have shown an increased risk of RCC in pregnant women with co-existing risk factors like: parity greater than five, obesity, hypertension and diabetes (Chow, WH., et al., 1995). It has been speculated that pregnancy-associated hormonal changes, particularly high oestrogen levels, may act as promoters of malignant change by stimulating renal cell proliferation either directly or via paracrine growth factors (Concolino, G., et al., 1993). Whether these observations have any implications for the biological behavior of malignant renal cells in pregnancy is not clear, but a tendency towards immediate rather than delayed surgery seems to be appropriate. However, as neonatal survival rates increase with increasing gestation at delivery, immediate surgery at early stages of pregnancy is potentially deleterious to fetal health. Therefore, it is extremely important to define whether pregnancy has to be interrupted or allowed to continue if radical nephrectomy is carried out (Fynn, J., & Venyo, AK., 2004).

If the RCC is discovered in the first trimester, immediate surgery is recommended by majority of the authors (Loughlin, KR., 1995; Gladman, MA., et al., 2002). Whether pregnancy should be terminated at this gestation or not is debatable. The decision should be based on the patient's wishes and medical indications. It is important to consider that the risks of miscarriage and teratogenesis are high at this age, making termination a better option for some authors (Fynn, J., & Venyo, AK., 2004). Others however, disagree with this approach (Usta, IM., et al., 1998).

Management of the disease in the second trimester is more challenging. In the late second trimester surgery should be delayed to at least 28 weeks, when the fetal survival of over 90% is achievable (Loughlin, KR., 1995). In the early second trimester however, immediate surgery is recommended by some of the authors due to the low risk of the fetal loss (Fazeli-Matin, S., et al., 1998; Gnessin, E., et al., 2002; Jenkins, TM., et al., 2003).

In the third trimester the fetal lung maturity is established and immediate surgery seems convenient. It has been suggested that CS should not be performed at the time of RN as the kidney is removed through different incision (Walker, JL. & Knight, EL., 1986). If the diagnosis is made in the late third trimester the surgery can be postponed until delivery (Loughlin, KR., 1995).

In case of the metastatic disease the pregnancy should be terminated (Hendry, WF., 1997). There are no reports of patients or fetal metastases so far.

The most frequent form of treatment of RCC in pregnancy is open or laparoscopic RN followed-up by spontaneous delivery. Gladman, MA., et al. reported 2 cases of RCC diagnosed in the second trimester. RN was performed without termination of pregnancy. One patient gave birth to healthy child and the second one underwent emergency CS for fetal distress at forty weeks' of gestation (Gladman, MA., et al., 2002). Two cases of successful open RN in the second trimester have been reported by Gnessin, E., et al., Both patients gave full term spontaneous delivery to healthy children (Gnessin, E., et al., 2002).

Qureshi, F., et al. detected RCC in the first trimester. Immediate RN was performed through a thoraco-abdominal approach. The patient gave birth to a healthy infant at full term by spontaneous vaginal delivery (Qureshi, F., et al., 2002). Lee, D. & Abraham, N., and O'Connor, J., et al., reported the case of RCC discovered in the first trimester. The operation was delayed till the second trimester. Laparoscopic transperitoneal nephrectomy was performed at 19 weeks' gestation in both cases. Both patients delivered a healthy child vaginally at 39 weeks' gestation (Lee, D., & Abraham, N., 2008; O'Connor, J., et al., 2004).

Simon, I., et al. reported a rare case of Von Hippel-Lindau disease in pregnant women presented with haematuria in the first trimester. RN was carried out after pregnancy interruption (Simon, I., et al., 2008).

Pearson, GAH., & Eckford, SD., detected RCC in the third trimester of pregnancy. CS was performed at 32 weeks of gestation followed-up by RN two weeks later. The same approach has been reported by Stojnić, J., et al. (Stojnić, J., et al., 2009).

Simultaneous RN and CS has also been performed for the treatment of RCC detected in the second trimester (Kobayashi, T., et al, 2000). There are no reports on the simultaneous NSS and CS in the literature.

The data on the effect of pregnancy on long-term survival of RCC is very limited. The same is true for the effect of future pregnancies on tumor recurrence. Some authors have reported good clinical results and survival in pregnant women with RCC (Walker, JL. & Knight, EL., 1986). More data on the outcomes of different treatment options, including the effect of subsequent pregnancies on the disease recurrence are needed to answer these questions.

4. Conclusion

The management of a pregnant woman with a malignant solid renal mass should follow certain principles: 1) the welfare of the mother should be main concern, unless she wishes otherwise; 2) management of the patient has to take place in a multidisciplinary setting involving: urologist, neonatologist, obstetrician, radiologist, anaesthetist, and morphologist; 3) the standard surgical treatment of the most stages of RCC is RN or NSS; 4) timing of the surgery depends on biological behavior of the tumor and the neonatal survival rates for the different gestations; 5) In case of widespread metastatic disease, the pregnancy should probably be terminated and the woman has to be treated according to the guidelines recommended for non-pregnant patients. Here we repot the first case of NSS performed simultaneously with CS for the treatment of pregnant woman with RCC. This approach can be considered feasible in women in the second and third trimesters of pregnancy.

5. References

Concolino, G., et al. (1993). Acquired cystic kidney disease: the hormonal hypothesis. *Urology,* Vol. 41, No. 2, (February 1993), pp. 170 – 175.

Chow, W., et al. (1995). Reproductive factors and risk of renal cell carcinoma among women. *International Journal of Cancer,* 1995; Vol. 60, No. 3, (January 1995), pp.321–324.

Fazeli-Matin, S., et al. (1998). Renal and adrenal surgery during pregnancy. *Urology,* Vol. 52, No. 3, (September 1998), pp. 510 – 511.

Fynn, J., & Venyo, AK. (2004). Renal cell carcinoma presenting as hypertension in pregnancy. *Journal of Obstetics and Gynaecology,* Vol. 24, No. 7, (October 2004), pp. 821-822.

Gnessin, E., et al. (2002). Renal cell carcinoma in pregnancy. *Urology,* Vol. 60, No. 6, (December 2002), p. 1111.

Hendry, WF. (1997). Management of urological tumours in pregnancy. *British Journal of Urology,* Vol. 80, Supplement 1, (July 1997), pp. 24 - 28.

Jenkins, TM., et al. (2003). Non-obstetric surgery during gestation: risk factors for lower birthweight. *Australian and New Zealand Journal of Obstetrics and Gynaecology,* Vol. 43, No.1, (February 2003), pp. 27 - 31.

Kobayashi, T., et al. (2000). A case of renal cell carcinoma during pregnancy: simultaneous cesarean section and radical nephrectomy. *Journal of Urology,* Vol. 163, No. 5, (May 2000), pp. 1515-1516.

Lambe, M., et al. (2002). Pregnancy and risk of renal cell cancer: a population-based study in Sweden. *British Journal of Cancer,* Vol. 86, No. 9, (May 2002), pp. 1425 - 1429.

Lee, D. & Abraham, N. (2008). Laparoscopic radical nephrectomy during pregnancy: case report and review of the literature. *Journal of Endourology,* Vol. 22, No. 3, (March 2008), pp. 517-519.

Loughlin, KR. (1995). The management of urological malignancies during pregnancy. *British Journal of Urology,* Vol. 76, No. 5, (November 1995), pp. 639-644.

Monga, M., et al., (1995). Renal cell carcinoma presenting as hemolytic anemia in pregnancy. *American Journal of Perinatology,* Vol. 12, No. 2, (March 1995), pp. 84-86.

O'Connor, JP., et al. (2004). Laparoscopic nephrectomy for renal-cell carcinoma during pregnancy. *Journal of Endourology,* Vol. 18, No. 9, (November 2004), pp. 871-874.

Pearson, GA., & Eckford, SD., Renal cell carcinoma in pregnancy. *Journal of Obstetrics and Gynaecology,* Vol. 29, No. 1, (January 2009), pp. 53-54.

Qureshi, F., et al. (2002). Renal cell carcinoma (chromophobe type) in the first trimester of pregnancy. *Scandinavian Journal of Urology and Nephrology,* Vol. 36, No. 3, pp. 228–230.

Ronchi, E., et al. (1984). Steroid hormone receptors in normal and malignant human renal tissue: relationship with progestin therapy. *Journal of Steroid Biochemistry and Molecular Biology,* Vol. 21, No. 3, (September 1984), pp. 329 - 335.

Silverman, SG., et al., (2009). Renal masses in the adult patient: the role of percutaneous biopsy. *Radiology,* Vol. 240, No. 1, (July 2009), pp. 6-22.

Simon, I., et al, (2008). Clear cell renal carcinoma presenting as a bleeding cyst in pregnancy: inaugural manifestation of a von Hippel-Lindau disease. *Clinical Nephrology.* Vol. 69, No. 3, (March 2008), pp. 224-228.

Stojnić, J., et al. (2009). Renal cell carcinoma in pregnancy: a case report. *European Journal of Gynaecological Oncology,* Vol. 30, No. 3, pp. 347-349.

Usta, IM., et al. (1998). Renal cell carcinoma with hypercalcemia complicating a pregnancy: case report and review of the literature. *European Journal of Gynaecological Oncology,* Vol. 19, No. 6, pp. 584 - 587.

Walker, JL. & Knight, EL. (1986) Renal cell carcinoma in pregnancy. *Cancer,* Vol. 58, No. 10, (November 1986), pp. 2343 - 2347.

Warshauer, DM., et al. (1988). Detection of renal masses: sensitivities and specificities of excretory urography/linear tomography, US, and CT. *Radiology,* Vol. 169, No. 2, 363–365.